Understanding Neurological Diseases

Understanding Neurological Diseases

Edited by Ian Glover

hayle
medical

New York

Hayle Medical,
750 Third Avenue, 9th Floor,
New York, NY 10017, USA

Visit us on the World Wide Web at:
www.haylemedical.com

ISBN: 978-1-63241-670-4

Cataloging-in-publication Data

Understanding neurological diseases / edited by Ian Glover.
    p. cm.
Includes bibliographical references and index.
ISBN 978-1-63241-670-4
1. Nervous system--Diseases. 2. Neurology. 3. Nervous system. I. Glover, Ian.
RC346 .U54 2019
616.8--dc23

Contents

Preface

The world is advancing at a fast pace like never before. Therefore, the need is to keep up with the latest developments. This book was an idea that came to fruition when the specialists in the area realized the need to coordinate together and document essential themes in the subject. That's when I was requested to be the editor. Editing this book has been an honour as it brings together diverse authors researching on different streams of the field. The book collates essential materials contributed by veterans in the area which can be utilized by students and researchers alike.

Any disorder of the nervous system comprising of the structural, electrical and biochemical abnormalities of the brain, spinal cord or other nerves may be termed as a neurological disorder. They can be divided into brain dysfunction and brain damage, spinal cord disorders, cranial nerve disorders, peripheral neuropathy, seizure disorders, central neuropathy, neuropsychiatric illnesses, etc. Loss of sensation, paralysis, poor coordination, confusion, muscle weakness and altered levels of consciousness are some symptoms of neurological diseases. Some of the causes of neurological disorders include congenital abnormalities, genetic disorders, lifestyle or environmental health problems including malnutrition, or brain, nerve or spinal cord injury. A neurological examination seeks to assess the impact of neurological disease and the damage incurred on brain function relative to memory, behavior or cognition. This book brings forth some of the most innovative concepts and elucidates the unexplored aspects of neurological diseases. It includes some of the vital pieces of work being conducted across the world, on neurological conditions. Those in search of information to further their knowledge will be greatly assisted by this book.

Each chapter is a sole-standing publication that reflects each author's interpretation. Thus, the book displays a multi-facetted picture of our current understanding of application, resources and aspects of the field. I would like to thank the contributors of this book and my family for their endless support.

Editor

Akt and mTORC1 signaling as predictive biomarkers for the EGFR antibody nimotuzumab in glioblastoma

Michael W. Ronellenfitsch[1,2,3*] , Pia S. Zeiner[1,2,3,4], Michel Mittelbronn[4,5,6,7], Hans Urban[1,2,3], Torsten Pietsch[8], Dirk Reuter[9], Christian Senft[10], Joachim P. Steinbach[1,2,3], Manfred Westphal[11] and Patrick N. Harter[2,3,4*]

Abstract

Glioblastoma (GB) is the most frequent primary brain tumor in adults with a dismal prognosis despite aggressive treatment including surgical resection, radiotherapy and chemotherapy with the alkylating agent temozolomide. Thus far, the successful implementation of the concept of targeted therapy where a drug targets a selective alteration in cancer cells was mainly limited to model diseases with identified genetic drivers. One of the most commonly altered oncogenic drivers of GB and therefore plausible therapeutic target is the epidermal growth factor receptor (EGFR). Trials targeting this signaling cascade, however, have been negative, including the phase III OSAG 101-BSA-05 trial. This highlights the need for further patient selection to identify subgroups of GB with true EGFR-dependency. In this retrospective analysis of treatment-naïve samples of the OSAG 101-BSA-05 trial cohort, we identify the EGFR signaling activity markers phosphorylated PRAS40 and phosphorylated ribosomal protein S6 as predictive markers for treatment efficacy of the EGFR-blocking antibody nimotuzumab in MGMT promoter unmethylated GBs. Considering the total trial population irrespective of MGMT status, a clear trend towards a survival benefit from nimotuzumab was already detectable when tumors had above median levels of phosphorylated ribosomal protein S6. These results could constitute a basis for further investigations of nimotuzumab or other EGFR- and downstream signaling inhibitors in selected patient cohorts using the reported criteria as candidate predictive biomarkers.

Keywords: Epidermal growth factor receptor, Mammalian target of rapamycin, Glioblastoma, Nimotuzumab, Biomarker, Targeted therapy

Introduction

Glioblastoma (GB) is an incurable brain cancer and the most common primary brain tumor in adults [33]. The epidermal growth factor receptor (EGFR) is frequently genetically altered in GB by gene amplification and mutations including a variant where deletion of exons 2–7 causes activated signaling termed EGFRvIII. EGFR gene alterations can be found in 45.1% of GBs [32], mutations in members of the receptor tyrosine kinase- Ras-PI3 Kinase-AKT signaling network are the most frequent

mutations (87.9% of cases) in GB [32]. Further, EGFR signaling is known to enhance proliferative signaling, resistance to cell death and reprogramming of energy metabolism [13, 38, 45]. Therefore, EGFR is a plausible target in GB therapy. Several clinical trials have been performed, with however rather disappointing results [39]. Strategies targeting EGFR in GB include small molecule inhibitors (e.g. erlotinib), antibodies or antibody-drug conjugates (e.g. depatuxizumab mafodotin (ABT-414)) as well as novel immunooncological approaches like a vaccine against EGFRvIII with rindopepimut. The depatuxizumab antibody portion of ABT-414 preferentially binds to cells with amplified EGFR or EGFRvIII [35]. After binding ABT-414 is internalized and can block microtubule formation via its mafodotin part [51]. Currently larger phase II and III clinical trials are underway evaluating ABT-414

* Correspondence: M.Ronellenfitsch@gmx.net; patrick.harter@kgu.de
[1]Dr. Senckenberg Institute of Neurooncology, University Hospital Frankfurt, Goethe University, Schleusenweg 2-16, 60528 Frankfurt am Main, Germany
[2]German Cancer Consortium (DKTK), Partner Site Frankfurt/Mainz, Frankfurt am Main, Germany
Full list of author information is available at the end of the article

in the primary (Intellance 1 phase III trial, ClinicalTrials.gov NCT02573324) and recurrent disease (Intellance 2 phase II trial, ClinicalTrials.gov NCT02343406) setting. In the ACT IV trial, the EGFRvIII vaccine rindopepimut did not prolong survival in GB patients [53]. It is noteworthy that the EGFRvIII mutation if present usually is only found in a fraction of tumor cells within a GB [54] and that even during the course of standard treatment EGFR-vIII is frequently lost [53]. Standard treatment for patients in sufficient clinical condition has been established in 2005 already and involves surgical resection, radiotherapy and chemotherapy with the alkylating agent temozolomide which led to median overall survival times of 14.6 months [47]. Many trials have been conducted in recent years, however, no new drugs have been approved [27, 39]. Histologically, GB is characterized by marked hypoxic areas, with typical histological features of neoangiogenesis and necrosis in a diffusely infiltrating growing glial tumor [25]. These areas reflect the metabolically challenging microenvironment where nutrient and oxygen supply can frequently not match demand of the tumor cells. The transcription factor hypoxia-inducible factor 1α (HIF-1α) is a major cellular regulator of adaptive programs to hypoxia and stabilization occurs when oxygen is low [42].

The current WHO classification further stratifies GB as either isocitrate dehydrohgenase (IDH) wildtype (wt) or IDH mutant (mut). The vast majority of primary GB harbors IDH wt status [24]. Further, current treatment relevant molecular stratification of GB mainly depends on the methylation status of the O(6)-methylguanine methyltransferase (MGMT)-promoter. MGMT-promoter methylation correlates with reduced expression of the DNA repair enzyme MGMT. Consequently, tumors with methylated MGMT promoter generally respond better to temozolomide treatment whereas MGMT expression in tumors with unmethylated gene promoter is a major mechanism of resistance and indicator for poor prognosis [15, 16, 46].

Many novel approaches to improve GB therapy rely on targeting specifically altered signal transduction cascades. However, these so called targeted therapies, including those targeting EGFR, thus far, have failed to show any benefit in GB treatment despite rational target selection and availability of potent drugs opening the quest for predictive biomarkers [39, 52]. One important downstream mediator of EGFR signaling is the kinase Akt (Fig. 1a) with numerous phosphorylation targets involved in proliferation, survival, cell motility and angiogenesis [49]. Proline rich Akt substrate of 40 kDa (PRAS40) has been identified as an inhibitory component of mTOR complex 1 (mTORC1). Akt is the main regulator of phosphorylation at Thr246 and relieves PRAS40-mediated inhibition of mTORC1 (Fig. 1a) [23, 41]. PRAS40-phosphorylation correlated with shorter time to progression in a smaller GB patient cohort [8]. Another study in low grade glioma found a trend towards shorter survival in tumors with higher phospho-PRAS40 levels; however, statistical significance was not reached [29]. Besides its regulation via PRAS40 phosphorylation, Akt also activates mTORC1 via inhibitory phosphorylation of a protein complex consisting of tuberin (TSC1), hamartin (TSC2) as well as the more recently discovered TBC1D7 (this complex will be termed in TSC1/2 in the following text for simplicity reasons) (Fig. 1a) [10, 19]. MTORC1 additionally integrates signals from the cellular energy status including oxygen availability [4], amino acid availability [2] and direct ATP content of the cell [20]. The ribosomal protein S6 (RPS6) is a downstream effector of mTORC1 and is part of the ribosomal machinery. RPS6 phosphorylation has been discovered many years ago, still its molecular and physiological effects especially with regard to the phosphorylation of the different serine sites are currently still under investigation [31]. RPS6 has several mTORC1-dependent phosphorylation sites including serines at position 235 and 236 as well as the highly specific position 240 and 244 (Fig. 1a) [31, 34].

Nimotuzumab is a blocking monoclonal antibody against EGFR [48] without intrinsic EGFR activating activity. It has shown promising results as a targeted therapy in the treatment of high grade gliomas in phase II studies [3] and pediatric brain stem gliomas [28, 57]. Therefore, a two arm phase III clinical trial (OSAG 101-BSA-05) involving 149 patients was performed comparing standard (radiotherapy and temozolomide) treatment with and without addition of nimotuzumab (EudraCT No. 2005–003101-85, ClinicalTrials.gov NCT00753246) [55]. Nimotuzumab was administered once weekly (400 mg) during the concomitant radio-temozolomide phase and afterwards continued biweekly (400 mg) for 12 weeks during the adjuvant temozolomide treatment phase. The trial was negative, and a benefit of nimotuzumab treatment was apparent neither in the whole population studied nor in patients with EGFR amplification. A post-hoc analysis of subgroups, however, revealed a trend for improved survival for MGMT unmethylated patients with residual tumor when treated with nimotuzumab (PFS 6.2 vs. 4.0 months; OS 19.0 vs. 13.8 months). This unplanned subgroup analysis, however, included only 28 patients and failed to reach statistical significance. The results of several recent trials suggest that for an effective targeted therapy, appropriate patients need to be identified [56]. With regard to signal transduction inhibitors it is plausible that genetic heterogeneity in GBs is also reflected by different degrees of dependence on certain signaling cascades [32]. The aim of this study

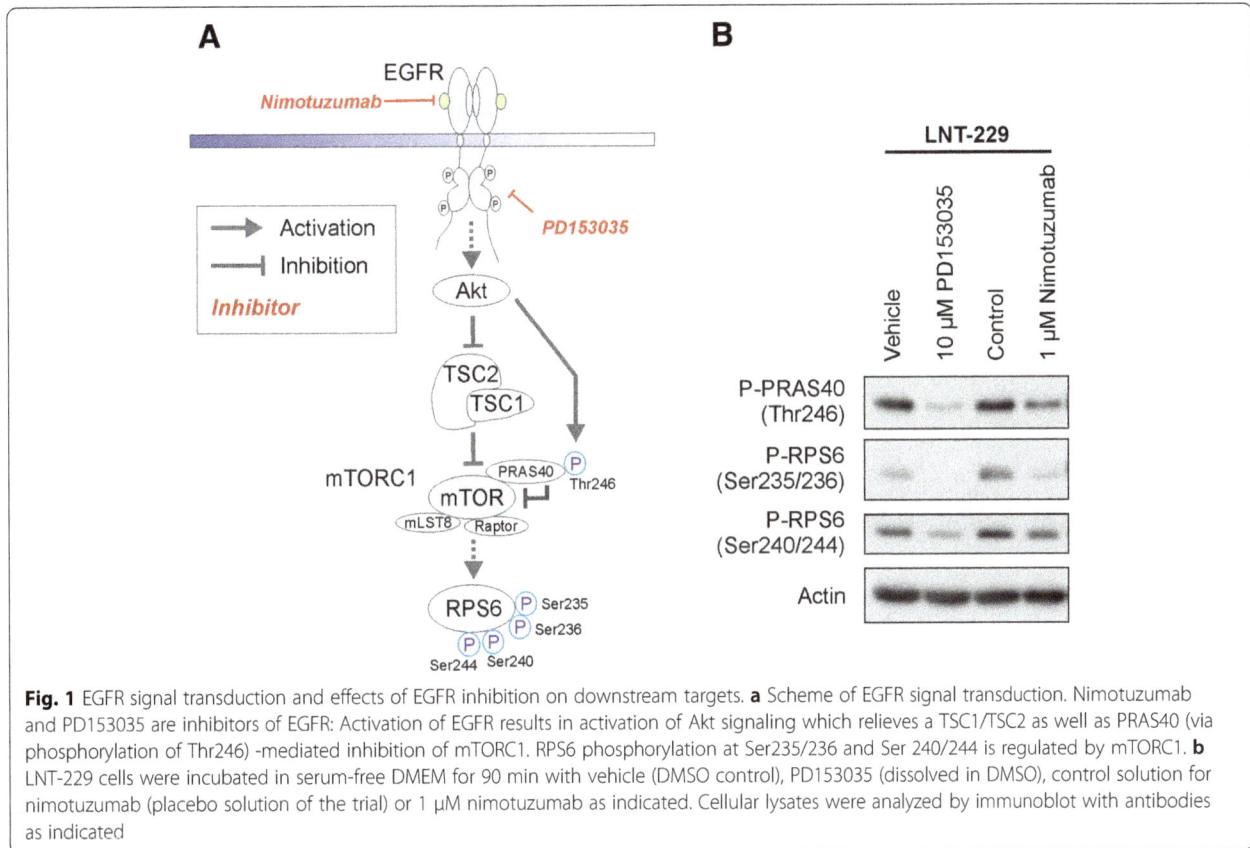

Fig. 1 EGFR signal transduction and effects of EGFR inhibition on downstream targets. **a** Scheme of EGFR signal transduction. Nimotuzumab and PD153035 are inhibitors of EGFR: Activation of EGFR results in activation of Akt signaling which relieves a TSC1/TSC2 as well as PRAS40 (via phosphorylation of Thr246) -mediated inhibition of mTORC1. RPS6 phosphorylation at Ser235/236 and Ser 240/244 is regulated by mTORC1. **b** LNT-229 cells were incubated in serum-free DMEM for 90 min with vehicle (DMSO control), PD153035 (dissolved in DMSO), control solution for nimotuzumab (placebo solution of the trial) or 1 μM nimotuzumab as indicated. Cellular lysates were analyzed by immunoblot with antibodies as indicated

was to analyze EGFR-dependent Akt and mTORC1 signaling in treatment-naïve tumor samples of the OSAG 101-BSA-05 patient cohort as a potential predictive biomarker of nimotuzumab efficacy. We analyzed the response to nimotuzumab therapy of molecular subgroups depending on activation of Akt and mTORC1 signaling, extent of necrosis, HIF-1α staining and MGMT-methylation status. We here report a predictive signature of RPS6 and PRAS40 phosphorylation in MGMT unmethylated patients. Furthermore, we describe a trend for a predictive value of RPS6 phosphorylation in all patients irrespective of MGMT promoter methylation status.

Materials and methods

Reagents

Nimotuzumab as well as the corresponding placebo control solution were provided by Oncoscience (Wedel, Germany). Nimotuzumab is an IgG subtype 1 kappa with a molecular weight of 147.613 kDa. The EGFR inhibitor PD153035 [11] was purchased from Sigma Aldrich (Taufkirchen, Germany).

Cell culture

LNT-229 GB cells have been described previously [38, 50] and were maintained in Dulbecco's modified eagle medium

(DMEM) containing 10% foetal calf serum (FCS) (Biochrom KG, Berlin, Germany), 100 IU/ml penicillin and 100 mg/ml streptomycin (Life Technologies, Darmstadt, Germany).

Immunoblot

Immunoblot was performed as described previously [14]. 10 μg of protein per condition were used for SDS-PAGE analysis. Membranes were incubated with antibodies against phospho-RPS6 (Ser 240/244) (D68F8; Cell Signaling), phospho-RPS6 (Ser 235/236) (D57.2.2.E; Cell Signaling), phospho-PRAS40 (Thr246) (C77D7, Cell signaling) or actin (# sc-1616 Santa Cruz Biotechnology, Dallas, Texas, USA). The secondary HRP-conjugated antibodies were purchased from Santa Cruz Biotechnology (Dallas, Texas, USA). A chemiluminescence solution was used for detection [50].

Patients, sample collection and immunohistochemistry

The OSAG 101-BSA-05 study (EudraCT No. is 2005–003101-85, ClinicalTrials.gov

NCT00753246) cohort included 149 patients with GB [55]. This open label, randomised phase III study was approved by the central and local ethics review boards. Informed consent was obtained from all patients. In case of availability, we obtained tissue sections from these tumors for further immunohistochemistry. We investigated the amount of necrosis (%) in hematoxylin and eosin (HE)-stained slides of the tissue sections ($n = 111$), HIF-1α expression (%) in the vital tumor centre ($n = 106$) as well as in perinecrotic areas ($n = 98$), P-PRAS40-positive cells (%) ($n = 101$), P-RPS6-positive cells (%) ($n = 109$) as well as Iba1-positive cells (%) ($n = 100$) using standard procedures on an automated IHC staining system. Stainings with antibodies against threonine 246-phosphorylated PRAS40 (P-PRAS40) and serine 240/244-phosphorylated RPS6 (P-RPS6) (Cell signaling, #2997 and #5364 respectively) were performed as recently reported [14]. Furthermore, the following antibodies were used: HIF-1α (Novus Biologicals, NB 100–134), Iba1 (Wako, 019–19,741). Samples that consisted of 100% necrosis were excluded from further analysis.

Statistical analyses

Statistical analyses were performed using JMP version 13 software (SAS Institute, Heidelberg, Germany). A p-value of $p < 0.05$ was chosen to declare statistical significance. Applied statistical test methods are either mentioned in the figure legend or in the flow content. For dichotomized univariate survival analyses we performed a median split to obtain a high and low group with regard to the investigated factor. The high group includes specimen with values above median, the low group includes specimen with median or below.

Results

Nimotuzumab inhibits EGFR downstream signaling

To test whether nimotuzumab inhibited signaling from the EGFR-downstream kinases Akt and mTORC1 (Fig. 1a), we exposed human LNT-229 glioblastoma cells to nimotuzumab or the intracellular EGFR inhibitor PD153035 [11]. Both substances caused effective inhibition of EGFR downstream signal transduction indicated by a similar degree of reduction in phosphorylation of the corresponding target proteins PRAS40 as well as RPS6 in an immunoblot experiment (Fig. 1b). We chose P-PRAS40 (Thr246) and P-RPS6 (Ser240/244) in our further tissue analysis due to the specificity of the phosphorylation site and the availability of robust, monoclonal antibodies for IHC. Effective Akt inhibition by nimotuzumab had also previously been reported in other cell lines including EGFR overexpressing U87 GB cells, lung and nasopharyngeal carcinoma cells [7, 18, 37].

Phosphorylation of PRAS40 and RPS6 is only detectable in a small proportion of tumor cells and does not correlate with EGFR gene amplification

For histological characterization of our cohort, we evaluated the extent of necrosis, P-PRAS40, P-RPS6 and HIF-1α in perinecrotic as well as in vital tumor areas.

Additionally, we analyzed Iba1 expression as a marker for glioma-associated microglia and macrophages (GAMs) and potential source of P-PRAS40 and P-RPS6 expression (Additional file 1: Figure S1). Extent of necrosis ranged from 0 to 100%, with a median of 10% (Fig. 2a). HIF-1α within central vital tumor areas was undetectable in most tumors but ranged up to 20% in one tumor with a median of 0% (Fig. 2b). In contrast, perinecrotic HIF-1α ranged from 0 to 80% with a median of 10% (Fig. 2c) and correlated with necrosis extent (Additional file 2: Figure S2). P-PRAS40 was detectable in a fraction of cells with a range of 0 to 80% and a median of 10% (Fig. 2d). P-RPS6 was similarly detectable in a fraction of tumor cells with a similar range of 0 to 60% however the median was lower at 3% (Fig. 2e). Besides the actual GB tumor cells, GAMs can account for a relevant fraction of intratumoral cells and potentially influence signal transduction of cancer cells or constitute a potential source of mTORC1 or AKT signaling. Therefore, we stained the samples for the pan-microglia and macrophage (M/M) marker Iba1. Staining frequency ranged from 3 to 70% with a median of 20% (Fig. 2f). Neither P-PRAS40 nor P-RPS6 correlated with Iba1 (Fig. 2g, h). In contrast, P-PRAS40 and P-RPS6 expression as markers of EGFR signal transduction correlated (Fig. 2i). Besides being downstream of EGFR, mTORC1 is also regulated by the cellular energy charge and nutrient supply [20, 40]. GB necrosis occurs where demand exceeds supply of the fast growing tumor cells and the perinecrotic area is where nutrient and oxygen deprivation are most severe within the tumor. Interestingly, P-RPS6 as a target of mTORC1 was increased in necrotic tumors potentially indicating a defective nutrient sensing as a cause of increased necrosis [50] (Fig. 2j). An inverse correlation was found for P-PRAS40 (Fig. 2k). Neither P-PRAS40 nor P-RPS6 correlated with Hif-1α staining (data not shown).

Information on EGFR amplification and vIII mutation was available for 88 and 81 cases respectively [55]. EGFR gene amplification correlates with increased expression of EGFR [43] and was found in 43 cases. An inverse effect was detectable on downstream Akt but not mTORC1 signal transduction (Fig. 2l). However, with only 7 cases of vIII mutation in our cohort, the number was too small to derive any conclusions in this regard. Notably, there was also no difference in the end points for patients with and without EGFR amplification or vIII mutation in the OSAG 101-BSA-05 trial [55].

Necrosis extent and HIF-1α staining is not associated with patient survival

While necrosis as a surrogate of hypoxia or ischemia is a common histological feature in GB, a more outspread or increased necrosis extent or hypoxia could indicate a

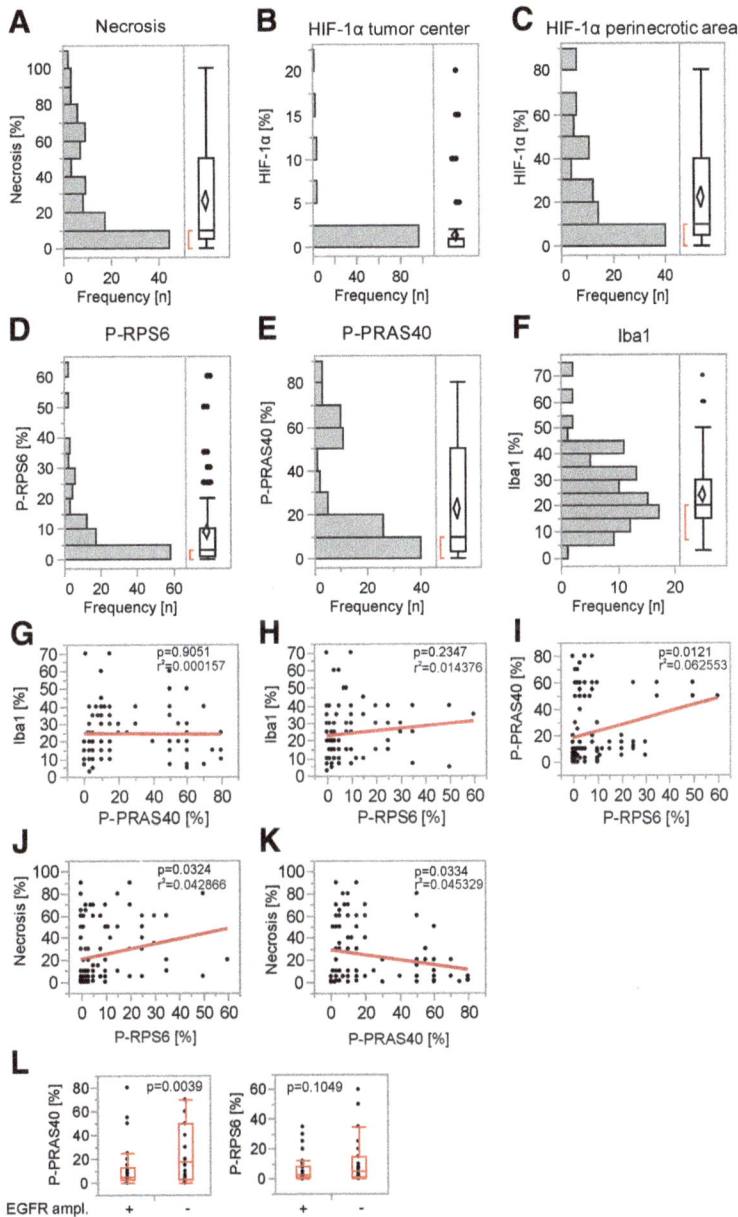

Fig. 2 Histological characterization of the patient cohort. **a-f**, outlier box plot for the distribution of necrosis, HIF-1α in vital, central or perinecrotic tumor areas, phosphorylated (P-)RPS6, P-PRAS40 and Iba1 in samples as indicated (horizontal line within the box is the median sample value; confidence diamond contains the mean and the upper and lower 95% of the mean; ends of the box represent the 25th and 75th quantiles; bracket outside of the box is the shortest half, which is the most dense 50% of observations). **g-k**, correlations of histological markers as indicated in a bivariate plot with a linear regression analysis. P and r^2 values as indicated. **l** one way analysis with outlier box plot of P-PRAS40 and P-RPS6 in EGFR amplified vs. non-amplified tumor specimens. *P*-value calculated using Student's *t*-test

particularly aggressive tumor subtype. A relationship between patient survival and intratumoral hypoxia has e.g. been reported for uterine cancer [17]. In our cohort, we did not find an association between necrosis extent or HIF-1α staining and patient survival in univariate Weibull parametric survival analysis (Table 1). EGFR signaling is known to promote many components of a more aggressive tumor phenotype and P-PRAS40 has been reported as an independent prognostic marker with regard to time to progression in a small glioma cohort [8]. Neither P-RPS6 nor P-PRAS40 staining correlated with overall survival (Table 1).

Treatment of hypoxic tumors with nimotuzumab is not detrimental

We have previously shown that inhibition of EGFR or mTORC1 signal transduction can protect human glioblastoma cells from hypoxia-induced cell death [38, 45].

Table 1 Correlation of histology markers with survival

Treatment arm	Parametric survival Weibull p					
	Necrosis	HIF-1α perinecrotic area	HIF-1α vital tumor	P-PRAS40	P-RPS6	Iba1
Nimotuzumab	0.7360	0.3733	0.6135	0.2365	0.6078	0.5149
Control	0.1003	0.4436	0.7257	0.6929	0.2967	0.0275

Univariate Weibull parametric survival analysis was performed for the listed parameters

Therefore, we hypothesized that in tumors with increased necrosis or HIF-1α staining, nimotuzumab could mediate tumor-protective effects resulting in decreased survival of patients. Necrosis extent, HIF-1α staining, P-PRAS40, P-RPS6 and Iba1 staining were well-balanced between the two treatment arms (Additional file 3: Figure S3A). Using a median split, we dichotomized tumors into two groups (high and low) (Additional file 1: Figure S1). Within the group of above median value necrotic tumors, nimotuzumab treatment resulted in a slight trend towards improved survival, whereas no trend was detectable in below or median value necrotic tumors (Fig. 3a). Also, no trend was detectable with regard to HIF-1α high and low tumors (Fig. 3b). Even though P-PRAS40 and P-RPS6 were not associated with patient survival in the treatment arms (Table 1), tumors with activated downstream signaling might define a patient subgroup more addicted to EGFR signaling and thus more prone to respond to nimotuzumab. There was no trend in overall survival in tumors with high or low P-PRAS40 with regard to nimotuzumab therapy (Fig. 3c). In contrast in P-RPS6 high tumors, we observed a clear trend towards improved survival when nimotuzumab treatment was administered (Fig. 3d).

Unmethylated MGMT promoter status defines a subgroup in which high necrosis, P-RPS6 or P-PRAS40 tumors benefit from nimotuzumab treatment

In accordance with previous results, MGMT promoter methylation status was associated with patient survival in the OSAG 101-BSA-05 study cohort [55]. To test if the difference in biological behavior was also reflected by different activities of Akt and mTORC1 signaling, we investigated P-PRAS40 and P-RPS6 in both tumor subgroups. There was no difference in staining frequency for P-PRAS40 and P-RPS6 in MGMT promoter methylated vs. unmethylated tumors (Additional file 3: Figure S3B). In MGMT unmethylated GBs a treatment effect might be to a lesser extent concealed by temozolomide efficacy. When considering only the MGMT unmethylated cohort, the clear trend in favor of nimotuzumab therapy already detectable in the whole cohort regardless of MGMT promoter methylation status, now became significant when using a median split for P-RPS6 in tumors with above median value (p value of 0.02, Wilcoxon) (Fig. 4a). Additionally, the same effect was also detectable when using a P-PRAS40 median split in the

MGMT promoter unmethylated tumor cohort ($p = 0.03$, Wilcoxon) (Fig. 4a). Also, there was a trend towards an efficacy of nimotuzumab in MGMT promoter unmethylated tumors with above median extent of necrosis (Fig. 4a). No effect was detectable in tumors with below or median values for necrosis, P-RPS6 and P-PRAS40 (Fig. 4b).

P-RPS6 expression predicts survival depending on the treatment group in MGMT promoter unmethylated GBs

We wondered whether P-RPS6 was also relevant for survival of patients within the treatment arms in MGMT promoter unmethylated GBs. In patients treated with nimotuzumab, an above median expression of P-RPS6 was associated with improved survival (Fig. 5a, left panel). In contrast in patients with control treatment, above median P-RPS6 expression was associated with reduced survival (Fig. 5a, right panel). No association of P-PRAS40 with patient survival within the treatment arms was detectable when using a median split (Fig. 5b).

Increased GAM levels correlate with improved survival in patients treated with nimotuzumab

GAMs constitute relevant portions of a GB and the assumption that GAMs might be associated with an adverse prognosis in GB patients is under debate [44]. Interestingly, in tumors with above median Iba1 staining frequency (Iba1 high), nimotuzumab treatment was associated with a prolonged survival (Fig. 6, right panel). In contrast no effect of nimotuzumab was detectable for tumors with below median Iba1 staining frequency (Iba1 low) (Fig. 6, left panel).

Discussion

The experience with targeted therapies in recent GB trials has been overall disappointing highlighting the need for predictive biomarkers. In this retrospective analysis of samples of the OSAG 101-BSA-05 trial [55], we investigated histological subgroups based on necrosis and hypoxia as markers for a nutrient-deprived tumor microenvironment as well as for phosphorylation of PRAS40 and RPS6 as downstream markers of EGFR signaling. We hypothesized a reduced efficacy of EGFR inhibition therapy in tumors with pronounced necrosis or hypoxia due to potential protective effects of inhibitor therapy in this context [38, 45]. Tumor hypoxia as indicated by HIF-1α staining as well as necrosis were not associated

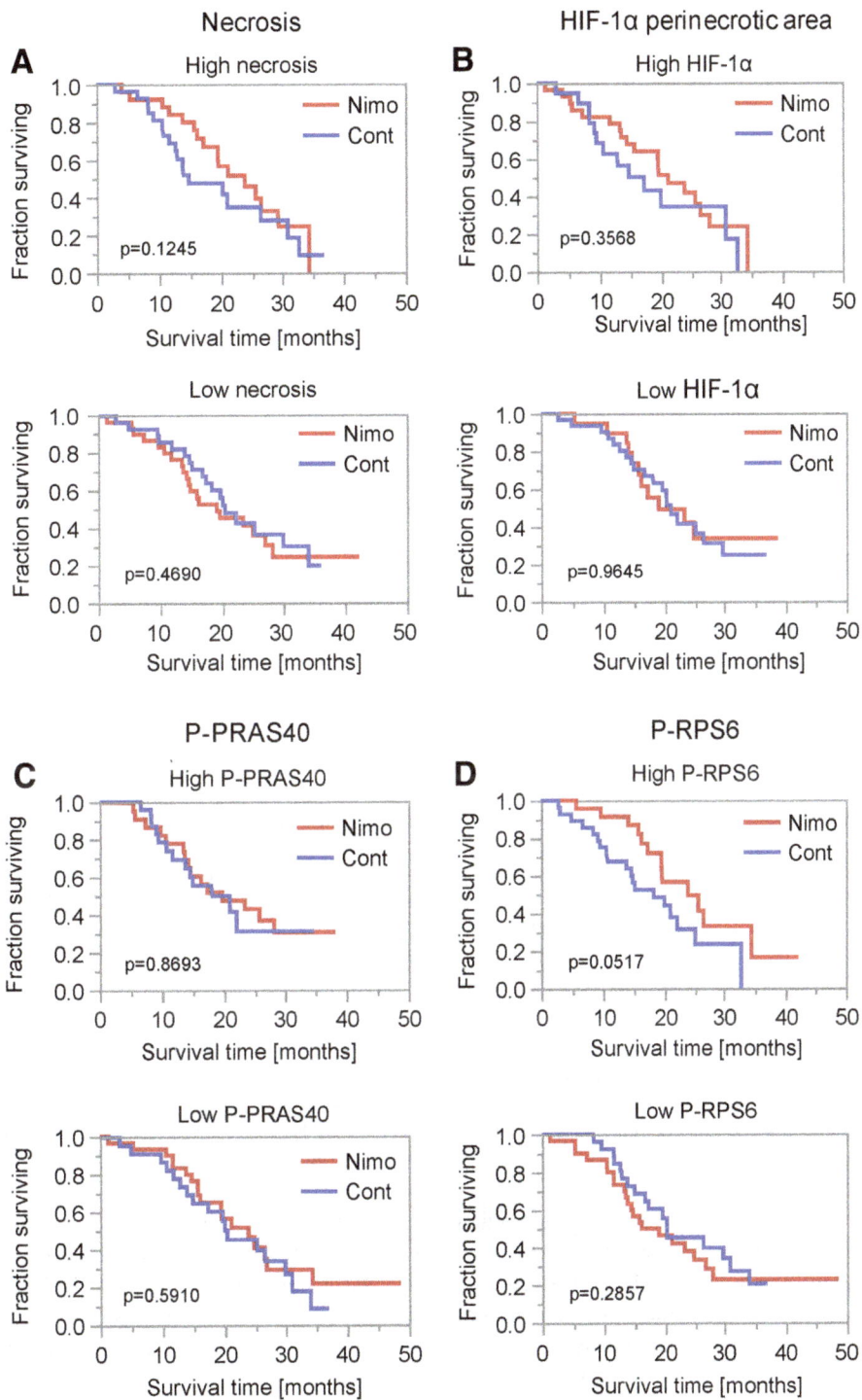

Fig. 3 Survival analyses depending on treatment in histological subgroups. **a-d** Kaplan-Meier survival curves for patients treated with nimotuzumab (nimo) or placebo (cont) in dichotomized histological subgroups (median split, above median: high, below and equal to median low) for necrosis (**a**), HIF-1α in perinecrotic regions (**b**), P-PRAS40 (**c**) and P-RPS6 (**d**). *P* values were calculated using the Wilcoxon test

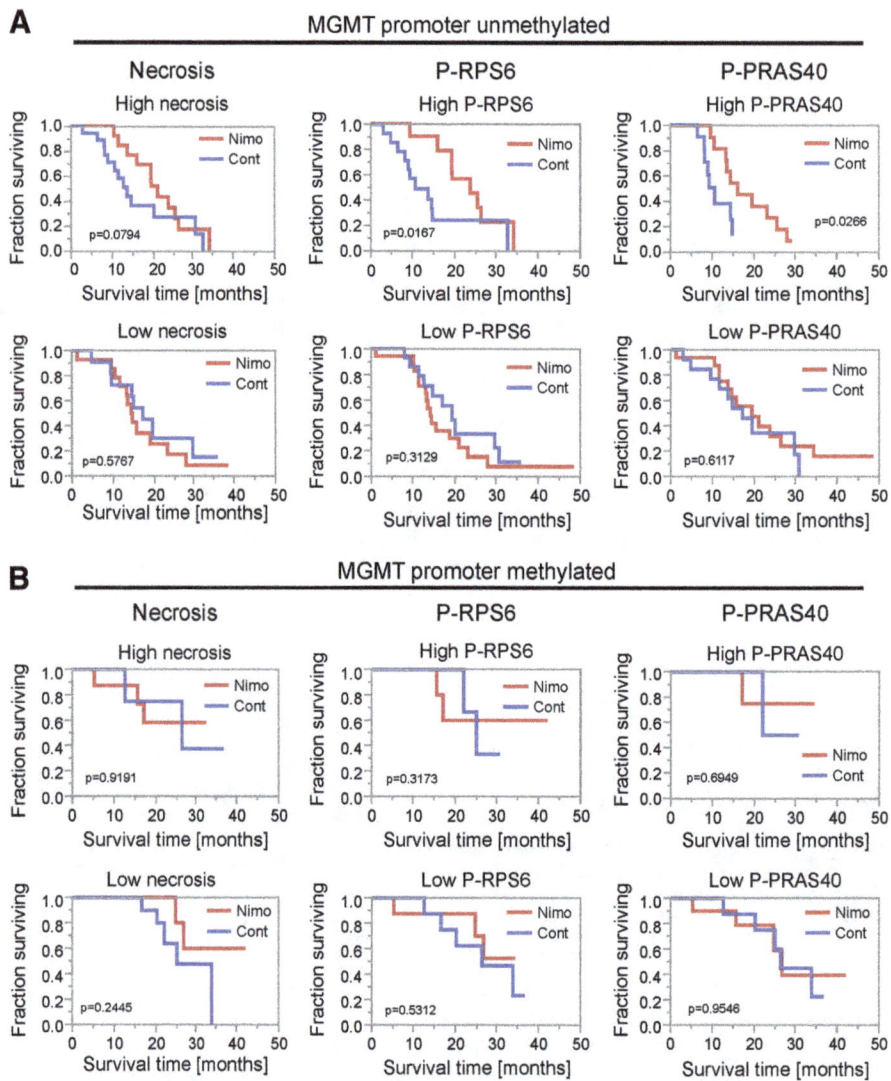

Fig. 4 Survival analyses depending on treatment in histological subgroups for the MGMT-promoter unmethylated and methylated tumor cohort. **a-b** Kaplan-Meier survival curves for patients treated with nimotuzumab (nimo) or placebo (cont) in dichotomized histological subgroups (median split, above median: high, below and equal to median low) for necrosis, P-PRAS40 and P-RPS6 in the MGMT-promoter unmethylated (**a**) and methylated (**b**) tumor cohort. P values were calculated using the Wilcoxon test

with patient survival (Table 1). When using a median split for necrosis extent, on the contrary to our hypothesis, there was a slight trend towards improved efficacy of nimotuzumab in patients with tumors with above median necrosis (Fig. 3a). No trend was detectable using a median split for perinecrotic HIF-1α staining frequency (Fig. 3b). HIF-1α staining frequency in vital tumor tissue was low with a median of 0%, therefore we did not include a dichotomized analysis in our study. GBs with increased signaling from EGFR and downstream kinases might constitute a collective with oncogene addiction exposing an Achilles heel for targeted therapies. Dichotomizing for P-PRAS40 high and low tumors had no effect on nimotuzumab treatment efficacy (Fig. 3c), in contrast to P-RPS6 where a clear trend towards

nimotuzumab efficacy was detectable in tumors with high P-RPS6 (Fig. 3d). Neither P-PRAS40 nor P-RPS6 was associated with patient survival (Table 1). However, when testing for time to progression, P-PRAS40 was associated with a shorter interval (Additional file 4: Figure S4A) similar to a previous report [8].

The majority of GB (approximately 55–65%) has an unmethylated MGMT promoter defining a subgroup that is especially difficult to treat due to the reduced efficacy of temozolomide [9, 15, 22]. When investigating only MGMT unmethylated tumors, above median P-RPS6 was associated with nimotuzumab efficacy (Fig. 4a) which has already been detectable as a trend in the whole study cohort (Fig. 3a, d). In addition, above median P-PRAS40 was associated with improved survival in patients treated

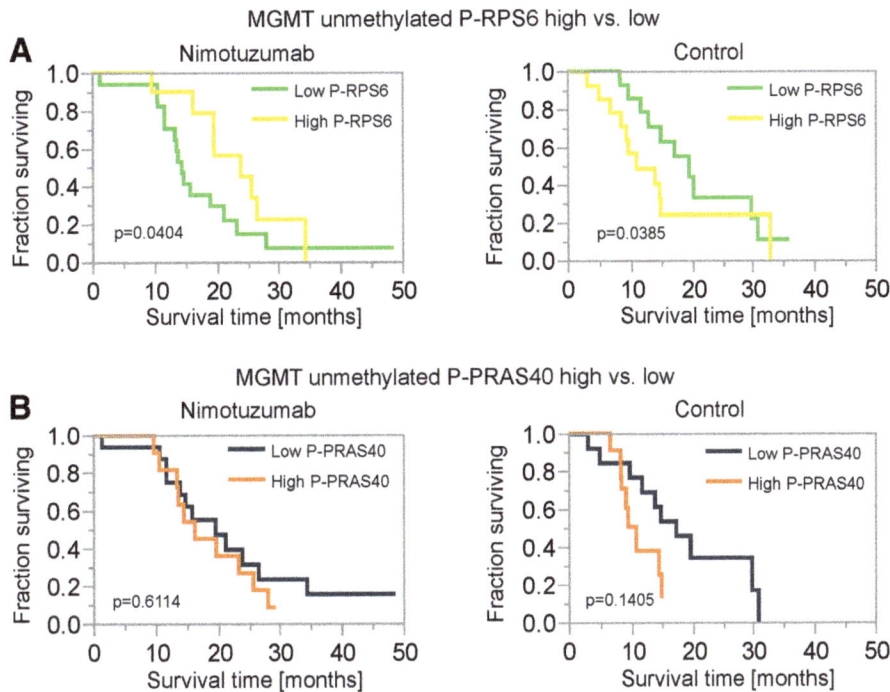

Fig. 5 Prognostic relevance of P-RPS6 and P-PRAS40 in treatment groups of MGMT-promoter unmethylated tumors. **a-b** Kaplan-Meier survival curves for patients with MGMT promoter unmethylated GBs treated with nimotuzumab or placebo (control) for dichotomized histological subgroups (median split, above median: high, below and equal to median low) for P-RPS6 (**a**) and P-PRAS40 (**b**). P values were calculated using the Wilcoxon test

with nimotuzumab (Fig. 4a). The positive correlation between necrosis extent and P-RPS6 (Fig. 2j) was unexpected considering that mTORC1 is also a component of central cellular nutrient sensing pathways and cells with intact nutrient sensing inhibit mTORC1 in nutrient deplete conditions [50]. This indicates a potentially dysregulated mTORC1 sensor in our cohort resulting in higher extent necrosis as has been suggested recently (Additional file 4: Figure S4B) [50]. The efficacy of

nimotuzumab in patients with high P-RPS6 (as a trend in the whole study cohort and statistically significant only in MGMT unmethylated GBs) points to a potentially higher degree of addiction to mTORC1 and ultimately EGFR signaling in this subgroup. While the homogeneous patient cohort of a registered randomized phase III trial adhering to central monitoring standards was a major strength of our study, introducing subgroups naturally shrunk patient numbers and our results need to be

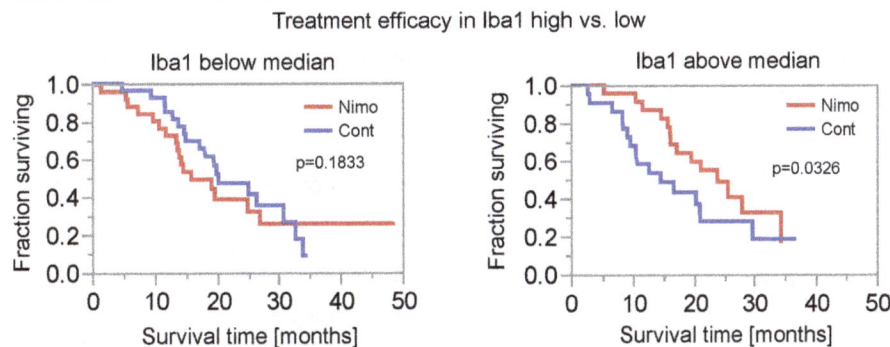

Fig. 6 Survival analysis depending on treatment in subgroups based on microglial prevalence. Kaplan-Meier survival curves for patients treated with nimotuzumab (nimo) or placebo (cont) in dichotomized subgroups based on Iba1 staining frequency (median split, above median: high, below and equal to median low). P values were calculated using the Wilcoxon test

validated prospectively in a larger patient cohort using our EGFR signaling markers as entry criteria. Additionally, PTEN and PI3 Kinase loss/mutation are frequent events in GB (~ 36% and ~ 6% of GB samples respectively) [32] and most likely partly impact nimotuzumab efficacy. Therefore, it is remarkable that P-RPS6 dichotomization was sufficient to define a subgroup with a clear trend towards nimotuzumab efficacy in samples of unknown PTEN and PI3 Kinase status (Fig. 3). In an upcoming prospective analysis, it would be important to include these markers and PTEN and PI3 Kinase wildtype status would most likely define an even more nimotuzumab-susceptible subgroup of tumors. Accordingly, in a previously published retrospective analysis of tissue of 26 GB patients treated with the non-antibody EGFR inhibitors erlotinib or gefitinib response in the recurrent disease setting correlated with expression of vIII-mutated EGFR and PTEN [30]. No evaluation of downstream phosphorylation events in the tumor tissue was included in this analysis, still these results suggest that tumors with high EGFR signaling activity and intact signal transduction are sensitive to EGFR inhibitors. In the recent phase II EORTC 26082 trial, similar to our results, mTORC1 activation as indicated by phosphorylation of the mTOR protein itself at Ser2448 was a marker to predict response to treatment with the mTOR inhibitor temsirolimus in MGMT unmethylated GBs [56]. The relevant kinase that mediates phosphorylation of mTOR at Ser2448 is S6 Kinase [5] which is exactly the same kinase that mediates RPS6 phosphorylation and therefore is responsible for P-RPS6 in our cohort (Additional file 4: Figure S4C). Additionally, in multivariate analyses, PRAS40 phosphorylation was associated with survival in the temsirolimus treatment arm [56]. The authors propose phosphorylated mTOR (Ser2448) and P-PRAS40 as potential biomarkers for mTOR inhibitor therapy in MGMT-promoter unmethylated GBs. Our results confirm this notion with nimotuzumab as an indirect mTORC1 inhibitor (Fig. 1b). Integrating the results of the analyses of predictive signatures for EGFR [30] and mTOR inhibitors [56] and our analysis points to a signature where a high (er) degree of activation and an intact EGFR signaling axis defines GBs susceptible to inhibitors of this pathway in general. Accurate analysis of the in vivo phosphorylation status of proteins by IHC to monitor EGFR signaling activity requires special caution. E.g. time to processing and several other factors can have a major influence on phosphorylation and dephosphorylation events [14]. Therefore, for a prospective analysis of biomarkers in a clinical trial, standardized tissue asservation will be an important topic to include in the protocol.

The need for and potential adverse effects of neglecting potential predictive biomarkers is highlighted by the recently published results of the thus far largest randomized phase II trial evaluating the efficacy of the mTORC1 inhibitor everolimus in newly diagnosed GB that randomized 171 patients [6]. Patients receiving everolimus in addition to standard radiochemotherapy in this trial had a reduced survival in comparison to sole standard radiochemotherapy [1, 6]. One potential explanation of these results demonstrating reduced survival when an mTOR inhibitor was added to the therapeutic regimen in GB could be protective effects of mTOR inhibition in the context of the tumor microenvironment that we have previously shown in cell culture models [38].

Data regarding the prognostic impact of the innate immune system including GAMs in GBs is conflicting [12, 21]. In our study cohort, we found a positive effect on prolonged overall survival in patients treated with nimotuzumab with GBs of above median Iba1 frequency (Fig. 6). Investigating the whole patient cohort irrespective of treatment arm, we found no association with survival when dichotomizing for high vs. low GAM infiltration (Additional file 4: Figure S4D). These results contrast the notion that GAM subpopulations might have negative effects on GB patient survival [36]. However, similar findings as in our cohort regarding the prognostic role of GAMs are described, likewise demonstrating a positive prognostic impact of at least a GAM subpopulation in GB [58]. Currently we can only speculate on the underlying reasons for this positive effect of intratumoral GAMs on overall survival in GB patients treated with nimotuzumab. It is interesting to note that microglia express receptors for binding of the Fc part of antibodies and might therefore react with nimotuzumab-bound GB cells similar to mechanistic hypotheses of antibody mediated plaque clearance in Alzheimer's models [26]. Further clarifying potential antibody effects on GAMs is beyond the scope of this article and should be investigated elsewhere.

Conclusions

The quest for new treatment options in GB has been cumbersome at best with no new drugs gaining approval since the introduction of temozolomide. In this current study, we investigated tissue samples of yet another negative phase III trial. The EGFR is one of the most plausible treatment targets in this cancer entity. We here report markers for the selection of patients that might benefit from the EGFR-blocking antibody nimotuzumab. Considering the majority of GB patients with unmethylated MGMT promoter status, activation of Akt or mTORC1 signaling was associated with a benefit from nimotuzumab treatment. A clear trend towards a benefit from nimotuzumab therapy was also detectable in the whole study cohort using activation of mTORC1 as a marker for dichotomy. We believe that our results constitute a basis for further investigation of nimotuzumab or other EGFR- and mTOR-inhibitors in selected patient cohorts using the reported criteria as candidate predictive biomarkers.

Additional files

Additional file 1: Figure S1. Representative images of histological subclassifications. Representative images of immunohistochemical staining for HIF-1α, P-PRAS40, P-RPS6 and Iba1 from FFPE tumor specimens of below and equal to (low) and above (high) median marker frequency. (TIF 13094 kb)

Additional file 2: Figure S2. Correlation of perinecrotic HIF-1α and necrosis. Correlation of perinecrotic HIF-1α and necrosis in a bivariate plot with a linear regression analysis. P and r^2 values as indicated. (TIF 64 kb)

Additional file 3: Figure S3. Distribution of histology markers in treatment arms. A, one way analysis with outlier box plot of necrosis, HIF-1α in perinecrotic or in vital central tumor regions, P-RPS6, P-PRAS40 and Iba1 in tumors of patients treated with nimotuzumab (nimo) or placebo (cont). B, one way analysis with outlier box plot of P-RPS6 and P-PRAS40 in tumors with methylated or unmethylated MGMT promoter. P-value calculated using Student's t-test. (TIF 495 kb)

Additional file 4: Figure S4. Survival analyses and schemes of signal transduction. A, Weibull parametric analysis of P-PRAS40 and time to progression in patients treated with nimotuzumab (left panel) or placebo (control, right panel). B, scheme of a nutrient sensing via mTORC1 and effects on cellular adaptation and necrosis. Cells with an intact mTORC1 sensor inhibit mTORC1 signaling during nutrient deprivation and hypoxia, despite signaling from EGFR preventing widespread necrosis (left panel). In contrast cells with a defective mTORC1 sensor fail to adequately inhibit mTORC1 in response to nutrient deprivation or hypoxia resulting in more widespread areas of necrosis (right panel). C, scheme of mTORC1 signal transduction to S6 kinase 1 (S6 K1). S6 K1 phosphorylates both RPS6 at Ser 240/244 as well as mTOR at Ser 2448. D, survival analysis depending on Iba1 staining frequency (median split, above median: high, below and equal to median low). P values were calculated using the Wilcoxon test. (TIF 559 kb)

Acknowledgements
The Dr. Senckenberg Institute of Neurooncology is supported by the Dr. Senckenberg Foundation and the Hertie Foundation. J.P.S. is "Hertie Professor of Neurooncology". P.S.Z. has received funding by the Frankfurt Research Funding (FFF) (program "Nachwuchswissenschaftler"). M.W.R. and P.N.H. have received a fellowship by the University Cancer Centre Frankfurt (UCT). M.W.R. has also received funding by the Frankfurt Research Funding (FFF) 'Clinician Scientists Program'. M.M. would like to thank the Luxembourg National Research Fond (FNR) for the support (FNR PEARL P16/BM/11192868 grant).

Authors' contributions
Study design and writing of the manuscript: MWR, PSZ, MM, JPS, MW, PNH. Provided material, data collection and data analyses: MWR, PSZ, MM, TP, DR, CS, JPS, MW, PNH. Performed experiments: MWR, PSZ, HU, PNH. All authors read and approved the final manuscript.

Competing interests
MWR, JPS and PNH received a grant to purchase materials necessary for immunohistochemistry from Oncoscience, the pharmaceutical company that owns nimotuzumab. DR is an employee and managing director of Oncoscience.

Author details
[1]Dr. Senckenberg Institute of Neurooncology, University Hospital Frankfurt, Goethe University, Schleusenweg 2-16, 60528 Frankfurt am Main, Germany. [2]German Cancer Consortium (DKTK), Partner Site Frankfurt/Mainz, Frankfurt am Main, Germany. [3]German Cancer Research Center (DKFZ), Heidelberg, Germany. [4]Institute of Neurology (Edinger-Institute), University Hospital Frankfurt, Goethe University, Heinrich-Hoffmann-Str. 7, 60528 Frankfurt am Main, Germany. [5]Luxembourg Centre for Systems Biomedicine (LCSB), University of Luxembourg, Dudelange, Luxembourg. [6]Laboratoire national de santé (LNS), Dudelange, Luxembourg. [7]Luxembourg Centre of Neuropathology (LCNP), Dudelange, Luxembourg. [8]Department of Neuropathology, University of Bonn, Bonn, Germany. [9]Oncoscience GmbH, Schenefeld, Germany. [10]Department of Neurosurgery, University Hospital Frankfurt, Goethe University, Frankfurt am Main, Germany. [11]Department of Neurosurgery, University Hospital Hamburg Eppendorf, Martinistrasse 52, 20246 Hamburg, Germany.

References
1. Babak S, Mason WP (2018) mTOR inhibition in glioblastoma: requiem for a dream? Neuro-oncology: noy034-noy034. https://doi.org/10.1093/neuonc/noy034
2. Bar-Peled L, Sabatini DM (2014) Regulation of mTORC1 by amino acids. Trends Cell Biol 24:400–406. https://doi.org/10.1016/j.tcb.2014.03.003
3. Bode U, Massimino M, Bach F, Zimmermann M, Khuhlaeva E, Westphal M, Fleischhack G (2012) Nimotuzumab treatment of malignant gliomas. Expert Opin Biol Ther 12:1649–1659. https://doi.org/10.1517/14712598.2012.733367
4. Brugarolas J, Lei K, Hurley RL, Manning BD, Reiling JH, Hafen E, Witters LA, Ellisen LW, Kaelin WG Jr (2004) Regulation of mTOR function in response to hypoxia by REDD1 and the TSC1/TSC2 tumor suppressor complex. Genes Dev 18:2893–2904
5. Chiang GG, Abraham RT (2005) Phosphorylation of mammalian target of rapamycin (mTOR) at Ser-2448 is mediated by p70S6 kinase. J Biol Chem 280:25485–25490. https://doi.org/10.1074/jbc.M501707200
6. Chinnaiyan P, Won M, Wen PY, Rojiani AM, Werner-Wasik M, Shih HA, Ashby LS, Michael Yu H-H, Stieber VW, Malone SC et al (2017) A randomized phase II study of everolimus in combination with chemoradiation in newly diagnosed glioblastoma: results of NRG oncology RTOG 0913. Neuro-oncology: nox209-nox209. https://doi.org/10.1093/neuonc/nox209
7. Chong DQ, Toh XY, Ho IA, Sia KC, Newman JP, Yulyana Y, Ng WH, Lai SH, Ho MM, Dinesh N et al (2015) Combined treatment of Nimotuzumab and rapamycin is effective against temozolomide-resistant human gliomas regardless of the EGFR mutation status. BMC Cancer 15:255. https://doi.org/10.1186/s12885-015-1191-3
8. Cloughesy TF, Yoshimoto K, Nghiemphu P, Brown K, Dang J, Zhu S, Hsueh T, Chen Y, Wang W, Youngkin D et al (2008) Antitumor activity of rapamycin in a phase I trial for patients with recurrent PTEN-deficient glioblastoma. PLoS Med 5:e8
9. Combs SE, Rieken S, Wick W, Abdollahi A, von Deimling A, Debus J, Hartmann C (2011) Prognostic significance of IDH-1 and MGMT in patients with glioblastoma: one step forward, and one step back? Radiat Oncol 6:115. https://doi.org/10.1186/1748-717X-6-115
10. Dibble CC, Elis W, Menon S, Qin W, Klekota J, Asara JM, Finan PM, Kwiatkowski DJ, Murphy LO, Manning BD (2012) TBC1D7 is a third subunit of the TSC1-TSC2 complex upstream of mTORC1. Mol Cell 47:535–546. https://doi.org/10.1016/j.molcel.2012.06.009
11. Fry DW, Kraker AJ, McMichael A, Ambroso LA, Nelson JM, Leopold WR, Connors RW, Bridges AJ (1994) A specific inhibitor of the epidermal growth factor receptor tyrosine kinase. Science 265:1093–1095
12. Gieryng A, Pszczolkowska D, Walentynowicz KA, Rajan WD, Kaminska B (2017) Immune microenvironment of gliomas. Lab Investig 97:498–518. https://doi.org/10.1038/labinvest.2017.19
13. Hanahan D, Weinberg RA (2011) Hallmarks of cancer: the next generation. Cell 144:646–674. https://doi.org/10.1016/j.cell.2011.02.013
14. Harter PN, Jennewein L, Baumgarten P, Ilina E, Burger MC, Thiepold AL, Tichy J, Zornig M, Senft C, Steinbach JP et al (2015) Immunohistochemical assessment of phosphorylated mTORC1-pathway proteins in human brain tumors. PLoS One 10:e0127123. https://doi.org/10.1371/journal.pone.0127123
15. Hegi ME, Diserens AC, Gorlia T, Hamou MF, de Tribolet N, Weller M, Kros JM, Hainfellner JA, Mason W, Mariani L et al (2005) MGMT gene silencing and benefit from temozolomide in glioblastoma. N Engl J Med 352:997–1003
16. Hegi ME, Liu L, Herman JG, Stupp R, Wick W, Weller M, Mehta MP, Gilbert MR (2008) Correlation of O6-methylguanine methyltransferase (MGMT) promoter methylation with clinical outcomes in glioblastoma and clinical strategies to modulate MGMT activity. J Clin Oncol Off J Am Soc Clin Oncol 26:4189–4199. https://doi.org/10.1200/JCO.2007.11.5964

17. Hockel M, Knoop C, Schlenger K, Vorndran B, Baussmann E, Mitze M, Knapstein PG, Vaupel P (1993) Intratumoral pO2 predicts survival in advanced cancer of the uterine cervix. Radiother Oncol 26:45–50

18. Huang J, Yuan X, Pang Q, Zhang H, Yu J, Yang B, Zhou L, Zhang F, Liu F (2018) Radiosensitivity enhancement by combined treatment of nimotuzumab and celecoxib on nasopharyngeal carcinoma cells. Drug Des Devel Ther 12:2223–2231. https://doi.org/10.2147/DDDT.S163595

19. Inoki K, Li Y, Zhu T, Wu J, Guan KL (2002) TSC2 is phosphorylated and inhibited by Akt and suppresses mTOR signalling. Nat Cell Biol 4:648–657

20. Inoki K, Zhu T, Guan KL (2003) TSC2 mediates cellular energy response to control cell growth and survival. Cell 115:577–590

21. Kennedy BC, Showers CR, Anderson DE, Anderson L, Canoll P, Bruce JN, Anderson RC (2013) Tumor-associated macrophages in glioma: friend or foe? J Oncol 2013:486912. https://doi.org/10.1155/2013/486912

22. Kessler T, Sahm F, Sadik A, Stichel D, Hertenstein A, Reifenberger G, Zacher A, Sabel M, Tabatabai G, Steinbach J et al (2018) Molecular differences in IDH wildtype glioblastoma according to MGMT promoter methylation. Neuro-Oncology 20:367–379. https://doi.org/10.1093/neuonc/nox160

23. Kovacina KS, Park GY, Bae SS, Guzzetta AW, Schaefer E, Birnbaum MJ, Roth RA (2003) Identification of a proline-rich Akt substrate as a 14-3-3 binding partner. J Biol Chem 278:10189–10194. https://doi.org/10.1074/jbc. M210837200

24. Louis DN, Perry A, Reifenberger G, von Deimling A, Figarella-Branger D, Cavenee WK, Ohgaki H, Wiestler OD, Kleihues P, Ellison DW (2016) The 2016 World Health Organization classification of tumors of the central nervous system: a summary. Acta Neuropathol 131:803–820. https://doi.org/10.1007/s00401-016-1545-1

25. Louis DNC, Webster K, Ohgaki H (2007) WHO classification of Tumours of the central nervous system. In: IARC WHO classification of Tumours, 4th edn. World health organization, City

26. Luo W, Liu W, Hu X, Hanna M, Caravaca A, Paul SM (2015) Microglial internalization and degradation of pathological tau is enhanced by an anti-tau monoclonal antibody. Sci Rep 5:11161. https://doi.org/10.1038/srep11161

27. Mandel JJ, Yust-Katz S, Patel AJ, Cachia D, Liu D, Park M, Yuan Y, Kent TA, de Groot JF (2018) Inability of positive phase II clinical trials of investigational treatments to subsequently predict positive phase III clinical trials in glioblastoma. Neuro-Oncology 20:113–122. https://doi.org/10.1093/neuonc/nox144

28. Massimino M, Bode U, Biassoni V, Fleischhack G (2011) Nimotuzumab for pediatric diffuse intrinsic pontine gliomas. Expert Opin Biol Ther 11:247–256. https://doi.org/10.1517/14712598.2011.546341

29. McBride SM, Perez DA, Polley MY, Vandenberg SR, Smith JS, Zheng S, Lamborn KR, Wiencke JK, Chang SM, Prados MD et al (2010) Activation of PI3K/mTOR pathway occurs in most adult low-grade gliomas and predicts patient survival. J Neuro-Oncol 97:33–40. https://doi.org/10.1007/s11060-009-0004-4

30. Mellinghoff IK, Wang MY, Vivanco I, Haas-Kogan DA, Zhu S, Dia EQ, Lu KV, Yoshimoto K, Huang JH, Chute DJ et al (2005) Molecular determinants of the response of glioblastomas to EGFR kinase inhibitors. N Engl J Med 353: 2012–2024

31. Meyuhas O (2015) Ribosomal protein S6 phosphorylation: four decades of research. Int Rev Cell Mol Biol 320:41–73. https://doi.org/10.1016/bs.ircmb. 2015.07.006

32. Network TCGAR (2008) Comprehensive genomic characterization defines human glioblastoma genes and core pathways. Nature 455:1061–1068

33. Ostrom QT, Gittleman H, Liao P, Rouse C, Chen Y, Dowling J, Wolinsky Y, Kruchko C, Barnholtz-Sloan J (2014) CBTRUS statistical report: primary brain and central nervous system tumors diagnosed in the United States in 2007-2011. Neuro-oncology 16(Suppl 4):iv1–i63. https://doi.org/10.1093/neuonc/nou223

34. Pende M, Um SH, Mieulet V, Sticker M, Goss VL, Mestan J, Mueller M, Fumagalli S, Kozma SC, Thomas G (2004) S6K1(−/−)/S6K2(−/−) mice exhibit perinatal lethality and rapamycin-sensitive 5′-terminal oligopyrimidine mRNA translation and reveal a mitogen-activated protein kinase-dependent S6 kinase pathway. Mol Cell Biol 24:3112–3124

35. Phillips AC, Boghaert ER, Vaidya KS, Mitten MJ, Norvell S, Falls HD, DeVries PJ, Cheng D, Meulbroek JA, Buchanan FG et al (2016) ABT-414, an antibody-drug conjugate targeting a tumor-selective EGFR epitope. Mol Cancer Ther 15:661–669. https://doi.org/10.1158/1535-7163.MCT-15-0901

36. Poon CC, Sarkar S, Yong VW, Kelly JJP (2017) Glioblastoma-associated microglia and macrophages: targets for therapies to improve prognosis. Brain J Neurol 140:1548–1560. https://doi.org/10.1093/brain/aww355

37. Qu YY, Hu SL, Xu XY, Wang RZ, Yu HY, Xu JY, Chen L, Dong GL (2013) Nimotuzumab enhances the radiosensitivity of cancer cells in vitro by inhibiting radiation-induced DNA damage repair. PLoS One 8:e70727. https://doi.org/10.1371/journal.pone.0070727

38. Ronellenfitsch MW, Brucker DP, Burger MC, Wolking S, Tritschler F, Rieger J, Wick W, Weller M, Steinbach JP (2009) Antagonism of the mammalian target of rapamycin selectively mediates metabolic effects of epidermal growth factor receptor inhibition and protects human malignant glioma cells from hypoxia-induced cell death. Brain 132:1509–1522

39. Ronellenfitsch MW, Steinbach JP, Wick W (2010) Epidermal growth factor receptor and mammalian target of rapamycin as therapeutic targets in malignant glioma: current clinical status and perspectives. Target Oncol 5: 183–191

40. Sancak Y, Bar-Peled L, Zoncu R, Markhard AL, Nada S, Sabatini DM (2010) Ragulator-rag complex targets mTORC1 to the lysosomal surface and is necessary for its activation by amino acids. Cell 141:290–303. https://doi.org/10.1016/j.cell.2010.02.024

41. Sancak Y, Thoreen CC, Peterson TR, Lindquist RA, Kang SA, Spooner E, Carr SA, Sabatini DM (2007) PRAS40 is an insulin-regulated inhibitor of the mTORC1 protein kinase. Mol Cell 25:903–915. https://doi.org/10.1016/j. molcel.2007.03.003

42. Semenza GL (2013) HIF-1 mediates metabolic responses to intratumoral hypoxia and oncogenic mutations. J Clin Invest 123:3664–3671. https://doi. org/10.1172/JCI67230

43. Shinojima N, Tada K, Shiraishi S, Kamiryo T, Kochi M, Nakamura H, Makino K, Saya H, Hirano H, Kuratsu J et al (2003) Prognostic value of epidermal growth factor receptor in patients with glioblastoma multiforme. Cancer Res 63:6962–6970

44. Sorensen MD, Dahlrot RH, Boldt HB, Hansen S, Kristensen BW (2018) Tumour-associated microglia/macrophages predict poor prognosis in high-grade gliomas and correlate with an aggressive tumour subtype. Neuropathol Appl Neurobiol 44:185–206. https://doi.org/10.1111/nan.12428

45. Steinbach JP, Klumpp A, Wolburg H, Weller M (2004) Inhibition of epidermal growth factor receptor signaling protects human malignant glioma cells from hypoxia-induced cell death. Cancer Res 64:1575–1578

46. Stupp R, Hegi ME, Mason WP, van den Bent MJ, Taphoorn MJ, Janzer RC, Ludwin SK, Allgeier A, Fisher B, Belanger K et al (2009) Effects of radiotherapy with concomitant and adjuvant temozolomide versus radiotherapy alone on survival in glioblastoma in a randomised phase III study: 5-year analysis of the EORTC-NCIC trial. Lancet Oncol 10:459–466. https://doi.org/10.1016/S1470-2045(09)70025-7

47. Stupp R, Mason WP, van den Bent MJ, Weller M, Fisher B, Taphoorn MJ, Belanger K, Brandes AA, Marosi C, Bogdahn U et al (2005) Radiotherapy plus concomitant and adjuvant temozolomide for glioblastoma. N Engl J Med 352:987–996

48. Talavera A, Friemann R, Gomez-Puerta S, Martinez-Fleites C, Garrido G, Rabasa A, Lopez-Requena A, Pupo A, Johansen RF, Sanchez O et al (2009) Nimotuzumab, an antitumor antibody that targets the epidermal growth factor receptor, blocks ligand binding while permitting the active receptor conformation. Cancer Res 69:5851–5859. https://doi.org/10.1158/0008-5472. CAN-08-4518

49. Testa JR, Tsichlis PN (2005) AKT signaling in normal and malignant cells. Oncogene 24:7391–7393. https://doi.org/10.1038/sj.onc.1209100

50. Thiepold AL, Lorenz NI, Foltyn M, Engel AL, Dive I, Urban H, Heller S, Bruns I, Hofmann U, Drose S et al (2017) Mammalian target of rapamycin complex 1 activation sensitizes human glioma cells to hypoxia-induced cell death. Brain J Neurol 140:2623–2638. https://doi.org/10.1093/brain/awx196

51. van den Bent M, Gan HK, Lassman AB, Kumthekar P, Merrell R, Butowski N, Lwin Z, Mikkelsen T, Nabors LB, Papadopoulos KP et al (2017) Efficacy of depatuxizumab mafodotin (ABT-414) monotherapy in patients with EGFR-amplified, recurrent glioblastoma: results from a multi-center, international study. Cancer Chemother Pharmacol 80:1209–1217. https://doi.org/10.1007/s00280-017-3451-1

52. van den Bent MJ, Brandes AA, Rampling R, Kouwenhoven MC, Kros JM, Carpentier AF, Clement PM, Frenay M, Campone M, Baurain JF et al (2009) Randomized phase II trial of erlotinib versus temozolomide or carmustine in recurrent glioblastoma: EORTC brain tumor group study 26034. J Clin Oncol 27.1268–1274

53. Weller M, Butowski N, Tran DD, Recht LD, Lim M, Hirte H, Ashby L, Mechtler L, Goldlust SA, Iwamoto F et al (2017) Rindopepimut with temozolomide for patients with newly diagnosed, EGFRvIII-expressing glioblastoma (ACT IV): a

randomised, double-blind, international phase 3 trial. Lancet Oncol 18:1373–1385. https://doi.org/10.1016/S1470-2045(17)30517-X

54. Weller M, Kaulich K, Hentschel B, Felsberg J, Gramatzki D, Pietsch T, Simon M, Westphal M, Schackert G, Tonn JC et al (2014) Assessment and prognostic significance of the epidermal growth factor receptor vIII mutation in glioblastoma patients treated with concurrent and adjuvant temozolomide radiochemotherapy. Int J Cancer 134:2437–2447. https://doi.org/10.1002/ijc.28576

55. Westphal M, Heese O, Steinbach JP, Schnell O, Schackert G, Mehdorn M, Schulz D, Simon M, Schlegel U, Senft C et al (2015) A randomised, open label phase III trial with nimotuzumab, an anti-epidermal growth factor receptor monoclonal antibody in the treatment of newly diagnosed adult glioblastoma. Eur J Cancer. https://doi.org/10.1016/j.ejca.2014.12.019

56. Wick W, Gorlia T, Bady P, Platten M, van den Bent MJ, Taphoorn MJ, Steuve J, Brandes AA, Hamou MF, Wick A et al (2016) Phase II study of radiotherapy and Temsirolimus versus Radiochemotherapy with Temozolomide in patients with newly diagnosed glioblastoma without MGMT promoter Hypermethylation (EORTC 26082). Clin Cancer Res 22:4797–4806. https://doi.org/10.1158/1078-0432.CCR-15-3153

57. Wolff JE, Rytting ME, Vats TS, Zage PE, Ater JL, Woo S, Kuttesch J, Ketonen L, Mahajan A (2012) Treatment of recurrent diffuse intrinsic pontine glioma: the MD Anderson Cancer Center experience. J Neuro-Oncol 106:391–397. https://doi.org/10.1007/s11060-011-0677-3

58. Zeiner PS, Preusse C, Blank AE, Zachskorn C, Baumgarten P, Caspary L, Braczynski AK, Weissenberger J, Bratzke H, Reiss S et al (2015) MIF receptor CD74 is restricted to microglia/macrophages, associated with a M1-polarized immune milieu and prolonged patient survival in gliomas. Brain Pathol 25:491–504. https://doi.org/10.1111/bpa.12194

2

Glycoprotein NMB: a novel Alzheimer's disease associated marker expressed in a subset of activated microglia

Melanie Hüttenrauch[1], Isabella Ogorek[2], Hans Klafki[1], Markus Otto[3], Christine Stadelmann[4], Sascha Weggen[2], Jens Wiltfang[1,5] and Oliver Wirths[1*]

Abstract

Alzheimer's disease (AD) is an irreversible, devastating neurodegenerative brain disorder characterized by the loss of neurons and subsequent cognitive decline. Despite considerable progress in the understanding of the pathophysiology of AD, the precise molecular mechanisms that cause the disease remain elusive. By now, there is ample evidence that activated microglia have a critical role in the initiation and progression of AD. The present study describes the identification of Glycoprotein nonmetastatic melanoma protein B (GPNMB) as a novel AD-related factor in both transgenic mice and sporadic AD patients by expression profiling, immunohistochemistry and ELISA measurements. We show that GPNMB levels increase in an age-dependent manner in transgenic AD models showing profound cerebral neuron loss and demonstrate that GPNMB co-localizes with a distinct population of IBA1-positive microglia cells that cluster around amyloid plaques. Our data further indicate that GPNMB is part of a microglia activation state that is only present under neurodegenerative conditions and that is characterized by the up-regulation of a subset of genes including *TREM2*, *APOE* and *CST7*. In agreement, we provide in vitro evidence that soluble Aβ has a direct effect on *GPNMB* expression in an immortalized microglia cell line. Importantly, we show for the first time that GPNMB is elevated in brain samples and cerebrospinal fluid (CSF) of sporadic AD patients when compared to non-demented controls.

The current findings indicate that GPNMB represents a novel disease-associated marker that appears to play a role in the neuroinflammatory response of AD.

Keywords: Alzheimer's disease (AD), Glycoprotein nonmetastatic melanoma protein B (GPNMB), Neuroinflammation, Activated microglia, Sporadic AD patients, Transgenic mice, 5XFAD

Introduction

Alzheimer's disease (AD) is a progressive, age-associated neurodegenerative disorder and the most frequent cause of dementia among the elderly population. Major neuropathological hallmarks of AD include an abnormal accumulation of extracellular β-amyloid (Aβ) peptides and intraneuronal neurofibrillary tangles composed of hyperphosphorylated tau protein. The disease involves extensive loss of synapses and neuronal death in the cerebral cortex and hippocampus, leading to gradual memory loss and cognitive decline. Despite considerable efforts during the last decades to find an efficacious therapy to halt or reverse AD pathology, currently available drugs allow at best an alleviation of the symptoms but do not affect the underlying cause of the disease [44].

Apart from amyloid plaques and intracellular tau aggregates, neuroinflammation represents an additional hallmark of AD. An increase in neuroinflammatory markers such as nitric oxide, interleukin-1β (IL-1β) and tumor necrosis factor (TNF-α) has been widely reported in brains of both Alzheimer's disease patients and transgenic AD models (reviewed in [14]). Emerging evidence suggests that instead of solely being a passive response to aberrant protein aggregation in the brain, persistent neuroinflammation might play a causal role in the

* Correspondence: owirths@gwdg.de
[1]Department of Psychiatry and Psychotherapy, University Medical Center (UMG), Georg-August-University, Von-Siebold-Str. 5, 37075 Göttingen, Germany
Full list of author information is available at the end of the article

pathogenesis of AD. This hypothesis is supported by recent genome-wide association studies (GWAS) linking specific polymorphisms in inflammation-associated genes such as complement receptor-1 (*CR1*) [26], CD33 [13, 31] or triggering receptor expressed on myeloid cells-2 (*TREM2*) [8] to an increased risk for AD. Therefore, a detailed understanding of immunological processes associated with the disease has become a major goal in Alzheimer's research in order to evaluate modulation of neuroinflammation as a new therapeutic modality.

In a previous project, we performed a whole-brain transcriptome study to identify genes differentially expressed in the brains of 6-month-old APP/PS1KI mice compared to age-matched PS1KI and WT controls [51]. APP/PS1KI mice are a widely used AD model showing profound neuron loss in several brain regions, as well as working memory deficits and disturbed long-term potentiation [3, 5, 55]. The majority of genes that we discovered to be upregulated in APP/PS1KI mice compared to both control groups were implicated in inflammation-associated pathways and included intensively studied genes such as *TREM2*. Intriguingly, one of the most strongly up-regulated genes in the APP/PS1KI model was Glycoprotein nonmetastatic melanoma protein B (*GPNMB*), a gene that so far has not been implicated in AD [51].

GPNMB (also known as osteoactivin, OA) is a type I transmembrane glycoprotein that was initially described in a poorly metastatic melanoma cell line [52]. GPNMB is at least partially localized to the cell surface and ectodomain shedding by ADAM10 can release its large N-domain into the extracellular space [40]. Since its identification, GPNMB expression has been detected in multiple tissues such as bone, kidney and skeletal muscle where it is implicated in various cellular processes like cell differentiation, tumor progression and tissue regeneration [1, 25, 34, 53]. Furthermore, there is profound evidence that GPNMB has a function as a negative regulator of inflammatory processes. In macrophages, overexpression of GPNMB reduced the secretion of proinflammatory cytokines in vitro [39]. More recent data (in peripheral tissues) further indicate that GPNMB promotes the polarization of macrophages into an anti-inflammatory "M2" status, which results in the secretion of anti-inflammatory cytokines such as IL-10 and TGF-β [59, 61]. Interestingly, in the central nervous system, GPNMB expression was identified within motor neurons, radial glia and most abundantly in microglia cells, which are the resident immune cells of the brain. Therefore, it has been proposed that GPNMB might also play a role in inflammatory processes in the CNS [15]. Furthermore, GPNMB has been shown to be elevated in brain and/or plasma of numerous neurodegenerative diseases such as Gaucher disease [23, 62], Niemann-Pick Type C disease [28] and amyotrophic lateral sclerosis (ALS) [48]. However, the impact of GPNMB overexpression on the pathophysiology of these diseases has not been elucidated.

The aim of the present work was to investigate a potential role of GPNMB in transgenic AD mouse models and human patients with sporadic AD. We demonstrate an age-dependent increase in *GPNMB* mRNA and protein levels in different AD mouse models. In addition, we discovered that GPNMB expression increases in parallel with Aβ plaque deposition, therefore reflecting disease severity. Moreover, increased GPNMB levels were observed in the cerebrospinal fluid (CSF) and brains of human patients with sporadic AD.

Material and methods
Transgenic mice
The generation of 5XFAD mice (Tg6799) has been described previously [33]. In brief, 5XFAD mice overexpress APP695 carrying the Swedish, Florida and London mutations under the control of the murine Thy-1 promoter. Additionally, human presenilin-1 (PSEN1), carrying the familial Alzheimer's disease (FAD)-linked mutations M146 L and L286 V, is also expressed under the control of the murine Thy-1 promoter. 5XFAD mice used in this study were backcrossed for more than 10 generations to C57Bl/6 J wild-type mice (WT) from the Jackson Laboratory (Jackson Laboratories, Bar Harbor, ME, USA) to obtain an incipient congenic line on a C57BL/6 J genetic background.

The generation of APP/PS1KI mice has also been described [5]. APP/PS1KI mice express human mutant APP751 carrying the Swedish and London mutations under the control of the murine Thy-1 promoter. In addition, murine PSEN1 containing the M233 T and L235P mutations is expressed under the control of the endogenous mouse PSEN1 promoter. The APP/PS1KI mouse model was a generous gift of Dr. Laurent Pradier, Sanofi-Aventis, Paris, France.

The APP23 model was originally described by Sturchler-Pierrat and colleagues [46]. In this AD mouse model, human APP751 with the Swedish double-point mutation K670 M/N671 L is overexpressed under the control of the murine Thy-1 promoter. APP23 mice were a generous gift of Dr. Mathias Staufenbiel, Novartis, Basel, Switzerland. All animals were handled according to German guidelines for animal care.

Patient samples
Human brain samples
Human frozen brain samples from sporadic AD ($n = 9$, mean age 79.78 ± 11.28 years, Braak stage V-VI) and non-demented control subjects (NDC, $n = 9$, mean age 82 ± 9.77 years, Braak stage I-II), as well as paraffin-embedded AD and NDC samples for immunohistochemistry were obtained from the Netherlands Brain Bank. The present study was approved by the ethics committee of the University Medical Center Göttingen (12/1/15). Details regarding autopsy procedure can be found at www.brainbank.nl.

Characteristics of the study cohort are presented in Additional file 1.

Human CSF samples

Human cerebrospinal fluid (CSF) and corresponding serum samples from patients suffering from sporadic AD ($n = 10$, mean age 70.4 ± 7.56 years) and NDC subjects ($n = 10$, mean age 62.5 ± 9.32) were obtained by lumbar puncture, centrifuged, aliquoted and stored within 2 h at -80 °C until analysis. All patients were seen at the Department of Neurology in Ulm (Ethical approval number 20/10). Characteristics of the study cohort are presented in Additional file 1.

Cell culture and treatment conditions

Murine immortalized microglial BV-2 cells were grown in DMEM/F-12 media supplemented with 10% heat-inactivated fetal bovine serum (FBS, Biochrom), 2 mM L-Alanyl-L-Glutamine (Sigma-Aldrich) and non-essential amino acids (Sigma-Aldrich). SH-SY5Y cells stably overexpressing APP695 containing the Swedish mutation K670 N/M671 L and carrying a Myc tag and a carboxy-terminal Flag tag [29] were cultured in DMEM/F-12 media supplemented with 10% heat-inactivated FBS, 2 mM L-Alanyl-L-Glutamine, non-essential amino acids, and 50 μg/ml Hygromycin B (Carl Roth). Cells were maintained at 37 °C in a humidified atmosphere containing 5% CO_2. BV-2 cells were seeded into 9.6 cm^2 petri dishes (3×10^5 cells/dish; $n = 6$/treatment group), cultured for 24 h, and then stimulated with lipopolysaccharide (LPS) (0.1 μg/ml), conditioned media of SH-SY5Y cells, or $A\beta_{1-42}$ (5 μM) for 24 h at 37 °C with 5% CO_2. Then cells were collected for RNA extraction. $A\beta_{1-42}$ peptides were purchased from Peptide Speciality Laboratory (PSL) and resuspended in 20 mM NaOH (final concentration, 1 mg/ml) directly before treatment of BV-2 cells. To obtain Aβ-containing conditioned SH-SY5Y media, cells were plated in a 175cm^2 cell culture flask w/o Hygromycin B and incubated for 48 h. The conditioned media were collected, centrifuged for 5 min at 1400 rpm, and applied to BV-2 cells for the indicated period of time.

Immunohistochemistry and immunofluorescence analyses

Mice were killed by CO_2 anesthetization followed by cervical dislocation. Brains and spinal cords were carefully dissected and post fixation for at least one week was carried out in 4% phosphate-buffered formalin at 4 °C before the tissue was embedded in paraffin. Immunohistochemistry was performed on 4 μm paraffin sections as described previously [38]. The following antibodies were used: anti-Aβ antibody 24311 (1:500, [41]), IBA1 (1:500; #234004, Synaptic Systems) and GPNMB (1:500, Santa Cruz). Biotinylated secondary anti-rabbit, anti-guinea pig and anti-goat antibodies (1:200) were purchased from

Dako or Jackson Immunoresearch. The staining was visualized using the avidin-biotin complex method with a VECTASTAIN kit (Vector Laboratories) and diaminobenzidine (DAB) as a chromogen providing a reddish-brown color with hematoxylin as nuclear counterstain.

For double-immunofluorescence staining, polyclonal goat anti-GPNMB antibody (1:500, AF2330, R&D Systems) was combined with IC16 (1:1000, against the N-terminus of Aβ), GFAP (1:500, #173004, Synaptic Systems), NeuN (1:300, MAB377, Millipore) and IBA1 (1:500, #234004, Synaptic Systems), respectively. The staining was visualized using Alexa Fluor 594- and Alexa Fluor 488-conjugated secondary antibodies (1:750, Jackson Immunoresearch) and analyzed using a Nikon Eclipse Ti-E fluorescent microscope.

Elisa

GPNMB levels were measured in human and mouse brain tissue, mouse spinal cord tissue and in human CSF and serum samples using commercially available mouse (DY2330) or human Osteoactivin/GPNMB ELISA (DY2550) sets according to the manufacturer's instructions (R&D systems, Abingdon, UK).

Proteins were extracted from human and mouse brain samples as well as from mouse spinal cord samples. Frozen tissue was weighed and homogenized in 0.7 ml Tris-buffered saline (TBS) buffer (120 mM NaCl, 50 mM Tris, pH 8.0 supplemented with complete protease inhibitor cocktail (Roche Diagnostics, Indianapolis, IN, USA)), per 100 mg tissue by using a Dounce homogenizer (800 rpm). The resulting homogenate was centrifuged at 17,000 x g for 20 min at 4 °C. The supernatant containing TBS-soluble proteins was stored at -80 °C. The pellet was dissolved in 2% sodium dodecyl sulfate (SDS) and sonicated followed by a centrifugation step at 17,000 x g for 20 min at 4 °C. The supernatant, which contained SDS-soluble proteins, was incubated with 1 μl of Benzonase under rotating conditions for 10 min at room temperature in order to reduce viscosity and stored at -80 °C.

Real-time PCR

For real-time RT-PCR analysis, WT, 5XFAD, APP/PS1KI and APP23 mice ($n = 3$–6 per group) or RNA extracts from BV2 cells ($n = 6$) were used. For RNA isolation, deep-frozen brain hemispheres or spinal cord tissue were homogenized in TriFast reagent (Peqlab) essentially as described previously [16]. Deep frozen liver samples were homogenized in 1 ml TriFast reagent (Peqlab) per 100 mg tissue using a glas-teflon homogenizer. BV2 cell pellets were homogenized manually in 1 ml TriFast reagent by repetitive pipetting. DNAse digestion and reverse transcription of the purified RNA samples were carried out according to the protocol of the manufacturer (Thermo Fisher). RT-PCR was performed using a Stratagene MX3000 Real-time Cycler. The SYBR green based FastStart Universal SYBR Green (Roche) containing ROX as an internal reference dye was used for amplification. Relative expression levels were calculated using the $2^{-\Delta\Delta Ct}$ method and normalized to the housekeeping gene β-actin [43]. Primer sequences can be found in Additional file 2.

Statistical analysis

Differences between groups were tested by either one-way analysis of variance followed by Tukey's multiple comparisons test or unpaired t-tests. All data were expressed as mean ± SD. Significance levels are indicated as follows: ***$p < 0.001$; **$p < 0.01$; *$p < 0.05$. All calculations were performed using GraphPad Prism version 6.07 for Windows (GraphPad Software, La Jolla, CA, USA).

Results

GPNMB expression levels increase with disease progression in distinct transgenic AD mouse models

As previously reported, we initially found GPNMB mRNA levels to be significantly up-regulated in 6-month-old APP/PS1KI mice when compared to control mice in a whole-brain deep sequencing analysis [51]. In order to test whether GPNMB mRNA up-regulation occurs during normal aging or if GPNMB expression is regulated in a disease-state dependent manner, RNA of whole brain hemispheres from 3-, 7- and 10-month-old APP/PS1KI and PS1KI control mice was extracted and GPNMB expression levels were analyzed using RT-PCR. We observed a disease-state dependent upregulation of GPNMB mRNA levels in APP/PS1KI mice but not in PS1KI mice. In good agreement with our previous study, GPNMB mRNA expression was significantly increased in 7-month-old APP/PS1KI mice compared to controls ($p < 0.01$) [51]. At 12 months of age, GPNMB expression increased even further when compared to 7-month-old APP/PS1KI mice ($p < 0.01$; Fig. 1a).

To determine whether GPNMB mRNA up-regulation also occurs in other AD mouse models, potentially indicating a general event during AD pathology progression, RT-PCR analyses of brain hemispheres of 3-, 7- and 12-month-old 5XFAD and age-matched WT control animals were performed. While GPNMB expression was unchanged in 3-month-old 5XFAD mice when compared to WT animals, mRNA levels were significantly upregulated at 7 months of age ($p < 0.05$). At 12 months of age, GPNMB mRNA levels in 5XFAD mice were even further increased compared to WT mice ($p < 0.001$), where no age-dependent changes were detectable (Fig. 1b). Interestingly, in APP23 mice, another frequently studied mouse model of AD, no GPNMB up-regulation was detected in 12-month-old APP23 mice as compared to WT control animals (Fig. 1c).

Cellular localization and distribution of GPNMB in the CNS of AD mouse models

Next, we aimed to investigate the cellular localization of GPNMB using double staining with cellular marker proteins such as NeuN for neurons, GFAP for astrocytes and IBA1 as a marker for microglia and macrophages. While no co-localization of GPNMB was observed with NeuN or GFAP, abundant GPNMB immunoreactivity could be detected in cells positive for the microglia/macrophage marker IBA1 in 5XFAD mice (Fig. 2).

In order to better characterize the localization of GPNMB in the CNS of AD transgenic mice, further immunohistochemical stainings were performed in brain and spinal cord of 12-month-old 5XFAD mice compared to age-matched WT controls. In 5XFAD mice, GPNMB immunoreactivity was observed throughout the whole brain with particular abundance in regions known for high Aβ plaque load in this model, such as subiculum (Fig. 3a, b), cortex or thalamus, while no signal could be detected in APP23 or WT control mice (Additional files 3 , 4). 5XFAD

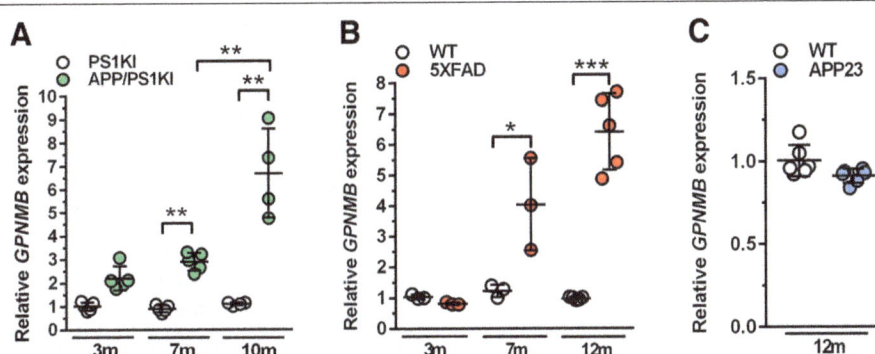

Fig. 1 GPNMB mRNA expression increases in an age- and dose-dependent manner in some Alzheimer's disease mouse models. (a) Cerebral GPNMB mRNA levels increased in an age-dependent manner in APP/PS1KI compared to PS1KI control mice. (b) In 5XFAD mice, levels of GPNMB mRNA started to be significantly increased at 7 months of age when compared to wild-type (WT) control mice. 12-month-old 5XFAD mice showed even higher GPNMB levels. (c) In 12-month-old APP23 mice, GPNMB gene expression levels were not increased compared to WT animals. All data are given as mean ± SD. ***$P < 0.001$; **$P < 0.01$; *$P < 0.05$

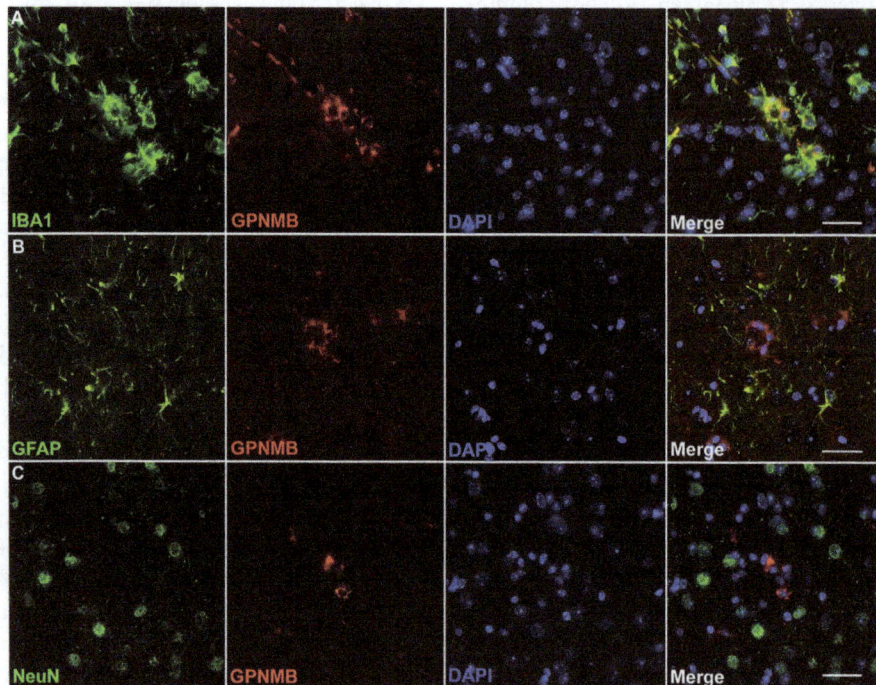

Fig. 2 GPNMB co-localizes with IBA1-positive microglia cells in 5XFAD brains. (**a-c**) Double immunostaining with antibodies against GPNMB and IBA1 revealed a cellular co-localization in 12-month-old 5XFAD brains, while no co-localization was seen with the astrocytic marker GFAP or the neuronal marker NeuN. Scale bar: A-C = 33 μm

mice start to develop amyloid pathology as early as two months of age in the subiculum and deep cortical layers. At 12 months of age, the model shows a massive Aβ plaque load in various brain regions, which is accompanied by extensive astro- and microgliosis [19, 33]. To investigate whether GPNMB accumulates in parallel with amyloid plaque deposition in this model, GPNMB and Aβ immunoreactivity were quantified in 2.5-, 7- and 12-month-old 5XFAD mice in the cortex, subiculum, dentate gyrus and thalamus. Compared to 2.5-month-old mice, aged mice (7 m and 12 m, respectively) revealed a significant increase in GPNMB levels in all regions analyzed. The same was true for extracellular amyloid deposition as demonstrated with antibody 24311 detecting a variety of different Aβ isoforms (Additional file 3). Hence, cerebral GPNMB accumulation increases in an age-dependent manner in 5XFAD mice, resembling β-amyloid accumulation.

In order to more accurately quantify whether the increased *GPNMB* mRNA expression in the brains of 5XFAD mice correlated with an elevation in GPNMB protein levels, a sandwich ELISA was used to measure GPNMB levels in TBS-soluble and SDS-soluble brain fractions from both 5XFAD and APP23 mice. Analysis of 12-month-old 5XFAD mice revealed a highly significant elevation of GPNMB protein levels when compared to age-matched WT or APP23 mice ($p < 0.001$). A similar pattern was seen in the SDS-soluble fraction, showing

significantly increased GPNMB protein levels in 12-month-old 5XFAD mice ($p < 0.001$) when compared to age-matched WT or APP23 animals, respectively (Fig. 3c). These measurements also confirmed that GPNMB protein levels were not increased in 12-month-old APP23 mice as compared to WT control animals.

As GPNMB has been previously implicated in motor neuron diseases [4], spinal cord samples from aged 5XFAD mice were analyzed where Aβ pathology has been previously demonstrated [19]. As seen in the brain, abundant GPNMB-immunoreactivity was observed throughout the whole spinal cord, largely resembling the IBA1 staining profile (Fig. 3d). Furthermore, a comparison of *GPNMB* mRNA expression levels in the spinal cord revealed a highly significant increase in 5XFAD compared to age-matched WT mice ($p < 0.001$). Liver samples were used as a control peripheral tissue and did not show any induction of GPNMB levels in aged 5XFAD mice (Fig. 3e). Likewise, protein extracts from 5XFAD and age-matched WT spinal cord samples revealed a significant elevation of GPNMB protein levels in both TBS- and SDS-soluble spinal cord fractions of 5XFAD mice ($p < 0.001$, respectively) (Fig. 3f). For a subset of analyzed animals, both RNA and protein samples from the same mouse was available. Statistical analysis revealed a high correlation for GPNMB RNA and protein levels (Additional file 5).

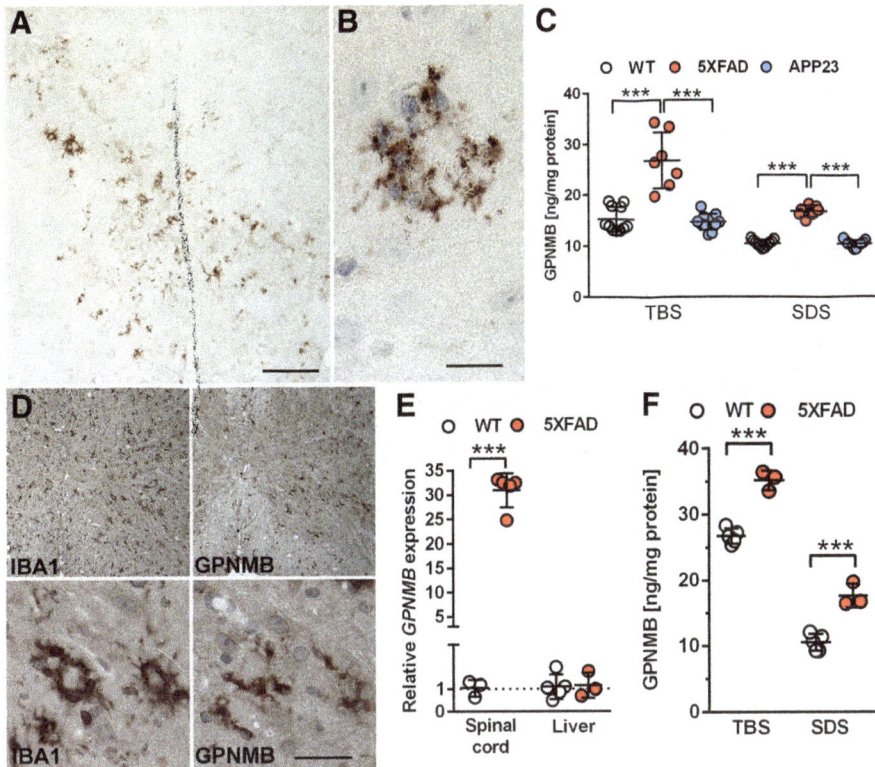

Fig. 3 Increased GPNMB protein levels and cerebral expression pattern in 5XFAD mice. (**a**) Abundant GPNMB staining was detected throughout the whole brain in 12-month-old 5XFAD mice, e.g. in the subiculum. (**b**) High-power view of GPNMB-positive cells surrounding an amyloid plaque core. (**c**) Quantitative analysis of GPNMB protein levels in TBS- and SDS-soluble brain fractions of 12-month-old WT, 5XFAD and APP23 mice revealed a highly significant increase in GPNMB levels in 5XFAD mice compared to WT animals, while no elevated levels could be observed in APP23 mice. (**d**) GPNMB immunoreactivity was also demonstrated in the spinal cord (SC) of 12-month-old 5XFAD mice. GPNMB was abundantly expressed throughout the whole SC tissue and showed co-localization with IBA1-positive microglia cells (parallel sections). (**e**) As demonstrated by RT-PCR analyses, 5XFAD mice showed a highly significant increase in *GPNMB* mRNA levels in the SC when compared to WT controls. However, no such differences were observed in peripheral liver samples serving as a non-neuronal control tissue. Enzyme-linked immunosorbent assay revealed highly increased GPNMB protein level in 5XFAD SC tissue compared to WT controls (**f**). All data are given as mean ± SD. ***$P < 0.001$. Scale bar: A = 133 µm, B = 25 µm; D = 200 µm (upper panel), 20 µm (lower panel)

As GPNMB immunoreactivity was mainly present in brain areas known for robust amyloid deposition in 5XFAD mice, co-immunofluorescence stainings for GPNMB, IBA1 and Aβ were performed in 12-month-old animals in order to study spatial co-localization. Triple-labeling with GPNMB (red), IBA1 (green) and pan-Aβ (magenta) demonstrated that GPNMB protein was mainly detectable around amyloid plaque cores (Fig. 4a-d). In order to further investigate whether elevated GPNMB expression is a common phenomenon in AD transgenic mice, 12-month-old APP23 were analyzed using immunohistochemistry. Although abundant IBA1-positive microglia surrounded extracellular Aβ deposits in both 5XFAD and APP23 mice, GPNMB-immunoreactivity was restricted to the 5XFAD model, where it clustered around the central dense plaque core (Additional file 6) with microglia being consistently negative in 12-month-old APP23 mice (Fig. 4e-h and Additional file 4).

GPNMB expression correlates with markers for disease-associated microglia

We further analyzed markers that have been proposed to be indicative of a subgroup of microglia cells under disease conditions, so called disease-associated microglia (DAMs) or microglial neurodegenerative phenotype (MGnD), but are absent or scarcely expressed in healthy animals [22, 24]. Indeed, levels of genes such as *CST7*, *TREM2*, *APOE*, *CLEC7a* or *CCL2* were found significantly up-regulated in 12-month-old 5XFAD mice compared to both WT and APP23 mice, while levels of homeostatic microglia genes like *AIF1* or *TMEM119* were unchanged (Fig. 4i). Significant correlations between *GPNMB* and *CST7*, *AIF1*, *TREM2*, *APOE*, *CLEC7a* and *CCL2* were observed while no correlation could be detected between *GPNMB* and the homeostatic microglia marker *TMEM119* (Additional file 7).

Next, we assessed whether Aβ peptides were able to trigger *GPNMB* expression in vitro. To this end, the

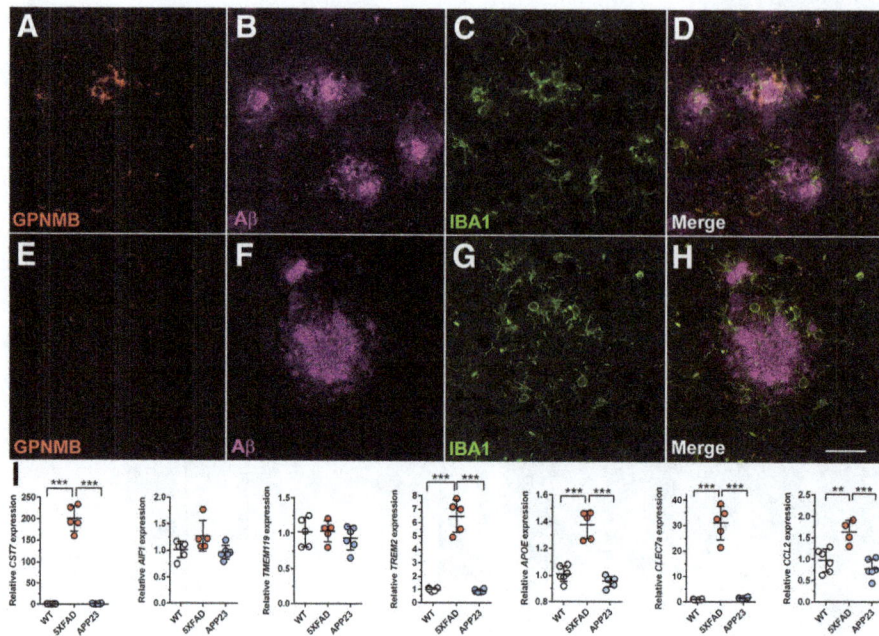

Fig. 4 GPNMB/IBA-1-positive microglia cells cluster around individual plaque cores in 5XFAD brains. Triple immunofluorescence staining using antibodies against GPNMB (**a**), Aβ (**b**) and IBA1 (**c**) demonstrated the spatial co-localization of GPNMB-positive microglia cells around amyloid plaque cores in 12-month-old 5XFAD brains (**d**). Even though APP23 mice showed numerous activated microglia cells (**g**) clustered around amyloid plaques (**f**), no GPNMB signal could be detected (**e,h**). (**i**) RT-PCR analyses revealed significantly increased mRNA levels of *CST7*, *TREM2*, *APOE*, *CLEC7A* and *CCL2* in 5XFAD brains when compared to WT and APP23 mice. However, levels of *AIF1* and *TMEM119* were comparable in all groups tested. All data are given as mean ± SD. ***$P < 0.001$; **$P < 0.01$. Scale bar: A–H = 33 μm

immortalized murine microglial cell line BV-2 was treated with 5 μM synthetic Aβ$_{1-42}$ or conditioned medium derived from SH-SY5Y cells overexpressing human APP695 with the Swedish mutation. This medium was harvested after 48 h and contained mainly Aβ$_{1-40}$ and Aβ$_{1-42}$ (Additional file 8). Treatment with LPS was employed as a control condition to trigger an inflammatory reaction. Quantification of mRNA expression levels revealed a significant up-regulation of *GPNMB* in cells treated with Aβ$_{1-42}$ or Aβ-conditioned medium while LPS treatment did not change *GPNMB* expression (Fig. 5a). Instead, LPS treatment led to a typical microglia activation pattern as indicated by up-regulation of genes encoding for pro-inflammatory cytokines such as *IL-1β* and *TNF* (Fig. 5b-c). *CLEC7A* and *APOE* representing DAM markers showed a significantly increased expression only after treatment with conditioned medium containing Aβ peptides (Fig. 5d-e). Surprisingly, the expression levels of the transcription factor MITF, which has been reported as an important regulator of *GPNMB* [9], was unchanged in conditions with elevated *GPNMB* expression (Fig. 5f).

GPNMB in sporadic Alzheimer's disease cases
Finally, we investigated whether our findings in mouse models of AD can be translated to human AD patients. Thus, brain samples from AD and NDC subjects were

stained with a GPNMB antibody. The specificity of the antibody used for immunohistochemical staining of human brain tissues was verified with a blocking peptide which entirely abolished GPNMB immunoreactivity (Additional file 9). Interestingly, abundant GPNMB immunoreactivity was observed throughout cortical tissue samples from sporadic AD patients. In particular, intense GPNMB staining was detected in vessel walls and around amyloid plaque cores, confirming our observations in AD mouse models (Fig. 6a, b, e). However, also non-plaque-associated GPNMB-positive cells were frequently detected showing an amoeboid phenotype reminiscent of lipid-laden microglia in tissue samples from human patients (Fig. 6c, f). In non-demented controls, considerably less GPNMB immunoreactivity was observed and only occasionally GPNMB-positive cells were detected throughout the cortex (Fig. 6d).

We next measured TBS- and SDS-soluble GPNMB protein levels in lysates of the medial frontal gyrus of human patients with sporadic AD and non-demented controls. Quantification using a GPNMB-specific sandwich ELISA revealed that TBS-soluble GPNMB protein levels tended to be increased in AD patients in comparison to non-demented control individuals, but the difference did not reach statistical significance ($p = 0.06$; Fig. 6g). In the SDS-soluble fraction, no difference in GPNMB protein levels was noted between the two groups (Fig. 6h).

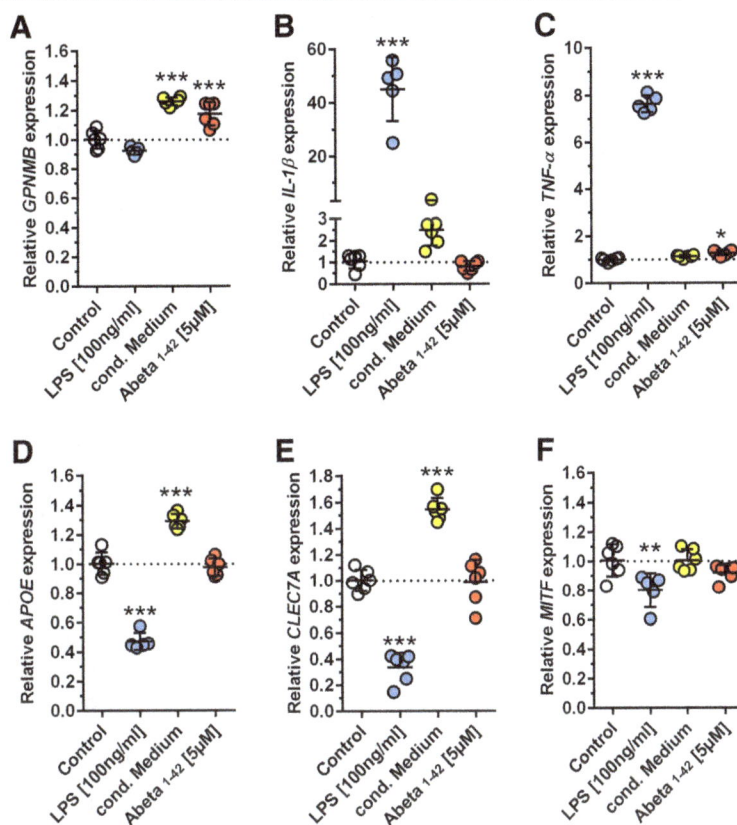

Fig. 5 Soluble Aβ induces *GPNMB* mRNA expression in immortalized microglia cells. (**a**) Treatment of BV2 cells with Aβ-containing medium or synthetic Aβ$_{1-42}$ peptides resulted in a highly significant increase in *GPNMB* mRNA expression, while LPS treatment had no effect on *GPNMB* levels. In contrast, LPS treatment caused microglia activation as shown by upregulation of the pro-inflammatory cytokines *IL1-β* and *TNFα* (**b**, **c**). While LPS treatment led to decreased expression of *APOE* and *CLEC7A*, conditioned Aβ-containing media induced these DAM phenotype-associated genes (**d**, **e**). *MITF* levels did not change following treatment with Aβ-conditioned medium or synthetic Aβ although *GPNMB* levels were clearly elevated (**f**). All data are given as mean ± SD. * $P < 0.05$; **$P < 0.01$; ***$P < 0.001$

In addition, GPNMB protein levels were measured in the CSF and sera of a distinct cohort of patients suffering from sporadic AD as well as in non-demented controls. Importantly, GPNMB protein levels were found to be significantly increased in the CSF of sporadic AD patients when compared to non-demented controls ($p < 0.05$). (Fig. 6i). No differences in GPNMB levels between non-demented controls and sporadic AD patients were found in serum samples (Fig. 6j). In order to validate the GPNMB ELISA measurements presented in the current study intra-assay coefficients of variation (relative standard deviations) between duplicate reads (technical replicates on the same assay plate) were calculated for the different sample matrices and are summarized in Additional file 10. In addition, TBS- and SDS-soluble brain extracts from WT mice ($n = 11$) were measured on 2 different days. The mean inter-assay coefficients of variation were 4.7% (median 3.4%, range 0.8–19.9%) for TBS- and 15.7% (median 16.8%, range 8.9–20.3%) for SDS-soluble fractions.

Discussion

Since therapeutic approaches against long established AD targets such as amyloid plaques and NFTs have so far not been successful, more recent therapeutic strategies try to tackle alternative targets, among which neuroinflammation is one of the most promising. Accumulating evidence suggests a critical role for microglia in the pathogenesis of AD, and latest human genetics data have identified several novel AD risk genes such as CD33 or CR1, which are highly expressed by these brain resident immune cells (reviewed in [21]). Two main hypotheses have been put forward regarding the role of reactive microglia in brain diseases. One is claiming that microglia is protective against CNS insults such as aggregated β-amyloid by promoting their clearance through phagocytosis. On the other hand, many findings indicate that chronic activation of microglia is harmful to neurons and contributes to disease progression and severity. In AD, while the detrimental effects of microglia activation seem to manifest in later stages of the

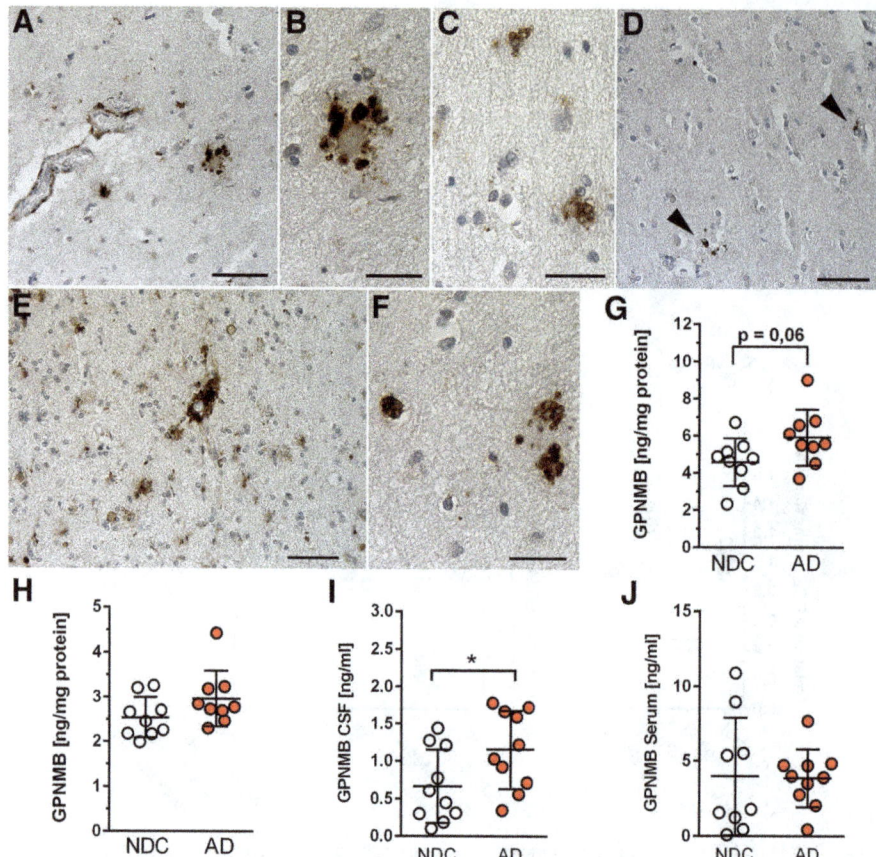

Fig. 6 Increased GPNMB protein levels in brain tissue and cerebrospinal fluid (CSF) of sporadic Alzheimer's disease cases. GPNMB immunoreactivity was detected in microglial cells surrounding amyloid plaque cores and in the vicinity of blood vessel walls (**a, e**). (**b**) High-power view of the plaque core in (**a**). In addition, GPNMB-positive amoeboid microglia were detected in plaque-free areas (**c, f**), while GPNMB-positive microglia were only occasionally observed in samples from non-demented control patients (**d**). (**g**) In the TBS-soluble brain fractions, higher levels of GPNMB were detected in AD cases when compared to non-demented controls (NDC), however, without reaching statistical significance ($p = 0.06$). (**h**) No differences were detected between the two groups in SDS-soluble brain fractions. (**i**) The amount of GPNMB in the CSF of AD patients was significantly higher than in control patients. (**j**) No significant difference in GPNMB serum levels could be detected between controls and AD. All data are given as mean ± SD. *$P < 0.05$. Scale bar: A,D,E = 50 µm; B,C,F = 20 µm

disease, protective microglial activities supposedly occur in the early disease stages [10]. In order to develop therapeutic approaches that target microglia and modulate their behaviour, a better understanding of the proteins and molecular mechanisms involved in their activation and potential dysfunction in AD brains is required.

In our recent transcriptome analysis of the APP/PS1KI transgenic AD mouse model, which develops severe neurodegeneration, a variety of genes implicated in the neuroinflammatory response were identified as overexpressed [51]. One of the most strongly up-regulated genes was *GPNMB*, a transmembrane type I protein also known as osteoactivin. We here describe GPNMB as a novel AD-associated marker in both transgenic AD models and sporadic AD patients. Using immunohistochemical analyses, RT-PCR experiments and ELISA measurements, we were able to show that *GPNMB* is overexpressed in the APP/PS1KI and

5XFAD transgenic mouse models of AD in an age-dependent manner, with age-matched WT animals being consistently negative. Double-immunofluorescent staining using GPNMB and the microglia/macrophage marker IBA1 revealed a distinct co-localization, corroborating previous results in the inflamed rat brain, where GPNMB was found to co-localize with the microglia/macrophage marker OX42 [15]. Co-stainings with markers against GFAP to detect astrocytes or NeuN to detect neurons were consistently negative, underscoring the restricted microglial localization. This result is also in good agreement with recent data from a RNA-sequencing study, which demonstrated GPNMB expression primarily in microglia and, to a lesser extent, in oligodendrocyte precursor cells [60]. It is further supported by a recent transcriptome study demonstrating an upregulation of GPNMB in major histocompatibility complex (MHC) II-positive microglial cells isolated from the 5XFAD mouse model [58].

Employing multi-fluorescent staining using antibodies against GPNMB, IBA1 and Aβ, we found that GPNMB-positive microglia were primarily located in the close vicinity of extracellular plaques in the 5XFAD mouse model. In contrast, no GPNMB-immunoreactivity could be detected in APP23 mice, although this model also showed abundant extracellular plaque pathology surrounded by numerous IBA1-positive microglia cells [45]. This is also reflected in an earlier RNA microarray analysis of APP23 mice, in which no overexpression of GPNMB was reported [49]. In contrast, GPNMB was found to be up-regulated in a longitudinal gene profiling analysis of the 5XFAD mouse model [27], as well as in a transcriptome study investigating gene expression changes in CD11c-positive microglia isolated from the amyloid-depositing APPswe/PS1dE9 mouse model [20, 35]. While 5XFAD mice show cortical neuron loss at 12 months of age [7, 19], even higher cortical neuron numbers have been reported in 8-month-old APP23 compared to WT mice, which decrease in 27-month-old APP23 mice back to WT levels [2]. In addition, the amyloid plaque composition in APP23 mice is much different compared to human AD with Aβ$_{1-40}$ representing the main component in APP23 while Aβ$_{1-42}$ is the predominant species in human AD brain [42].

Activated microglia are characteristic for numerous neurodegenerative diseases aside from AD [50]. Studies integrating microglial/myeloid expression data sets from diverse neurodegenerative disease models, including AD transgenic mice, multiple sclerosis and ALS models, have suggested the presence of a particular microglia activation state, which has been termed either "microglial neurodegenerative phenotype" (MGnD) [24] or "disease-associated microglia" (DAM) [22]. Together with other genes (e.g. CLEC7A, CCL2 or FABP5), GPNMB was found to be up-regulated in the MGnD profile. In addition, it has been proposed that Trem2 and ApoE are intimately linked to a switch from a homeostatic to a neurodegenerative microglial phenotype [24]. Based on these findings, we tested whether other MGnD genes might be induced in 5XFAD mice with elevated GPNMB levels, but not in APP23 mice, in which GPNMB expression was not increased. Indeed, the strong transcriptional activation of GPNMB and CST7 in 12-month-old 5XFAD but not in APP23 mice, together with the unchanged expression levels of the microglia homeostatic genes AIF1 and TMEM119 was consistent with the idea that GPNMB might be regulated as part of the MGnD response. The exact role of the MGnD activation state is not clear. However, it has been shown that the injection of apoptotic neurons into the cortex and hippocampus of adult mice resulted in the induction of APOE and the up-regulation of other genes implicated in the MGnD profile, including GPNMB [24]. APOE expression was also up-regulated in our 5XFAD but not in the APP23 mice, together with additional MGnD-associated markers

such as CLEC7A or CCL2. This could mean that the MGnD activation state is only triggered in the presence of dead or dying neurons, and fits well to the observation of abundant GPNMB-immunoreactivity in 5XFAD mice. In contrast to APP23 mice, which show no neocortical neuron loss even at 27 months of age [2], significantly reduced neuron numbers have been reported in deep cortical layers of 5XFAD mice beginning at nine months of age [7, 19, 54]. Similarly, APP/PS1KI mice also show a strong age-dependent induction of GPNMB expression, together with the up-regulation of several MGnD-associated genes such as CLEC7A, ITGAX or CSF1 [51] and with robust hippocampal and cortical neuron loss [3, 6].

Additionally, we provide in vitro evidence that soluble Aβ might promote the switch in microglia gene expression from a "homeostatic" to a "disease-associated" state. Upon treatment of an immortalized microglial cell line with synthetic Aβ$_{1-42}$ or Aβ-containing conditioned media, the expression levels of GPNMB as well as other MGnD-associated markers such as APOE and CLEC7A were highly increased. This indicates that soluble Aβ peptides are also capable of inducing GPNMB expression, in addition to aggregated Aβ as found in brain tissues from human AD or transgenic AD mice. In contrast, treatment of microglia cells with LPS induced a typical pro-inflammatory gene expression profile, with GPNMB levels being unchanged. Surprisingly, expression levels of the transcription factor MITF, which has been reported to be a critical regulator of GPNMB expression [9], was found to be down-regulated following LPS treatment. However, it has also been shown that LPS is capable of suppressing gene expression in macrophages by down-regulating factors such as MITF [18].

We suggest that Aβ itself could be partially responsible for the phenotypic switch of microglia to a neurodegenerative state during AD progression, although it is clearly not sufficient in vivo as shown by the lack of MGnD markers in APP23 mice. In conclusion, our findings in transgenic AD mouse models support that GPNMB is part of a microglial activation state that occurs in advanced disease stages and only in AD models showing profound cerebral neuron loss. Besides elevated GPNMB levels, this microglial activation state under neurodegenerative conditions is characterized by the upregulation of a subset of genes including APOE, TREM2, CLEC7A and CST7. Whether GPNMB has a protective or detrimental role in this context has to be elucidated, but available in vitro evidence would argue for an anti-inflammatory, regenerative role of GPNMB [32, 39, 59, 61] (Fig. 7).

Importantly, we also found GPNMB to be elevated in both brain tissue and CSF samples of sporadic AD patients. To the best of our knowledge, the current study is the first to report elevated GPNMB levels in human AD subjects. At present, due to the small group sizes, the current results have to be interpreted with caution. Further studies with

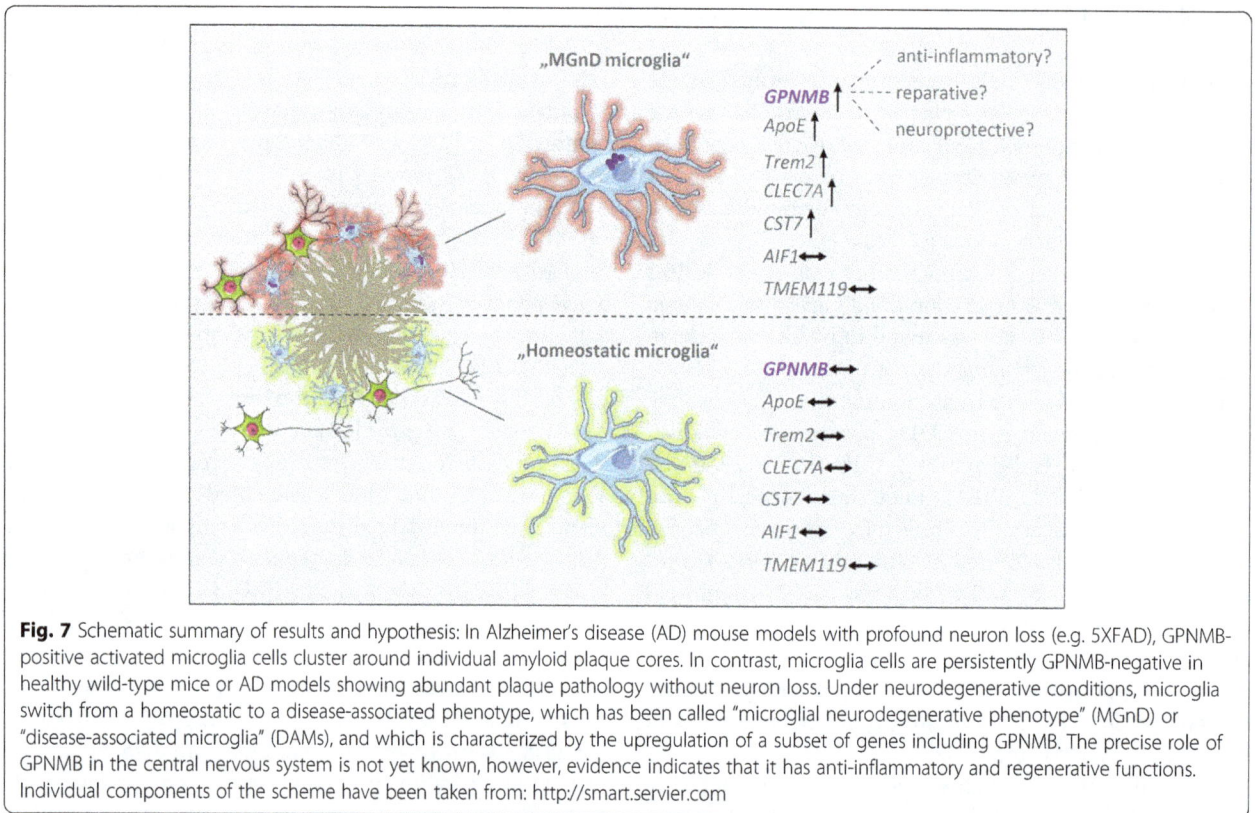

Fig. 7 Schematic summary of results and hypothesis: In Alzheimer's disease (AD) mouse models with profound neuron loss (e.g. 5XFAD), GPNMB-positive activated microglia cells cluster around individual amyloid plaque cores. In contrast, microglia cells are persistently GPNMB-negative in healthy wild-type mice or AD models showing abundant plaque pathology without neuron loss. Under neurodegenerative conditions, microglia switch from a homeostatic to a disease-associated phenotype, which has been called "microglial neurodegenerative phenotype" (MGnD) or "disease-associated microglia" (DAMs), and which is characterized by the upregulation of a subset of genes including GPNMB. The precise role of GPNMB in the central nervous system is not yet known, however, evidence indicates that it has anti-inflammatory and regenerative functions. Individual components of the scheme have been taken from: http://smart.servier.com

larger cohorts will be required to confirm these observations. Nevertheless, our findings are partially similar to studies of TREM2, which has been proposed as a potential microglia-associated biomarker for AD progression and therapy monitoring. TREM2 is also a type-I transmembrane protein localized to the cell surface that can undergo ecto-domain shedding by ADAM proteases, and soluble TREM2 (sTREM2) has been detected in body fluids including the CSF. Although not consistent between all published studies, elevated sTREM2 levels have been reported in CSF samples of sporadic AD patients versus non-demented controls [11, 12, 36, 47]. Taken together, these studies provide proof of concept evidence that a microglia-derived protein that is detectable in body fluids like TREM2 or GPNMB could be used as a biomarker to monitor disease onset and progression, and might even function as a prognostic marker.

Elevated GPNMB levels were also reported in several other neurodegenerative disorders apart from AD. In patients with sporadic ALS, a disease characterized by the degeneration of motor neurons in the cerebral cortex and spinal cord, extracellular GPNMB aggregates were found in the grey and white matter of spinal cord tissue [30]. Consistent with this finding, the same group reported increased levels of GPNMB in the CSF and serum of ALS patients [48]. Elevated levels of GPNMB have also been shown in brains, CSF and plasma of Gaucher disease patients [23, 62]. Furthermore, the glycoprotein has been

reported to be increased in Niemann-Pick Type C disease as well as in Tay-Sachs- and Sandhoff disease [28]. These diseases belong to the group of lysosomal storage disorders (LSDs), which are characterized by the abnormal accumulation of cellular debris in lysosomes and subsequent neuro-degeneration [37]. Interestingly, a two-stage genome-wide association (GWA) meta-analysis associated GPNMB with a higher risk for Parkinson's disease (PD) [17]. However, follow-up studies with independent cohorts of patients did not corroborate these initial findings [56, 57]. Given the involvement of GPNMB in other neurodegenerative diseases besides AD, it is unlikely to serve as a disease-specific biomarker. However, this does not exclude the possibility that multiplexing putative microglia-derived markers such as TREM2 and GPNMB with other proteins that might be discovered in future studies could result in disease-specific marker signatures. Apart from that, CSF GPNMB levels could potentially be used to monitor disease progression. In mice, we could demonstrate that GPNMB levels increased with age and disease progression. As the transgenic mouse models employed in the current study address in particular amyloid pathology, other models reflecting further pathological hallmarks have to be considered in future studies. In addition, longitudinal studies will be required to translate these findings into human patients and to prove that GPNMB levels correlate with the onset and course of human AD.

Conclusions

Finally, as GPNMB has been shown to negatively regulate inflammatory responses [39], it is tempting to speculate that the protein is induced in neurodegenerative conditions such as AD or LSDs to restrain inflammation and to protect neurons. Therefore, increasing GPNMB levels in the CNS might be a potential future therapeutic strategy. However, more research to elucidate the precise role of GPNMB in the inflammatory responses associated with neurodegenerative diseases is clearly required.

Funding

Oliver Wirths is supported by the Alzheimer Forschung Initiative (grant 16013) and Gerhard-Hunsmann-Stiftung. The study was also supported by grants from the German Federal Ministry of Education and Research (project FTLDc 01GI1007A, the EU Joint Programme–Neurodegenerative Diseases networks PreFrontAls (01ED1512) and the foundation of the state of Baden-Wuerttemberg (D.3830) and BIU (D.5009) to Markus Otto. Jens Wiltfang is supported by an Ilídio Pinho professorship and iBiMED (UID/BIM/04501/2013) at the University of Aveiro, Portugal. Figure 7 was modified from Smart Servier Medical Art website (https://smart.servier.com), licensed under a Creative Common Attribution 3.0 Unported License.

Author contributions

MH performed experiments, analyzed data and wrote the manuscript. IO performed experiments, MO and JW provided reagents and samples and HK, CS and SW analyzed data and contributed to the interpretation of findings and revision of the manuscript. OW designed the study, performed experiments, analyzed data and wrote the manuscript. All authors read and approved the final manuscript.

Competing interests

The authors declare that they have no competing interests.

Author details

[1]Department of Psychiatry and Psychotherapy, University Medical Center (UMG), Georg-August-University, Von-Siebold-Str. 5, 37075 Göttingen, Germany. [2]Department of Neuropathology, Heinrich-Heine-University, Düsseldorf, Germany. [3]Department of Neurology, University of Ulm, Ulm, Germany. [4]Department of Neuropathology, University Medical Center, Georg-August-University, Göttingen, Germany. [5]German Center for Neurodegenerative Diseases (DZNE), Göttingen, Germany.

References

1. Abdelmagid SM, Barbe MF, Rico MC, Salihoglu S, Arango-Hisijara I, Selim AH, Anderson MG, Owen TA, Popoff SN, Safadi FF (2008) Osteoactivin, an anabolic factor that regulates osteoblast differentiation and function. Exp Cell Res 314:2334–2351
2. Bondolfi L, Calhoun M, Ermini F, Kuhn HG, Wiederhold KH, Walker L, Staufenbiel M, Jucker M (2002) Amyloid-associated neuron loss and gliogenesis in the neocortex of amyloid precursor protein transgenic mice. J Neurosci 22:515–522
3. Breyhan H, Wirths O, Duan K, Marcello A, Rettig J, Bayer TA (2009) APP/PS1KI bigenic mice develop early synaptic deficits and hippocampus atrophy. Acta Neuropathol 117:677–685
4. Budge KM, Neal ML, Richardson JR, Safadi FF (2018) Glycoprotein NMB: an emerging role in neurodegenerative disease. Mol Neurobiol 55:5167–5176
5. Casas C, Sergeant N, Itier JM, Blanchard V, Wirths O, van der Kolk N, Vingtdeux V, van de Steeg E, Ret G, Canton T et al (2004) Massive CA1/2 neuronal loss with intraneuronal and N-terminal truncated Abeta42 accumulation in a novel Alzheimer transgenic model. Am J Pathol 165:1289–1300
6. Christensen DZ, Kraus SL, Flohr A, Cotel MC, Wirths O, Bayer TA (2008) Transient intraneuronal Abeta rather than extracellular plaque pathology correlates with neuron loss in the frontal cortex of APP/PS1KI mice. Acta Neuropathol 116:647–655
7. Eimer WA, Vassar R (2013) Neuron loss in the 5XFAD mouse model of Alzheimer's disease correlates with intraneuronal Abeta42 accumulation and Caspase-3 activation. Mol Neurodegener 8:2
8. Guerreiro R, Wojtas A, Bras J, Carrasquillo M, Rogaeva E, Majounie E, Cruchaga C, Sassi C, Kauwe JSK, Younkin S et al (2013) TREM2 variants in Alzheimer's disease. N Engl J Med 368:117–127
9. Gutknecht M, Geiger J, Joas S, Dörfel D, Salih HR, Müller MR, Grünebach F, Rittig SM (2015) The transcription factor MITF is a critical regulator of GPNMB expression in dendritic cells. Cell Communication and Signaling 13:19
10. Hansen DV, Hanson JE, Sheng M (2018) Microglia in Alzheimer's disease. J Cell Biol 217:459–472
11. Henjum K, Almdahl IS, Årskog V, Minthon L, Hansson O, Fladby T, Nilsson LNG (2016) Cerebrospinal fluid soluble TREM2 in aging and Alzheimer's disease. Alzheimers Res Ther 8:17
12. Heslegrave A, Heywood W, Paterson R, Magdalinou N, Svensson J, Johansson P, Öhrfelt A, Blennow K, Hardy J, Schott J et al (2016) Increased cerebrospinal fluid soluble TREM2 concentration in Alzheimer's disease. Mol Neurodegener 11:3
13. Hollingworth P, Harold D, Sims R, Gerrish A, Lambert J-C, Carrasquillo MM, Abraham R, Hamshere ML, Pahwa JS, Moskvina V, et al: Common variants at ABCA7, MS4A6A/MS4A4E, EPHA1, CD33 and CD2AP are associated with Alzheimer's disease. Nat Genet 2011, 43:429
14. Hopperton KE, Mohammad D, Trépanier MO, Giuliano V, Bazinet RP (2018) Markers of microglia in post-mortem brain samples from patients with Alzheimer's disease: a systematic review. Mol Psychiatry 23:177–198
15. Huang J-J, Ma W-J, Yokoyama S (2012) Expression and immunolocalization of Gpnmb, a glioma-associated glycoprotein, in normal and inflamed central nervous systems of adult rats. Brain and Behavior 2:85–96
16. Hüttenrauch M, Baches S, Gerth J, Bayer TA, Weggen S, Wirths O (2015) Neprilysin deficiency alters the neuropathological and behavioral phenotype in the 5XFAD mouse model of Alzheimer's disease. J Alzheimers Dis 44:1291–1302
17. International Parkinson's Disease Genomics C, Wellcome Trust Case Control C (2011) A Two-Stage Meta-Analysis Identifies Several New Loci for Parkinson's Disease. PLoS Genet 7:e1002142
18. Ishii J, Kitazawa R, Mori K, McHugh KP, Morii E, Kondo T, Kitazawa S (2008) Lipopolysaccharide suppresses RANK gene expression in macrophages by down-regulating PU.1 and MITF. J Cell Biochem 105:896–904
19. Jawhar S, Trawicka A, Jenneckens C, Bayer TA, Wirths O (2012) Motor deficits, neuron loss, and reduced anxiety coinciding with axonal degeneration and intraneuronal Abeta aggregation in the 5XFAD mouse model of Alzheimer's disease. Neurobiol Aging 33(196):e129–e196 e140
20. Kamphuis W, Kooijman L, Schetters S, Orre M, Hol EM (2016) Transcriptional profiling of CD11c-positive microglia accumulating around amyloid plaques in a mouse model for Alzheimer's disease. Biochim Biophys Acta (BBA) - Mol Basis Dis 1862:1847–1860
21. Karch CM, Goate AM (2015) Alzheimer's disease risk genes and mechanisms of disease pathogenesis. Biol Psychiatry 77:43–51
22. Keren-Shaul H, Spinrad A, Weiner A, Matcovitch-Natan O, Dvir-Szternfeld R, Ulland TK, David E, Baruch K, Lara-Astaiso D, Toth B et al (2017) A Unique Microglia Type Associated with Restricting Development of Alzheimer's Disease. Cell 169:1276–1290 e1217
23. Kramer G, Wegdam W, Donker-Koopman W, Ottenhoff R, Gaspar P, Verhoek M, Nelson J, Gabriel T, Kallemeijn W, Boot RG et al (2016) Elevation of glycoprotein nonmetastatic melanoma protein B in type 1 Gaucher disease patients and mouse models. FEBS Open Bio 6:902–913
24. Krasemann S, Madore C, Cialic R, Baufeld C, Calcagno N, El Fatimy R, Beckers L, O'Loughlin E, Xu Y, Fanek Z et al (2017) The TREM2-APOE Pathway Drives the Transcriptional Phenotype of Dysfunctional Microglia in Neurodegenerative Diseases. Immunity 47:566–581 e569
25. Kuan C-T, Wakiya K, Dowell JM, Herndon JE, Reardon DA, Graner MW, Riggins GJ, Wikstrand CJ, Bigner DD (2006) Glycoprotein nonmetastatic melanoma protein B, a potential molecular therapeutic target in patients with glioblastoma Multiforme. Clin Cancer Res 12:1970–1982
26. Lambert J-C, Heath S, Even G, Campion D, Sleegers K, Hiltunen M, Combarros O, Zelenika D, Bullido MJ, Tavernier B, et al: Genome-wide association study identifies variants at CLU and CR1 associated with Alzheimer's disease. Nat Genet 2009, 41:1094
27. Landel V, Baranger K, Virard I, Loriod B, Khrestchatisky M, Rivera S, Benech P, Feron F (2014) Temporal gene profiling of the 5XFAD transgenic mouse

model highlights the importance of microglial activation in Alzheimer's disease. Mol Neurodegener 9:33

28. Marques ARA, Gabriel TL, Aten J, van Roomen CPAA, Ottenhoff R, Claessen N, Alfonso P, Irún P, Giraldo P, Aerts JMFG, van Eijk M (2016) Gpnmb is a potential marker for the visceral pathology in Niemann-pick type C disease. PLoS One 11:e0147208

29. Munter LM, Voigt P, Harmeier A, Kaden D, Gottschalk KE, Weise C, Pipkorn R, Schaefer M, Langosch D, Multhaup G (2007) GxxxG motifs within the amyloid precursor protein transmembrane sequence are critical for the etiology of Aβ42. EMBO J 26:1702–1712

30. Nagahara Y, Shimazawa M, Ohuchi K, Ito J, Takahashi H, Tsuruma K, Kakita A, Hara H (2017) GPNMB ameliorates mutant TDP-43-induced motor neuron cell death. J Neurosci Res 95:1647–1665

31. Naj AC, Jun G, Beecham GW, Wang L-S, Vardarajan BN, Buros J, Gallins PJ, Buxbaum JD, Jarvik GP, Crane PK, et al: Common variants at MS4A4/MS4A6E, CD2AP, CD33 and EPHA1 are associated with late-onset Alzheimer's disease. Nat Genet 2011, 43:436

32. Neal ML, Boyle AM, Budge KM, Safadi FF, Richardson JR (2018) The glycoprotein GPNMB attenuates astrocyte inflammatory responses through the CD44 receptor. J Neuroinflammation 15:73

33. Oakley H, Cole SL, Logan S, Maus E, Shao P, Craft J, Guillozet-Bongaarts A, Ohno M, Disterhoft J, Van Eldik L et al (2006) Intraneuronal beta-amyloid aggregates, neurodegeneration, and neuron loss in transgenic mice with five familial Alzheimer's disease mutations: potential factors in amyloid plaque formation. J Neurosci 26:10129–10140

34. Ogawa T, Nikawa T, Furochi H, Kosyoji M, Hirasaka K, Suzue N, Sairyo K, Nakano S, Yamaoka T, Itakura M et al (2005) Osteoactivin upregulates expression of MMP-3 and MMP-9 in fibroblasts infiltrated into denervated skeletal muscle in mice. Am J Phys Cell Phys 289:C697–C707

35. Orre M, Kamphuis W, Osborn LM, Jansen AHP, Kooijman L, Bossers K, Hol EM (2014) Isolation of glia from Alzheimer's mice reveals inflammation and dysfunction. Neurobiol Aging 35:2746–2760

36. Piccio L, Deming Y, Del-Águila JL, Ghezzi L, Holtzman DM, Fagan AM, Fenoglio C, Galimberti D, Borroni B, Cruchaga C (2016) Cerebrospinal fluid soluble TREM2 is higher in Alzheimer disease and associated with mutation status. Acta Neuropathol 131:925–933

37. Plotegher N, Duchen MR (2017) Mitochondrial dysfunction and neurodegeneration in lysosomal storage disorders. Trends Mol Med 23:116–134

38. Reinert J, Richard BC, Klafki HW, Friedrich B, Bayer TA, Wiltfang J, Kovacs GG, Ingelsson M, Lannfelt L, Paetau A et al (2016) Deposition of C-terminally truncated Aβ species Aβ37 and Aβ39 in Alzheimer's disease and transgenic mouse models. Acta Neuropathologica Communications 4:1–12

39. Ripoll VM, Irvine KM, Ravasi T, Sweet MJ, Hume DA (2007) Gpnmb is induced in macrophages by IFN-γ and lipopolysaccharide and acts as a feedback regulator of Proinflammatory responses. J Immunol 178:6557–6566

40. Rose AAN, Annis MG, Dong Z, Pepin F, Hallett M, Park M, Siegel PM (2010) ADAM10 releases a soluble form of the GPNMB/Osteoactivin extracellular domain with Angiogenic properties. PLoS One 5:e12093

41. Saul A, Sprenger F, Bayer TA, Wirths O (2013) Accelerated tau pathology with synaptic and neuronal loss in a novel triple transgenic mouse model of Alzheimer's disease. Neurobiol Aging 34:2564–2573

42. Schieb H, Kratzin H, Jahn O, Mobius W, Rabe S, Staufenbiel M, Wiltfang J, Klafki HW (2011) Beta-amyloid peptide variants in brains and cerebrospinal fluid from amyloid precursor protein (APP) transgenic mice: comparison with human Alzheimer amyloid. J Biol Chem 286:33747–33758

43. Schmittgen TD, Livak KJ (2008) Analyzing real-time PCR data by the comparative C(T) method. Nat Protoc 3:1101–1108

44. Selkoe DJ, Hardy J (2016) The amyloid hypothesis of Alzheimer's disease at 25 years. EMBO Molecular Medicine 8:595–608

45. Stalder M, Phinney A, Probst A, Sommer B, Staufenbiel M, Jucker M (1999) Association of microglia with amyloid plaques in brains of APP23 transgenic mice. Am J Pathol 154:1673–1684

46. Sturchler-Pierrat C, Abramowski D, Duke M, Wiederhold KH, Mistl C, Rothacher S, Ledermann B, Burki K, Frey P, Paganetti PA et al (1997) Two amyloid precursor protein transgenic mouse models with Alzheimer disease-like pathology. Proc Natl Acad Sci U S A 94:13287–13292

47. Suárez-Calvet M, Kleinberger G, Araque Caballero MÁ, Brendel M, Rominger A, Alcolea D, Fortea J, Lleó A, Blesa R, Gispert JD et al (2016) sTREM2 cerebrospinal fluid levels are a potential biomarker for microglia activity in early-stage Alzheimer's disease and associate with neuronal injury markers. EMBO Molecular Medicine 8:466–476

48. Tanaka H, Shimazawa M, Kimura M, Takata M, Tsuruma K, Yamada M, Takahashi H, Hozumi I (2012) Niwa J-i, Iguchi Y, et al: The potential of GPNMB as novel neuroprotective factor in amyotrophic lateral sclerosis. Sci Rep 2:573

49. Tseveleki V, Rubio R, Vamvakas S-S, White J, Taoufik E, Petit E, Quackenbush J, Probert L (2010) Comparative gene expression analysis in mouse models for multiple sclerosis, Alzheimer's disease and stroke for identifying commonly regulated and disease-specific gene changes. Genomics 96:82–91

50. Walker DG, Lue L-F (2015) Immune phenotypes of microglia in human neurodegenerative disease: challenges to detecting microglial polarization in human brains. Alzheimers Res Ther 7:56

51. Weissmann R, Huttenrauch M, Kacprowski T, Bouter Y, Pradier L, Bayer TA, Kuss AW, Wirths O (2016) Gene expression profiling in the APP/PS1KI mouse model of familial Alzheimer's disease. J Alzheimers Dis 50:397–409

52. Weterman MAJ, Ajubi N, van Dinter IMR, Degen WGJ, van Muijen GNP, Ruiter DJ (1995) Bloemers HPJ: nmb, a novel gene, is expressed in low-metastatic human melanoma cell lines and xenografts. Int J Cancer 60:73–81

53. Williams MD, Esmaeli B, Soheili A, Simantov R, Gombos DS, Bedikian AY, Hwu P (2010) GPNMB expression in uveal melanoma: a potential for targeted therapy. Melanoma Res 20:184–190

54. Wirths O, Bayer TA (2012) Intraneuronal Abeta accumulation and neurodegeneration: lessons from transgenic models. Life Sci 91:1148–1152

55. Wirths O, Breyhan H, Schafer S, Roth C, Bayer TA (2008) Deficits in working memory and motor performance in the APP/PS1ki mouse model for Alzheimer's disease. Neurobiol Aging 29:891–901

56. Wu H-C, Chen C-M, Chen Y-C, Fung H-C, Chang K-H, Wu Y-R (2018) DLG2, but not TMEM229B, GPNMB, and ITGA8 polymorphism, is associated with Parkinson's disease in a Taiwanese population. Neurobiology of Aging 64(158):e151–e158 e156

57. Xu Y, Chen Y, Ou R, Wei Q-Q, Cao B, Chen K, Shang H-F (2016) No association of GPNMB rs156429 polymorphism with Parkinson's disease, amyotrophic lateral sclerosis and multiple system atrophy in Chinese population. Neurosci Lett 622:113–117

58. Yin Z, Raj D, Saiepour N, Van Dam D, Brouwer N, Holtman IR, Eggen BJL, Möller T, Tamm JA, Abdourahman A et al (2017) Immune hyperreactivity of Aβ plaque-associated microglia in Alzheimer's disease. Neurobiol Aging 55: 115–122

59. Yu B, Alboslemy T, Safadi F, Kim M-H (2018) Glycoprotein nonmelanoma clone B regulates the crosstalk between macrophages and mesenchymal stem cells toward wound repair. J Investig Dermatol 138:219–227

60. Zhang Y, Chen K, Sloan SA, Bennett ML, Scholze AR, O'Keeffe S, Phatnani HP, Guarnieri P, Caneda C, Ruderisch N et al (2014) An RNA-sequencing transcriptome and splicing database of glia, neurons, and vascular cells of the cerebral cortex. J Neurosci 34:11929–11947

61. Zhou L, Zhuo H, Ouyang H, Liu Y, Yuan F, Sun L, Liu F, Liu H (2017) Glycoprotein non-metastatic melanoma protein b (Gpnmb) is highly expressed in macrophages of acute injured kidney and promotes M2 macrophages polarization. Cell Immunol 316:53–60

62. Zigdon H, Savidor A, Levin Y, Meshcheriakova A, Schiffmann R, Futerman AH (2015) Identification of a biomarker in cerebrospinal fluid for Neuronopathic forms of Gaucher disease. PLoS One 10:e0120194

3

Degeneration of human photosensitive retinal ganglion cells may explain sleep and circadian rhythms disorders in Parkinson's disease

Isabel Ortuño-Lizarán[1†], Gema Esquiva[1†], Thomas G. Beach[2], Geidy E. Serrano[2], Charles H. Adler[3], Pedro Lax[1] and Nicolás Cuenca[1*] (iD)

Abstract

Parkinson's disease (PD) patients often suffer from non-motor symptoms like sleep dysregulation, mood disturbances or circadian rhythms dysfunction. The melanopsin-containing retinal ganglion cells are involved in the control and regulation of these processes and may be affected in PD, as other retinal and visual implications have been described in the disease. Number and morphology of human melanopsin-containing retinal ganglion cells were evaluated by immunohistochemistry in eyes from donors with PD or control. The Sholl number of intersections, the number of branches, and the number of terminals from the Sholl analysis were significantly reduced in PD melanopsin ganglion cells. Also, the density of these cells significantly decreased in PD compared to controls. Degeneration and impairment of the retinal melanopsin system may affect to sleep and circadian dysfunction reported in PD pathology, and its protection or stimulation may lead to better disease prospect and global quality of life of patients.

Keywords: Retina, Parkinson's disease, Circadian rhythms, Sleep disorders, Melanopsin retinal ganglion cell, Human

Introduction

The retina is an accessible and visible tissue, part of the central nervous system (CNS). Its well defined and highly characterized layered structure, together with the extensive knowledge about its neurons, synaptic contacts and physiology, make the retina an ideal material for pathophysiological studies of the CNS. In fact, neurodegenerative diseases mainly observed in the brain such as Parkinson's disease (PD), Alzheimer's disease, or Multiple Sclerosis present similar signs of degeneration in the retina [14], which is considered as a "window to the brain".

Intrinsically photosensitive melanopsin-containing retinal ganglion cells (mRGCs) are, together with cones and rods, retinal photoreceptors. While cones and rods are responsible for vision forming pathways, mRGCs are also in charge of the non-image forming pathways that primarily control and measure light irradiance detection [27, 48]. Melanopsin, an opsin protein containing a vitamin A-based chromophore maximally sensitive at 479 nm [40, 47], is the photopigment contained within mRGCs. Melanopsin-containing RGCs project to different CNS regions and regulate physiological and behavioral responses as important as circadian rhythms, pupillary reflex, melatonin production or mood [28, 30].

PD is the second most common neurological disorder and affects over 10 million people worldwide (http://parkinson.org/understanding-parkinsons/causes-and-statistics). Its main motor clinical features are rigidity, tremor and bradykinesia [19, 21, 46], but people with PD may also have several non-motor symptoms including cognitive decline and dementia [11], gastrointestinal and cardiovascular problems [43], mood disturbance [50], visual disruption [2, 55], impairment of the pupillary reflex response [54], and

* Correspondence: cuenca@ua.es
†Isabel Ortuño-Lizarán and Gema Esquiva contributed equally to this work.
[1]Department of Physiology, Genetics and Microbiology, University of Alicante, 03690 San Vicente del Raspeig, Spain
Full list of author information is available at the end of the article

sleep disorders [19, 46]. Sleep disorders including REM sleep behavior disorder (RBD), altered sleep, and hypersomnolence are extremely common in PD patients, affecting up to a 90% [10, 56]. Moreover, people with PD also exhibit alterations in the circadian secretion pattern of melatonin [9]. Dysfunction of circadian rhythms in PD is thought to be one of the causes of sleep disturbances and it can lead to cognitive and metabolic deficits, psychiatric and mood symptoms, or cardiovascular problems, negatively impacting quality of life [56].

The defining pathological lesions of PD are Lewy bodies and associated neurites with cytoplasmic accumulation of α-synuclein phosphorylated at serine-129 (p-α-syn), and the loss of dopaminergic neurons in the *substantia nigra pars compacta* [5, 13, 19]. The latter has traditionally been considered the cause of the motor clinical manifestations. Nevertheless, PD is today mostly considered as a multisystem disorder in which other different nervous system subdivisions are affected. Brain regions involved in vision are affected in PD, including the hypothalamic suprachiasmatic nucleus [16] and the retina [6, 45], both of which exhibit p-α-syn deposits. This visual system pathology in PD is accompanied by clinical findings including reduced electroretinography response and reduced visual evoked potentials, lower contrast sensitivity and impaired color and motion perception [3, 39]. These all suggest that vision is strongly affected at a cellular level.

As retinal mRGCs innervate the suprachiasmatic nucleus [20] and are jointly responsible for regulating circadian rhythms, which are in turn involved in mood and sleep behaviors, mRGCs dysfunction may be at least partially involved in the PD pathological process. Others have previously proposed a link between mRGCs, circadian rhythms and sleep regulation [1, 32], and a relationship between sleep disturbances and morphological impairment of mRGCs in human with aging has been described [18]. Therefore, the aim of this study was to evaluate the morphological changes of human mRGCs in PD, hypothesizing an involvement in sleep and circadian dysfunction. In this work, we show that the retinal melanopsin system is impaired in PD. We demonstrate that mRGCs degenerate in PD, as revealed by its number reduction and their morphological alterations, and this fact may be linked to the circadian and sleep disturbances suffered by PD patients.

Materials and methods
Human retinas
Human retinas from 11 donors were obtained postmortem, within 6 h of death, from the Arizona Study of Aging and Neurodegenerative Disorders (AZSAND), the

Banner Sun Health Research Institute Brain and Body Donation Program (BBDP; http://www.brainandbodydonationprogram.org/). All procedures were in accordance with the Declaration of Helsinki and with the recommendations and protocols approved by the Ethics Committee of the University of Alicante. Signed written informed consent was provided by all the participants in the study. Human donors, both men and women, were not significantly different in age, ranging from 70 to 82 years at death, and did not report any past history of retinal diseases.

The control group consisted of patients without neurodegenerative diseases ($n = 5$) and the Parkinson's disease group ($n = 6$) included subjects with a typical clinicopathological profile, diagnosed from the BBDP. Standard tests and neuropathological examinations were performed in deceased subjects as previously described [7].

Retinal histology
The human enucleated eyes were fixed in formaldehyde (3,75–4%) for 2 h at room temperature or 24–72 h at 4 °C, washed in PBS and then successively cryoprotected in increasing sucrose solutions of 15%, 20% and 30%. After removing the iris, lens and vitreous body, the retina was extracted and dissected, obtaining eight quadrants. The superior-nasal portion was used for further analysis.

Immunoperoxidase labeling
Wholemount retinas were stained using the immunoperoxidase labeling technique described by Esquiva et al. [17, 18]. Following inactivation of endogenous peroxidase activity with 1% H_2O_2 (H1009; Sigma, St. Louis, MO, USA), retinas were incubated in 2.28% $NaIO_4$ (S1878; Sigma) and later in 0.02% $NaBH_4$ (163314; Panreac, Barcelona, Spain). Then, flat-mount retinas were incubated in the anti-melanopsin primary antibody (1:5000; UF028) for 3 days at 4 °C. This antibody, raised against the 15 N-terminal amino acids of human melanopsin, was kindly provided by Dr. Ignacio Provencio (University of Virginia, Charlottesville, VA, USA). After the incubation time, they were washed in PBS, incubated for 2 days in a goat anti-rabbit biotinylated secondary antibody (1:100; 111–064-9144; Jackson ImmunoResearch Laboratories, West Grove, PA, USA), and then incubated 2 more days in an avidin-biotin peroxidase complex solution (0.9% avidin + 0.9% biotin; PK-6100, Vectastain Elite ABC Kit; Vector Laboratories Ltd., Cambridgeshire, UK). Retinas were finally washed and incubated in a fresh solution of 0.1% 3,3′-diaminobenzidine tetrahydrochloride (DAB, D5637; Sigma) plus 0.01% H_2O_2 and 0.025% ammonium nickel (II) sulfate hexahydrate (A1827; Sigma) until the staining was revealed as a brown precipitate. After DAB reaction, flat retinas were prepared with

the ganglion cell layer side up, and coverslipped for optical microscopy (Leica DMR; Leica Microsystems).

To determine their type and morphology, immunostained mRGCs were traced by hand in all flat-mounted retinas using a camera lucida connected to a Leica DMR microscope (Leica Microsystems). Images were then digitized, using image-editing software (Adobe Photoshop 10.0; Adobe Systems, Inc., San Jose, CA, USA). Total number of cells expressing melanopsin was counted and density of mRGCs per mm^2 was calculated.

Morphological analysis

Representative mRGCs were traced by hand in order to recreate their soma and dendritic profiles using a camera lucida (120 cells analyzed in total, 60 cells of controls and 60 of PD, 15 cells of each morphological subtype and group).

To analyze the morphology of mRGCs the Bonfire program developed in the Firestein laboratory at Rutgers University [33] was used. From digitized neuritic arbors, this software allowed us to perform a Sholl analysis and to estimate the number of branch points, the terminal neurite tips and the total number of Sholl intersections per cell [49].

Statistical analysis

Statistical analysis was performed using Prism 6 for Windows (Graphpad Software, Inc., La Jolla, CA, USA). To assess the differences of the studied variables, both globally or per mRGC subtype (M1, M1d, M2 and M3),

between PD and control patients a non-parametric two-tailed Mann-Whitney test was used. Differences of the Sholl curve representing the number of intersections per distance between PD and controls were evaluated using a paired non-parametric Wilcoxon signed rank test. In all cases, a p-value lower than 0.05 was considered statistically significant.

Results

Types of mRGCs in the human retina

In the human retina, four types of mRGCs are found. They are classified in accordance with their soma location and dendritic stratifications: M1, M1d, M2, and M3. As the diagram of Fig. 1 shows, M1, M2 and M3 cells have their soma located in the ganglion cell layer, while their dendrites stratify in different strata of the inner plexiform layer (IPL). M1 cells stratify in the S1 plexus of the IPL, M2 stratify in S5 plexus, and M3 has dendrites in both strata: S1 and S5. M1d cell is a displaced M1 cell, with its soma located in the inner nuclear layer (INL) and its dendrites in the S1 plexus of the IPL, near the INL [8]. M1d mRGC is the predominant type in the human retina, accounting for about half of all mRGCs [18, 25]. An example of control and PD DAB immunostained M1d mRGC is shown in Fig. 1a and b respectively. Notice the lower dendrite complexity in PD mRGC (Fig. 1b) and its lower staining intensity when compared to controls (Fig. 1a). Identification of S1 and S5 strata can be done changing the microscope focus and using the

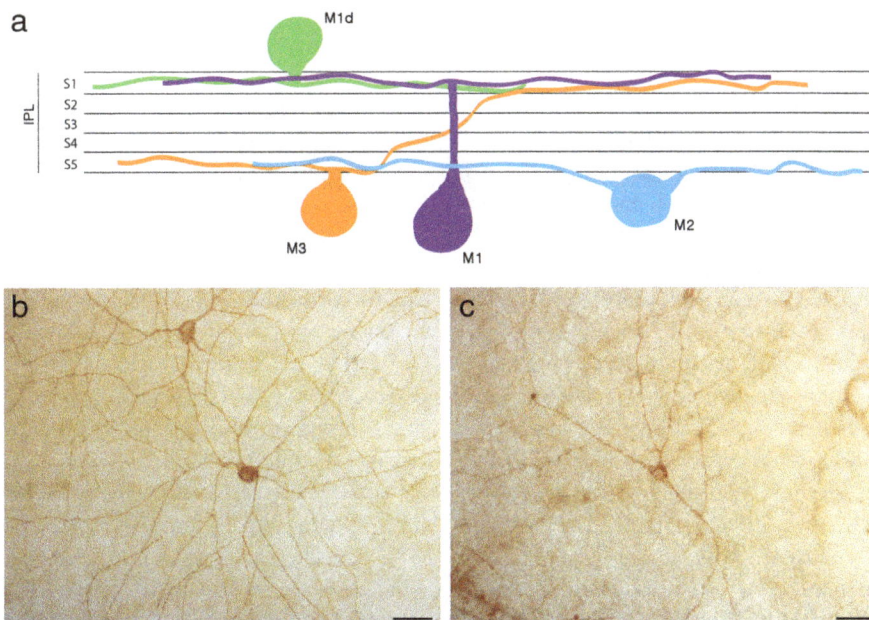

Fig. 1 Melanopsin retinal ganglion cells in the human retina. **a** Diagram showing the structure and classification of mRGC depending on their soma location and dendrites stratification in IPL S1 or S5. **b**, **c** Immunostaining of human melanopsin using the DAB method in flat wholemount retinas of control (**b**) and PD (**c**) subjects. Scale bar, 50 μm

Nomarski technique of differential interference contrast. This technique allows us to identify and differentiate the INL, the IPL, and the ganglion cell layer (GCL). Thus, S1 and S5 strata can be differentiated, without need of counterstaining, because S1 is near the INL and S5 in the opposite side of the IPL, near the GCL.

Decrease of mRGC density in PD retinas

Cell density quantification and morphological analysis were performed to evaluate differences in mRGCs between PD and control subjects. These studies were made considering the total mRGCs as well as differentiating by mRGC type. A reduction in the mRGC density and in the complexity of the melanopsin plexus was found. Fig. 2a and b are drawings representing retinal fields that show mRGCs and its plexus in control and PD. Fig. 2c and d show the density of mRGCs, expressed as number of mRGCs per mm^2, both totally and by mRGC type. A reduction in number of mRGCs, accompanied by a drastic reduction in their plexus complexity, can be clearly seen in the drawings. The decrease in mRGC number is statistically significant (control: 4.8 ± 1.3 cells/mm^2; PD: 3.2 ± 0.8 cells/mm^2; p-value = 0.05) and it mostly affects the M1d and M2 mRGC types. In normal conditions, mRGCs make contacts to other mRGCs creating a dense plexus and have numerous dendritic beads, as the control drawing shows. In PD, the plexus is highly reduced and there are very few contacts between cells and fewer dendritic beads.

Morphological impairment of mRGCs in PD

Apart from cell density decline, morphological changes were also found in PD mRGCs. Morphology, dendritic arborization and dendritic tree size of normal and PD cells can be observed in Fig. 3. Red drawings show the elements that are placed in the IPL S5 stratum and blue represent the elements from S1 stratum, allowing the differentiation of the mRGC types. Visually, structure, size and dendritic trees are altered in PD compared to controls: dendritic area is reduced and cells have fewer and shorter ramifications. Dendritic beads, which are thought to represent synaptic contact points, are also reduced in PD (control: 44.7 ± 25.8 beads per cell; PD: 19.3 ± 10.9 beads per cell; p-value < 0.0001), what could be a sign of functional alteration. These morphological alterations are drastic in M1, M1d and M2 cells, while M3 cells seem to be the least affected by the disease.

Morphological changes were measured using the Sholl analysis, that includes the total number of intersections, the number of intersections per distance, and terminal points and branch points numbers. Results are shown in Fig. 4 and corroborate the differences described above.

The three analyzed measures are significantly reduced in PD, compared to controls: terminal points decrease from 16 ± 5 (controls) to 13 ± 4 (PD) (p-value < 0.001); branch points from 13 ± 5 to 9 ± 4 (p-value < 0.0001); and Sholl total number of intersections from $137,2 \pm 41,3$ to $106,8 \pm 38,2$ (p-value < 0.001). When comparing these parameters in each cell type, M1d and M2 cells show statistically significant reduced values in PD in the three measures, M1 cells show a statistically significant decrease in Sholl analysis and terminal points, and M3 were not significantly affected, although they present a tendency for fewer terminal and branch points. The Sholl analysis curve (Fig. 4g) shows the number of intersections per distance from the cell soma. Less intersections have been found in PD until a distance from the soma of 340 µm, what indicates a lower cell complexity and less ramifications of PD mRGCs, as concluded also by the less branches, terminal points, and number of total intersections that they present in comparison to controls.

Discussion

In recent years, a huge effort has been made to study the state and health of brain regions related to circadian rhythms disturbances and sleep dysregulation, like the suprachiasmatic nucleus, but these alterations are not yet completely understood and some regions are found not to be affected until advanced states of the disease [22]. The study of the retinal mRGCs is a new approach in trying to understand the cellular mechanisms underlying circadian rhythms dysfunctions in PD and may add valuable information to the current knowledge of the disease.

This study demonstrates a loss of melanopsin-immunoreactive RGCs in Parkinson's disease compared to control subjects. The density of mRGCs is significantly decreased in PD patients, and the remaining cells exhibit morphological alterations like decreased Sholl area, fewer ramifications and terminal points, and a reduced melanopsin-immunoreactive plexus. These morphological changes and numerical reduction demonstrate that mRGCs are affected in PD, probably by dying or losing melanopsin production, and it is likely that both of these would lead to functional impairment. To the best of our knowledge, this is the first study that describes alterations of mRGCs in PD.

A recent study in humans show that the mRGC density and plexus decrease with age and correlate it with the circadian rhythm dysfunction observed with aging [18]. In the present study, the mRGC type most affected is M1d, the main mRGC type in the human retina; that is also the type most affected by age [18]. M2 cells also have lower cell densities and both M1 and M2 show altered morphological parameters. These differences are not significant in the aging retina, but in

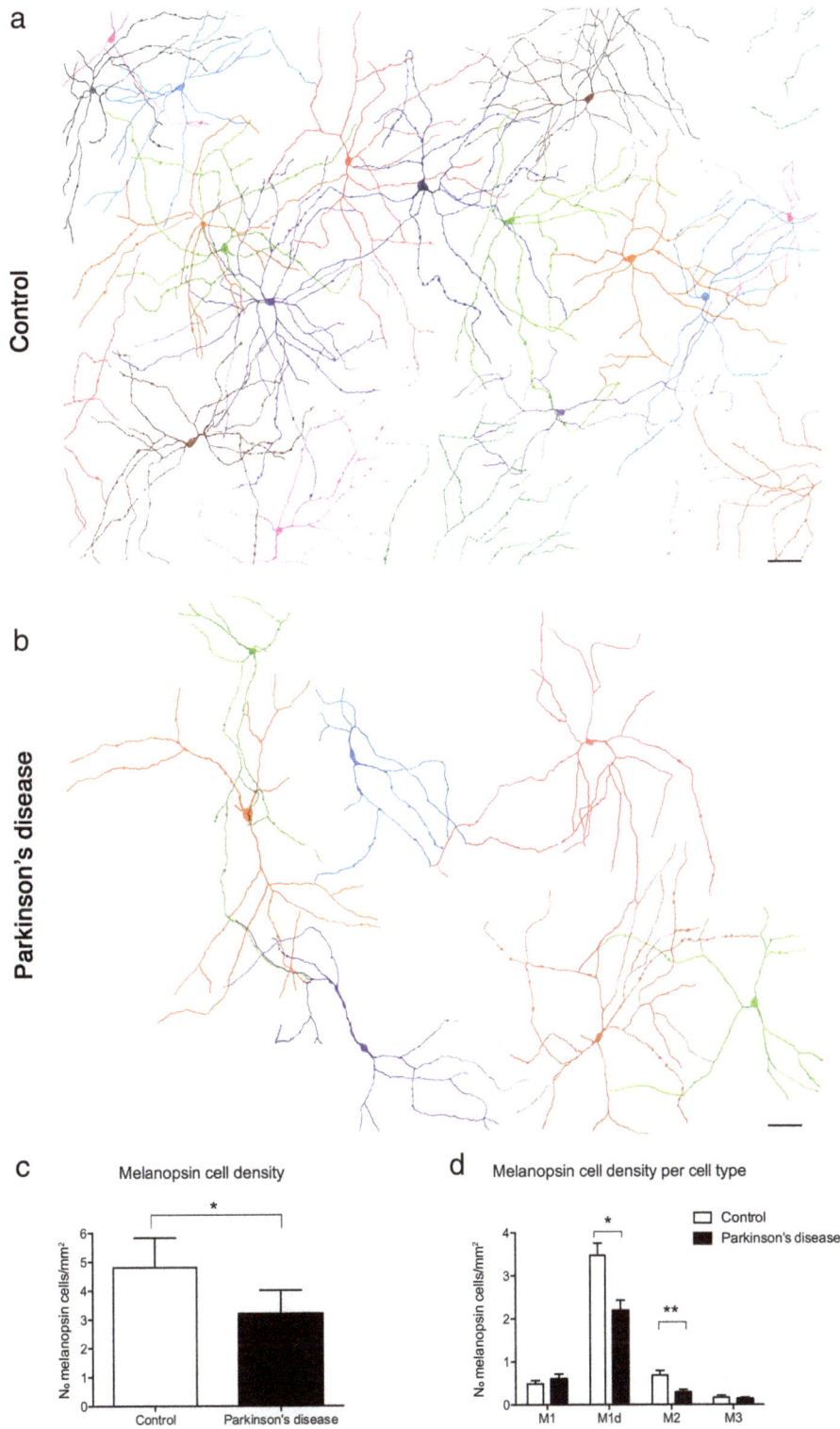

Fig. 2 Representative drawings of control and PD retinal fields. Each color defines an individual mRGC. **a** Melanopsin plexus in a control wholemount retina. **b** Melanopsin plexus in a PD wholemount retina. **c** Total mRGC quantification (number of mRGCs per mm^2) and comparison between control and PD subjects. **d** Comparison of the mRGC density per cell type in control and PD subjects. Scale bar, 100 µm. Data is presented as mean ± s.d. *$P < 0.05$, **$P < 0.01$

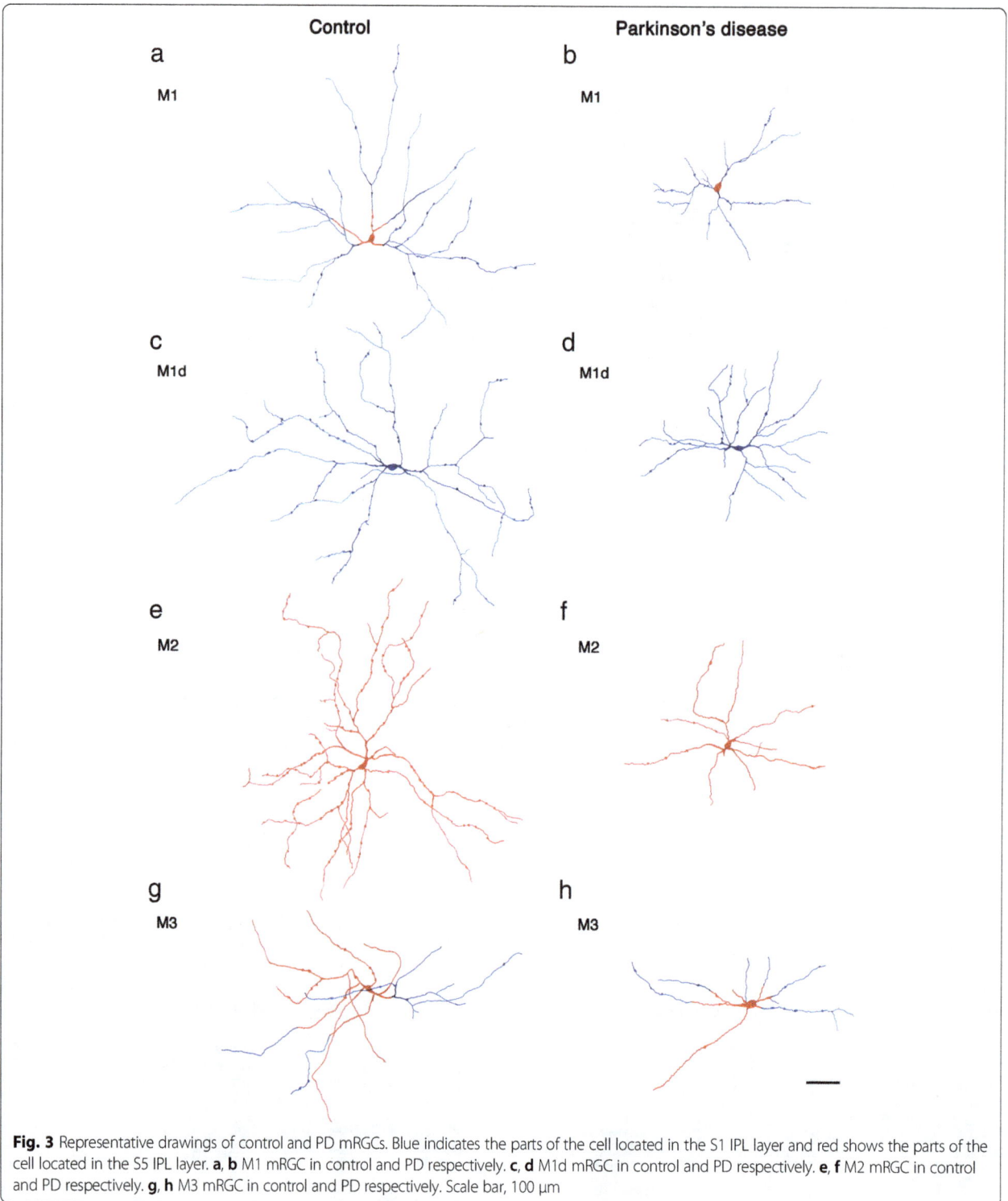

Fig. 3 Representative drawings of control and PD mRGCs. Blue indicates the parts of the cell located in the S1 IPL layer and red shows the parts of the cell located in the S5 IPL layer. **a**, **b** M1 mRGC in control and PD respectively. **c**, **d** M1d mRGC in control and PD respectively. **e**, **f** M2 mRGC in control and PD respectively. **g**, **h** M3 mRGC in control and PD respectively. Scale bar, 100 μm

PD it seems that almost all mRGCs show morphological abnormalities as well as a numerical decline. As mRGCs innervate the suprachiasmatic nucleus [20], it is expected that these morphological alterations lead to a dysfunction mostly related with circadian rhythms, mood, and sleep; and also with the pupillary reflex: the major mRGC functions. Morphological and connectivity studies about mRGCs have also demonstrated its relationship with dopaminergic cells, which make contacts in the S1 strata of the IPL with mRGC somas and dendrites, mainly with

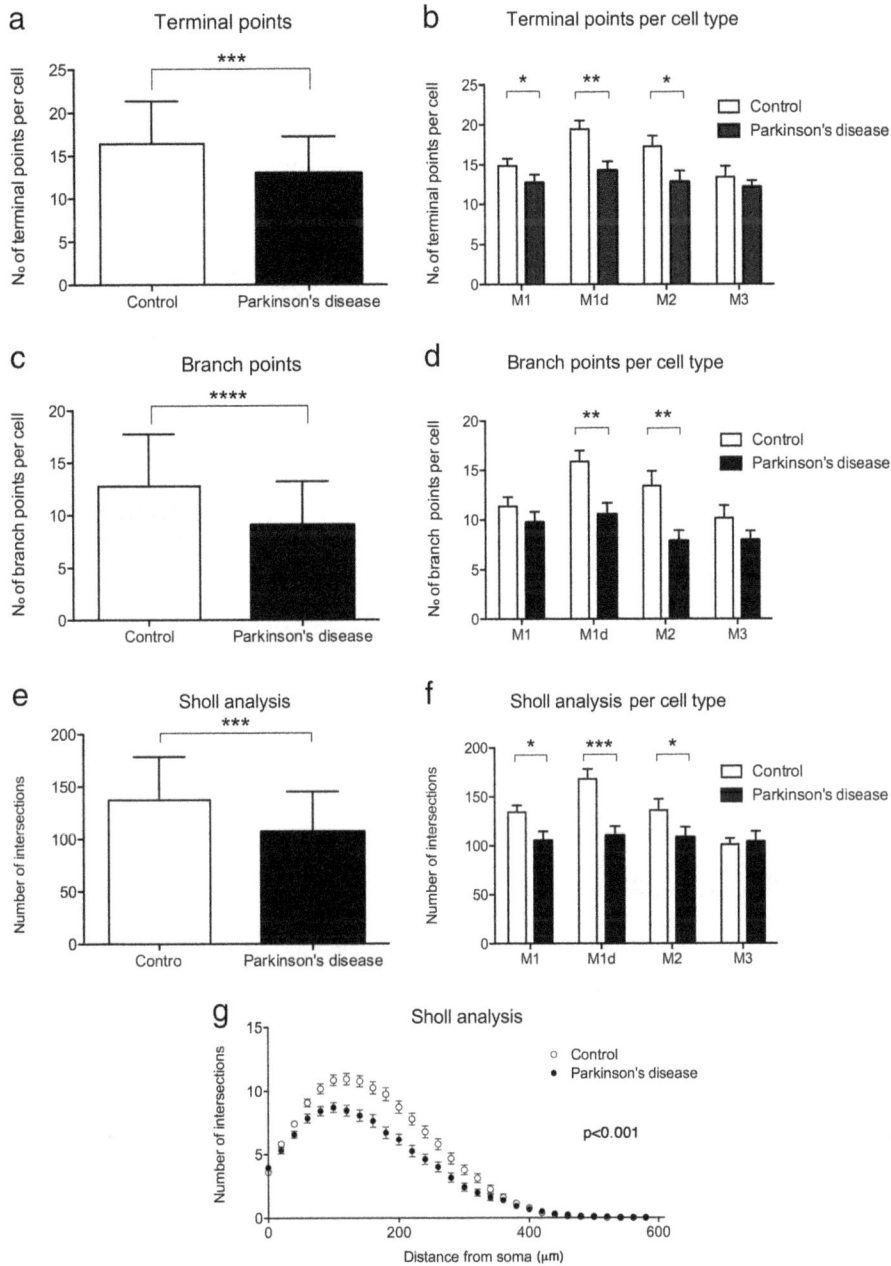

Fig. 4 Morphological Sholl analysis of mRGCs in PD and controls. **a**, **b** Comparison of terminal points number per cell in PD and controls considering total mRGC (**a**) or per cell type (**b**). **c**, **d** Comparison of the number of branch points in all mRCGs (**c**) and per cell type (**d**) in PD and controls. **e**, **f** Sholl area comparison of PD and control mRGCs globally (**e**) and per cell type (**f**). Data is presented as mean ± s.d. *$P < 0.05$, **$P < 0.01$, ***$P < 0.001$, ****$P < 0.0001$. **g** Sholl analysis curve representing number of intersections per distance from soma, comparing total controls and PD mRGCs. Data is presented as mean ± s.e.m.

the M1d type [38]. Diminution of dopamine levels in the retina in PD [26] may be one of the causes of M1d cell degeneration, as this would represent a loss of one of their main synaptic inputs.

In animal models, MPTP-treated monkeys exhibit dopaminergic system impairment and circadian rhythm disruption with altered sleep/wake cycle, REM sleep impairment and daytime sleepiness [15, 23, 51, 56]. Also, in P23H blind rats, degeneration of mRGCs statistically correlates with circadian rhythms impairment [34]. Other existing works that analyzed the effect of parkinsonism in circadian rhythms described changes in the expression of the "clock genes" [12], in circadian melatonin secretion [9], in pupillary reflex [4, 54], depression [57] and in REM sleep [10, 52], all directly or indirectly controlled and affected by mRGCs. But the suprachiasmatic nucleus has been found to be un-affected until advanced stages of the disease, suggesting that there are other components of the circadian system causing circadian abnormalities in PD [22]. Thus, it is easy to question the implication of the retina, and specifically of the mRGCs, in circadian dysfunction in PD, but until now no cellular studies were available to determine its real con-tribution. The retinal melanopsin system abnormalities de-tected in PD in the present study help to explain some of the circadian and sleep problems that are common in the disease, as it probably contributes to or worsens them. The loss of mRGCs have also been described in other neuro-logical pathologies like Alzheimer's disease and diabetic ret-inopathy [31, 44] where its impairment is related to circadian rhythm alterations and sleep disorders [32, 35].

There is growing evidence that circadian rhythm disor-ders, normally accompanied by sleep disruption, not only negatively affect the patients' quality of life but may also accelerate the progression of neurodegenerative dis-ease pathology [41]. The identification and management of these symptoms is therefore important not only for a clinical benefit but perhaps also for modulation of dis-ease progression. In this sense, knowing the effect that the retina and mRGCs may have in the progression of circadian disorders, eye protection should be recom-mended to patients. Additionally, novel therapies using light stimulation to synchronize circadian rhythms are demonstrating beneficial results in PD [24, 29, 36]. Martino et al. found that long-term light therapy im-proves sleep quality, reduces awakenings during the night and increases the total sleep time [42]. Light ther-apy was also found to be effective for excessive daytime sleepiness and global sleep quality [53]. A cellular explanation of this light therapy success might possibly invoke the stimulation of mRGCs, leading to dopamine release and to circadian rhythms synchronization, glo-bally improving PD pathology [37].

Conclusions

In summary, the present work demonstrates that the retinal melanopsin system is affected in PD. This fact has clinical implications for PD-related circadian rhythm alteration as well as for mood and sleep disor-ders. Protecting the retina to prolong mRGC health and using light therapies could be beneficial for the maintenance of circadian rhythms and for improving global life quality of patients.

Acknowledgements
This work was supported by the Michael J. Fox Foundation for Parkinson's Research. I.O.L. acknowledges financial support from the Ministerio de Educación, Spain (FPU 14/03166). N.C. acknowledges financial support from the Ministerio de Economía y Competitividad, Spain (MINECO-FEDER-BFU2015-67139-R), Generalitat Valenciana (Prometeo 2016/158), and Instituto Carlos III (ISCIII RETICS-FEDER RD16/0008/0016). The Brain and Body Donation Program has been supported by the National Institute of Neurological Disorders and Stroke (U24 NS072026), the National Institute on Aging (P30 AG19610), the Arizona Department of Health Services, the Arizona Biomedical Research Commission, and the Michael J. Fox Foundation for Parkinson's Research.

Authors' contributions
NC and PL conceived the concept and designed the experiments. GES, TGB and CHA were in charge of the eye donation program. IOL and GE performed the experiments, analyzed data and drafted the manuscript. NC, PL, TGB and CHA obtained funding and revised the manuscript. All authors read and approved the final manuscript.

Competing interests
The authors declare that they have no competing interests.

Author details
[1]Department of Physiology, Genetics and Microbiology, University of Alicante, 03690 San Vicente del Raspeig, Spain. [2]Banner Sun Health Research Institute, Sun City, AZ 85351, USA. [3]Mayo Clinic Arizona, Scottsdale, AZ 85259, USA.

References
1. Altimus CM, Güler AD, Villa KL, McNeill DS, Legates TA, Hattar S (2008) Rods-cones and melanopsin detect light and dark to modulate sleep independent of image formation. Proc Natl Acad Sci U S A 105:19998–20003. https://doi.org/10.1073/pnas.0808312105
2. Archibald NK, Clarke MP, Mosimann UP, Burn DJ (2009) The retina in Parkinsons disease. Brain 132:1128–1145. https://doi.org/10.1093/brain/awp068
3. Archibald NK, Clarke MP, Mosimann UP, Burn DJ (2011) Visual symptoms in Parkinson's disease and Parkinson's disease dementia. Mov Disord 26:2387–2395. https://doi.org/10.1002/mds.23891
4. Armstrong RA (2017) Visual dysfunction in Parkinson's disease. Int Rev Neurobiol 134:921–946. https://doi.org/10.1016/bs.irn.2017.04.007
5. Beach TG, Adler CH, Lue L, Sue LI, Bachalakuri J, Henry-Watson J, Sasse J, Boyer S, Shirohi S, Brooks R, Eschbacher J, White CL 3rd, Akiyama H, Caviness J, Shill HA, Connor DJ, Sabbagh MN, Walker DG (2009) Unified staging system for Lewy body disorders: correlation with nigrostriatal degeneration, cognitive impairment and motor dysfunction. Acta Neuropathol 117:613–634. https://doi.org/10.1007/s00401-009-0538-8
6. Beach TG, Carew J, Serrano G, Adler CH, Shill HA, Sue LI, Sabbagh MN, Akiyama H, Cuenca N, Caviness J, Driver-Dunckley E, Jacobson S, Belden C, Davis K (2014) Phosphorylated α-synuclein-immunoreactive retinal neuronal elements in Parkinson's disease subjects. Neurosci Lett 571:34–38. https://doi.org/10.1016/j.neulet.2014.04.027
7. Beach TG, Sue LI, Walker DG, Roher AE, Lue L, Vedders L, Connor DJ, Sabbagh MN, Rogers J (2008) The Sun Health Research Institute Brain Donation Program: description and experience, 1987–2007. Cell Tissue Bank 9:229–245. https://doi.org/10.1007/s10561-008-9067-2
8. Berson DM, Castrucci AM, Provencio I (2010) Morphology and mosaics of melanopsin-expressing retinal ganglion cell types in mice. J Comp Neurol 518:2405–2422. https://doi.org/10.1002/cne.22381
9. Bordet R, Devos D, Brique S, Touitou Y, Guieu JD, Libersa C, Destée A (2003) Study of circadian melatonin secretion pattern at different stages of Parkinson's disease. Clin Neuropharmacol 26:65–72
10. Breen DP, Vuono R, Nawarathna U, Fisher K, Shneerson JM, Reddy AB, Barker RA (2014) Sleep and circadian rhythm regulation in early Parkinson disease. JAMA Neurol 71:589. https://doi.org/10.1001/jamaneurol.2014.65
11. Caballol N, Martí MJ, Tolosa E (2007) Cognitive dysfunction and dementia in Parkinson disease. Mov Disord 22:358–366. https://doi.org/10.1002/mds.21677
12. Cai Y, Liu S, Sothern RB, Xu S, Chan P (2010) Expression of clock genes Per1 and Bmal1 in total leukocytes in health and Parkinson's disease. Eur J Neurol 17:550–554. https://doi.org/10.1111/j.1468-1331.2009.02848.x
13. Campello L, Esteve-Rudd J, Cuenca N, Martín-Nieto J (2013) The ubiquitin–proteasome system in retinal health and disease. Mol Neurobiol 47:790–810. https://doi.org/10.1007/s12035-012-8391-5

14. Cuenca N, Fernández-Sánchez L, Campello L, Maneu V, De la Villa P, Lax P, Pinilla I (2014) Cellular responses following retinal injuries and therapeutic approaches for neurodegenerative diseases. Prog Retin Eye Res 43:17–75. https://doi.org/10.1016/j.preteyeres.2014.07.001

15. Cuenca N, Herrero MT, Angulo A, De Juan E, Martínez-Navarrete GC, López S, Barcia C, Martín-Nieto J (2005) Morphological impairments in retinal neurons of the scotopic visual pathway in a monkey model of Parkinson's disease. J Comp Neurol 493:261–273. https://doi.org/10.1002/cne.20761

16. De Pablo-Fernández E, Courtney R, Warner TT, Holton JL (2018) A histologic study of the circadian system in Parkinson disease, multiple system atrophy, and progressive supranuclear palsy. JAMA Neurol 75:1008. https://doi.org/10.1001/jamaneurol.2018.0640

17. Esquiva G, Lax P, Cuenca N (2013) Impairment of intrinsically photosensitive retinal ganglion cells associated with late stages of retinal degeneration. Invest Ophthalmol Vis Sci 54:4605–4618. https://doi.org/10.1167/iovs.13-12120

18. Esquiva G, Lax P, Pérez-santonja JJ, García-fernández JM, Cuenca N (2017) Loss of melanopsin-expressing ganglion cell subtypes and dendritic degeneration in the aging human retina. Front Aging Neurosci 9:79. https://doi.org/10.3389/fnagi.2017.00079

19. Fahn S (2006) Description of Parkinson's disease as a clinical syndrome. Ann N Y Acad Sci 991:1–14. https://doi.org/10.1111/j.1749-6632.2003.tb07458.x

20. Fernandez DC, Chang Y-T, Hattar S, Chen S-K (2016) Architecture of retinal projections to the central circadian pacemaker. Proc Natl Acad Sci 113: 6047–6052. https://doi.org/10.1073/pnas.1523629113

21. Ferreira M, Massano J (2017) An updated review of Parkinson's disease genetics and clinicopathological correlations. Acta Neurol Scand 135:273–284. https://doi.org/10.1111/ane.12616

22. Fifel K (2017) Alterations of the circadian system in Parkinson's disease patients. Mov Disord 32:682–692. https://doi.org/10.1002/mds.26865

23. Fifel K, Vezoli J, Dzahini K, Claustrat B, Leviel V, Kennedy H, Procyk E, Dkhissi-Benyahya O, Gronfier C, Cooper HM (2014) Alteration of daily and circadian rhythms following dopamine depletion in MPTP treated non-human primates. PLoS One 9:e86240. https://doi.org/10.1371/journal.pone.0086240

24. Fifel K, Videnovic A (2018) Light therapy in Parkinson's disease: towards mechanism-based protocols. Trends Neurosci 41:252–254. https://doi.org/10.1016/j.tins.2018.03.002

25. Hannibal J, Christiansen AT, Heegaard S, Fahrenkrug J, Kiilgaard JF (2017) Melanopsin expressing human retinal ganglion cells: subtypes, distribution, and intraretinal connectivity. J Comp Neurol 525:1934–1961. https://doi.org/10.1002/cne.24181

26. Harnois C, Di Paolo T (1990) Decreased dopamine in the retinas of patients with Parkinson's disease. Invest Ophthalmol Vis Sci 31:2473–2475

27. Hattar S (2002) Melanopsin-containing retinal ganglion cells: architecture, projections, and intrinsic photosensitivity. Science 295:1065–1070. https://doi.org/10.1126/science.1069609

28. Hattar S, Kumar M, Park A, Tong P, Tung J, Yau K-W, Berson DM (2006) Central projections of melanopsin-expressing retinal ganglion cells in the mouse. J Comp Neurol 497:326–349. https://doi.org/10.1002/cne.20970

29. Högl B (2017) Circadian rhythms and chronotherapeutics - underappreciated approach to improving sleep and wakefulness in Parkinson disease. JAMA Neurol 74:387–388. https://doi.org/10.1001/jamaneurol.2016.5519

30. Ksendzovsky A, Pomeraniec IJ, Zaghloul KA, Provencio JJ, Provencio I (2017) Clinical implications of the melanopsin-based non–image-forming visual system. Neurology 88:1282–1290. https://doi.org/10.1212/WNL.0000000000003761

31. La Morgia C, Ross-Cisneros FN, Koronyo Y, Hannibal J, Gallassi R, Cantalupo G, Sambati L, Pan BX, Tozer KR, Barboni P, Provini F, Avanzini P, Carbonelli M, Pelosi A, Chui H, Liguori R, Baruzzi A, Koronyo-Hamaoui M, Sadun AA, Carelli V (2016) Melanopsin retinal ganglion cell loss in Alzheimer disease. Ann Neurol 79:90–109. https://doi.org/10.1002/ana.24548

32. La Morgia C, Ross-Cisneros FN, Sadun AA, Carelli V (2017) Retinal ganglion cells and circadian rhythms in Alzheimer's disease, Parkinson's disease, and beyond. Front Neurol 8:1–8. https://doi.org/10.3389/fneur.2017.00162

33. Langhammer CG, Previtera ML, Sweet ES, Sran SS, Chen M, Firestein BL (2010) Automated Sholl analysis of digitized neuronal morphology at multiple scales: whole-cell Sholl analysis vs. Sholl analysis of arbor sub-regions. Cytometry A 77:1160–1168. https://doi.org/10.1002/cyto.a.20954

34. Lax P, Esquiva G, Fuentes-Broto L, Segura F, Sánchez-Cano A, Cuenca N, Pinilla I (2016) Age-related changes in photosensitive melanopsin-expressing retinal ganglion cells correlate with circadian rhythm

impairments in sighted and blind rats. Chronobiol Int 33:374–391. https://doi.org/10.3109/07420528.2016.1151025

35. Lazzerini Ospri L, Prusky G, Hattar S (2017) Mood, the circadian system, and melanopsin retinal ganglion cells. Annu Rev Neurosci 40:539–556. https://doi.org/10.1146/annurev-neuro-072116-031324

36. Li S, Wang Y, Wang F, Hu L-F, Liu C-F (2017) A new perspective for Parkinson's disease: circadian rhythm. Neurosci Bull 33:62–72. https://doi.org/10.1007/s12264-016-0089-7

37. Li Z, Tian T (2017) Light therapy promoting dopamine release by stimulating retina in Parkinson disease. JAMA Neurol 74:1267. https://doi.org/10.1001/jamaneurol.2017.1906

38. Liao HW, Ren X, Peterson BB, Marshak DW, Yau KW, Gamlin PD, Dacey DM (2016) Melanopsin-expressing ganglion cells on macaque and human retinas form two morphologically distinct populations. J Comp Neurol 524: 2845–2872. https://doi.org/10.1002/cne.23995

39. Lin TP, Rigby H, Adler JS, Hentz JG, Balcer LJ, Galetta SL, Devick S, Cronin R, Adler CH (2015) Abnormal visual contrast acuity in Parkinson's disease. J Parkinsons Dis 5:125–130. https://doi.org/10.3233/JPD-140470

40. Lucas RJ, Douglas RH, Foster RG (2001) Characterization of an ocular photopigment capable of driving pupillary constriction in mice. Nat Neurosci 4:621–626. https://doi.org/10.1038/88443

41. Malhotra RK (2018) Neurodegenerative Disorders and Sleep. Sleep Med Clin 13:63–70. https://doi.org/10.1016/j.jsmc.2017.09.006

42. Martino JK, Freelance CB, Willis GL (2018) The effect of light exposure on insomnia and nocturnal movement in Parkinson's disease: an open label, retrospective, longitudinal study. Sleep Med 44:24–31. https://doi.org/10.1016/j.sleep.2018.01.001

43. Micieli G, Tosi P, Marcheselli S, Cavallini A (2003) Autonomic dysfunction in Parkinson's disease. Neurol Sci 24:32–34. https://doi.org/10.1007/s100720300035

44. Obara EA, Hannibal J, Heegaard S, Fahrenkrug J (2017) Loss of melanopsin-expressing retinal ganglion cells in patients with diabetic retinopathy. Investig Opthalmology Vis Sci 58:2187. https://doi.org/10.1167/iovs.16-21168

45. Ortuño-Lizarán I, Beach TG, Serrano GE, Walker DG, Adler CH, Cuenca N (2018) Phosphorylated α-synuclein in the retina is a biomarker of Parkinson's disease pathology severity. Mov Disord. https://doi.org/10.1002/mds.27392

46. Postuma RB, Berg D, Stern M, Poewe W, Olanow CW, Oertel W, Obeso J, Marek K, Litvan I, Lang AE, Halliday G, Goetz CG, Gasser T, Dubois B, Chan P, Bloem BR, Adler CH, Deuschl G (2015) MDS clinical diagnostic criteria for Parkinson's disease. Mov Disord 30:1591–1601. https://doi.org/10.1002/mds.26424

47. Provencio I, Rodriguez IR, Jiang G, Hayes WP, Moreira EF, Rollag MD (2000) A novel human opsin in the inner retina. J Neurosci 20:600–605

48. Provencio I, Rollag MD, Castrucci AM (2002) Photoreceptive net in the mammalian retina. This mesh of cells may explain how some blind mice can still tell day from night. Nature 415:493. https://doi.org/10.1038/415493a

49. Sholl DA (1953) Dendritic organization in the neurons of the visual and motor cortices of the cat. J Anat 87:387–406

50. Tan LCS (2012) Mood disorders in Parkinson's disease. Parkinsonism Relat Disord 18(Suppl 1):S74–S76. https://doi.org/10.1016/S1353-8020(11)70024-4

51. Vezoli J, Fifel K, Leviel V, Dehay C, Kennedy H, Cooper HM, Gronfier C, Procyk E (2011) Early presymptomatic and long-term changes of rest activity cycles and cognitive behavior in a MPTP-monkey model of Parkinson's disease. PLoS One 6:e23952. https://doi.org/10.1371/journal.pone.0023952

52. Videnovic A, Golombek D (2013) Circadian and sleep disorders in Parkinson's disease. Exp Neurol 243:45–56. https://doi.org/10.1016/j.expneurol.2012.08.018

53. Videnovic A, Klerman EB, Wang W, Marconi A, Kuhta T, Zee PC (2017) Timed light therapy for sleep and daytime sleepiness associated with Parkinson disease a randomized clinical trial. JAMA Neurol 74:411–418. https://doi.org/10.1001/jamaneurol.2016.5192

54. Wang C-A, McInnis H, Brien DC, Pari G, Munoz DP (2016) Disruption of pupil size modulation correlates with voluntary motor preparation deficits in Parkinson's disease. Neuropsychologia 80:176–184. https://doi.org/10.1016/J.NEUROPSYCHOLOGIA.2015.11.019

55. Weil RS, Schrag AE, Warren JD, Crutch SJ, Lees AJ, Morris HR (2016) Visual dysfunction in Parkinson's disease. Brain 139:2827–2843. https://doi.org/10.1093/brain/aww175

4

Expression of renal cell markers and detection of 3p loss links endolymphatic sac tumor to renal cell carcinoma and warrants careful evaluation to avoid diagnostic pitfalls

Rachel Jester[1], Iya Znoyko[1], Maria Garnovskaya[1], Joseph N Rozier[1], Ryan Kegl[1], Sunil Patel[2], Tuan Tran[3], Malak Abedalthagafi[4], Craig M Horbinski[5], Mary Richardson[1], Daynna J Wolff[1], Razvan Lapadat[6], William Moore[7], Fausto J Rodriguez[8], Jason Mull[9] and Adriana Olar[1,2,10*]

Abstract

Endolymphatic sac tumor (ELST) is a rare neoplasm arising in the temporal petrous region thought to originate from endolymphatic sac epithelium. It may arise sporadically or in association with Von-Hippel-Lindau syndrome (VHL). The ELST prevalence in VHL ranges from 3 to 16% and may be the initial presentation of the disease. Onset is usually in the 3rd to 5th decade with hearing loss and an indolent course. ELSTs present as locally destructive lesions with characteristic computed tomography imaging features. Histologically, they show papillary, cystic or glandular architectures. Immunohistochemically, they express keratin, EMA, and variably S100 and GFAP. Currently it is recommended that, given its rarity, ELST needs to be differentiated from other entities with similar morphologic patterns, particularly other VHL-associated neoplasms such as metastatic clear cell renal cell carcinoma (ccRCC). Nineteen ELST cases were studied. Immunohistochemistry (18/19) and single nucleotide polymorphism microarray testing was performed (12/19). Comparison with the immunophenotype and copy number profile in RCC is discussed. Patients presented with characteristic bone destructive lesions in the petrous temporal bones. Pathology of tumors showed characteristic ELST morphology with immunoexpression of CK7, GFAP, S100, PAX-8, PAX-2, CA-9 in the tumor cells. Immunostaines for RCC, CD10, CK20, chromogranin A, synaptophysin, TTF-1, thyroglobulin, and transthyretin were negative in the tumor cells. Molecular testing showed loss of 3p and 9q in 66% (8/12) and 58% (7/12) cases, respectively. Immunoreactivity for renal markers in ELST is an important diagnostic caveat and has not been previously reported. In fact, renal markers are currently recommended in order to rule out metastatic RCC although PAX gene complex and CA-9 have been implicated in the development of the inner ear. Importantly copy number assessment of ELST has not been previously reported. Loss of 3p (including the *VHL* locus) in ELST suggests similar mechanistic origins as ccRCC.

Keywords: Endolymphatic sac tumor, Renal cell carcinoma, VHL, PAX-8, PAX-2, CA-9, Copy number profiles

* Correspondence: adriana_olar@yahoo.com; olar@musc.edu
Preliminary results of this work have been presented at the 2018 USCAP annual meeting, Vancouver, BC, Canada.
[1]Department of Pathology and Laboratory Medicine, Medical University of South Carolina, 171 Ashley Ave, Charleston 29425, SC, USA
[2]Department of Neurosurgery, Medical University of South Carolina, 171 Ashley Ave, Charleston 29425, SC, USA
Full list of author information is available at the end of the article

Introduction

Von-Hippel Lindau (VHL) is an autosomal dominant hereditary cancer predisposition syndrome characterized by abberations in the *VHL* tumor supressor gene at chromosome location 3p25.3. Patients with VHL are at increased risk of developing a variety of neoplasasms such as central nervous system (CNS) hemangioblastomas, clear cell renal cell carcinomas (ccRCC), pheochromocytomas and extra-adrenal paragangliomas, pancreatic neuroendocrine tumors and adenomas, and endolymphatic sac tumors (ELST) of the inner ear [7, 32].

ELST are very rare tumors of neuroectodermal origin, thought to arise from the rugose, intraosseous portion of the endolymphatic sac. The endolymphatic sac represents an extension of the membranous labyrinth that follows the endolymphatic duct. It has both intraosseous and extraosseous components and ends in a blind pouch in the dura mater lining the posterior surface of the temporal bone. Histologically, the endolymphatic sac is composed of a single layer of flat to cuboidal to low and tall columnar cells resting on a basement membrane with folds and papillae formation in the inferomedial aspect of the intraosseous portion [1, 3, 18]. ELSTs more commonly arise sporadically, but also may arise in association with VHL, with a prevalence of up to approximately 16%. ELST typically occur around the 3rd to 5th decade and present with sensorineural hearing loss, tinnitus, and cranial nerve palsies on the affected side [2, 7]. Radiographically on computed tomography (CT), the tumors are characterized by heterogenous bone destruction centered on the posterior portion of the temporal bone. On magnetic resonance imaging (MRI), ELST demostrate T1 post-contrast enhancement and bright T2 signal [3, 7]. Grossly, tumors are described as blue to red in color and hypervascular [7, 37]. The histologic appearance of ELST ranges from a follicular growth pattern with colloid-filled cystic spaces to a papillary arrangement with solid and hypercellular areas, and occasionally an epithelioid clear cell pattern. The neoplastic cells are arranged in a single cuboidal layer with uniform nuclei and minimal pleomorphism, mitotic activity, or necrosis. Tumors are cytokeratin positive and immunoexpress epithelial membrane antigen (EMA), vimentin, neuron specific enolase (NSE), glialfibrillary acidic protein (GFAP), and variable S100, vascular endothelial growth factor (VEGF), and synaptophysin [14, 39].

The radiographic and histologic appearance of ELST raises a broad differential diagnosis and one must be aware of other more common conditions that may mimic such in order to avoid diagnostic pitfalls [18]. In fact, ELSTs are often not diagnosed until after the initial interpretation is questioned clinically [3]. Entities to consider in the work-up of suspected ELST include choroid plexus tumors, paragaganglioma, and metastatic papillary thyroid carcinoma, tumors which would be expected to immunoexpress transthyretin, chromogranin/synapthophysin, and TTF-1/thyroglobulin, respectively [7, 39]. Of particular importance to rule out are other VHL-associated neoplasms such as metastatic ccRCC. Immunohistochemistry for paired box (PAX) transcription factors PAX-8 and PAX-2, carbonic anhydrase 9 (CA-9), RCC, and CD10 has been suggested for this purpose and are reportedly negative in ELST [7, 25, 32, 39].

In this paper we characterize a cohort of ELST and demostrate immunoreactivity for renal cell markers as well as molecular evidence of predominant 3p and 9q loss which has not been previously described. Loss of 3p (including the *VHL* locus) in ELST suggests similar mechanistic origins as ccRCC. These findings are important, both to correct the previous assumption that renal cell immunohistochemical markers should not be expressed by ELST, which is important for diagnosis, and also to further characterize this rare neoplasm in order to better understand its pathogenesis.

Materials and Methods

Cases of ELST were identified via search of the laboratory information system and details regarding patient demographics, presentation, and imaging were collected through electronic medical record review with the approval of the institutional review board from all institutions. Hematoxylin and eosin (H&E) stained slides were reviewed and the diagnosis confirmed. The best tumor block was selected for DNA extraction. All immunohistochemical and molecular testing was performed on formalin-fixed, paraffin embedded (FFPE) tissues except in one case where only fresh frozen tumor tissue was available.

Immunohistochemistry

Antibodies were validated according to protocol with appropriate tissue controls. Four μm sections were prepared for immunohistochemical evaluation with the following antibodies (clone, dilution, antigen retrieval, supplier): CK7 (OV-TL 12/30, 1:500, citrate, Cell Marque, Rocklin, California, USA), CK20 (Ks20.8, 1:500, EDTA, Cell Marque, Rocklin, CA, USA), PAX-8 (MRQ-50, 1:3000, EDTA, Cell Marque, Rocklin, CA, USA), RCC (PN-15, 1:500, protease, Cell Marque, Rocklin, CA, USA), CD10 (56C6, 1:1000, EDTA, Cell Marque, Rocklin, CA, USA), CA-9 (MRQ-54, 1:2000, EDTA, Cell Marque, Rocklin, CA, USA), GFAP (EP672Y, 1:200, EDTA, Cell Marque, Rocklin, CA, USA), thyroglobulin (2H11+6E1, 1:5000, EDTA, Cell Marque, Rocklin, CA, USA), S100 (4C4.9, 1:4000, EDTA, Cell Marque, Rocklin, CA, USA), chromogranin A (LK2H10, 1:6000, citrate, Cell Marque, Rocklin, CA, USA), synaptophysin (MRQ-40, 1:5000, citrate, Cell Marque, Rocklin, CA, USA), PAX-2 (EP235, 1:1000, citrate, Cell

Marque, Rocklin, CA, USA), transthyretin (rabbit poly-clonal, 1:15000, citrate, Boster Biological Technology, Pleasanton, CA, USA), TTF-1 (EP229, 1:500, EDTA, Cell Marque, Rocklin, CA, USA), and Ki-67 (SP6, 1:500, EDTA, Cell Marque, Rocklin, CA, USA). Visualization was performed using the HiDef Detection™ HRP Polymer System (Cell Marque, Rocklin, CA, USA) with diamino-benzidine substrate (Cell Marque, Rocklin, CA, USA) and with hematoxylin counterstain in order to visualize the antibody-antigen complex and background tissue, respectively.

Single nucleotide polymorphism (SNP)-microarray
Genomic DNA extraction for SNP-microarray analysis was performed using the Maxwell® CSC DNA FFPE Kit (Promega, Madison, WI, USA) as detailed by the manu-facturer. Microarray-based chromosome analysis of copy number and genotype data was performed according to the manufacturer's protocol using the IScan System with the Infinium CytoSNP-850 K v1.1 BeadChip (Illumina, Inc., San Diego, CA, USA) and analyzed using Geno-meStudio (Illumina, Inc), and Nexus, version 9.0 (Bio-Discovery, Inc., El Segundo, CA, USA) software. The signal intensity was determined using the $\log_2$ ratio and was used along with the specific allele (B-allele) fre-quency to evaluate copy number patterns of aberrations (clonal changes in less than 100% of cells including deletion, duplication, loss of heterozygosity, ploidy) and genotype, and assessed visually using the KaryoStudio and Nexus files, by comparing with standard curve data charts generated by computer modeling of mosaicism (SiDCoN [simulated DNA copy number]) [26]. Non-mosaic aberrations (those found in 100% of cells) were not included in data analysis as they were consid-ered to represent constitutional changes.

Statistical methods and bioinformatics
Descriptive statistics were performed in Microsoft® Excel® 2013 (15.0.4971.1000), 64-bit. Gene mapping and visualization was performed using the hg19 assembly, UCSC Genome Browser tool suite [17, 19]. Pathway analysis and protein interactions was performed using Ingenuity Pathway Analysis (IPA) v. 01–07 (Qiagen Inc., https://www.qiagenbioinformatics.com/products/ingenuity-pathway-analysis/) [20].

Results
Clinical data
Nineteen ESLT from 10 males and 9 females were ana-lyzed. The median age at diagnosis was 45.1 years (mean: 42.8, range: 14.7–63.3). One patient had known VHL dis-ease confirmed by sequencing (VHL exon 2 heterozygous deletion identified) with multiple small nodular cerebellar lesions on imaging suggestive of hemangioblastomas

(biopsy not performed). None of the patients had clinical history of RCC. Abdominal imaging when available (9/19) showed no evidence of a renal mass. Patients presented with symptoms including hearing loss, balance difficulties, and unilateral facial paralysis.

Imaging
On CT, all patients showed unilateral expansile bone-destructive lesions involving the posterior petrous segment of the temporal bones. Tumors reached up to 6.4 cm in largest dimension (Case 10). Larger lesions were complex in nature with combined solid and cystic patterns (Fig. 1, Case 10 and 17) and mass effect in the posterior cranial fossa (Case 17). On MRI the lesions showed het-erogeneous T1 and T2 signal and post-contrast enhance-ment on T1-weighted sequences (Fig. 1, Cases 1, 4, 10, 17). Some tumors demonstrated regions of intrinsic T1 hyperintensity, which has been described and is thought to correlate with internal hemorrhage or proteinaceous material (Fig. 1Ab, Db, Hb) [6, 23].

Gross features
Tumors were tan-pink to red in color and many were described intraoperatively as "vascular" appearing. Some were pulsating intraoperatively, and were initially thought to represent glomus jugulare tumors.

Microscopy
The histopathological appearance of ELST displayed characteristic papillary architecture with a single-cell epithelial lining and central fibrovascular cores. The sur-face epithelial cells were cuboidal to cylindrical, bland in appearance, with vacuolated to clear cytoplasm and round to elongated nuclei. Several cases showed cystic growth with glandular spaces filled with an eosinophilic colloid-like material (Fig. 2). Immunohistochemically, the neoplastic cells showed diffuse expression of CK7 (18/18, 100%), CA-9 (19/19, 100%), focal to regional GFAP (15/18, 83.33%), PAX-8 (18/18, 100%), PAX-2 (15/18, 83.33%), and S100 (15/18, 83.33%). The tumor cells were negative for CK20, synaptophysin, chromogranin A, transthyretin, TTF-1, RCC, thyroglobulin, and CD10. Ki-67 (MIB-1) showed a < 10% proliferative index for all cases (1000 tumor nuclei counted) (median: 1.1, mean: 1.97, range: 0–9.4) (Figs. 2 and 3).

Copy number alterations
Of 12 cases tested by SNP-microarray, 8 demonstrated loss of 3p of which 7 also showed loss of 9q. A detailed summary of the chromosomal regions involved in pre-sented in Figs. 3, 4 and Table 1. Four cases had no ab-normalities detected on SNP-microarray.

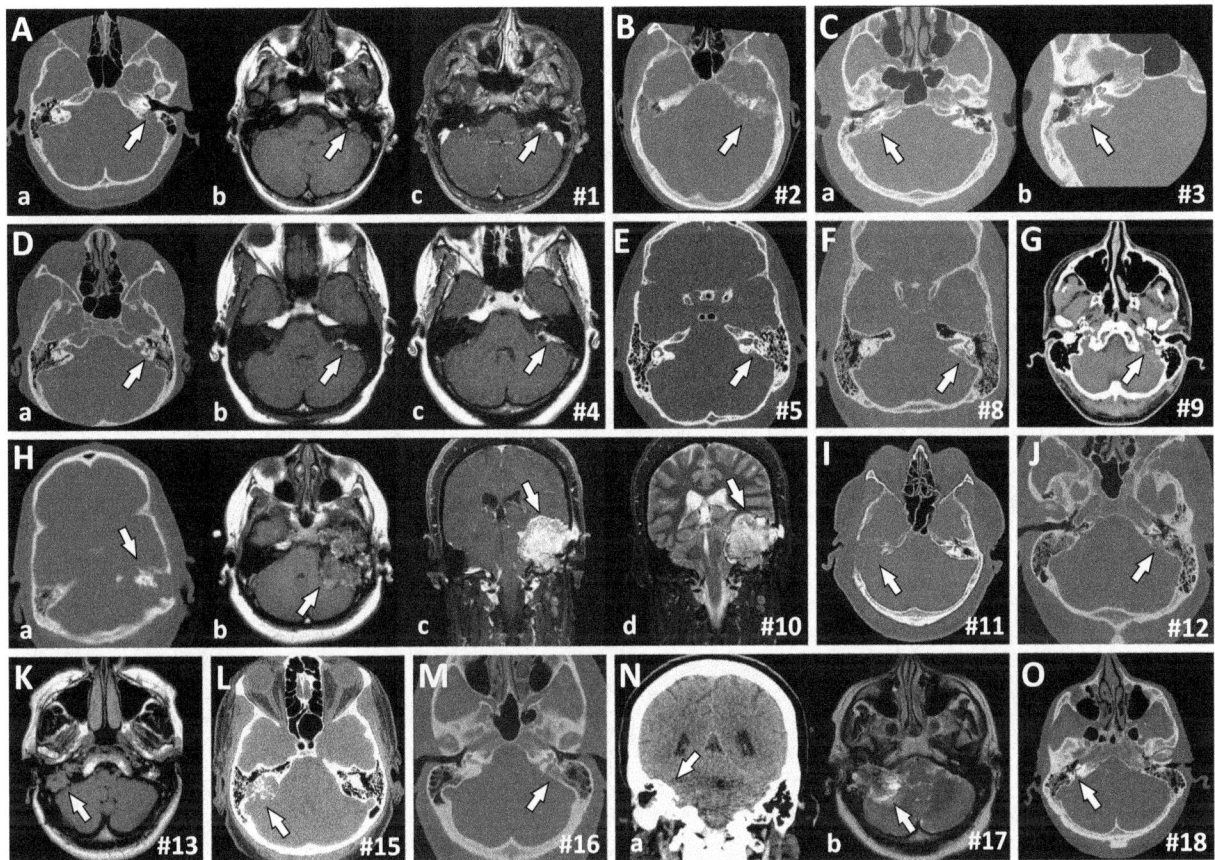

Fig. 1 Imaging Findings: Computed tomography shows bone destructive lesions involving the posterior aspect of the petrous temporal bones (**Aa, B, C, Da, E-G, Ha, I, J, L, M, Na, O**). Magnetic resonance imaging shows expansile complex partially solid and cystic masses centered on the petrous segment of the temporal bones demonstrating heterogeneous intrinsic T1 (**Ab, Db, Hb**) and T2 signal (**Hd, Nb**) and post-contrast enhancement (**Ac, Dc, Hc**). (# represents case number). Note: All images are pre-operative except K which is an axial T1-weighted post-operative (at recurrence) image

Pathway and protein interaction analyses

Using 584 and 686 genes mapped on 3p and 9q chromosomal regions, respectively, we investigated which of the encoded proteins potentially interact with PAX-2, PAX-8, CA-9, HIF-1, and GFAP. Relevant genes on chromosome 3p were: *CTNNB1, CAND2, VHL, MIFT, WNT7A, PDCD6IP, TGFBR2, PRKCD,* and *MST1.* Relevant genes on chromosome 9q were: *LMX1B, GOLGA2, HSPA5, LCN2, RAD23B, TLR4, KLF4,* and *NOTCH1.* The protein products of these genes are involved in cancer activation pathways like WNT, mTOR, HIF-1alpha, renal cell carcinoma, and p53 signaling, regulation of epithelial to mesenchymal transition, and neuroinflammation signaling (Additional file 1). Based on interactions with PAX-2, PAX-8, and CA-9 the main candidates for ELST tumorigenesis were *VHL* (on 3p), *KLF4* (on 9q), and *CTNNB1* (*beta-catenin*) (on 3p).

Treatment and follow-up

Treatment involved surgical resection of the mass in all except 2 cases (3 and 12) that underwent biopsy only

(Fig. 3). None of the patients with complete medical records (15/19) received chemotherapy. Two patients received radiation therapy. One patient (case 9) received gamma knife radiotherapy to what was considered to be an intraoperative macroscopic glomus jugulare tumor (tissue was not sent to pathology), 8 and 5 years before a histologic diagnosis of ELST was rendered. Another patient (case 11) received radiation at initial diagnosis and at recurrence. Seven patients experienced recurrence of the ELST (Fig. 3), 4 of which required additional surgery (cases 6, 7, 13, and 19), and three of which underwent radiation therapy (cases 6, 11, and 18). One of the patients who experienced tumor recurrence passed away (case 7); however, it is not known with certainty whether this was related to disease or not. One patient was lost to follow-up after his initial resection (case 15) (Fig. 3).

Discussion

In this paper we present a cohort of patients with ELSTs and show that the majority of tumors immunoexpress renal cell markers. This novel finding is an important

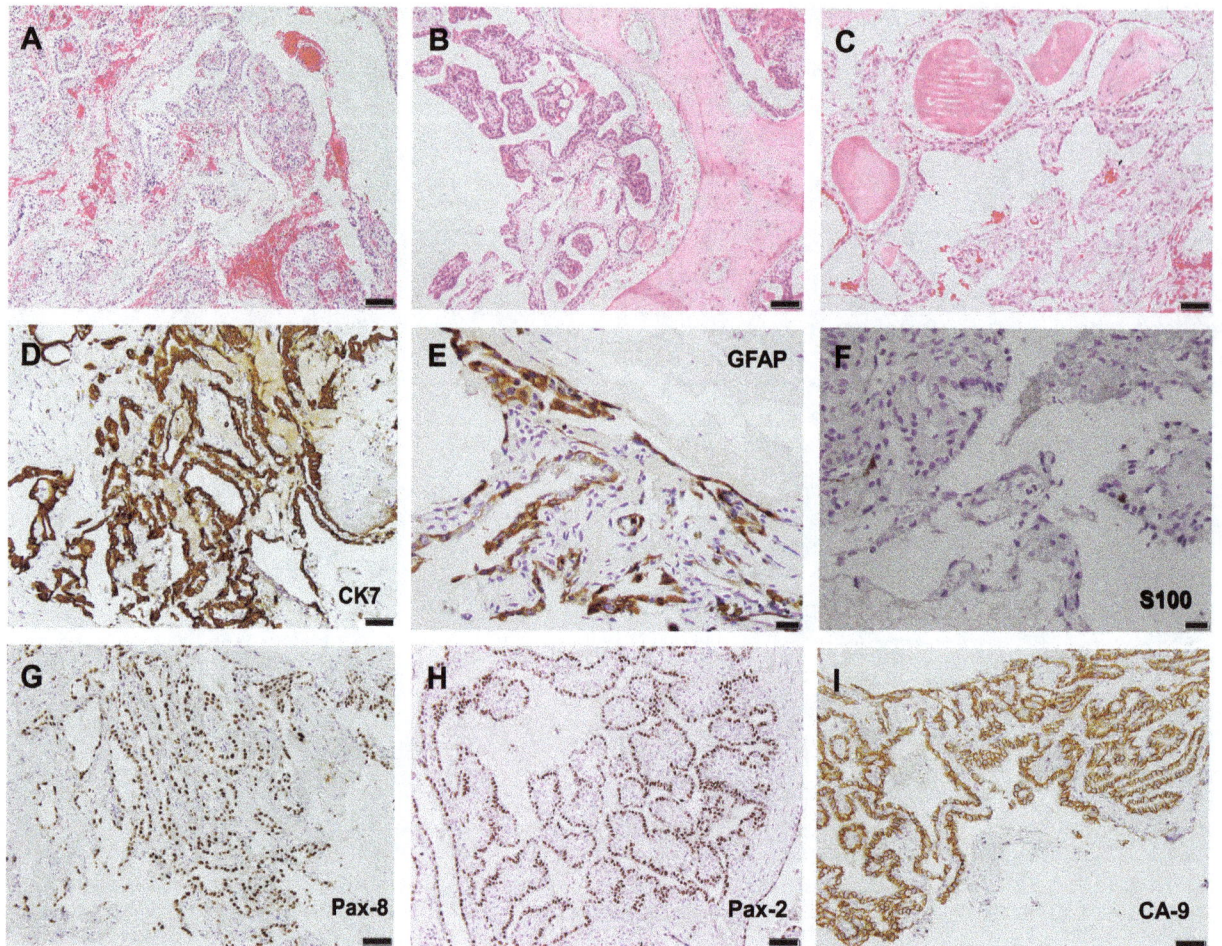

Fig. 2 Histological and immunophenotypical findings: All tumors showed the characteristic papillary architecture (**a, b, 100X**) with bone invasion (**b**) and some showed follicular morphology (**c, 200X**). All tumors immunoexpressed GFAP (**d, 400X**), CK7 (**e, 200X**), PAX-8 (**f, 200X**), PAX-2 (**g, 200X**), and CA-9 (**h, 200X**). S100 was focally immunoexpressed (**i, 400X**) in all but one case

diagnostic caveat for general surgical pathology practice and we emphasize the importance of correlating the clinical pathological and radiological findings before rendering a final diagnosis for tumors involving the posterior temporal bone. In addition, we demonstrate combined loss of 3p (including the *VHL* locus) and 9q in the majority (58%, 7/12) of the tested cases by SNP-microarray analysis. These novel molecular findings suggest similar mechanistic origins between sporadic ELST and ccRCC with *VHL* likely playing a central role.

Immunoexpression of CA-9, PAX-8, and PAX-2 prove an important diagnostic caveat when attempting to rule out metastatic RCC in the work-up of suspected ELST. While these markers are more commonly associated with RCC, there are a number of syndromes that link the kidney to the inner ear suggesting certain embryological and functional similarities between the two organ systems [12, 36]. Torban et al. investigated the parallel functions between these two organ systems and

categorized diseases affecting both the kidney and ear into groups that A) arose from mutations in shared developmental genes [e.g. Branchio-Oto-renal (BOT) syndrome, Hypoparathyroidism, Deafness, and Renal Dysplasia (HDR) syndrome, Townes-Brocks syndrome (TBS), Kallmann syndrome], B) involved defective ciliary function (e.g. Bardet-Biedl syndrome–associated hearing loss, Alstrom syndrome, nephronophthisis-associated inner ear dysfunction) and C) were due to disruption of specialized transport or structural proteins [e.g. Distal Renal Tubular Acidosis with Deafness (dRTA), Alport syndrome, Bartter syndrome with deafness] [36].

Paired box genes encode a family of transcription factors with roles in organogenesis [12]. PAX-8 activation is tightly linked to PAX-2 (Additional file 1) and these proteins are essential for proper ear [4] and kidney development [27]. In particular, *PAX-2* has been shown to play a role in the induction of inner ear development and commitment of progenitor cells to the formation of the otic

SUMMARY OF CLINICAL, EXPRESSION, AND COPY NUMBER DATA

	Case #	1	2	3	4	5	6	7	8	9	10	11	12	13	14	15	16	17	18	19
Clinical data	Sex																			
	Age (yr.)	14	21	30	31	35	38	39	41	45	49	49	50	50	51	51	52	55	57	63
	VHL syndrome?																			
	Specimen type																			
	Recurrence? (Y/N)																			
	Time to recurrence (mo.)			10.4			75	20.8				155		159					31.8	159
	Patient alive? (Y/N)																			
Immunohistochemistry	CK7																			
	GFAP	FR	F	R	R	FR	F	*	FR	R	R	F	FR			R	F	F	*	
	S100	F	F	F	F			*	F	F	F	F	F	F		F	F	F	*	
	Pax-8		FR				FR	R	F*	F			F	FR						R
	Pax-2		FR		F	F	FR	*					R	FR		R		R	R	
	CA-9																			
	CK20																			
	RCC																			
	CD10																			
	TTF-1																			
	Thyroglobulin																			
	Chromogranin A																			
	Synaptophysin																			
	Transthyretin																			
	Ki-67 (MIB-1) (%)	9.4	0.6	1.6	1.2	1	1	0	0.3	1.3	5	0.5	0.4	2		0.2	0.4	6	3.8	1.4
SNP-array	1p																			
	2																			
	3p																			
	4q																			
	8																			
	9q																			
	14q																			
	15q																			
	16																			
	17q																			
	19																			

Legend

- Yes
- Negative/No
- Not available/applicable
- Male
- Female
- Resection
- Biopsy
- Immunoexpressed
  F-focally
  R-regionally
  *small tissue
- Gain
- Loss

Fig. 3 Overview of the clinical, immunohistochemical, and molecular results. Abbreviations: mo.-months; N-no; Y-yes; yr.-years

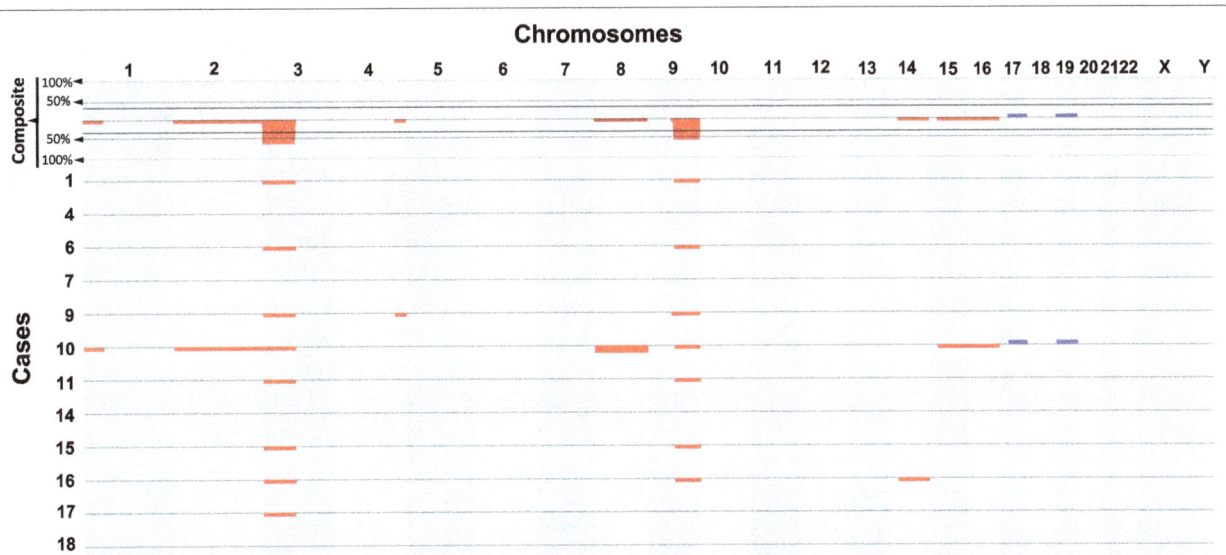

Fig. 4 Overview of the SNP-microarray findings: Loss of 3p in 8/12 cases and loss of 9q in 7/12 cases, copy number changes present in clear cell renal cell carcinoma. Legend: chromosomal gains are depicted in blue, losses are depicted in red

Table 1 SNP-microarray results

Case #	Summary	ISCN 2016
1	-3p, −9q	arr[GRCh37] 3p26.3p11.1(1_90450511)×1[0.3],9q21.11q34.3(70715485_141213431)×1[0.3]
4		arr(1−22,X)×2 normal female
6	-3p, −9q	arr[GRCh37] 3p26.3q11.1(1_91025539)×1[0.2],9q21.11q34.3(70726185_141213431)×1[0.2]
7		arr(1−22)×2,(X,Y)× 1 normal male
9	-3p, −4q, −9q	arr[GRCh37] 3p26.3p11.1(1_89605910)×1[0.1],4q32.1q35.2(160067846_191154276)×1[0.1], 9q12q34.3(63455393_141011985)×1[0.1]
10	-1p, −2, −3p, −4q, −8, −9q, −14q, −15q, −16, −17q, − 19	arr[GRCh37] 1p36.33p32.2(1_56794840)×1[0.2],2p25.3-q37.3(1_243199373)×1[0.2],3p26.3p11.1(1_91000000)×1[0.5], 8p23.3-q24.3(1_146364022)×0[0.2],9q21.11q34.3(70965125_141213431)×1[0.5],15q11.2-q26.3(22437778_102531392) ×1[0.2],16p13.3-q24.3(1_90354753)×1[0.2],17q11.1-q25.3(25295032_81195210)×3[0.2],19p13.3-q13.43(0_59128983)×3[0.2]
11	-3p, −9q	arr[GRCh37] 3p26.3p11.1(1_89317847)×1[0.5],9q21.11q34.3(69901656_141213431)×1[0.5]
14		arr(1−22)×2,(X,Y)×1 normal male
15	-3p, −9q	arr[GRCh37] 3p26.3p11.1(1_89189701)×1[0.2],9q21.11q34.3(70251958_141213431)×1[0.2]
16	-3p, −9q, −14q	arr[GRCh37] 3p26.3p11.1(1_90311584)×1[0.2],9q21.11q34.3(70618596_141213431)×1[0.2], 14q11.2q32.33(19754766_107349540)×1[0.2]
17	-3p	arr[GRCh37] 3p26.3p11.1(1_88135518)×1[0.15]
18		arr(1−22)×2,(X,Y)×1 normal male

Abbreviations: *ISCN* the International System for Human Cytogenomic Nomenclature

placode, the earliest structure identified in the morphogenesis of the inner ear, calling into question its anecdotic specificity for the kidney in the surgical pathology community [9]. PAX-2 is highly expressed in proliferating areas of the early developing inner ear (otic placode and otic vesicle) and is downregulated in areas of apoptosis at later stages of development and in maturing, differentiated hair cells [21, 22]. Its important role in cochlear development has been demonstrated using knockout mice [4, 5]. PAX-8 is one of the earliest markers for the ectodermally-derived otic placode and intermediate mesoderm, having a central role in auditory and urinary system development [12, 27]. It seems that in the neoplastic cells of ELSTs PAX-2 and PAX-8 become upregulated, reproducing the proliferative stages of early development. We speculate the role of an upstream activation mechanism which possibly involves VHL-KLF4-CTNNB1 protein interactions (Additional file 1). *VHL* is a tumor suppressor with known roles in tumorigenesis [7, 32]. VHL physically interacts with Krüppel-like factor 4 (KLF4), a transcription factor with roles in tumorigenesis [8]. Human KLF4 induces increased mouse *PAX-2* and *CTNNB1* mRNA expression [31] and, importantly, KLF4 binds to CTNNB1 inhibiting WNT signaling [13, 34]. In addition, it has been shown that gain-of-function CTNNB1 mutant protein promotes increased expression of *PAX-8* mRNA in mice [28].

The enzyme carbonic anhydrase is distributed in a wide variety of organ systems, including the renal tubules and the inner ear. Within the ear, carbonic anhydrase has activity in the cochlear hair cells, supporting cells surrounding the sensory hair cells in the vestibule,

in the stria vascularis, and in the epithelial cells of the rugose portion of the endolymphatic sac. It is thought to play a role in regulating the pH and ionic balance of the endolymph [15]. CA-9 is upregulated in hypoxic conditions and has been shown to play a role in tumorigenesis by altering pH to promote tumor growth and survival in a number of tumors, notably renal cell carcinoma [24, 29]. CA-9 expression is regulated by VHL. Briefly, under normal conditions VHL binds HIF-1alpha and degrades it, preventing its binding to HIF-1beta. Mutant VHL or normal VHL under hypoxic conditions facilitates HIF-1alpha binding to HIF1-beta and HIF-1 protein complex formation which causes downstream transcription of hypoxia-inducible genes such as CA-9. CA-9 is a marker of hypoxia [16, 29, 30, 32, 33]. CA-9 immunoexpression in ELST along with 3p loss provides supporting evidence of *VHL* deficiency in the mechanism of ELST development.

Furthermore, both syndromic and sporadic ELSTs have been shown to harbor mutations in the *VHL* gene [35, 38]; however, to the best of our knowledge molecular profiling of ELST has not yet been attempted [3, 18]. Our finding of 3p loss in ELST links it to ccRCC, which is characterized by variably sized deletions in the short arm of chromosome 3, including the *VHL* tumor suppressor gene [10, 11, 29]. Loss of 9q is also frequently seen in ccRCC, where it, along with 14q deletions, denote a poorer prognosis [10]. In our cohort, only one ELST patient had combined 3p/9q/14q losses but no tumor recurrence after 1.6 years of follow-up (Case 16). While 3p deletions in ccRCC may encompass the entire chromosome arm or only a small portion around the *VHL* locus, the 8 ELST cases in our cohort harboring 3p alterations showed whole p arm losses. Moreover, the 7 cases with concurrent 9q deletions showed large partial chromosomal losses of similar size among all tested tumors. From this, we can speculate the possibility of a derivative (3;9) resulting from an unbalanced translocation as the common mechanism of chromosomal alteration in ELST.

The molecular similarities between ccRCC and ELST may make the diagnosis of ELST even more challenging and we emphasize the importance of integrating the clinical presentation with the radiological features of this tumor. Certainly, the presence of 3p loss in both tumors suggests a similar mechanistic origin of tumorigenesis between the two entities that warrants further investigation. Furthermore, ELST may benefit from therapies targeting the same molecular pathways that lead to RCC development including HIF-1 and its targets such as VEGF, CA-9, and platelet derived growth factor (PDGF) [24, 29].

While this study is limited by small sample size due to the rarity of ELST, we believe the novelty of our findings and the implications for avoiding diagnostic pitfalls lend its strength. Additionally, the opportunity to better understand the pathogenesis of such a rare neoplasm as ELST make this a unique and meaningful investigation. Other potential limitations of the study include the small amount of tissue available for testing in some cases, the age of some samples impairing the quality of DNA, and the unavailability of tissue for more extensive molecular testing in several cases.

Although ELST are uncommon tumors, generally associated with VHL disease, the majority of cases in our cohort had no history of VHL disease or other associated neoplasms. While ELST may be the initial presentation of the disease, it is more likely that these are sporadic cases of ELST. As such, our findings may be generalizable to both sporadic and syndromic ELST cases. Furthermore, loss of 3p has been seen in a number of other human cancers and our findings of 3p loss in ELST further support the presence of one or more tumor suppressor genes including *VHL* in this region of the chromosome.

Conclusion

In conclusion, our findings dispel the previously reported misconception that ESLT are negative for expression of PAX-2, PAX-8, and CA-9. Likewise, copy number profiling will not help differentiate ELST from metastatic ccRCC. Based on our panel of immunohistochemical stains, CD10 and RCC may prove more useful in discriminating between the two entities. These noteworthy findings have important implications for the diagnosis, study, and possibly treatment of ELST and further investigation into the molecular pathways involved in tumorigenesis is warranted.

Abbreviations

CA-9: Carbonic anhydrase 9; ccRCC: clear cell renal cell carcinoma; CNS: Central nervous system; CT: Computed tomography; ELST: Endolymphatic sac tumor; EMA: Epithelial membrane antigen; FFPE: Formalin-fixed paraffin embedded; GFAP: Glial fibrillary acidic protein; H&E: Hematoxylin and eosin; MRI: Magnetic resonance imaging; NSE: Neuron specific enolase; PAX: Paired box; PDGF: Platelet derived growth factor; RCC: Renal cell carcinoma; SNP: Single nucleotide polymorphism; VEGF: Vascular endothelial growth factor; VHL: Von-Hippel-Lindau

Funding

This research was funded by an intramural grant from the MUSC Department of Pathology and Laboratory Medicine to support research by residents and clinical fellows.

Authors' contributions

Study conception and design: AO. Data collection/organization: RJ, IZ, MG, SP, TT, MA, CMH, MR, DJW, RL, WM, FJR, JM, AO. Bench work and experiments: RJ, IZ, MG, JNR, RK. Data analysis: RJ, IZ, AO. Writing of manuscript: RJ, AO. Critical manuscript review: IZ, MG, JNR, RK, SP, TT, MA, CMH, MR, DJW, RL, WM, FJR, JM. All authors read and approved the final manuscript.

Competing interests

The authors declare that they have no competing interests.

Author details

[1]Department of Pathology and Laboratory Medicine, Medical University of South Carolina, 171 Ashley Ave, Charleston 29425, SC, USA. [2]Department of Neurosurgery, Medical University of South Carolina, 171 Ashley Ave, Charleston 29425, SC, USA. [3]Department of Pathology, Baylor University Medical Center, 3500 Gaston Ave, Dallas 75246, TX, USA. [4]Genomics Research Department, Saudi Humane Genome Project, King Fahad Medical City and King Abdulaziz City for Science and Technology, Riyadh, Saudi Arabia. [5]Department of Pathology and Neurosurgery, Feinberg School of Medicine, Northwestern University, 251 E. Huron St, Chicago 60611, IL, USA. [6]Department of Pathology, Loyola University Medical Center, 2160 S 1st Ave, Maywood 60153, IL, USA. [7]Department of Radiology, UT Southwestern Medical Center, 5323 Harry Hines Blvd, Dallas 75390, TX, USA. [8]Department of Pathology, Johns Hopkins Hospital, 1800 Orleans St, Baltimore 21287, MD, USA. [9]Department of Pathology, UT Southwestern Medical Center, 5323 Harry Hines Blvd, Dallas 75390, TX, USA. [10]Hollings Cancer Center, 86 Jonathan Lucas Street, Charleston 29425, SC, USA.

References

1. Bagger-Sjöbäck D, Friberg U, Rask-Anderson H (1986) The human endolymphatic sac. An ultrastructural study. Arch Otolaryngol Head Neck Surg 112:398–409. https://doi.org/10.1001/archotol.1986.03780040038008
2. Bausch B, Wellner U, Peyre M, Boedeker CC, Hes FJ, Anglani M, de Campos JM, Kanno H, Maher ER, Krauss T et al (2016) Characterization of endolymphatic sac tumors and von Hippel-Lindau disease in the international endolymphatic sac tumor registry. Head Neck 38(Suppl 1): E673–E679. https://doi.org/10.1002/hed.24067
3. Bell D, Gidley P, Levine N, Fuller GN (2011) Endolymphatic sac tumor (aggressive papillary tumor of middle ear and temporal bone): sine qua non radiology-pathology and the University of Texas MD Anderson Cancer Center experience. Ann Diagn Pathol 15:117–123. https://doi.org/10.1016/j.anndiagpath.2010.08.009
4. Bouchard M, de Caprona D, Busslinger M, Xu P, Fritzsch B (2010) Pax2 and Pax8 cooperate in mouse inner ear morphogenesis and innervation. BMC Dev Biol 10:89. https://doi.org/10.1186/1471-213x-10-89
5. Burton Q, Cole LK, Mulheisen M, Chang W, Wu DK (2004) The role of Pax2 in mouse inner ear development. Dev Biol 272:161–175. https://doi.org/10.1016/j.ydbio.2004.04.024
6. Choyke PL, Glenn GM, Walther MM, Patronas NJ, Linehan WM, Zbar B (1995) von Hippel-Lindau disease: genetic, clinical, and imaging features. Radiology 194:629–642. https://doi.org/10.1148/radiology.194.3.7862955

7. Devaney KO, Ferlito A, Rinaldo A (2003) Endolymphatic sac tumor (low-grade papillary adenocarcinoma) of the temporal bone. Acta Otolaryngol 123:1022–1026

8. Gamper AM, Qiao X, Kim J, Zhang L, DeSimone MC, Rathmell WK, Wan Y (2012) Regulation of KLF4 turnover reveals an unexpected tissue-specific role of pVHL in tumorigenesis. Mol Cell 45:233–243. https://doi.org/10.1016/j.molcel.2011.11.031

9. Groves AK, Bronner-Fraser M (2000) Competence, specification and commitment in otic placode induction. Development 127:3489–3499

10. Hagenkord JM, Gatalica Z, Jonasch E, Monzon FA (2011) Clinical genomics of renal epithelial tumors. Cancer Genet 204:285–297. https://doi.org/10.1016/j.cancergen.2011.06.001

11. Hamilton HH, McDermott A, Smith MT, Savage SJ, Wolff DJ (2015) Clinical utility of concurrent single-nucleotide polymorphism microarray on fresh tissue as a supplementary test in the diagnosis of renal epithelial neoplasms. Am J Clin Pathol 144:731–737. https://doi.org/10.1309/ajcpjt7f5vnrxxpf

12. Heller N, Brandli AW (1999) Xenopus Pax-2/5/8 orthologues: novel insights into Pax gene evolution and identification of Pax-8 as the earliest marker for otic and pronephric cell lineages. Dev Genet 24:208–219. https://doi.org/10.1002/(sici)1520-6408(1999)24:3/4<208::Aid-dvg4>3.0.Co;2-j

13. Hoffmeyer K, Raggioli A, Rudloff S, Anton R, Hierholzer A, Del Valle I, Hein K, Vogt R, Kemler R (2012) Wnt/beta-catenin signaling regulates telomerase in stem cells and cancer cells. Science 336:1549–1554. https://doi.org/10.1126/science.1218370

14. Horiguchi H, Sano T, Toi H, Kageji T, Hirokawa M, Nagahiro S (2001) Endolymphatic sac tumor associated with a von Hippel-Lindau disease patient: an immunohistochemical study. Mod Pathol 14:727–732. https://doi.org/10.1038/modpathol.3880380

15. Hsu CJ, Nomura Y (1985) Carbonic anhydrase activity in the inner ear. Acta Otolaryngol Suppl 418:1–42

16. Ivanov SV, Kuzmin I, Wei MH, Pack S, Geil L, Johnson BE, Stanbridge EJ, Lerman MI (1998) Down-regulation of transmembrane carbonic anhydrases in renal cell carcinoma cell lines by wild-type von Hippel-Lindau transgenes. Proc Natl Acad Sci U S A 95:12596–12601

17. Karolchik D, Hinrichs AS, Furey TS, Roskin KM, Sugnet CW, Haussler D, Kent WJ (2004) The UCSC table browser data retrieval tool. Nucleic Acids Res 32:D493–D496. https://doi.org/10.1093/nar/gkh103

18. Kempermann G, Neumann HP, Volk B (1998) Endolymphatic sac tumours. Histopathology 33:2–10

19. Kent WJ, Sugnet CW, Furey TS, Roskin KM, Pringle TH, Zahler AM, Haussler D (2002) The human genome browser at UCSC. Genome Res 12:996–1006. https://doi.org/10.1101/gr.229102

20. Kramer A, Green J, Pollard J Jr, Tugendreich S (2014) Causal analysis approaches in ingenuity pathway analysis. Bioinformatics 30:523–530. https://doi.org/10.1093/bioinformatics/btt703

21. Kwan KY, Shen J, Corey DP (2015) C-MYC transcriptionally amplifies SOX2 target genes to regulate self-renewal in multipotent otic progenitor cells. Stem Cell Reports 4:47–60. https://doi.org/10.1016/j.stemcr.2014.11.001

22. Li H, Liu H, Corrales CE, Mutai H, Heller S (2004) Correlation of Pax-2 expression with cell proliferation in the developing chicken inner ear. J Neurobiol 60:61–70. https://doi.org/10.1002/neu.20013

23. Lo WW, Applegate LJ, Carberry JN, Solti-Bohman LG, House JW, Brackmann DE, Waluch V, Li JC (1993) Endolymphatic sac tumors: radiologic appearance. Radiology 189:199–204. https://doi.org/10.1148/radiology.189.1.8372194

24. McDonald PC, Winum JY, Supuran CT, Dedhar S (2012) Recent developments in targeting carbonic anhydrase IX for cancer therapeutics. Oncotarget 3:84–97. https://doi.org/10.18632/oncotarget.422

25. Megerian CA, Pilch BZ, Bhan AK, McKenna MJ (1997) Differential expression of transthyretin in papillary tumors of the endolymphatic sac and choroid plexus. Laryngoscope 107:216–221

26. Nancarrow DJ, Handoko HY, Stark MS, Whiteman DC, Hayward NK (2007) SiDCoN: a tool to aid scoring of DNA copy number changes in SNP chip data. PLoS One 2:e1093. https://doi.org/10.1371/journal.pone.0001093

27. Narlis M, Grote D, Gaitan Y, Boualia SK, Bouchard M (2007) Pax2 and pax8 regulate branching morphogenesis and nephron differentiation in the developing kidney. J Am Soc Nephrol 18:1121–1129. https://doi.org/10.1681/asn.2006070739

28. Park JS, Valerius MT, McMahon AP (2007) Wnt/beta-catenin signaling regulates nephron induction during mouse kidney development. Development 134:2533–2539. https://doi.org/10.1242/dev.006155

29. Rathmell WK, Chen S (2008) VHL inactivation in renal cell carcinoma: implications for diagnosis, prognosis and treatment. Expert Rev Anticancer Ther 8:63–73. https://doi.org/10.1586/14737140.8.1.63

30. Shen T, Shi Q, Velosa C, Bai S, Thompson L, Simpson R, Wei S, Brandwein-Gensler M (2015) Sinonasal renal cell-like adenocarcinomas: robust carbonic anhydrase expression. Hum Pathol 46:1598–1606. https://doi.org/10.1016/j.humpath.2015.06.017

31. Shu J, Wu C, Wu Y, Li Z, Shao S, Zhao W, Tang X, Yang H, Shen L, Zuo X et al (2013) Induction of pluripotency in mouse somatic cells with lineage specifiers. Cell 153:963–975. https://doi.org/10.1016/j.cell.2013.05.001

32. Sommaruga SAOV (2014) Neuropathology of von Hippel Lindau disease. J Transl Med Epidemiol 2:1011

33. Stillebroer AB, Mulders PF, Boerman OC, Oyen WJ, Oosterwijk E (2010) Carbonic anhydrase IX in renal cell carcinoma: implications for prognosis, diagnosis, and therapy. Eur Urol 58:75–83. https://doi.org/10.1016/j.eururo.2010.03.015

34. Thylur RP, Senthivinayagam S, Campbell EM, Rangasamy V, Thorenoor N, Sondarva G, Mehrotra S, Mishra P, Zook E, Le PT et al (2011) Mixed lineage kinase 3 modulates beta-catenin signaling in cancer cells. J Biol Chem 286:37470–37482. https://doi.org/10.1074/jbc.M111.298943

35. Tibbs RE Jr, Bowles AP Jr, Raila FA, Fratkin JD, Hutchins JB (1997) Should endolymphatic sac tumors be considered part of the von Hippel-Lindau complex? Pathology case report. Neurosurgery 40:848–855 discussion 855

36. Torban E, Goodyer P (2009) The kidney and ear: emerging parallel functions. Annu Rev Med 60:339–353. https://doi.org/10.1146/annurev.med.60.052307.120752

37. Virk JS, Randhawa PS, Saeed SR (2013) Endolymphatic sac tumour: case report and literature review. J Laryngol Otol 127:408–410. https://doi.org/10.1017/s0022215113000327

38. Vortmeyer AO, Huang SC, Koch CA, Governale L, Dickerman RD, McKeever PE, Oldfield EH, Zhuang Z (2000) Somatic von Hippel-Lindau gene mutations detected in sporadic endolymphatic sac tumors. Cancer Res 60:5963–5965

39. Wenig BM (2016) Atlas of head and neck pathology. Philadelphia: Elsevier Inc.

5

A de novo variant in *ADGRL2* suggests a novel mechanism underlying the previously undescribed association of extreme microcephaly with severely reduced sulcation and rhombencephalosynapsis

Myriam Vezain[1†], Matthieu Lecuyer[1†], Marina Rubio[2], Valérie Dupé[3], Leslie Ratié[3], Véronique David[3], Laurent Pasquier[4], Sylvie Odent[3,4], Sophie Coutant[1], Isabelle Tournier[1], Laetitia Trestard[5], Homa Adle-Biassette[6,7], Denis Vivien[2], Thierry Frébourg[1,8], Bruno J Gonzalez[1], Annie Laquerrière[1,9†] and Pascale Saugier-Veber[1,8*†] [ID]

Abstract

Extreme microcephaly and rhombencephalosynapsis represent unusual pathological conditions, each of which occurs in isolation or in association with various other cerebral and or extracerebral anomalies. Unlike microcephaly for which several disease-causing genes have been identified with different modes of inheritance, the molecular bases of rhombencephalosynapsis remain unknown and rhombencephalosynapsis presents mainly as a sporadic condition consistent with de novo dominant variations. We report for the first time the association of extreme microcephaly with almost no sulcation and rhombencephalosynapsis in a fœtus for which comparative patient-parent exome sequencing strategy revealed a heterozygous de novo missense variant in the *ADGRL2* gene. *ADGRL2* encodes latrophilin 2, an adhesion G-protein-coupled receptor whose exogenous ligand is α-latrotoxin. Adgrl2 immunohistochemistry and in situ hybridization revealed expression in the telencephalon, mesencephalon and rhombencephalon of mouse and chicken embryos. In human brain embryos and fœtuses, Adgrl2 immunoreactivity was observed in the hemispheric and cerebellar germinal zones, the cortical plate, basal ganglia, pons and cerebellar cortex. Microfluorimetry experiments evaluating intracellular calcium release in response to α-latrotoxin binding showed significantly reduced cytosolic calcium release in the fœtus amniocytes vs amniocytes from age-matched control fœtuses and in HeLa cells transfected with mutant ADGRL2 cDNA vs wild-type construct. Embryonic lethality was also observed in constitutive *Adgrl2*[−/−] mice. In *Adgrl2*[+/−] mice, MRI studies revealed microcephaly and vermis hypoplasia. Cell adhesion and wound healing assays demonstrated that the variation increased cell adhesion properties and reduced cell motility. Furthermore, HeLa cells overexpressing mutant *ADGRL2* displayed a highly developed cytoplasmic F-actin network related to cytoskeletal dynamic modulation. *ADGRL2* is the first gene identified as being responsible for extreme microcephaly with rhombencephalosynapsis. Increased cell adhesion, reduced cell motility and cytoskeletal dynamic alterations induced by the variant therefore represent

(Continued on next page)

* Correspondence: Pascale.Saugier-Veber@chu-rouen.fr
[†]Myriam Vezain, Matthieu Lecuyer, Annie Laquerrière and Pascale Saugier-Veber contributed equally to this work.
[1]Normandie Univ, UNIROUEN, Inserm U1245, Normandy Centre for Genomic and Personalized Medicine, F 76000 Rouen, France
[8]Department of Genetics, Normandy Centre for Genomic and Personalized Medicine, Rouen University Hospital, F 76000 Rouen, France
Full list of author information is available at the end of the article

(Continued from previous page)

a new mechanism responsible for microcephaly.

Keywords: ADGRL2, LPHN2, Adhesion-GPCR, Alpha-latrotoxin, Human extreme microcephaly, Rhombencephalosynapsis,

Introduction

At the end of the 4th post-conception week (PCW), the neural tube closes and immediately undergoes drastic changes, which consist in the setting of several events regulated by multiple, often redundant, signalling pathways leading to anteroposterior and dorsoventral polarity and emergence of four curvatures that demarcate the primary cerebral vesicles—the prosencephalon, the mesencephalon, pons and myelencephalon—from the spinal cord. Concomitantly, other key events come into play to allow the proper growth, folding and differentiation of all brain structures and particularly of the cerebral cortex; these events are schematically divided into three main stages encompassing cell proliferation with expansion of the progenitor population, neuronal migration and post-migration developmental processes. The critical role of these events, which are necessary for appropriate development and function of the human six-layered cortex, is reflected by the wide range of disease phenotypes arising from their disruption, the most severe of them being polymicrogyria, lissencephaly, microcephaly and microlissencephaly.

Lissencephalies are usually single-gene disorders that affect neuronal migration during cortical development; polymicrogyria, which has been associated with genetic and environmental causes, is still often considered as secondary to abnormal post-migration development [9, 21, 22, 33]. Microlissencephaly is a rare condition characterized by severe congenital microcephaly with absent sulci and gyri with either a thinned or thickened cortical plate. Similar to polymicrogyria, microcephaly and microlissencephaly may be due to both genetic and environmental causes, the latter including infections, toxic insults (notably antiepileptic drugs, opioids or cocaine) and prenatal alcohol exposure. Genetic causes are multiple and result from abnormal neuronal proliferation or survival associated with defective neuronal migration [5, 21]. Whatever the cause, lissencephaly and microlissencephaly may be observed alone or in combination with various brainstem or cerebellar lesions.

Among the diverse cerebellar developmental abnormalities, rhombencephalosynapsis (RES) is an extremely rare malformation initially described by Obersteiner as complete or partial vermis agenesis with fusion of the cerebellar hemispheres and apposition or fusion of the deep cerebellar nuclei [55]. RES is thought to occur early during embryogenesis, between the 5th and 7th PCW,

but its pathophysiological mechanism remains a matter of debate, considered by some authors as resulting from a fusion and by others from a non-separation of cerebellar hemispheres over an absent or severely hypoplastic vermis [8, 32, 56]. RES occurs in a vast majority of cases as a sporadic condition consistent with de novo dominant variations, and to date, exceedingly rare syndromic forms have been described and comprise Gomez-Lopez-Hernandez syndrome (MIM#601853), Fanconi anaemia complementation group B (MIM#300514) and autosomal recessive (MIM#276950) or X-linked (MIM#314390) inherited condition designated VACTERL-H [19]. In sporadic forms, RES occurs in isolation or in combination with other central nervous system (CNS) and extra-CNS malformations; it has been described in association with mesencephalic lesions such as atresia forking of the aqueduct of Sylvius and fusion of the colliculi. Associated supratentorial lesions have also been reported, consisting in agenesis of the corpus callosum, atresia of the 3rd ventricle, holoprosencephaly and neural tube closure defects [56]. So far, however, the association of severe microcephaly with RES has never been reported to our knowledge.

Using comparative patient-parents exome sequencing strategy, a powerful method to detect de novo pathogenic variants involved in human Mendelian genetic diseases [52, 53], we identified the first molecular basis of this association of extreme microcephaly with severely reduced sulcation with RES in a fœtus, a deleterious variant in the *ADGRL2* gene, which encodes an adhesion G-Protein-Coupled Receptor (GPCR). Mechanistic and functional characterization of the variant provides compelling evidence that this deleterious variant causes early human developmental defects involving both supratentorial and infratentorial structures.

Materials and methods

Whole exome sequencing

The parents provided written informed consent for Whole Exome Sequencing (WES). High quality genomic DNA was extracted from the peripheral blood of the fœtus and her parents using QIAamp DNA Blood Midi Kit (Qiagen, Courtabœuf, France) and QuickGene DNA Whole Blood Kit L (Kurabo, Japan), respectively, according to the manufacturer's instructions. Approximately 3 µg was sheared with a Covaris E220 DNA Sonicator (Covaris, Inc., Woburn, MA, USA) and coding regions captured using a SureSelectXT Human All Exon V2 kit

(Agilent Technologies, Santa Clara, CA, USA) according to the manufacturer's instructions. The enriched libraries were sequenced on a Genome Analyzer IIx (GAIIx, Illumina, Inc., San Diego, CA, USA) with 76 bp paired-end reads. Image analysis and base calling were performed by Real-Time Analysis (RTA 1.10) and CASAVA software (v1.8, Illumina, Inc.). Reads were mapped to the human reference sequence (GRCh37, Hg19) with the Burrows-Wheeler Aligner (BWA v.0.6.2). Read duplicates were marked with Picard tools, local realignments around indels, base-quality-score recalibration and variant calling were performed with the Genome Analysis Toolkit (GATK 2.5). Single-nucleotide variants and small indels were identified with the GATK UnifiedGenotyper and were filtered according to the Broad Institute's best-practice guidelines (Additional file 1: Table S1). Variants were then annotated with ANNOVAR (version 2012). Filtration of unknown variations and differential exome analysis were achieved using the Exome Variation Analyzer (EVA 2.0), our in-house software [16]. To evaluate its pathogenic potential, the *ADGRL2* DNA sequence alteration was analysed in the following web-based programs: MutationTaster [60], SIFT [40] and PROVEAN [15].

Sanger sequencing analysis

The 20 *ADGRL2* exons, 100 bp exon-intron boundaries and UTRs were PCR amplified from 50 to 100 ng of genomic DNA extracted from peripheral blood (exome trio) and from fœtal tissues coming from the Department of Genetics, Rennes University Hospital. These DNA samples were first amplified using the Whole Genome Amplification GenomePlex2 kit (Sigma-Aldrich, St Louis, MO, USA). Sanger sequencing of these fragments was performed using the BigDye® Terminator v3.1 Cycle sequencing Kit (Applied Biosystems, Courtabœuf, France). Sequencing reactions were migrated on a 3100xl Genetic Analyzer (Applied Biosystems) and analysed using the Sequencing analysis software 5.2.0 (Applied Biosystems). PCR and sequencing primers are available upon request.

Adgrl2 mouse and chicken in situ hybridization

Chick (*Gallus gallus*) or mouse (C57Bl6) embryos were fixed overnight at 4 °C in 4% paraformaldehyde (PFA), rinsed and processed for whole-mount RNA in situ hybridization. Chick embryos were staged according to Hamburger and Hamilton (HH) [27]. For the hybridization step, embryos were permeabilized 5 min in proteinase K solution (10 μg/ml), then fixed for 20 min in 4% PFA/0,2% Glutaraldehyde. After several washes in PBT, the embryos were incubated in a prehybridization solution (50% formamide, 5× SSC pH 4.5, 2% SDS, 2% blocking reagent (Roche, Meylan, France), 250 μg/ml tRNA, 100 μg/ml Heparin) at 65 °C before the addition of 10 μg/ml of the *Adgrl2* probe, and overnight incubation at 65 °C. Probes were generated by PCR, subcloned in pCRII-TOPO® (Invitrogen, Saint Aubin, France), and used to transcribe the digoxigenin (DIG)-labelled antisense RNA probes. After incubation, embryos were washed 4 times for 30 min with a solution containing 50% formamide, 2× SSC and 1% SDS at 65 °C, then cooled down to room temperature in 1 M maleic acid buffer containing Tween 20 (MABT) and washed several times. For the antibody step, nonspecific binding was blocked by incubating 2 times for 30 min then 1 h in MABT containing a 2% blocking reagent solution and 20% normal calf serum. AP-conjugated anti-DIG antibody was added at a concentration of 1:3000 and incubated overnight at 4 °C. The embryos were washed 5 times for 1 h in MABT at room temperature, followed by 2 times for 10 min in a solution containing 100 mM NaCl, 100 mM Tris-HCL, 50 mM MgCl2 and 0.1% Tween20 at pH 9.5 (NTMT). The AP-conjugated anti-DIG antibody was detected by a mixture of NBT/BCIP in NTMT, pH 9.5. The reaction was stopped by washing in PBT once the required staining intensity was achieved.

ADGRL2 immunohistochemical studies in normal human embryos and fœtuses

A series of 3 embryos and 19 fœtuses were selected for this study (collection number DC-2015-2468, cession number AC-2015-2467). Detailed characteristics of the selected cases are presented in Additional file 2: Table S2. Gestational age was estimated according to biometric data, skeletal measurements and histological maturation of the brain and viscera. Six-μm paraffin-embedded sections from whole embryos (6–10 PCW) and from brains and gonads from fœtuses at 13 weeks of gestation (WG) to birth were mounted on coated slides (Superfrost Slides, Thermo Fisher Scientific, Illkirch, France) and dried overnight in a convection oven (37 °C). Induced epitope retrieval was performed by immersion in a citrate buffer solution pH 6 at 95 °C for 1 h. Incubations with the primary antibody ADGRL2 (diluted 1:200, Clinisciences, Nanterre, France) were carried out for 1 h at room temperature using the Benschmark Ultra system (Ventana Medical Systems, Tucson, AZ), the primary antibody being diluted in an antibody diluent reagent solution (Life technologies, Saint Aubin, France). After incubation, slides were processed by the detection kit Ultraview (Ventana Medical Systems). Peroxidase was visualized using the alkaline phosphatase detection kit (Ventana Medical Systems). Slides were rinsed in tap water, counterstained with hæmatoxylin and mounted in mounting medium. Negative controls were obtained by omission of the primary antibody or by the use of other antibodies of known reactivity.

Cell culture

Amniocytes from control and patient fœtuses were collected by amniocentesis at 19 WG in order to explore chromosomal abnormalities. HeLa and amniocytes cultures were grown as monolayer in T-75 flasks. Cells were incubated in Ham's F12 nutrient mixture (Gibco, Life Technologies, Saint-Aubin, France) containing 10% fœtal bovine serum (Gibco) and 2 mM L-Glutamin (Sigma-Aldrich) at 37 °C in an atmosphere of 5% CO_2.

Immunoblotting

Amniocytes were washed once with 1× phosphate saline buffer (PBS), trypsinized, centrifuged at 1,500 × rpm for 5 min, and solubilized in 100 µl of RIPA buffer (Thermo Fisher Scientific) with 1× Protease Inhibitor Cocktail (Sigma-Aldrich) and 1× Phosphatase Inhibitor Cocktail (Thermo Fisher Scientific) for 30 min at 4 °C. After 30 min of centrifugation at 14,000×g, 30 µg proteins were separated by denaturing sodium-dodecyl sulphate polyacrylamide gel electrophoresis (10%, SDS-PAGE) and transferred to nitrocellulose membrane (Hybond C-Extra; Amersham Biosciences, Arlington Heights, IL, USA). Blots were blocked for 1 h with 5% skimmed milk in PBS and incubated with anti-ADGRL2 polyclonal antibody (1:500, LifeSpan BioSciences, Seattle, WA, USA) or anti-GAPDH polyclonal antibody (1:1000, Abcam, Cambridge, UK) in 0.05% Tween-PBS (PBST) overnight at 4 °C under gentle agitation. Membranes were washed with PBST, and primary antibody was detected using peroxidase-labelled anti-rabbit or anti-goat antibodies (1:10,000, Jackson Immunoresearch Laboratories, West Grove, PA, USA). Signals were detected with chemiluminescence reagents (Pierce Biotechnology, Rockford, IL, USA) and acquired with a G:BOX (Syngene, Cambridge, UK), monitored by the Gene Snap software (Syngene). The signal intensity in each lane was quantified using the Genetools software (Syngene), and the ratio of ADGRL2 signal vs GAPDH was calculated. All immunoblotting experiments were carried out in triplicate.

Plasmids and cell transfection

The *Adgrl2* variation was introduced using Quick Change XL Site-Directed Mutagenesis Kit (Agilent Technologies), into previously published pcDCIRL-2 or pcDCIRL-2-GFP expression plasmids containing the full length rat Adgrl2 cDNA [31]. Owing to the fact that rat wild-type Adgrl2 protein contains a phenylalanine (TTC) instead of the leucine (CTC) at position 1262 in humans (same hydrophobic class, Grantham distance 22), we performed a double mutagenesis to introduce the mutant-related histidine (CAC) at position 1262. Wild-type and mutant pcDCIRL-2 expression plasmids (2 µg) were transiently transfected into HeLa cells, using fuGENE 6 transfection reagent (Promega, Madison, WI,

USA) according to the manufacturer's protocol. Cells were plated at 5×10^5 cells/well in 6-well plates in Ham's F12 medium, and transfections were incubated for 48–72 h to allow Adgrl2 addressing to the plasma membrane. All transfection experiments were carried out in triplicate.

Microfluorimetry and intracellular calcium measurements

For measurement of whole cell intracellular calcium levels, amniocytes or HeLa cells were grown in 6 well plates on glass coverslips (diameter 30 mm) coated with poly-L-lysine (Sigma-Aldrich). Cultured cells were rinsed in PBS and incubated in Ham's F12 culture medium containing 10 µM of the calcium probe Fura-2 AM, 0.3% pluronic F-127 (Molecular Probes, Life Technologies, Cergy-Pontoise, France) and 50 µM MK-571 sodium salt hydrate (Sigma Aldrich) for 30 min at 37 °C in the dark. After the loading step, cells were washed twice for 5 min in culture medium, and the coverslips supporting the cells were placed under an inverted fluorescence Leica DM 6000B microscope equipped with a rapid shutter wheel (Rueil-Malmaison, France) and continuously infused with Ham's F12-EDTA solution. The fluorescent signals associated with calcium-free and calcium-bound Fura-2 were acquired by alternately exciting the cells at 340 and 380 nm. The emitted fluorescence was collected at 510 nm and a ratio of both signals was calculated using the Metamorph software (Roper Scientific, Evry, France). Total recording time was 15 min, and the time interval between two acquisitions was 5 s. After 3 min baseline recording, α-latrotoxin (1 nM, Alomone Labs, Jerusalem, Israel) was added in the calcium-free perfusion medium. To allow dimer formation, α-latrotoxin was prepared in Ham's F12 calcium free medium 30 min before use. After a 3-min period under drug stimulation, the perfusion medium was replaced by Ham's F12 containing 1.2 mM calcium. The exogenous ligand α-latrotoxin induces intracellular Ca^{2+} (Ca^{2+}_i) elevation by two mechanisms that are not mutually exclusive, i.e., activation of phospholipase C (PLC) through specific ADGRL receptor activation [4, 42] and the ionophoric properties of α-latrotoxin [3, 30]. Culture media complemented with 4 nM EDTA were used to induce extracellular Ca^{2+} chelation and target intracellular calcium flux resulting from ADGRL receptor activation [71]. When required, cells were incubated during the loading step with 10 µM of the phospholipase C inhibitor U73122 (Sigma Aldrich) [10]. Data were then exported to the biostatistics Prism software (GraphPad Inc., San Diego, CA) and areas under the curve were quantified. For statistical analyses, experiments were performed three times on at least 20 cells per condition.

Cell cycle analyses in human fœtal ganglionic eminences

Since the germinal zone of the dorsal telencephalon disappears by 24WG, proliferative stem cells were evaluated on lateral ganglionic eminences (LGE), which are known to massively produce interneurons at this stage [50]. LGE were micro-dissected from the paraffin-embedded section passing through the diencephalon from the fœtus, from an age-matched control brain aged 26WG as well as from a fœtus interrupted for microcephaly due to homozygous pathogenic variant in the *MCPH1* gene, NM_024596.3:c.427dup;p.(Thr143Asnfs*5). *MCPH1* variations are responsible for delayed mitosis of cycling progenitors in the germinal zones, and in microlissencephaly brain lesions may also include extreme hypoplasia of the cerebellum and brainstem. The sections were treated using the technique described by Hedley et al. with minor modifications [29]. Briefly, 35-µm sections were dewaxed in xylene and rehydrated in decreasing concentrations of ethanol. Enzymatic digestion was carried out in a 0.5% pepsin PBS solution. The nuclear suspension, adjusted at a final concentration of 10^6 nuclei/ml were incubated in a 1 mg/ml ribonuclease solution for 30 min at 37 °C and stained with propidium iodide (6 µg/ml in a 40 µM trisodium citrate solution) for 1 h at 4 °C. Flow cytometric analyses of the cell cycle were performed on an XL Beckman Coulter flow cytometer (Coultronics, Hialeah, Florida, USA) with the 488-nm wavelength of an ion argon laser as an excitation source. The cytofluorograph was adjusted to maximal resolution with flow check microspheres (Coultronics) having a coefficient of variation lower than 1.5%. For each sample, 10^4 to 10^5 cells were analysed, and the proliferative index (PI) was estimated using the Multicycle software (Coultronics), calculated as the percentage of cells in phases S + G2/M.

Cytometric analyses of Adgrl2 transfected HeLa cells

HeLa cells were transfected with an empty vector or with plasmids encoding the wild-type or the mutant Adgrl2 cDNA. After a 3-day culture, cells were gently detached from their support using 1 mM EDTA in PBS and processed for cell cycle analysis according to the three steps method of Vindeløv [70]. Single cell suspensions were obtained after incubation in a 3% trypsin PBS buffer solution. Cell suspensions were filtered through a 48-µm pore nylon gauze. Cell count was adjusted to obtain a final concentration of at least 10^4 cells. The suspensions were mixed with chicken red blood cells (CRBC) used as internal standard, as described by Vindeløv et al. [70]. The concentration was adjusted to obtain a final ratio of CRBC to cultured cells of 1/10. An aliquot of 300 µL of these nuclear suspension samples was centrifuged at 500 g, then resuspended in 500 µl of a staining solution including RNase, propidium iodide and non-ionic detergent Nonidet P40 for 10 min at 4 °C.

Evaluation of the cell cycle was performed as described above. For evaluation of cell size and content, 5000 to 6000 cells were incubated in a PBS solution containing 0.3% saponin, 1% bovine serum albumin, 1% RNase and 0.005% propidium iodide. The size corresponding to the light emitted by the cells under exposition to the incident light of the laser (forward scatter) was arbitrarily expressed by the ratio number of cells vs fluorescence intensity on a scale of 1024 channels (AU, arbitrary units). The cellular content corresponding to the more or less heterogeneous cytoplasmic content (granulometry) was evaluated using emitted scattered light of the cell at 90° (side scatter) also expressed by the ratio number of cells vs fluorescence intensity on a scale of 1024 channels.

Confocal microscopy

To study the addressing of Adgrl2 to the plasma membrane, HeLa cells were grown in 6-well plates on glass coverslips (diameter 10 mm) coated with poly-L-lysin (Sigma-Aldrich). HeLa cells were transfected with 2 µg pcD-empty vectors or with pcD plasmids encoding Wt and mutant rat Adgrl2 (CIRL-2) constructs coupled with a GFP tag using the fuGENE 6 transfection reagent (Promega). After 72 h, glass coverslips were rinsed with PBS and cells were fixed with 4% paraformaldehyde in PBS for 15 min. After 3 gentle washes with PBS, coverslips were mounted in DAPI-containing Vectashield (Vector laboratories, Cambridgeshire, UK) and images were acquired with the Leica laser scanning confocal microscope TCS SP2 AOBS (Leica Microsystems, Wetzlar, Germany).

Cell-adhesion assays

Cell adhesion assays were performed in triplicate with HeLa cells as previously described [12]. HeLa cells were transfected with 2 µg pcDCIRL-2 Wt or pcDCIRL-2 Mt. coupled or not with a GFP tag using fuGENE 6 transfection reagent (Promega). After 72 h, the living and dead cells were respectively labelled with cell tracker green (Invitrogen) and 7-amino-actinomycin D (7-AAD, Sigma Aldrich). Cells were gently detached using 1 mM EDTA in PBS and 5.10^5 cells were resuspended in 330 µL of aggregation medium (Ham's F12 containing 10% FBS, 50 mM Hepes-NaOH, pH 7.4, 10 mM $CaCl_2$, and 10 mM $MgCl_2$) using a Countess Automated Cell Counter (Invitrogen). Cell suspensions were placed into 0.5-ml polypropylene tubes, leaving a small air bubble between the liquid and the lid and incubated under gentle agitation at 25 °C. Cell aggregation was addressed at T0 and T90 min by removing aliquots, spotting them onto culture slides (BD Falcon), and imaging the aggregates with a Leica DM 6000B microscope. Acquired images were then analysed by quantifying the number and size of aggregates using the Metamorph software (Roper Scientific). The mean aggregation index was calculated using the formula: (total aggregate area / aggregate number)$_{T90}$ − (total aggregate area / aggregate number)$_{T0}$. When required, the aggregation index of the HeLa cells was determined in the presence of 1 nM α-latrotoxin or 3 μM U73122 added in the aggregation medium.

Wound healing assay
HeLa cells transfected with 2 μg pcD-empty, pcDCIRL-2 Wt or pcDCIRL-2 Mt. plasmids were seeded in 6-well plates at a density of 5×10^5 cells per well. When cells reached confluence, a scratch was performed with a sterile tip to create an artificial wound. Tiff format images were acquired every 6 h during 72 h using an inverted microscope (Leica DM 6000B). Cell migration from the wound edge into the wound space was recorded and a time-course quantification of the scratch width was evaluated using the Metamorph software (Roper Scientific). Cell wound repair was calculated using wound width (expressed in percentage of the initial size).

Cytoskeletal network immunolabelling
HeLa cells were grown in 6-well plates on glass coverslips (10 mm diameter) coated with poly-L-lysin (Sigma-Aldrich). Cells were transfected with 2 μg pcD-empty or pcD plasmids encoding Wt or Mt. rat Adgrl2 (CIRL-2) using fuGENE 6 transfection reagent (Promega). After 72 h, glass coverslips were rinsed with PBS and fixed 15 min with 4% paraformaldehyde in PBS. HeLa cells were incubated overnight at 4 °C with an anti-acetylated α-tubulin monoclonal antibody (T-9026; Sigma-Aldrich) and Texas Red®-X Phalloidin (Molecular Probes) in the incubation buffer (PBS containing 1% bovine serum albumin (BSA) and 3% Triton X-100). Cells were rinsed twice with PBS for 20 min and incubated with the same incubation buffer containing the appropriate secondary antibody. Nuclei were visualized by incubating the cells for 5 min with a PBS solution containing 1 μg/mL Hœchst 33258. Fluorescent signals were observed with a Leica DMI 6000B microscope. The specificity of α-tubulin immunolabelling was controlled by omitting the primary antibody.

Mouse *Adgrl2* inactivation
$Adgrl2^{+/-}$ mice were purchased from INFRAFRONTIER (Neuherberg, Germany). *Adgrl2* was inactivated by insertion of a LacZ-neo cassette in the DNA sequence (strain B6;129P2-Adgrl2^{tm1Dgen}/H, Mary Lyon Centre, MRC Harwell, Oxfordshire, UK). Mice were maintained at the animal facility of the Rouen Medical University. All rodent work was performed with the consent of the Animal Ethics Committee, Rouen Faculty of Medicine.

All animals were fed a standard diet and maintained in a pathogen-free environment on a 12 h light/12 h dark cycle.

For genotyping, at least 3 mm of the mouse tail was cut, genomic DNA was then extracted using the NucleoSpin® Tissue kit (Macherey-Nagel, Hœrdt, France) and quantified using a NanoVue TM spectrophotometer (GE Healthcare Life Sciences, Pittsburgh, PA, USA). To make sure that mice were accurately genotyped, three genotyping assays were developed, the first multiplex PCR being designed to simultaneously detect the wild-type and targeted allele, the second being designed to detect the targeted allele only and the third to amplify the wild-type allele only. PCR primers and conditions are available upon request.

Magnetic resonance imaging (MRI)
To evaluate long-term brain lesions, MRI analyses were carried out on female and male adult (P45) mice using a Pharmascan 7 T (Bruker, Wissenbourg, France). T2-turboRARE 3D weighted images were acquired using a multislice multiecho sequence: TE/TR 31.5 ms/1500 ms. Quantification of morphometric brain characteristics was done using ImageJ (NIH software v1.45r, National Institute of Health, Bethesda, MD, USA) previously upgraded with the Bruker plugins. Image analyses provided access to qualitative and quantitative neuroanatomical criteria including cerebrum width, cerebrum volume, lateral ventricle volume and mid-sagittal anteroposterior vermis diameter.

Statistical analyses
Statistical analyses were performed using the biostatistics Prism software (GraphPad Inc.). Tests used for each experiment, the number of independent experiments and *p*-values are detailed in Additional file 3: Table S3.

Results
Neuropathological examination reveals extreme microcephaly and RES
A 26-year-old woman, gravida II, para I, underwent routine ultrasonography at 22WG which displayed intra-uterine growth retardation, polyhydramnios, decreased fœtal movements, and microcephaly with gyral abnormalities and pontocerebellar hypoplasia. An MRI carried out at 25WG confirmed these abnormalities, and a medical termination of the pregnancy was achieved at 26WG in accordance with the French law and after approval by our local ethical committee. Array CGH using an Agilent array 105 K performed on amniotic fluid cells revealed a normal female karyotype, 46,XX. Both unrelated parents had no personal or familial medical history. General autopsy confirmed growth failure (<5th percentile) with malposition of the extremities but with no visceral anomalies [24]. Brain weight was ≪ 3rd

centile (28.5 g, normal weight = 146.21 g +/− 21.69) with an infratentorial weight and a transverse cerebellar corresponding to 13WG [23, 34]. The brain surface was agyric. Sylvian fissures were short, dimple-shaped and vertically oriented (Fig. 1a and b). Olfactory tracts and optic chiasm were present. At the level of the cerebral peduncles, the aqueduct of Sylvius was identified and the cerebellum was replaced by a single non-foliated mass corresponding to RES (Fig. 1c), the vermis being indiscernible and the cerebellar hemispheres entirely fused across the midline. On coronal sections, the corpus callosum was identified, but the hippocampi were hypoplastic (Fig. 1d). Histological examination of the spinal cord revealed hypoplasia of the corticospinal tracts. In the mesencephalon, pons and medulla, neuronal density was diminished within the cranial nerve nuclei. Olivary nuclei were poorly convoluted and hypoplastic, but with no olivary ectopias (Fig. 2a). In the cerebellum, the dentate nuclei were non-convoluted but not fused. The cerebellar cortex was rudimentary, the transient external granular cell layer being particularly thin (Fig. 2b). Neither Purkinje cell nor internal granular cell layers were clearly identified (Fig. 2c) and calbindin immunohistochemistry revealed scattered Purkinje cells irregularly distributed throughout the cerebellar cortex (Fig. 2d). In the cerebral hemispheres, neuronal density was decreased in the cortical plate, particularly in layer II but with normal cortical lamination (Fig. 2e and f). Layer I was cellular, with abnormal persistence of the transient external granular cell layer and scarce reelin-positive Cajal-Retzius cells compared to the control case. The calretinin antibody also immunolabelled

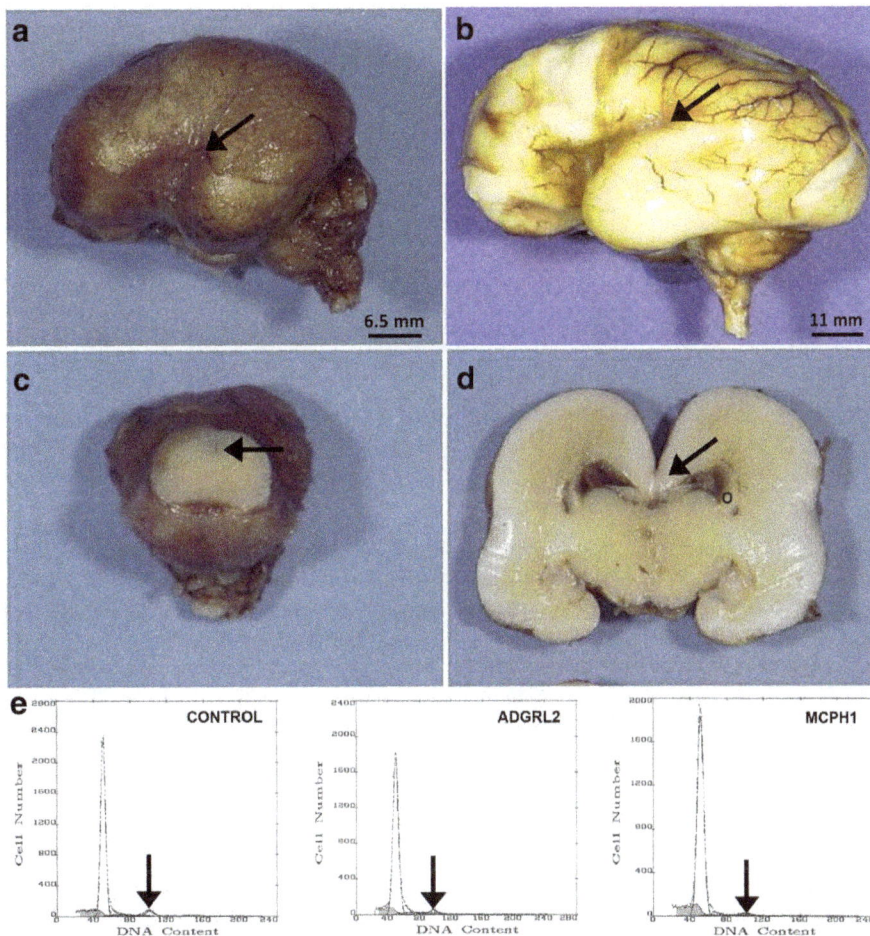

Fig. 1 Main macroscopic findings. **a** Left side of the brain showing lissencephaly with no gradient of severity, with a short Sylvian fissure reduced to a dimple (black arrow). **b** Comparison with an age-matched control brain aged 26WG, where all primary fissures are present, with a posteriorly closed Sylvian fissure (black arrow). **c** Macroscopic view of the mesencephalon, displaying a punctiform aqueduct of Sylvius (black arrow) beneath the cerebellum, which forms a single non-foliated mass corresponding to an RES. **d** On a coronal section passing through the cerebral hemispheres at the level of the hippocampi, the third ventricle is severely narrowed, the corpus callosum is present (black arrow) and the hippocampi appear hypoplastic. The circle represents the LGE. **e** Flow cytometry cell cycle profiles in the LGE at 26WG. Left: control fœtus, middle: *ADGRL2* mutated fœtus and right: *MCPH1* mutated fœtus. Arrows indicate G2/M phases

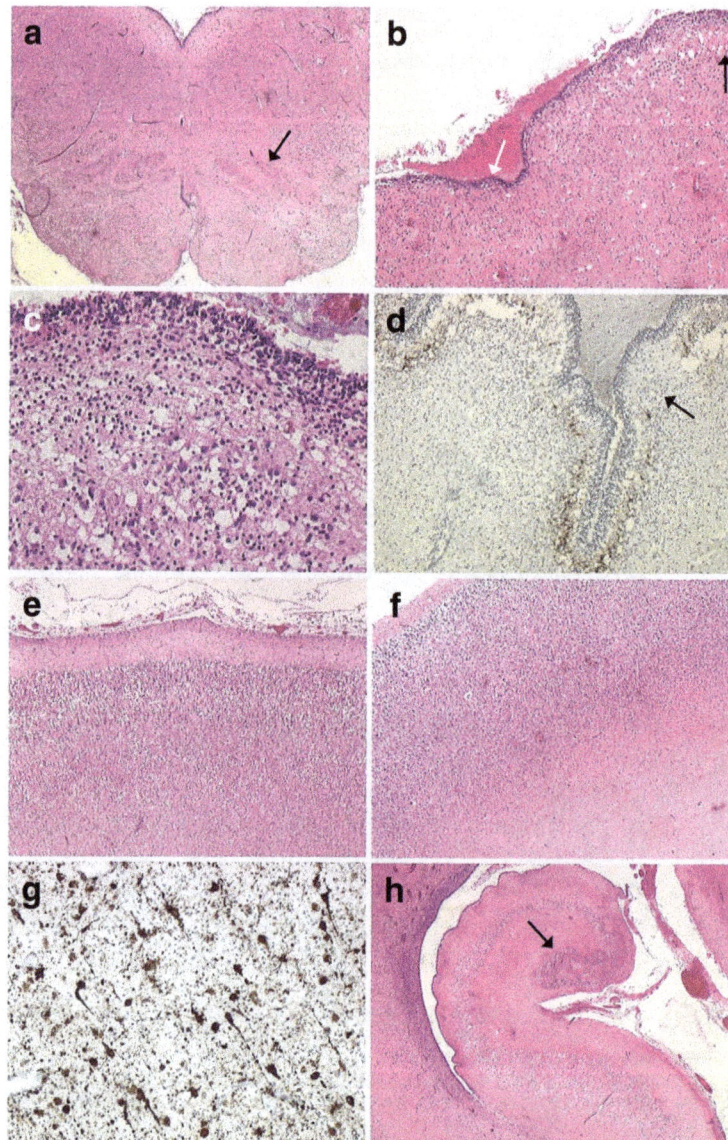

Fig. 2 Histological hallmarks of brain lesions. **a** Histological section passing through the medulla, where the olivary nuclei are poorly convoluted and hypoplastic (arrow) [H&E, OM × 15]. **b** In the most severely affected areas, the cerebellar cortex is rudimentary, with a strongly hypoplastic transient external granular cell layer (white arrow) [H&E, OM × 100]. **c** With higher magnification, almost no discernible Purkinje cell and internal granular cell layers [H&E, OM × 200]. **d** Focally missing Purkinje cells in the less affected areas (black arrow) [anti-calbindin immunolabelling, OM × 100]. **e** Thin six-layered cortical plate [H&E, OM × 25]. **f** Comparison with the control brain, where the cortical plate is thicker, with a higher density of neurons [H&E, OM × 25]. **g** Anti-MAP2 immunohistochemistry revealing numerous persistent migrating neurons in the intermediate zone [OM × 400]. **h** Hypoplastic hippocampi, the dentate gyrus being reduced to a small mass of granular neurons (arrow) [H&E, OM × 25]. H&E: haematoxylin-eosin staining. OM: original magnification

Cajal-Retzius cells, along with dispersed positive neurons distributed throughout the telencephalon. Layers IV, V and VI were made of immature neurons. Vimentin-positive radial glial fibres persisted in the intermediate zone, which contained numerous migrating MAP2-positive neurons and GFAP-positive astrocytes, with no axonal spheroids (Fig. 2g). The hippocampal uncus was also abnormal, the dentate gyrus being short and thick, but with a preserved pyramidal cell layer (Fig. 2h). No lesion was observed in the basal ganglia and thalami. Thus, histological lesions were suggestive of a defect in neural cell production along with abnormalities of radial and tangential migration. Proliferative indices (PI) evaluated by means of flow cytometry from LGE in normal control, *ADGRL2* mutated and *MCPH1* mutated fœtuses at the same term revealed that in the control brain, LGE cell PI was 9.6%, with 4.9% of cells in phase S. In the *ADGRL2* mutated patient, PI was measured at 9.1% that did not differ from the normal control, but with a slightly higher percentage of S-phase cells evaluated at 7%. Conversely, PI in the *MCPH1* mutated brain was severely decreased by a factor of 2, calculated at 5.1%, with a reduced S phase measured at 3.8% (Fig. 1e). These results clearly indicate that proliferative capacities to provide post-mitotic neuroblasts are not affected in the *ADGRL2* mutated fœtus.

Whole exome sequencing reveals a de novo variation in the *ADGRL2* gene

In the absence of clinical symptoms in the parents and because no genetic cause is known for this brain malformation association, a germline de novo variation was likely to be responsible for this very unusual neuropathological phenotype. To identify such variations, a comparative WES analysis of the fœtus and her healthy parents was performed (Fig. 3a). Parental links were verified by microsatellite analysis. Across the three exomes, an average of 5.6Gb with 97% of mappable sequences was obtained, a mean read depth of 61×, 89% of bases were covered to a minimum depth of 10 and 89% of the read bases had a Qscore above 30 (Additional file 1: Table S1). More than 65% of reads were On-target captured. On average, 17,500 exonic variants were identified per exome. First, variants with a read depth of less than 10× and a Qscore below 30 were filtered out. The resulting variants were filtered according to their null frequency in the general population from 1000 Genomes Project, Exome Aggregation Consortium (ExAC 0.3.1) and genome Aggregation Database (gnomAD r2.0.2). When the variants detected in the parents were subtracted from those encountered in the patient to identified de novo variations, only one variation remained: c.3785T>A;p.(Leu1262His) in exon 20 of the *ADGRL2* (NM_012302.4, MIM#607018). The missense

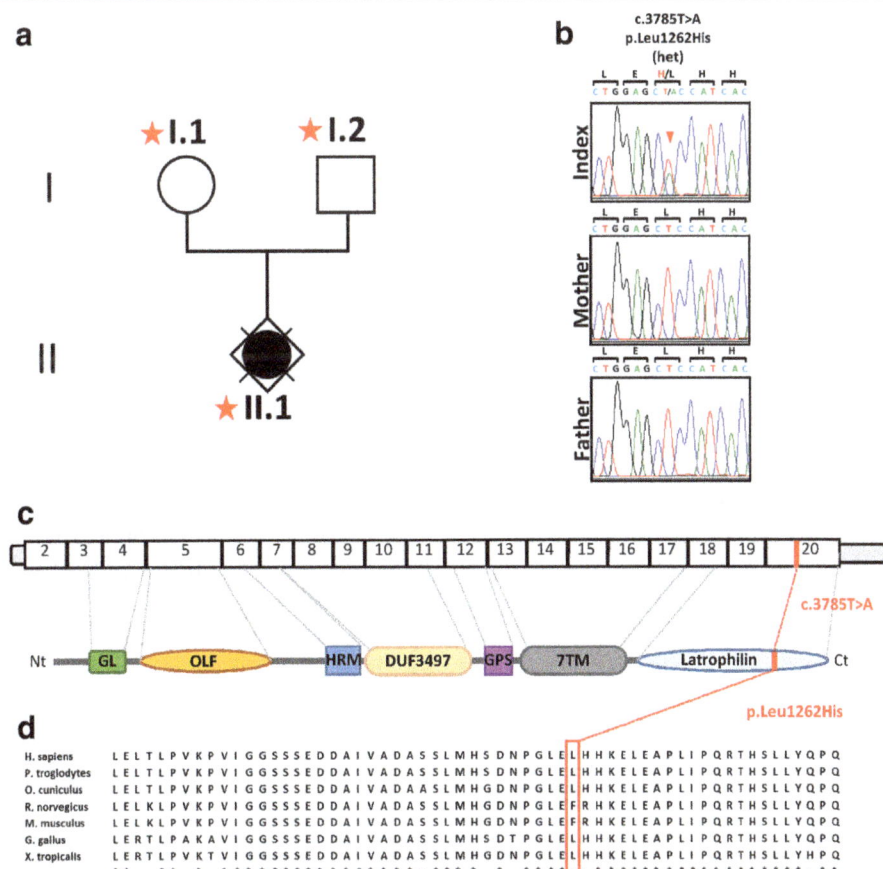

Fig. 3 Identification of a de novo heterozygous variant in *ADGRL2*. **a** Pedigree structure of the family. Red stars depict individuals subjected to WES. **b** WES identified a *ADGRL2* c.3785T>A heterozygous variant resulting in a p.(Leu1262His) amino acid substitution, confirmed de novo by Sanger sequencing of proband and parents. **c** Schematic representation of ADGRL2 mRNA and protein. ADGRL2 contains a galactose binding lectin domain (GL), an olfactomedin-like domain (OLF), a domain present in hormone receptors (HRM), a domain of unknown function (DUF), a G-protein coupled receptor proteolytic site domain (GPS), 7 transmembrane domains (TM) and a cytoplasmic latrophilin domain. The variant (red) was localized in the exon 20, the resulting amino acid substitution occurred in the latrophilin domain. **d** Phylogenic conservation of the C-terminal domain. The position of the amino acid substitution is indicated by the red rectangle. Nt: amino-terminal; Ct: carboxy-terminal

variation was predicted to be damaging by MutationTaster, SIFT, and PROVEAN, suggestive of its pathogenicity. According to the ExAC consortium, *ADGRL2* is loss-of-function intolerant (pLI = 1). No other variant was found when analysing trio data under recessive and X-linked hypotheses. This heterozygous variant was then validated by Sanger sequencing in the patient and its absence in the peripheral blood DNA of the parents indicating that the c.3785T>A variation occurred de novo (Fig. 3b). *ADGRL2* (adhesion G protein-coupled receptor L2) gene previously called *LPHN2* encodes the latrophilin 2 protein [26] and maps to chromosome 1, at 1p31.1. It belongs to the adhesion class G protein-coupled receptor (GPCR) family. The three human ADGRLs (1, 2 and 3) have previously been identified as the functional receptors of α-latrotoxin, the major neurotoxin of the black widow spider venom [64, 65, 69]. ADGRLs are evolutionary conserved across species and share similar protein architecture characterized by three major domains: a long glycosylated N-terminal extracellular domain, seven Trans Membrane Regions (TMRs), and a long cytoplasmic tail (Fig. 3c) [39, 42]. The de novo variation identified by comparative WES is located in the intracellular conserved domain (Fig. 3d).

ADGRL2 resequencing in a panel of 29 unrelated RES-affected individuals fails to detect any pathogenic variant

As RES was one of the main lesions observed in the foetus, the hypothesis that *ADGRL2* variants could be responsible for a wider phenotypic spectrum was raised. All coding exons of the *ADGRL2* gene by means of the Sanger technique were sequenced in 29 unrelated foetuses affected with RES alone or with associated mesencephalosynapsis (atresia-forking of the aqueduct of Sylvius and fusion of the colliculi), diencephalosynapsis (atresia of the 3rd ventricle with collapse of the thalami), holoprosencephaly or encephalocele [56]. No variant was detected in these 29 foetuses.

Adgrl2 is early expressed during chicken and mouse development

Aldgrl2 expression was investigated in chicken and mouse embryos just after brain segmentation has taken place (HH12-HH18 for chicken embryo and E9.5 for mouse embryo). In the HH12 chick embryo, *Adgrl2* was expressed along the neural tube with an intense expression in the telencephalic vesicles (both in the future cerebral mantle and in the germinal zones), in the mesencephalon and in the rhombencephalon. Low levels of in situ hybridization signals for *Adgrl2* were detected in the diencephalic vesicle and in the isthmic organizer region (rO), at the mesencephalon-metencephalon boundary (Fig. 4a). Significant expression was also observed along the notochord (Fig. 4a, b), with increased

expression at subsequent developmental stages. At HH18, on dissected brains, strong *Adgrl2* expression persisted in the telencephalon, mesencephalon and in the developing cerebellum, but remained weak in the diencephalon and at the level of isthmic organizer region (Fig. 4b). In the developing cerebellum, *Adgrl2* expression was observed in the rhombic lips and transient external granular cell layer.

Similar *Adgrl2* expression domains were observed in mouse embryos at E9.5. Mouse *Adgrl2* was strongly expressed in the telencephalon, mesencephalon and cerebellum, but absent in the diencephalon and at the mesencephalon-metencephalon boundary (Fig. 4c). These first expression studies of *Adgrl2* reveal that mouse and chicken *Adgrl2* display similar region-specific expression in the cephalic vesicles and that *Adgrl2* is involved in a highly conserved mechanism that is crucial during early development of the telencephalon and cerebellum.

ADGRL2 is expressed from early human development

In human embryos, at 6th, 9th and 10th PCW, strong immunoreactivity was observed in almost all organs and tissues, notably in the liver parenchyma, heart, primary bronchi, digestive epithelium, nephrogenic blastema, smooth and striated muscle cells, vascular endothelium, as well as in mesenchymal tissues, especially the cartilaginous cells of the head, neck, thorax and of the axial skeleton. ADGRL2 immunoreactivity was strong in the seminiferous cords of the testes and in the epithelium of the epididymis from the 6th PCW, and from the 10th PCW in ovary germ cells. From 14WG onward, oogonia and follicular cells were intensively immunoreactive along with the ovarian superficial epithelium. From 18WG to birth, diffuse immunolabelling persisted in the primordial follicles (oogonia and follicular cells, Additional file 4: Figure S1a, b), and in the Leydig cells of the ovarian hilum (Additional file 4: Figure S1c). In male foetuses, spermatogonia, Sertoli and Leydig cells, as well as interstitial mesenchymal testicular matrix, were strongly immunolabelled from 18WG to birth (Additional file 4: Figure S1d).

Apart from gonad immunohistochemistry, immunohistochemical analyses were restricted to brain anatomical structures from 13WG onwards. In the cerebral hemispheres, the neuroepithelium was intensively immunoreactive from the 6th PCW to 24WG, with a progressive increase in cell immunoreactivity in the subventricular zone (Fig. 5a). LGE were moderately positive from 13WG, became intensely immunolabelled until 24WG (Fig. 5b) and became negative by around 30WG, whereas ependymal cell lining was positive from 30 to 34WG. In the cortical plate, the tangential fibre network of layer I was positive as early as 6PCW, with few positive neurons in the developing cortical plate.

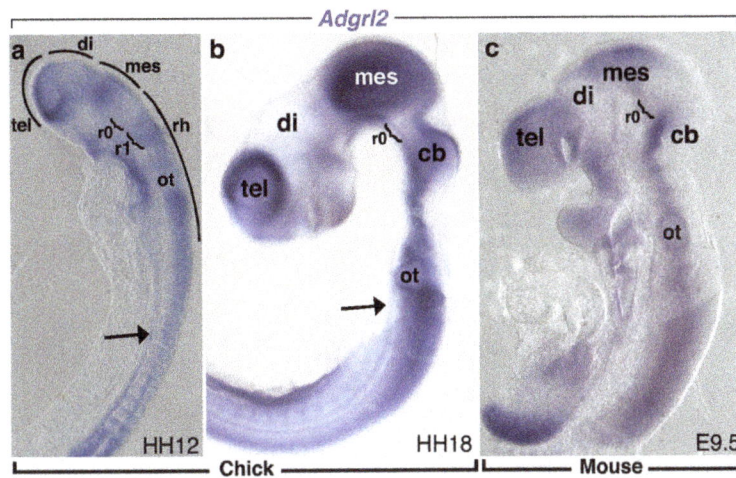

Fig. 4 Expression of the *Adgrl2* gene during early development in chicken and mouse embryos. **a, b** Spatiotemporal expression of *Adgrl2* on a HH12 whole chick embryo (**a**) and on an HH18 chick dissected neural tube (**b**). At HH12, strong expression is seen throughout the neural tube while weak expression is observed in the diencephalon and isthmocerebellar region (black bracket). At HH18, strong expression is still present in the telencephalon, mesencephalon and cerebellum. Very low expression is still observed in the diencephalon and isthmocerebellar region (black bracket). **c** Similar strong expression of *Adgrl2* is observed in the telencephalon, mesencephalon and cerebellum of a 9.5 mouse embryo. di: diencephalon; cb: cerebellum; mes: mesencephalon; ot: otic vesicle; r0: isthmic organizer region; r1: rhombomere 1; rh: rhombencephalon; tel.: telencephalon

From 16WG, Cajal-Retzius cells were positive (Fig. 5c), and from 22WG to 34WG pyramidal neurons differentiated from layers III and V (Fig. 5d), whereas ADGRL2 immunoreactivity remained weak in layers II and IV until birth. Radial glia was immunolabelled from 13WG to 30WG. Positive-ADGRL2 migrating neurons were observed in the intermediate zone until 24WG, a developmental stage corresponding to radial migration termination. At birth, a few migrating interneurons were still observed. ADGRL2-positive neurons were scattered throughout the basal ganglia, thalami and hypothalamic nuclei. At the infratentorial level, transiently immunoreactive fibres and neurons were observed within and around the colliculi, and in the substantia nigra between 13 and 30WG. A transient ADGRL2 immunoreactivity was also present in the pontine transverse fibres and pontine nuclei from 13WG to 22WG. In the cerebellum, the dorsal neuroepithelium of the 4th ventricle and the rhombic lips were strongly immunolabelled from the 6th PCW to 16WG (Fig. 5e), then gradually disappeared by 20WG. Bergman glia, migrating Purkinje and cerebellar deep nuclei positive neurons were apparent from 10 PCW. Purkinje cells were positive until birth (Fig. 5f). From 13WG onward, the transient external granular cell layer was strongly immunolabelled, and became negative at 34WG. In the internal granular cell layer, only Golgi II neurons were positive (Fig. 5g). Cranial nerve nuclei of the pons and medulla became positive from the 24th WG, as well as olivary nuclei, whose immunoreactivity persisted until birth (Fig. 5h). To summarize, ADGRL2 immunoreactivity was mainly observed in the germinal zones both at the supra- and infratentorial levels, and to a lesser degree, in some discrete migrating neuron populations and more mature anatomical structures.

ADGRL2 expression is normal in patient amniocytes carrying the c.3785T>A variant

ADGRL2 is post-transcriptionally processed, the full length precursor being autoproteolytically cleaved in two independent fragments (N-terminal fragment, 70-75 kDa and C-terminal fragment, 105-110 kDa) which are addressed to the plasma membrane [72]. To investigate whether the missense variant identified by WES could alter ADGRL2 protein stability or processing, protein expression was evaluated by western blot experiments on the patient amniocytes collected at the time of amniocentesis performed at 21WG, by comparison with amniocyte ADGRL2 expression from control fœtuses at the same developmental stage. As shown in Additional file 5: Figure S2, no differences in ADGRL2 expression and cleavage were observed between the patient's and the control amniocytes, indicating that the *ADGRL2* c.3785T>A variant does not alter ADGRL2 expression or processing, but rather impairs its functionality.

Intracellular Ca^{2+} release in response to ligand activation is altered in patient *ADGRL2* amniocytes

The exogenous ligand α-latrotoxin induces Ca$^{2+}_i$ elevation by two mechanisms, which are not mutually exclusive. The first is ADGRL2-receptor specific: the subsequent receptor transduction pathway involves a G protein coupled to activation of phospholipase C (PLC),

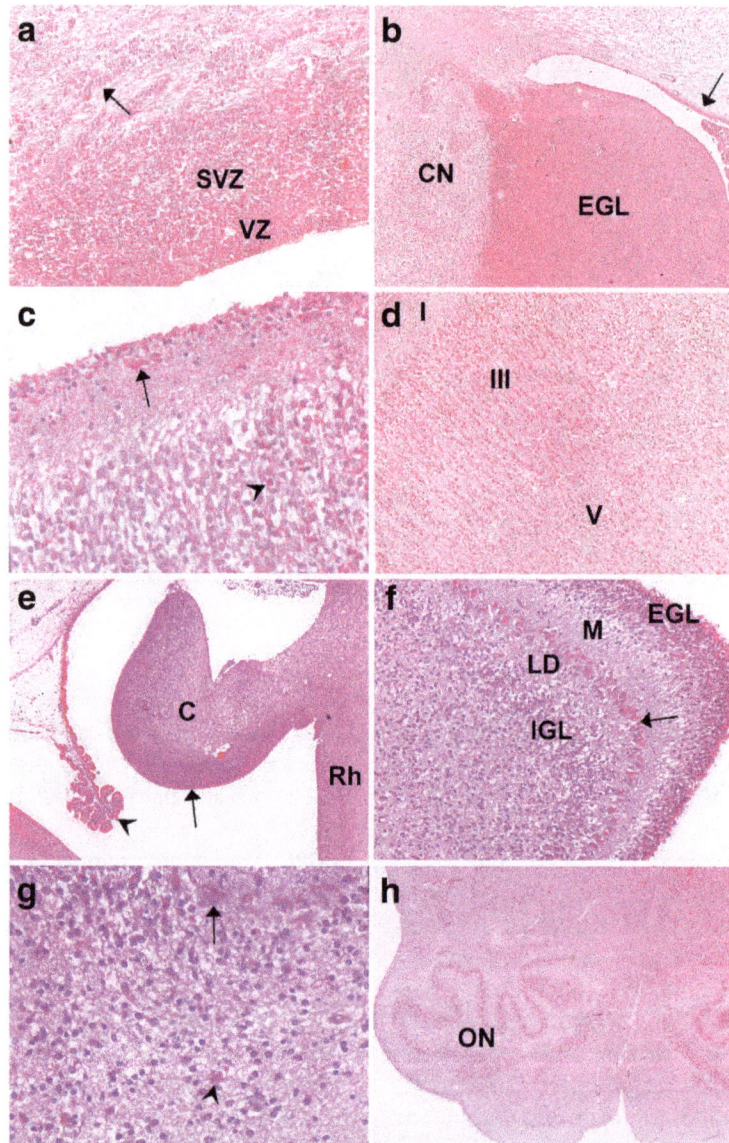

Fig. 5 ADGRL2 immunohistochemistry in the normal developing human brain. **a** Strong immunoreactivity of stem cells in the VZ and of intermediate progenitors in the SVZ, as well as in several migrating neurons (arrow) [OM × 100]. **b** Immunopositivity of LGE at 18WG [OM × 25]. **c** 18WG onward positive Cajal-Retzius cells in layer I (thick arrow) and cortical neurones (arrow head) [OM × 250]. **d** Immunoreactive differentiating pyramidal neurons of the layers III and V [OM × 25]. **e** Intense immunolabelling of the developing cerebellum at 6PCW, predominating in the ventricular zone (thick arrow) and in the choroid plexuses (arrow head) [OM × 25]. **f** At 24WG, strong immunoreactivity of the transient external granular cell layer and in Purkinje cells (arrow), but with no positivity in the developing internal granular cell layer [OM × 250]. **g** Only positive Golgi II neurons at 32WG in the internal granular cell layer (arrow head), Purkinje cells remaining strongly immunoreactive (thick arrow) [OM × 400]. **h** Diffuse neuronal immunoreactivity in the olivary nuclei from 25WG [OM × 25]. OM: original magnification; VZ: ventricular zone; SVZ: subventricular zone; CN: caudate nucleus; LGE: lateral ganglionic eminences; C: cerebellum; Rh: rhombencephalon; EGL: external granular cell layer of the cerebellar cortex; M: molecular layer; LD: lamina dissecans; IGL: internal granular cell layer of the cerebellar cortex, ON: olivary nucleus

production of inositol-triphosphate (IP3) and release of Ca^{2+} from intracellular stores [4, 42]. The second is a consequence of the ionophoric properties of α-latrotoxin [3, 30]. Toxin tetramers forming transmembrane pores induce passive extracellular Ca^{2+} (Ca^{2+}_e) influx into the cell. Moreover, α-latrotoxin binds to at least two types of receptors associated with Ca^{2+}_i release. Neurexins are exclusively activated by α-latrotoxin in a Ca^{2+}_e dependent manner [17, 38], whereas ADGRLs also bind the toxin in the absence of Ca^{2+}_e [4, 31]. To specifically study ADGRLs, media complemented with 4 nM EDTA (F12-EDTA condition) to induce Ca^{2+}_e chelation were used [3]. To study the functionality of the ADGRL2 receptor, an assay was carried out using microfluorimetry that reflected mutated receptor ability to transduce Ca^{2+}_i [66]. Alpha-latrotoxin was used as a ligand on fura-2 loaded amniocytes obtained from the fœtus carrying the *ADGRL2* variation and wild-type amniocytes from control fœtuses at the same term (Fig. 6). To discriminate between intra- and extra-cellular pools of calcium [3], amniocytes were cultured in F12 media in absence or presence of 4 mM EDTA in F12-EDTA condition. Application of 1 nM α-latrotoxin on control cells (Wt) induced a cytosolic Ca^{2+}_i increase within the first 30 s (Fig. 6a; full line). Three minutes after 1 nM α-latrotoxin exposure, EDTA removal from the perfusion medium was associated with another cytosolic Ca^{2+}_i increase, which reached a maximum stable value (Fig. 6a). The effect of 1 nM α-latrotoxin on cytosolic Ca^{2+}_i under F12-EDTA condition was more than two times lower in mutant cells (Mt) (Fig. 6a, d; dotted line). As found in Wt cells, a similar second phase of cytosolic Ca^{2+}_i increase was observed after removal of EDTA (Fig. 6a, d).

To investigate in greater details the Ca^{2+}_i mobilization associated with the ADGRL2 receptor, Wt and Mt. cells were co-incubated in the presence of the PLC inhibitor, U73122 (Fig. 6b, c) [10]. In F12-EDTA condition, 10 μM U73122 abrogated the cytosolic Ca^{2+}_i increase induced by α-latrotoxin in both Wt and Mt. cells (Fig. 6b, c). In contrast, U73122 had no significant impact on the late phase of Ca^{2+}_i increase resulting from EDTA removal (Fig. 6d).

ADGRL2 c.3785T>A variant is responsible for signal transduction alteration

To demonstrate the deleterious effect of the variant independently from the patient genetic background, HeLa cells were used as an exogenous cellular model in which the candidate gene was overexpressed, due to the very low expression of ADGRL2 in these cells. As human ADGRL2 cDNA is toxic to bacteria, cloning was not possible and a previously described construct derived from rat *Adgrl2* homolog, pcDCIRL-2 coupled to GFP, was used [31]. To generate mutant Adgrl2 clones, a histidine was introduced at position 1262 using site-directed mutagenesis. First, the correct processing and trafficking of the GFP coupled receptor to the plasma membrane of transfected HeLa cells was verified by confocal microscopy and transfection efficiency by western blot (Additional file 6: Figure S3a, b). However, in F-12 EDTA condition, microfluorimetry experiments performed with pcDCIRL-2-GFP cells did not display any cytosolic Ca^{2+}_i increase after α-latrotoxin exposure: only a late phase of Ca^{2+}_i increase was observed. Because C-terminal GFP could induce steric hindrance and inhibit Adgrl2 signal transduction coupled to G protein in response to ligand binding, the wild-type pcDCIRL-2 construct lacking the GFP sequence was transfected into

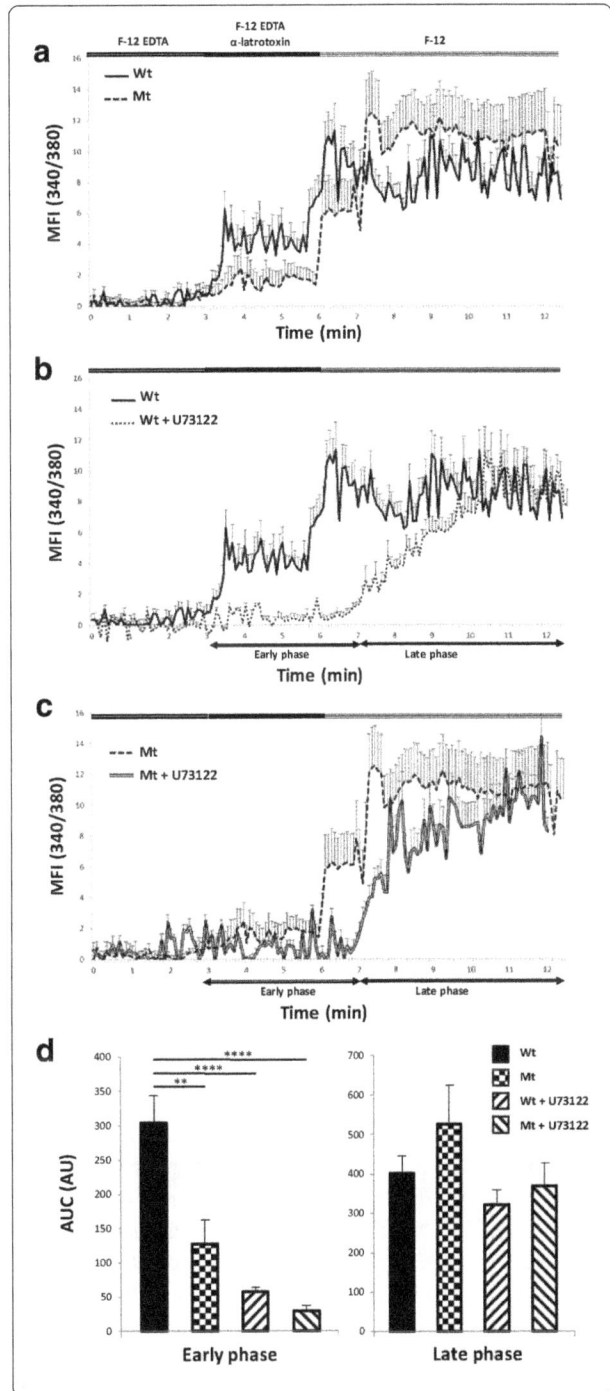

Fig. 6 Signal transduction coupled to G protein is altered in mutant *ADGRL2* amniocytes. Intracellular calcium levels were monitored by microfluorimetry using the ratiometric Fura-2 AM calcium probe and results expressed as mean fluorescence intensity (MFI). **a** α-latrotoxin (1 nM) was applied to wild-type (Wt) and mutant (Mt) cultured amniocytes under extracellular chelated-calcium conditions (EDTA 4 mM). Three minutes after α-latrotoxin administration, cells were perfused without EDTA to restore extracellular calcium levels. **b** α-latrotoxin (1 nM) was applied to Wt amniocytes under chelated-calcium conditions (EDTA 4 mM). Cultured cells were pre-incubated or not with the phospholipase C inhibitor U73122 (10 μM). Three minutes after α-latrotoxin administration, cells were perfused without EDTA to restore extracellular calcium levels. **c** α-latrotoxin (1 nM) was applied to Mt amniocytes under chelated-calcium conditions (EDTA 4 mM). Cultured cells were pre-incubated or not with the phospholipase C inhibitor U73122 (10 μM). Three minutes after α-latrotoxin administration, cells were perfused without EDTA to restore extracellular calcium levels. **d** Quantification and statistical analysis of intracellular calcium levels from the early and late phases in response to α-latrotoxin stimulation. Areas under the curves (AUC) were expressed in arbitrary units (AU). Each value represents the mean (±S.E.M.) of 30 cells. *, $p < 0.05$; **, $p < 0.01$, vs Wt amniocytes using one-way ANOVA test

HeLa cells. The resulting cytosolic Ca^{2+}_i profiles after α-latrotoxin exposure were very similar to those obtained with Wt amniocytes (Fig. 6a,). In contrast, HeLa cells overexpressing mutant Adgrl2 presented exclusively the late-phase Ca^{2+}_i increase (Additional file 6: Figure S3c), confirming that *ADGRL2* c.3785T>A variant is responsible for the alteration of the signal transduction coupled to G-protein in response to ligand binding.

Adgrl2−/− mice die at E15.5

An *Adgrl2* knock-out (KO) mouse model was used to outline the phenotype associated to *ADGRL2* inactivation. Adult heterozygous mice were fertile and survived for more than 1 year, but had a shorter fertility lifespan compared with wild-type mice, a few months vs 2 years, respectively. *Adgrl2*+/− F2 mice were mated in order to obtain *Adgrl2*−/−. A balanced sex ratio distribution was observed in the 15 litters analysed. Nevertheless, *Adgrl2* genotyping of mouse pups was not in agreement with the Hardy–Weinberg equilibrium, confirming embryo lethality of *Adgrl2*−/− mice as previously described by the provider, who suggested an embryonic lethality at ~E15.5 ($\chi^2 = 49.35$). In contrast, E15 embryos *Adgrl2* genotyping was concordant with the Hardy–Weinberg equilibrium ($\chi^2 = 1.81$), even if a slight deviation began to occur.

MRI findings in *Adgrl2*+/− adult mice confirm microcephaly, hypoplasia of the vermis and mesencephalon

Comparative analyses of horizontal T2-weighted images passing through the mesencephalon at the level of red nuclei revealed a defective growth of the tectum (consisting of less developed superior colliculi) and of the tegmentum (with narrowed cerebral peduncles) in *Adgrl2*+/− female adult mice compared to wild type female mice (Fig. 7a, b). A growth failure of the cerebellum was also observed, with a smaller cerebellar transverse diameter (Fig. 7a, b). On transversal planes passing though the widest cerebellar transverse diameter, para-flocculonodular lobes were visualized in *Adgrl2*+/− animals, reflecting a defect in anterior-posterior growth of the cerebellum. At the supratentorial level, a mild dilatation of the lateral ventricles due to insufficient expansion of the brain parenchyma (as reflected by a diminished bi-parietal diameter) was also noted, arguing for microcephaly. Quantitative measurements of cerebral volumes confirmed a significant reduction in brain volumes (wild-type mice: 392 ± 8 mm^3 vs *Adgrl2*+/−: 332 ± 7 mm^3; $p < 0.001$; Additional file 3: Table S3). Microcephaly extending to the parietal lobes was also present in males, with a moderate enlargement of the subarachnoid spaces in the anterior regions, but with no shape anomalies of the lateral ventricles. Examination of T2-weighted transversal planes passing through the optic chiasm revealed a defect in superior and middle frontal gyrus expansion, as well as abnormally-shaped lateral ventricles in female *Adgrl2*+/− adult mice (Fig. 7c, d). Quantitative analyses performed on vermis median sagittal planes (heights, anterior-posterior diameters and global vermis areas, Fig. 7e) revealed that, contrary to heights that did not significantly differ between wild-type and heterozygous males or females (Fig. 7f), anterior-posterior diameters were significantly reduced when comparing wild-type and heterozygous males and wild-type and heterozygous females (Fig. 7g). Significantly reduced vermis areas were observed in female *Adgrl2*+/− adult mice (Fig. 7h).

ADGRL2 c.3785T>A variant increases cell adhesion properties and reduces cell motility

Given the close relationship between Ca^{2+}_i concentration, cell adhesion and migration [36, 37, 74] and because latrophilin function as cell-adhesion molecules [12], an alteration of the ADGRL2 signal transduction could induce modifications in cell adhesive properties. A cell adhesion assay was therefore developed to allow measurement of the binding of cells to each other as a function of Adgrl2 plasma membrane expression in HeLa cells (adapted from Boucard et al. [12], Additional file 7: Figure S4). In line with microfluorimetry experiment results, when pcDCIRL-2 coupled to GFP was overexpressed, no cellular aggregates were observed, suggesting that absence of homophilic cell adhesion properties explained the calcimetry results (Fig. 8j, k, l) [12]. In contrast to pcD-empty plasmid, cells expressing wild-type pcDCIRL-2 assembled to each other to form

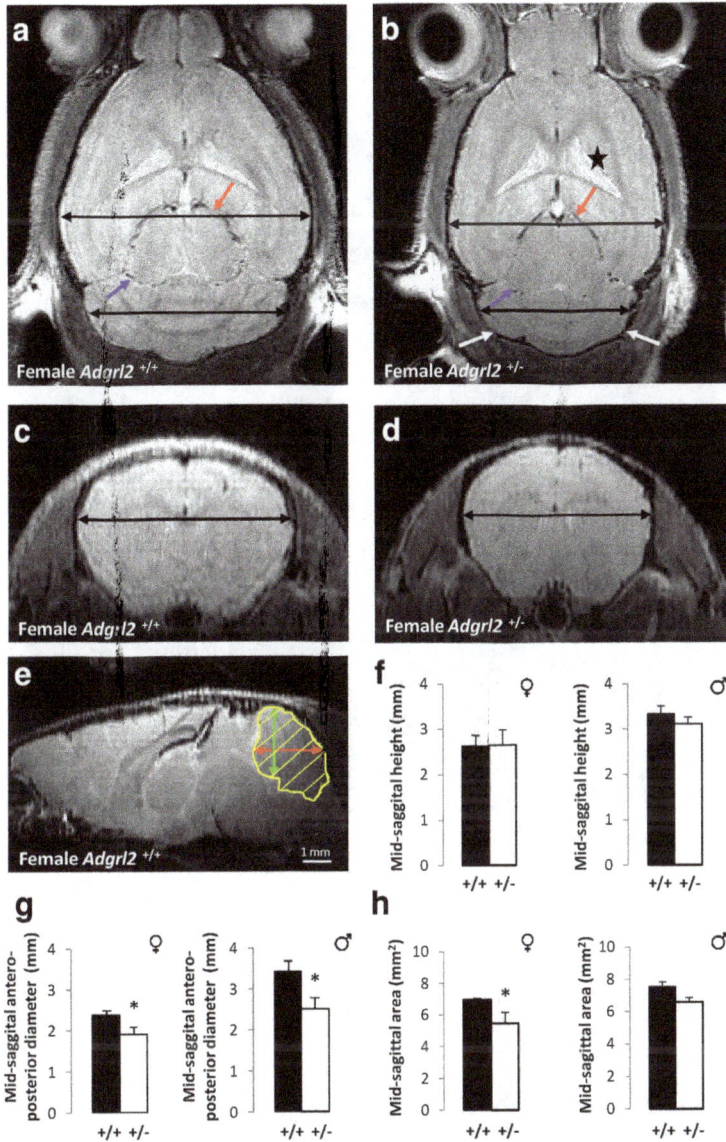

Fig. 7 Main representative images and quantitative findings obtained from MRI performed in Adgrl2$^{+/+}$ and Adgrl2$^{+/-}$ male and female adult mouse brains. **a-b** Horizontal T2-weighted images passing through the mesencephalon of Adgrl2$^{+/+}$ mice. **a** revealing in Adgrl2$^{+/-}$ mice **b** a defect in tectum growth with insufficiently developed colliculi (red arrow) and pes pedunculi (blue arrow) with a growth defect of the telencephalon (line corresponding to bi-parietal diameter) responsible for *a vacuo* ventricular dilatation (asterisk), and of the cerebellum (line corresponding to transverse diameter) with smaller cerebellar hemispheres (white arrows). **c** T2-weighted images passing through the optic chiasm in Adgrl2$^{+/+}$ mice. **d** Deficient frontal growth in Adgrl2$^{+/-}$ mice (thick line). **e** Schematic representation of the different measurements performed on Adgrl2$^{+/+}$ and Adgrl2$^{+/-}$ male and female adult mouse vermis (height in green, anterior-posterior diameter in red, and area in yellow) revealing no difference in heights in Adgrl2$^{+/+}$ and Adgrl2$^{+/-}$ females compared to males (**f**), whereas significant differences in anterior-posterior diameters were apparent both in females and males (**g**), but with significant differences in vermis areas between Adgrl2$^{+/+}$ and Adgrl2$^{+/-}$ female mice only contrary to Adgrl2$^{+/+}$ and Adgrl2$^{+/-}$ males (**h**)

aggregates after 90 min under gentle stirring, suggesting homophilic cell adhesion (Fig. 8a, b, m). The size of cell aggregates was two times larger for cells overexpressing the mutant pcDCIRL-2 construct (Fig. 8c). As rat Adgrl2 homolog CIRL-2 carrying the variation is unable to transduce any signal in response to its activation, a link between cell adhesion and G protein–mediated intracellular signalling is highly conceivable. To confirm this hypothesis, PLC was blocked by adding 10 μM U73122 in the aggregation medium (Fig. 8d, e, f). Under this condition, aggregate size of cells overexpressing CIRL-2 Wt reached the size of aggregates overexpressing CIRL-2 Mt. (Fig. 8e, f, m). Treatment by U73122 of cells transfected with the empty plasmid also

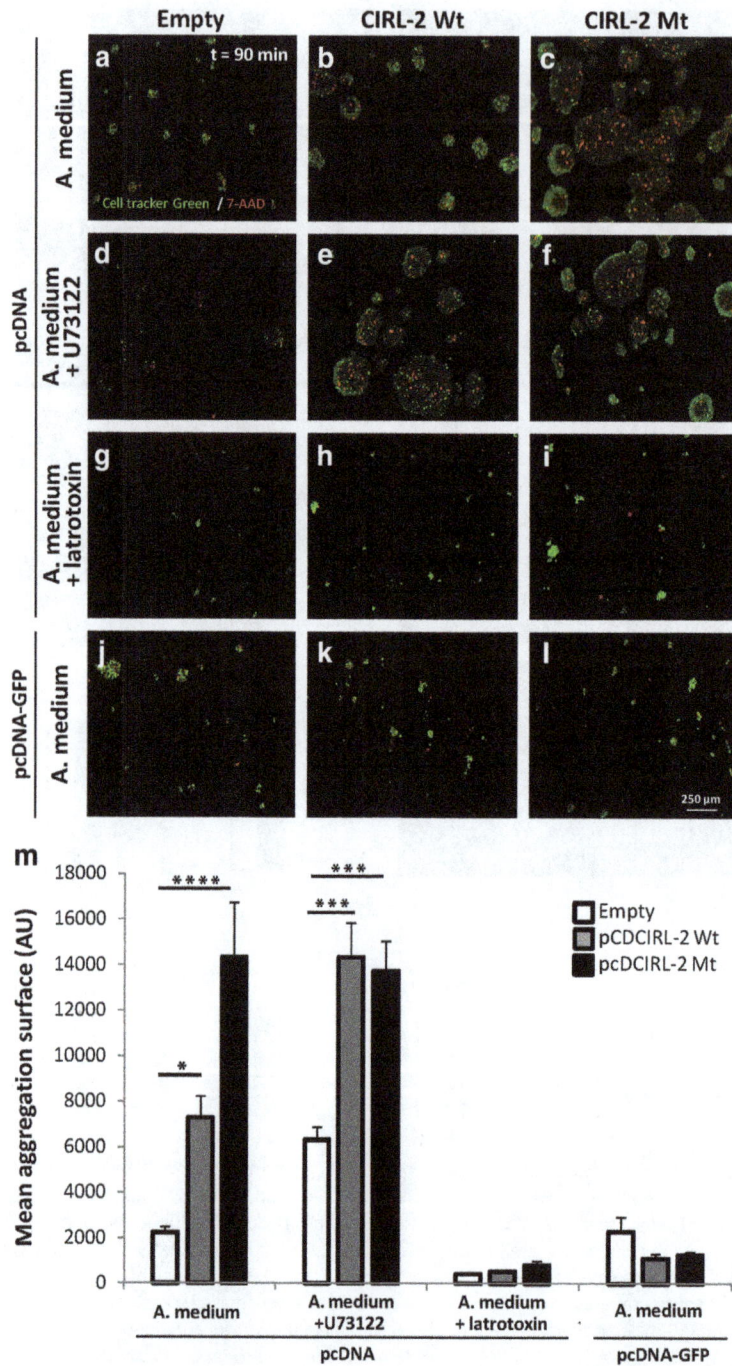

Fig. 8 HeLa cells overexpressing mutant *ADGRL2* present enhanced cell adhesive properties associated to signal transduction alteration. **a-c** HeLa cells expressing either pcD-Empty (**a**), CIRL2-Wt (**b**) or CIRL2-Mt (**c**) were labelled with the viability marker, cell tracker green (10 µM), and the mortality marker 7-AAD (50 µg/ml) and incubated at room temperature for 90 min in aggregation medium. Note the marked increase of aggregate sizes in CIRL2-Mt expressing cells. **d-f** HeLa cells expressing either pcD-Empty (**d**) CIRL2-Wt (**e**) or CIRL2-Mt (**f**) were incubated at room temperature for 90 min in aggregation medium containing the PLC inhibitor U73122 (3 µM). Note that inhibition of PLC enhanced homophilic binding of HeLa cells overexpressing CIRL2-Wt. **g-i** HeLa cells expressing either pcD-Empty (**g**), CIRL2-Wt (**h**) or CIRL2-Mt (**i**) were incubated at room temperature for 90 min in aggregation medium containing α-latrotoxin (1 nM) which prevented cell aggregation. **j-l** HeLa cells expressing either pcD-GFP-Empty (**j**), CIRL2-GFP-Wt (**k**) or CRL2-GFP-Mt (**l**) were incubated at room temperature for 90 min in aggregation medium. Cells expressing CIRL2 coupled to GFP in C-terminal were not able to aggregate. **m** Quantification and statistical analysis of the aggregation index. Each value represents the mean (±S.E.M.) of three independent cell-adhesion assays. **, $p < 0.01$; ***, $p < 0.001$, ****, $p < 0.0001$ using one-way ANOVA test

allowed for aggregate size increase (Fig. 8m). The effect on aggregate formation under massive increase of cytosolic Ca^{2+}_i was also investigated by adding α-latrotoxin in the aggregation medium. After 90 min, no cell aggregates were formed (Fig. 8g-i, m). These findings support that PLC coupling and Ca^{2+}_i concentrations affect cell adhesion properties, with higher Ca^{2+}_i concentration being correlated with the lower adhesion.

To determine if cell adhesion excess was associated with cell motility modulation when *Adgrl2* is overexpressed in HeLa cells, scratch assays were carried out (Fig. 9) [44]. In pcD-empty cells, the wound width was reduced by 56.6% after 72 h of culture. Although no differences were found between pcD-empty and pcDCIRL2-Wt cells, a dramatic reduction of wound healing was observed in cells overexpressing pcDCIRL2-Mt (Fig. 9a, b). To ensure that wound healing inhibition resulted from cell migration or proliferation alteration, cell cycle experiments were performed. Although the PI was evaluated at 48.8%, with 34.4% of cells in S phase in pcD-empty cells, PI was evaluated at 41.5% with 27.7% of cells in S phase in pcDCIRL2-Wt cells and PI was evaluated at 43.1% with 28.3% of cells in S phase in pcDCIRL2-Mt cells respectively. For each condition, the percentage of cells in G2/M phases was not significantly different and was between 13.8 and 15.1%. Cell cycle data were not different among the three transfected cell conditions, strongly suggesting that wound healing inhibition quantified in pcDCIRL2-Mt cells is unlikely to be due to effects on cell division or proliferation, which argues for delayed cell motility and migration due to an over-adhesion mechanism.

Mutant *ADGRL2* cells present size and cytoskeletal network alterations

One of the mechanisms required for cell adhesion consists in fluctuations of Ca^{2+}_i, which regulate the dynamic assembly of cytoskeletal elements [45, 62]. To visualize F-actin and microtubule network modifications, glass coverslips cultured HeLa cells overexpressing pcD-empty, pcDCIRL-2 Wt or pcDCIRL-2 Mt. were immunolabelled with phalloidin and acetylated α-tubulin (Additional file 8: Figure S5). Depending on the transfected plasmid, cells harboured various morphologies: pcD-empty cells possessed a fusiform shape (Additional file 8: Figure S5a) while pcDCIRL-2 Wt spread out on the substratum (Additional file 8: Figure S5b). In the pcDCIRL-2 Mt. condition, cells were significantly more spread out than pcDCIRL-2 Wt cells (Additional file 8: Figure S5c). However, when detached from their culture support, cells from these three conditions displayed only minor differences concerning their size and content. Using flow cytometry quantitative studies, HeLa cultured cells had a mean size of 234.2 ± 5.95 AU, HeLa

cells transfected with an empty vector a mean size of 241.7+/− 8.30 AU, HeLa cells transfected with the Wt *Adgrl2* a mean size of 238.7 ± 6.73 AU and cells transfected with the *ADGRL2* variant a mean value of 258.6 ± 13.49 AU. Regarding intracellular heterogeneity, some differences were observed between HeLa cells alone (236.7 ± 3.65 AU) and cells transfected with the *ADGRL2* variant (264.9 ± 5.70 AU). From these data, increased size of cells overexpressing Adgrl2 (Additional file 8: Figure S5b, c) appears to be directly associated with their over-adhesive properties. Similar to flow cytometry studies, which evidenced intracellular heterogeneity differences among the different conditions, immunohistochemistry revealed cytoskeleton architecture modifications (Additional file 8: Figure S5a-c). In the three conditions, the α-tubulin network was located in the perinuclear area, whereas the F-actin network appeared to be modified in the case of *Adgrl2* overexpression. In control cells, a well-defined F-actin filament network was essentially located at the periphery of the cell (Additional file 8: Figure S5a). When *Adgrl2* was overexpressed, cells displayed a highly developed cytoplasmic F-actin network with numerous anchoring points to the glass coverslip (Additional file 8: Figure S5b; arrows). Overexpression of the mutant *Adgrl2* exacerbated this phenomenon in the cell surface membrane of HeLa cells by homophilic Adgrl2 interaction activation (Additional file 8: Figure S5c). Thus, the *ADGRL2* c.3785T>A;p.(Leu1262His) variant that alters signal transduction coupled to G protein is responsible for excessive adhesion properties associated with abnormal cytoskeletal remodelling of cells overexpressing this variant.

Discussion

Within the large GPCR superfamily, ADGRL2 (previously named LPHN2) together with ADGRL1 (previously named LPHN1), ADGRL3 (previously named LPHN3) and ADGRL4 (previously named ELTD1) belong to the Adhesion family encompassing 33 mammalian members [26]. Adhesion-GPCRs are involved in several key molecular and cellular functions, including planar cell polarity, regulation of cytoskeleton organization, cell adhesion and migration, cell cycle, cell death and differentiation [26], but the precise mechanisms by which ADGRL2 acts remain elusive. An exogenous agonist for ADGRLs has long been identified: α-latrotoxin, the major neurotoxin in black widow spider venom, which attests a synaptic role for ADGRLs [47]. Endogenous ligands include Teneurin-2 (also known as Lasso), neurexins and FLRT1–3 (Fibronectin Leucine-Rich Transmembrane protein) [11, 48, 54, 63]. Contrary to ADGRL1 and ADGRL3, ADGRL2 does not bind to neurexins (neurexin-1a, −1b, −2b), binds only weakly to teneurin-2, and interacts with FLRT3, but not with FLRT1. Because ADGRLs were first identified as

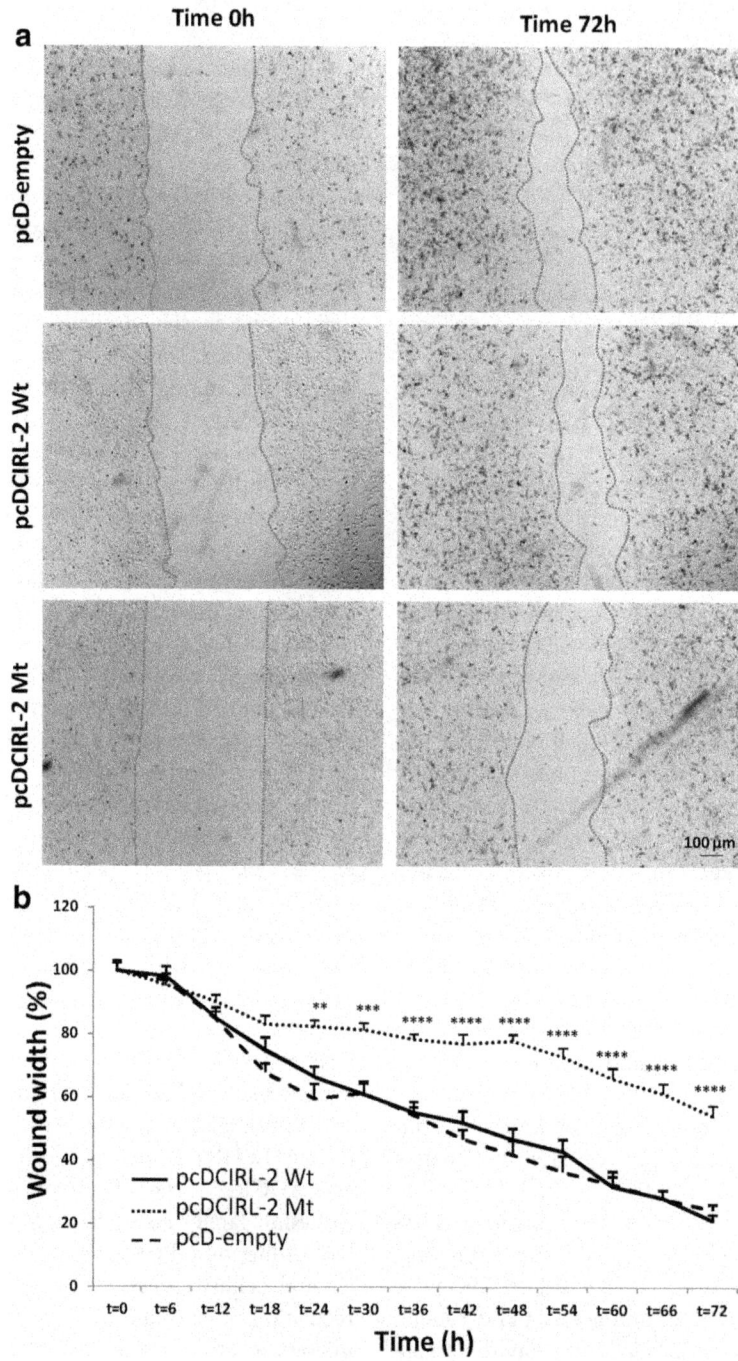

Fig. 9 Cell motility is altered in HeLa cells overexpressing mutant ADGRL2. **a** Wound healing experiments were performed on monolayer HeLa cells overexpressing pcD-empty, CIRL2-Wt or CIRL2-Mt. Microphotographs visualize wound healing images acquired 0 and 72 h after the scratch. **b** Time-course quantification of scratch width in monolayer HeLa cells overexpressing pcD-empty, CIRL2-Wt or CIRL2-Mt. Each value represents the mean (±S.E.M.) from three independent experiments. **, $p < 0.01$; ***, $p < 0.001$; ****, $p < 0.0001$ using two-way ANOVA test

putative synaptic receptors for α-latrotoxin, researchers initially focused their attention on the role of ADGRL2 in the synapse, showing that ADGRL2 could mediate synapse recognition and assembly and/or contribute to a synapse maintenance signal [2].

The c.3785T>A;p.(Leu1262His) variant is localized in the intracellular domain of ADGRL2, which exhibits 35% and 49% similarity between ADGRL1 and ADGRL3 proteins, respectively. G protein–mediated intracellular signalling has been demonstrated for ADGRL1 by its interaction with $G\alpha_o$ and its binding to teneurin-2, which induces Ca^{2+} signals [42, 63]. Microfluorimetry experiments confirmed that the c.3785T>A variant impairs the early stage of cytosolic Ca^{2+}_i release in response to α-latrotoxin binding, both in the patient's amniocytes and in HeLa cells transfected with the mutant Adgrl2 construct. Moreover, addition of the PLC inhibitor U73122 in wild-type amniocytes induced early step calcium release impairment. Thus ADGRL2 activation is necessary for G protein–mediated intracellular signalling. More precisely, ADGRL2 is required for this early step of calcium release, whereas α-latrotoxin tetramer pores are responsible for passive Ca^{2+}_e influx into the cell during the second step. Pure α-latrotoxin is a very stable homodimer, which further assembles into tetramers in the presence of Mg^{2+} or Ca^{2+} to form α-latrotoxin pores [3]. Cyclic nucleotide signalling and Ca^{2+} are known to be intracellular downstream targets for many extracellular guidance molecules. They convert the information from locally expressed guidance molecules to intracellular effectors, which control migration by regulating cytoskeleton dynamics, in particular the F-actin network. Using cerebellar granule cell cultures, Komuro et al. demonstrated that their migration speed from the transient external granule cell layer was correlated to both the amplitude and frequency of Ca^{2+} elevations, and that the reduction of the Ca^{2+} transients resulted in the termination of granule cell migration [37]. The modulation of intracellular Ca^{2+} release by the adhesion-GPCR ADGRL2 could therefore exert a role in the regulation of neuronal migration. Cell adhesion assay confirmed that the inhibition of the G protein–mediated intracellular signalling was correlated with enhanced adhesion and increase in size of aggregates overexpressing mutant Adgrl2. Transfection of either wild-type or mutant-type pcDCIRL-2, the rat homologue of ADGRL2, in HeLa cells induced a strongly developed microtubule network with many focal adhesion points, indicating that ADGRL2 inactivation leads to increased adhesion properties due to intracellular Ca^{2+} flux and cytoskeletal organization perturbations. Further characterisation of focal adhesions points could provide additional evidence of cell migration alteration as the recruitment of talin and vinculin is correlated with the mechanical force applied to the focal adhesion [18].

The causal effect of the c.3785T>A;p.(Leu1262His) variation in ADGRL2 on the foetal brain malformation in Adgrl2+/− mice, Adgrl2−/− genotype being lethal in utero at E15.5 was supported by MRI findings. Both male and female Adgrl2+/− adult mice displayed microcephaly, affecting mainly the telencephalon, although more severe in Adgrl2+/− female mice, with a defect in anteroposterior growth of the vermis, in line with ADGRL2 expression during telencephalic and cerebellar development

in human embryos and foetuses as well as in chicks and mice.

Our results suggest that this ADGRL2 variation impedes the proper development of the cerebellum resulting in RES which is thought to occur when the cerebellar primordium develops and probably results from abnormal function of genes expressed during initial patterning of the mesencephalon-rhombencephalon [43, 68]. For some authors, RES is thought to result from loss of anterior cerebellar anlage cells derived from the medial ventricular zone (VZ) of the cerebellar primordium destined to become the vermis, or from a shift of these anterior cells toward a more posterior and/or ventral hemispheric fate [56]. For others, RES results rather from a loss of posterior expansion of the medial region of the cerebellar primordium [61]. Expansion of the medial cerebellar primordium plays a considerable role in generating the vermis and the hemispheres, which grow together rapidly from the two other germinal zones, the rhombic lips. Although the precise mechanisms that lead to the proper individualisation of the vermis and the hemispheres (which are lacking in RES) remain unknown, ADGRL2 variation likely avoids expansion of the vermis and of the hemispheres from the medial VZ and EGL. Besides, the ADGRL2 ligand, FLRT3, has a strong specific expression in the isthmic organizer, whereas ADGRL2 is not expressed in this area [25]. This non-overlapping pattern of expression could be due to a specific dosage code to specify the boundaries of the future cerebellum along the rostrocaudal axis of the rhombencephalon. Interestingly, it has also been shown that lat-1, an orthologue of vertebrate ADGRLs in C. elegans, plays an essential role in anterior-posterior tissue polarity in the embryo [41, 51]. Moreover, in the absence of lat-1, stem cells display positioning defects as they remain clustered near their place of birth, highly reminiscent of what observed in ADGRL2 mutant cells using wound healing experiments [41]. Our results suggest that RES could result from abnormal positional cues along the anteroposterior axis.

Primary congenital microcephaly and microlissencephaly have classically been classified as disorders of neurogenesis, consisting above all in a severe decrease of symmetric and asymmetric divisions in the ventricular and subventricular zones resulting in neuronal cell production depletion. These disorders could be attributed to four major pathophysiological mechanisms, including first, early events (during the 5th gestational week) that have been postulated as being of major importance for the control of cell cycle and proper functioning of the primary cilium; second, abnormalities during the different phases of mitosis (prometaphase, metaphase and cytodieresis); third, anomalies of formation and positioning of the mitotic spindle; and fourth, abnormal structure and function of associated molecules that are involved in cytoskeletal dynamics.

A constellation of disease-causing genes have been described as affecting the early steps of neural tube development, i.e., planar polarity, primary cilium structure (such as kinesins) or functions involving in particular Wnt and Sonic hedgehog pathways, as well as cell cycle length controlling molecules, notably *PAX6* and *FLNA* [67].

As regards the different phases of mitosis, *WDR81* deleterious variants were shown to increase the number of mitotic cells with an accumulation of cells in prometaphase and metaphase resulting in mitotic delay without any impact on mitotic spindle or primary cilia organization [13]. Variations in the *CIT* gene encoding citron kinase localizes to the cleavage furrow and midbody, where it functions in cytodieresis. The neuropathological phenotype includes extreme microcephaly or microlissencephaly [28].

In fact, the vast majority of genes responsible for microcephaly encode centrosomal proteins involved in spindle orientation or proteins regulating these centrosomal proteins. To date, bi-allelic deleterious variations in 13 genes (*MCPH1, WDR62, CDK5RAP2, CASC5, ASPM, CENPJ, STIL, CEP135, CEP152, ZNF335, PHC1, CDK6, CENPE* [20, 57]) which are normally expressed in ventricular (apical) and subventricular (basal) radial glial cells, impair proper spindle positioning and orientation leading to a drastic decrease in the generation of intermediate progenitors and of post-mitotic neuroblasts due to a lack of maintenance of centrosome asymmetry [73]. In these pathological conditions, brain lesions range from microcephaly with simplified gyral pattern to microlissencephaly. Pathogenic variations in *NDE1* which interacts directly with LIS1 and is expressed in the neuroepithelium of the cerebral and cerebellar cortices where it contributes to interkinetic nuclear migration and also localized at the centrosome and on the mitotic spindle, result in early failure of neuron production and microlissencephaly [1, 7].

Microtubule structure alterations as well as alterations of binding partners necessary for proper microtubule dynamics resulting from pathogenic variants in *TUBA1A, TUBB2A, TUBB2B, TUBB3, TUBB5, TUBG1* and *TUBA8* genes are also responsible microcephaly and microlissencephaly. These lesions are constantly associated with several brain abnormalities due to defects in progenitor proliferation with decreased symmetric divisions, impaired neuronal radial migration and abnormal neuronal differentiation resulting in deficient neurite outgrowth, axon path-finding and connectivity. It is worth noting that in all these conditions, various brainstem and cerebellar abnormalities have been described, but RES has never been identified [5, 14].

Other pathophysiological mechanisms that may cause primary microcephaly have been recently identified, among others microRNAs and Golgi trafficking defects [46, 58]. But to our knowledge, microcephaly due to excessive adhesion of progenitors in the germinal zones (VZ, inner SVZ and outer SVZ) has never reported so far.

In the present case, no lesions that could argue for one of the above mentioned pathophysiological mechanisms were identified. Although lat-1, the orthologue of vertebrate ADGRLs in *C. elegans*, is required for cell division plane orientation in the *C. elegans* embryo [41, 51], normal proliferative indices in the LGE indicate that neither symmetric nor asymmetric divisions are altered by comparison with the fœtus harbouring a deleterious variant in the *MCPH1* gene and in which the proliferative index was reduced by a factor of two. Also due to normal proliferative indices, extreme microcephaly with no sulcation associated with this *ADGRL2* variant is unlikely to be connected to mitotic spindle dysfunction. The variation in the *ADGRL2* gene is responsible for Ca^{2+}_i release alteration that constitutes the step before the modulation of microtubule organization. Furthermore, neuronal cells acquire abnormal adhesion and aggregation properties that make them stay in the subventricular zone and probably thereafter prompt them to die. All these data highlight a new mechanism for microcephaly that results from an excess of cell adhesion of neuronal progenitors in the germinal zones, which could also at least partly explain the co-occurrence of RES.

Unlike *ADGRL2* variations that have never been reported to be responsible for human pathologies, variants in other adhesion-GPCR have been recognized, notably *ADGRG1* (previously named *GPR56*), which is responsible for an autosomal recessive condition associated with the presentation of bilateral fronto-parietal polymicrogyria associated with cerebellar hypoplasia, dysgenesis and pseudo-cysts [6, 59]. Similar to humans, *Adgrg1/Gpr56* null mice display a malformed cerebral cortex resembling cobblestone lissencephaly with similar cerebellar lesions [49]. The rostral cerebellar defects result from specific failure of adhesion of the late migrating granule cells to extracellular molecules of the glia limitans whose structural integrity is disrupted with subsequent overmigration of granule cells into the subarachnoid spaces, but not from intrinsic defects in neuronal proliferation and migration [35]. In contrast to ADGRG1/GPR56, which promotes cell adhesion of developing neurons to basal lamina molecules, ADGRL2 promotes cell migration by controlling Ca^{2+}_i release.

Conclusions

In conclusion, we have identified an *ADGRL2* variation very likely responsible for severe microcephaly with almost no sulcation highlighting a new mechanism for the two associated malformations related to excessive adhesion of neuron progenitors within the germinal zones at least mediated by reduction of Ca^{2+} transients. Given its role in the determination of the anteroposterior axis suggested by its orthologue lat-1 [41, 51], we also hypothesize that RES results from abnormal positional cue alterations and defective expansion of the medial VZ in the cerebellar primordium. The identification of ADGRL2 ligands and/or of pathogenic variations in other genes associated with RES will shed more light on the role of ADGRL2 in the pathophysiology of this rare condition. Finally, in addition to its role in synapse assembly, our observations reveal the role of ADGRL2 in development, as already shown for other adhesion GPCRs.

Additional files

Additional file 1: Table S1. Whole Exome Sequencing qualities. For the three exomes performed on Illumina GAIIx (2x76pb) are summarized: the number of sequenced reads, the yield in Gigagabase, the number and the percentage of reads mapped on the human reference sequence (Hg19), the mean depth of the exome, the percentage of base that have been read more than 10 or 50 times, the percentage of bases with a Qscore of at least 30, the mean quality score and the percentage of reads on target captured. (DOCX 16 kb)

Additional file 2: Table S2. Age and cause of death in human cases for ADGRL2 Immunohistochemical. (DOCX 16 kb)

Additional file 3: Table S3. Statistical analysis (DOCX 23 kb)

Additional file 4: Figure S1. ADGRL2 immunoreactivity in the fœtal female and male gonads. a Clustered primordial follicles in the superficial ovarian cortex, containing strongly immunoreactive oocytes (arrow) surrounded by a single layer of flattened granulosa cells at 24WG [OM × 250]. b At birth, some primary follicles are present, with a centrally placed oocytes (arrow head) surrounded by multilayered ADGRL2-positive granulosa cells (thick arrow) [OM × 400] with weaker immunoreactivity of interstitial cells. c Numerous Leydig cells (arrow) being positive in the ovarian hilum at 36WG [OM × 400]. d Multiple seminiferous tubules composed of moderately immunoreactive Sertoli cells (arrow head) and strongly immunolabelled spermatogonia (thick arrow) in a testis at 32WG. Interstitial Leydig and mesenchymal cells are also moderately immunoreactive (asterisk) [OM × 100]. (TIF 22156 kb)

Additional file 5: Figure S2. Expression of ADGRL2 in patient amniocytes and control amniocytes cells. a Western blot analyses of amniocytes cells lysates obtained from patient (P) and two control fœtuses (C1 and C2) of the same development stage. Blot was probed with an antibody that recognizes ADGRL2 or GAPDH protein (loading control). Anti-ADGRL2 antibody recognizes two forms of ADGRL2: 163 kDa (precursor) and 72 kDa (N-terminal fragment). b Quantification of ADGRL2 precursor and N-terminal fragments was performed using GAPDH as the loading control. The histogram represents mean values (±S.E.M.) of three independent experiences. (TIF 7407 kb)

Additional file 6: Figure S3. Signal transduction coupled to G protein is altered in HeLa cell overexpressing mutant *ADGRL2*. a, b Confocal fluorescence image of GFP-tagged CIRL-2 in transfected HeLa cells (a). Nuclei are labelled with Hœchst (b). CIRL2-GFP is expressed as a membrane protein in HeLa cells. c Intracellular calcium was monitored by microfluorimetry of Fura-2 loaded HeLa cells overexpressing wild-type or mutant pcDCIRL-2. Results are expressed as a mean fluorescence intensity (MFI) during time. Alpha-latrotoxin was applied (1 nM) to HeLa cells under calcium free conditions. Three minutes after treatment, extracellular calcium was added. d Quantification of the areas under the curves (UAC, arbitrary units) obtained by the measurement of intracellular calcium levels for the early and late phases in response to α-latrotoxin stimulation. Each value represents the mean (±S.E.M.) of 30 cells. (**, $p < 0.001$ vs Wt using the unpaired t test). (TIF 16017 kb)

Additional file 7: Figure S4. Mean aggregation index calculation. a, b For example, cells overexpressing pcDCIRL-2 Mt. were spotted onto culture slides after 0 (a) and 90 min (b) under gentle stirring in aggregation medium. Viable cells were labelled with cell tracker green (green) and dead cells with 7-AAD (red) to control cell viability. c The extent of cell aggregation was assessed by fluorescence microscopy and the resulting images were then analysed by quantifying the number and size of aggregates in the field. Practically, a basal aggregate size was determined on negative control condition and was set as a threshold for image segmentation. The mean aggregation index was calculated using this formula: (sum of aggregate areas / aggregate number)$_{T90}$ − (sum of aggregate areas / aggregate number)$_{T0}$. Scale bar = 250 μm. (TIF 5261 kb)

Additional file 8: Figure S5. Cytoskeletal organization is altered in HeLa cells overexpressing mutant ADGRL2. Seventy two hours after transfection, HeLa cells were processed for histochemistry using phalloidin conjugates for F-actin labelling (red), alpha-tubulin antibody (green) and Hœscht as a nucleic acid stain (blue). a HeLa cells overexpressing the pcD-empty plasmid present predominant fusiform shapes with few focal contacts. b HeLa cells overexpressing Wt pcDCIRL-2 are characterized by spread out cytoplasms with numerous focal contacts (arrows). c HeLa cells overexpressing Mt. pcDCIRL-2 present very large and spread out cytoplasms with a very high density of focal contacts (arrows). (TIF 7878 kb)

Acknowledgements
We would like to thank Pr. Alexander Petrenko for the pcDCIRL-2 plasmid constructs and anti-CIRL-2 rat antibodies. We would also like to acknowledge Dr. Géraldine Joly-Helas and Dr. Pascal Chambon for providing control amniocyte culture cells.

Grants
Co-supported by European Union and Région Normandie. Europe is involved in Normandy through the European Regional Development Fund (ERDF).

Authors' contributions
MV performed NGS experiments and analysis and drafted the manuscript. MV and ML carried out molecular and cellular studies. MR and DV performed MRI study. VD and LR carried out in situ hybridization. LP and SO made possible the RES collection study. SC and IT belongs to NGS facilities. LT followed mother's pregnancy. HA made possible the fetuses' collection study. TF and BG are the team directors. BG participated to the design of the study and coordination and perfomed the statistical analysis. PSV and AL conceived the study and drafted the manuscript. All authors read and approved the final manuscript.

Competing interests
The authors declare that they have no competing interest.

Author details
[1]Normandie Univ, UNIROUEN, Inserm U1245, Normandy Centre for Genomic and Personalized Medicine, F 76000 Rouen, France. [2]Normandie Univ, UNICAEN, Inserm U1237, F 14000 Caen, France. [3]Rennes1 University, Faculty of Medicine, UMR6290 CNRS IGDR, F 35000 Rennes, France. [4]Department of Genetics, Rennes University Hospital, F 35000 Rennes, France. [5]Belvedere Hospital, Department of Genetics, F 76130 Mont-Saint-Aignan, France. [6]Lariboisière Hospital, APHP, Department of Pathology, F 75000 Paris, France. [7]Paris Diderot University, Sorbonne Paris Cité, PROTECT INSERM, F 75019 Paris, France. [8]Department of Genetics, Normandy Centre for Genomic and Personalized Medicine, Rouen University Hospital, F 76000 Rouen, France. [9]Department of Pathology, Rouen University Hospital, F 76000 Rouen, France.

References

1. Alkuraya FS, Cai X, Emery C, Mochida GH, Al-Dosari MS, Felie JM, Hill RS, Barry BJ, Partlow JN, Gascon GG, Kentab A, Jan M, Shaheen R, Feng Y, Walsh CA (2011) Human mutations in NDE1 cause extreme microcephaly with lissencephaly [corrected]. Am J Hum Genet 88:536–547. https://doi.org/10.1016/j.ajhg.2011.04.003

2. Anderson GR, Maxeiner S, Sando R, Tsetsenis T, Malenka RC, Südhof TC (2017) Postsynaptic adhesion GPCR latrophilin-2 mediates target recognition in entorhinal-hippocampal synapse assembly. J Cell Biol 216:3831–3846. https://doi.org/10.1083/jcb.201703042

3. Ashton AC, Rahman MA, Volynski KE, Manser C, Orlova EV, Matsushita H, Davletov BA, van Heel M, Grishin EV, Ushkaryov YA (2000) Tetramerisation of alpha-latrotoxin by divalent cations is responsible for toxin-induced non-vesicular release and contributes to the ca(2+)-dependent vesicular exocytosis from synaptosomes. Biochimie 82:453–468

4. Ashton AC, Volynski KE, Lelianova VG, Orlova EV, Van Renterghem C, Canepari M, Seagar M, Ushkaryov YA (2001) Alpha-Latrotoxin, acting via two Ca2+ –dependent pathways, triggers exocytosis of two pools of synaptic vesicles. J Biol Chem 276:44695–44703. https://doi.org/10.1074/jbc.M108088200

5. Bahi-Buisson N, Cavallin M (2016) Tubulinopathies overview. In: Adam MP, Ardinger HH, Pagon RA, Wallace SE, Bean LJ, Mefford HC, Stephens K, Amemiya A, Ledbetter N (eds) GeneReviews(®). University of Washington, Seattle

6. Bahi-Buisson N, Poirier K, Boddaert N, Fallet-Bianco C, Specchio N, Bertini E, Caglayan O, Lascelles K, Elie C, Rambaud J, Baulac M, An I, Dias P, des Portes V, Moutard ML, Soufflet C, El Maleh M, Beldjord C, Villard L, Chelly J (2010) GPR56-related bilateral frontoparietal polymicrogyria: further evidence for an overlap with the cobblestone complex. Brain J Neurol 133:3194–3209. https://doi.org/10.1093/brain/awq259

7. Bakircioglu M, Carvalho OP, Khurshid M, Cox JJ, Tuysuz B, Barak T, Yilmaz S, Caglayan O, Dincer A, Nicholas AK, Quarrell O, Springell K, Karbani G, Malik S, Gannon C, Sheridan E, Crosier M, Lisgo SN, Lindsay S, Bilguvar K, Gergely F, Gunel M, Woods CG (2011) The essential role of centrosomal NDE1 in human cerebral cortex neurogenesis. Am J Hum Genet 88:523–535. https://doi.org/10.1016/j.ajhg.2011.03.019

8. Barkovich AJ (2012) Developmental disorders of the midbrain and hindbrain. Front Neuroanat 6:7. https://doi.org/10.3389/fnana.2012.00007

9. Barkovich AJ, Guerrini R, Kuzniecky RI, Jackson GD, Dobyns WB (2012) A developmental and genetic classification for malformations of cortical development: update 2012. Brain J Neurol 135:1348–1369. https://doi.org/10.1093/brain/aws019

10. Bleasdale JE, Thakur NR, Gremban RS, Bundy GL, Fitzpatrick FA, Smith RJ, Bunting S (1990) Selective inhibition of receptor-coupled phospholipase C-dependent processes in human platelets and polymorphonuclear neutrophils. J Pharmacol Exp Ther 255:756–768

11. Boucard AA, Ko J, Südhof TC (2012) High affinity neurexin binding to cell adhesion G-protein-coupled receptor CIRL1/latrophilin-1 produces an intercellular adhesion complex. J Biol Chem 287:9399–9413. https://doi.org/10.1074/jbc.M111.318659

12. Boucard AA, Maxeiner S, Südhof TC (2014) Latrophilins function as heterophilic cell-adhesion molecules by binding to teneurins: regulation by alternative splicing. J Biol Chem 289:387–402. https://doi.org/10.1074/jbc.M113.504779

13. Cavallin M, Rujano MA, Bednarek N, Medina-Cano D, Bernabe Gelot A, Drunat S, Maillard C, Garfa-Traore M, Bole C, Nitschké P, Beneteau C, Besnard T, Cogné B, Eveillard M, Kuster A, Poirier K, Verloes A, Martinovic J, Bidat L, Rio M, Lyonnet S, Reilly ML, Boddaert N, Jenneson-Liver M, Motte J, Doco-Fenzy M, Chelly J, Attie-Bitach T, Simons M, Cantagrel V, Passemard S, Baffet A, Thomas S, Bahi-Buisson N (2017) WDR81 mutations cause extreme microcephaly and impair mitotic progression in human fibroblasts and Drosophila neural stem cells. Brain J Neurol 140:2597–2609. https://doi.org/10.1093/brain/awx218

14. Chakraborti S, Natarajan K, Curiel J, Janke C, Liu J (2016) The emerging role of the tubulin code: from the tubulin molecule to neuronal function and disease. Cytoskelet Hoboken NJ 73:521–550. https://doi.org/10.1002/cm.21290

15. Choi Y, Sims GE, Murphy S, Miller JR, Chan AP (2012) Predicting the functional effect of amino acid substitutions and indels. PLoS One 7:e46688. https://doi.org/10.1371/journal.pone.0046688

16. Coutant S, Cabot C, Lefebvre A, Léonard M, Prieur-Gaston E, Campion D, Lecroq T, Dauchel H (2012) EVA: exome variation analyzer, an efficient and versatile tool for filtering strategies in medical genomics. BMC Bioinformatics 13(Suppl 14):S9. https://doi.org/10.1186/1471-2105-13-S14-S9

17. Davletov BA, Shamotienko OG, Lelianova VG, Grishin EV, Ushkaryov YA (1996) Isolation and biochemical characterization of a Ca2+–independent alpha-latrotoxin-binding protein. J Biol Chem 271:23239–23245

18. De Pascalis C, Etienne-Manneville S (2017) Single and collective cell migration: the mechanics of adhesions. Mol Biol Cell 28:1833–1846. https://doi.org/10.1091/mbc.E17-03-0134

19. Démurger F, Pasquier L, Dubourg C, Dupé V, Gicquel I, Evain C, Ratié L, Jaillard S, Beri M, Leheup B, Lespinasse J, Martin-Coignard D, Mercier S, Quelin C, Loget P, Marcorelles P, Laquerrière A, Bendavid C, Odent S, David V (2013) Array-CGH analysis suggests genetic heterogeneity in Rhombencephalosynapsis. Mol Syndromol 4:267–272. https://doi.org/10.1159/000353878

20. Faheem M, Naseer MI, Rasool M, Chaudhary AG, Kumosani TA, Ilyas AM, Pushparaj P, Ahmed F, Algahtani HA, Al-Qahtani MH, Saleh Jamal H (2015) Molecular genetics of human primary microcephaly: an overview. BMC Med Genomics 8(Suppl 1):S4. https://doi.org/10.1186/1755-8794-8-S1-S4

21. Fallet-Bianco C, Laquerrière A, Poirier K, Razavi F, Guimiot F, Dias P, Loeuillet L, Lascelles K, Beldjord C, Carion N, Toussaint A, Revencu N, Addor MC, Lhermitte B, Gonzales M, Martinovich J, Bessieres B, Marcy-Bonnière M, Jossic F, Marcorelles P, Loget P, Chelly J, Bahi-Buisson N (2014) Mutations in tubulin genes are frequent causes of various foetal malformations of cortical development including microlissencephaly. Acta Neuropathol Commun 2:69. https://doi.org/10.1186/2051-5960-2-69

22. Guerrini R, Dobyns WB (2014) Malformations of cortical development: clinical features and genetic causes. Lancet Neurol 13:710–726. https://doi.org/10.1016/S1474-4422(14)70040-7

23. Guihard-Costa AM, Larroche JC (1990) Differential growth between the fetal brain and its infratentorial part. Early Hum Dev 23:27–40

24. Guihard-Costa AM, Ménez F, Delezoide AL (2002) Organ weights in human fetuses after formalin fixation: standards by gestational age and body weight. Pediatr Dev Pathol 5:559–578. https://doi.org/10.1007/s10024-002-0036-7

25. Haines BP, Wheldon LM, Summerbell D, Heath JK, Rigby PWJ (2006) Regulated expression of FLRT genes implies a functional role in the regulation of FGF signalling during mouse development. Dev Biol 297:14–25. https://doi.org/10.1016/j.ydbio.2006.04.004

26. Hamann J, Aust G, Araç D, Engel FB, Formstone C, Fredriksson R, Hall RA, Harty BL, Kirchhoff C, Knapp B, Krishnan A, Liebscher I, Lin HH, Martinelli DC, Monk KR, Peeters MC, Piao X, Prömel S, Schöneberg T, Schwartz TW, Singer K, Stacey M, Ushkaryov YA, Vallon M, Wolfrum U, Wright MW, Xu L, Langenhan T, Schiöth HB (2015) International Union of Basic and Clinical Pharmacology. XCIV. Adhesion G protein-coupled receptors. Pharmacol Rev 67:338–367. https://doi.org/10.1124/pr.114.009647

27. Hamburger V, Hamilton HL (1992) A series of normal stages in the development of the chick embryo. 1951. Dev Dyn 195:231–272

28. Harding BN, Moccia A, Drunat S, Soukarieh O, Tubeuf H, Chitty LS, Verloes A, Gressens P, El Ghouzzi V, Joriot S, Di Cunto F, Martins A, Passemard S, Bielas SL (2016) Mutations in citron kinase cause recessive Microlissencephaly with multinucleated neurons. Am J Hum Genet 99:511–520. https://doi.org/10.1016/j.ajhg.2016.07.003

29. Hedley DW, Friedlander ML, Taylor IW, Rugg CA, Musgrove EA (1983) Method for analysis of cellular DNA content of paraffin-embedded pathological material using flow cytometry. J Histochem Cytochem 31:1333–1335. https://doi.org/10.1177/31.11.6619538

30. Hlubek MD, Stuenkel EL, Krasnoperov VG, Petrenko AG, Holz RW (2000) Calcium-independent receptor for alpha-latrotoxin and neurexin 1alpha [corrected] facilitate toxin-induced channel formation: evidence that channel formation results from tethering of toxin to membrane. Mol Pharmacol 57:519–528

31. Ichtchenko K, Bittner MA, Krasnoperov V, Little AR, Chepurny O, Holz RW, Petrenko AG (1999) A novel ubiquitously expressed alpha-latrotoxin receptor is a member of the CIRL family of G-protein-coupled receptors. J Biol Chem 274:5491–5498

32. Ishak GE, Dempsey JC, Shaw DWW, Tully H, Adam MP, Sanchez-Lara PA, Glass I, Rue TC, Millen KJ, Dobyns WB, Doherty D (2012) Rhombencephalosynapsis: a hindbrain malformation associated with incomplete separation of midbrain and forebrain, hydrocephalus and a broad spectrum of severity. Brain 135:1370–1386. https://doi.org/10.1093/brain/aws065

33. Judkins AR, Martinez D, Ferreira P, Dobyns WB, Golden JA (2011) Polymicrogyria includes fusion of the molecular layer and decreased neuronal populations but normal cortical laminar organization. J Neuropathol Exp Neurol 70:438–443. https://doi.org/10.1097/NEN.0b013e31821ccf1c

34. Keeling JW (1989) Development of the human fetal brain: an anatomical atlas. A. Feess-Higgins and J.-C. Larroche, Masson, Paris, 1988. No. of pages:

200. Price: Ffr 350. ISBN: 285598 337. J Pathol 158:178–178. https://doi.org/10.1002/path.1711580219

35. Koirala S, Jin Z, Piao X, Corfas G (2009) GPR56-regulated granule cell adhesion is essential for rostral cerebellar development. J Neurosci 29:7439–7449. https://doi.org/10.1523/JNEUROSCI.1182-09.2009

36. Komuro H, Yacubova E (2003) Recent advances in cerebellar granule cell migration. Cell Mol Life Sci CMLS 60:1084–1098. https://doi.org/10.1007/s00018-003-2248-z

37. Komuro Y, Galas L, Lebon A, Raoult E, Fahrion JK, Tilot A, Kumada T, Ohno N, Vaudry D, Komuro H (2015) The role of calcium and cyclic nucleotide signaling in cerebellar granule cell migration under normal and pathological conditions. Dev Neurobiol 75:369–387. https://doi.org/10.1002/dneu.22219

38. Krasnoperov VG, Beavis R, Chepurny OG, Little AR, Plotnikov AN, Petrenko AG (1996) The calcium-independent receptor of alpha-latrotoxin is not a neurexin. Biochem Biophys Res Commun 227:868–875. https://doi.org/10.1006/bbrc.1996.1598

39. Krasnoperov VG, Bittner MA, Beavis R, Kuang Y, Salnikow KV, Chepurny OG, Little AR, Plotnikov AN, Wu D, Holz RW, Petrenko AG (1997) Alpha-Latrotoxin stimulates exocytosis by the interaction with a neuronal G-protein-coupled receptor. Neuron 18:925–937

40. Kumar P, Henikoff S, Ng PC (2009) Predicting the effects of coding non-synonymous variants on protein function using the SIFT algorithm. Nat Protoc 4:1073–1081. https://doi.org/10.1038/nprot.2009.86

41. Langenhan T, Prömel S, Mestek L, Esmaeili B, Waller-Evans H, Hennig C, Kohara Y, Avery L, Vakonakis I, Schnabel R, Russ AP (2009) Latrophilin signaling links anterior-posterior tissue polarity and oriented cell divisions in the C. elegans embryo. Dev Cell 17:494–504. https://doi.org/10.1016/j.devcel.2009.08.008

42. Lelianova VG, Davletov BA, Sterling A, Rahman MA, Grishin EV, Totty NF, Ushkaryov YA (1997) Alpha-latrotoxin receptor, latrophilin, is a novel member of the secretin family of G protein-coupled receptors. J Biol Chem 272:21504–21508

43. Leto K, Arancillo M, Becker EBE, Buffo A, Chiang C, Ding B, Dobyns WB, Dusart I, Haldipur P, Hatten ME, Hoshino M, Joyner AL, Kano M, Kilpatrick DL, Koibuchi N, Marino S, Martinez S, Millen KJ, Millner TO, Miyata T, Parmigiani E, Schilling K, Sekerková G, Sillitoe RV, Sotelo C, Uesaka N, Wefers A, Wingate RJT, Hawkes R (2016) Consensus Paper: Cerebellar Development. Cerebellum Lond Engl 15:789–828. https://doi.org/10.1007/s12311-015-0724-2

44. Liang CC, Park AY, Guan JL (2007) In vitro scratch assay: a convenient and inexpensive method for analysis of cell migration in vitro. Nat Protoc 2:329–333. https://doi.org/10.1038/nprot.2007.30

45. Liu G, Dwyer T (2014) Microtubule dynamics in axon guidance. Neurosci Bull 30:569–583. https://doi.org/10.1007/s12264-014-1444-6

46. Liu X, Sun T (2016) microRNAs and molecular pathogenesis of microcephaly. Curr Mol Pharmacol 9:300–304

47. Longenecker HE, Hurlbut WP, Mauro A, Clark AW (1970) Effects of black widow spider venom on the frog neuromuscular junction. Effects on end-plate potential, miniature end-plate potential and nerve terminal spike. Nature 225:701–703

48. Lu YC, Nazarko OV, Sando R, Salzman GS, Li NS, Südhof TC, Araç D (2015) Structural Basis of Latrophilin-FLRT-UNC5 interaction in cell adhesion. Struct Lond Engl 23:1678–1691. https://doi.org/10.1016/j.str.2015.06.024

49. Luo R, Jeong SJ, Jin Z, Strokes N, Li S, Piao X (2011) G protein-coupled receptor 56 and collagen III, a receptor-ligand pair, regulates cortical development and lamination. Proc Natl Acad Sci U S A 108:12925–12930. https://doi.org/10.1073/pnas.1104821108

50. Verloes A, Elmaleh M, Gonzales M, Laquerrière A, Gressens P (2007) Genetic and clinical aspects of lissencephaly. Rev Neurol (Paris) 163:533–547. https://doi.org/10.1016/S0035-3787(07)90460-9

51. Müller A, Winkler J, Fiedler F, Sastradihardja T, Binder C, Schnabel R, Kungel J, Rothemund S, Hennig C, Schöneberg T, Prömel S (2015) Oriented cell division in the C. elegans embryo is coordinated by G-protein signaling dependent on the adhesion GPCR LAT-1. PLoS Genet 11:e1005624. https://doi.org/10.1371/journal.pgen.1005624

52. Ng SB, Buckingham KJ, Lee C, Bigham AW, Tabor HK, Dent KM, Huff CD, Shannon PT, Jabs EW, Nickerson DA, Shendure J, Bamshad MJ (2010) Exome sequencing identifies the cause of a mendelian disorder. Nat Genet 42:30–35. https://doi.org/10.1038/ng.499

53. Nicolas G, Pottier C, Maltête D, Coutant S, Rovelet-Lecrux A, Legallic S, Rousseau S, Vaschalde Y, Guyant-Maréchal L, Augustin J, Martinaud O, Defebvre L, Krystkowiak P, Pariente J, Clanet M, Labauge P, Ayrignac X, Lefaucheur R, Le Ber I, Frébourg T, Hannequin D, Campion D (2013)

54. Mutation of the PDGFRB gene as a cause of idiopathic basal ganglia calcification. Neurology 80:181–187. https://doi.org/10.1212/WNL.0b013e31827ccf34

54. O'Sullivan ML, de Wit J, Savas JN, Comoletti D, Otto-Hitt S, Yates JR, Ghosh A (2012) FLRT proteins are endogenous latrophilin ligands and regulate excitatory synapse development. Neuron 73:903–910. https://doi.org/10.1016/j.neuron.2012.01.018

55. Obersteiner H (1914) Ein Kleinhirn ohne Wurm. Arb Neurol Inst Wien 21:124–126

56. Pasquier L, Marcorelles P, Loget P, Pelluard F, Carles D, Perez MJ, Bendavid C, de La Rochebrochard C, Ferry M, David V, Odent S, Laquerrière A (2009) Rhombencephalosynapsis and related anomalies: a neuropathological study of 40 fetal cases. Acta Neuropathol (Berl) 117:185–200. https://doi.org/10.1007/s00401-008-0469-9

57. Passemard S, Laquerrière A, Journiac N, Gressens P (2018) Microcephaly. Dev Neuropathol. https://doi.org/10.1002/9781119013112.ch4

58. Passemard S, Perez F, Colin-Lemesre E, Rasika S, Gressens P, El Ghouzzi V (2017) Golgi trafficking defects in postnatal microcephaly: the evidence for "Golgipathies". Prog Neurobiol 153:46–63. https://doi.org/10.1016/j.pneurobio.2017.03.007

59. Piao X, Hill RS, Bodell A, Chang BS, Basel-Vanagaite L, Straussberg R, Dobyns WB, Qasrawi B, Winter RM, Innes AM, Voit T, Ross ME, Michaud JL, Déscarie JC, Barkovich AJ, Walsh CA (2004) G protein-coupled receptor-dependent development of human frontal cortex. Science 303:2033–2036. https://doi.org/10.1126/science.1092780

60. Schwarz JM, Cooper DN, Schuelke M, Seelow D (2014) MutationTaster2: mutation prediction for the deep-sequencing age. Nat Methods 11:361–362. https://doi.org/10.1038/nmeth.2890

61. Sgaier SK, Millet S, Villanueva MP, Berenshteyn F, Song C, Joyner AL (2005) Morphogenetic and cellular movements that shape the mouse cerebellum; insights from genetic fate mapping. Neuron 45:27–40. https://doi.org/10.1016/j.neuron.2004.12.021

62. Sheng L, Leshchyns'ka I, Sytnyk V (2013) Cell adhesion and intracellular calcium signaling in neurons. Cell Commun Signal CCS 11:94. https://doi.org/10.1186/1478-811X-11-94

63. Silva JP, Lelianova VG, Ermolyuk YS, Vysokov N, Hitchen PG, Berninghausen O, Rahman MA, Zangrandi A, Fidalgo S, Tonevitsky AG, Dell A, Volynski KE, Ushkaryov YA (2011) Latrophilin 1 and its endogenous ligand lasso/teneurin-2 form a high-affinity transsynaptic receptor pair with signaling capabilities. Proc Natl Acad Sci U S A 108:12113–12118. https://doi.org/10.1073/pnas.1019434108

64. Silva JP, Suckling J, Ushkaryov Y (2009) Penelope's web: using alpha-latrotoxin to untangle the mysteries of exocytosis. J Neurochem 111:275–290. https://doi.org/10.1111/j.1471-4159.2009.06329.x

65. Silva JP, Ushkaryov YA (2010) The latrophilins, "split-personality" receptors. Adv Exp Med Biol 706:59–75

66. Srikanth S, Kim KD, Gwack Y (2014) Methods to measure cytoplasmic and mitochondrial ca(2+) concentration using ca(2+)-sensitive dyes. Methods Enzymol 543:1–20. https://doi.org/10.1016/B978-0-12-801329-8.00001-5

67. Sun T, Hevner RF (2014) Growth and folding of the mammalian cerebral cortex: from molecules to malformations. Nat Rev Neurosci 15:217–232. https://doi.org/10.1038/nrn3707

68. ten Donkelaar HJ, Lammens M, Wesseling P, Thijssen HOM, Renier WO (2003) Development and developmental disorders of the human cerebellum. J Neurol 250:1025–1036. https://doi.org/10.1007/s00415-003-0199-9

69. Ushkaryov YA, Rohou A, Sugita S (2008) alpha-Latrotoxin and its receptors. Handb Exp Pharmacol:171–206. https://doi.org/10.1007/978-3-540-74805-2_7

70. Vindeløv LL, Christensen IJ, Nissen NI (1983) A detergent-trypsin method for the preparation of nuclei for flow cytometric DNA analysis. Cytometry 3:323–327. https://doi.org/10.1002/cyto.990030503

71. Voccoli V, Tonazzini I, Signore G, Caleo M, Cecchini M (2014) Role of extracellular calcium and mitochondrial oxygen species in psychosine-induced oligodendrocyte cell death. Cell Death Dis 5:e1529. https://doi.org/10.1038/cddis.2014.483

72. Volynski KE, Silva JP, Lelianova VG, Atiqur Rahman M, Hopkins C, Ushkaryov YA (2004) Latrophilin fragments behave as independent proteins that associate and signal on binding of LTX(N4C). EMBO J 23:4423–4433. https://doi.org/10.1038/sj.emboj.7600443

73. Wollnik B (2010) A common mechanism for microcephaly. Nat Genet 42:923–924. https://doi.org/10.1038/ng1110-923

74. Zheng JQ, Poo MM (2007) Calcium signaling in neuronal motility. Annu Rev Cell Dev Biol 23:375–404. https://doi.org/10.1146/annurev.cellbio.23.090506.123221

6

Rapid dissemination of alpha-synuclein seeds through neural circuits in an in-vivo prion-like seeding experiment

Ayami Okuzumi[1], Masaru Kurosawa[2], Taku Hatano[1], Masashi Takanashi[3], Shuuko Nojiri[4], Takeshi Fukuhara[1], Tomoyuki Yamanaka[5], Haruko Miyazaki[5], Saki Yoshinaga[5], Yoshiaki Furukawa[6], Tomomi Shimogori[7], Nobutaka Hattori[1*] and Nobuyuki Nukina[1,5*] (iD)

Abstract

Accumulating evidence suggests that the lesions of Parkinson's disease (PD) expand due to transneuronal spreading of fibrils composed of misfolded alpha-synuclein (a-syn), over the course of 5–10 years. However, the precise mechanisms and the processes underlying the spread of these fibril seeds have not been clarified in vivo. Here, we investigated the speed of a-syn transmission, which has not been a focus of previous a-syn transmission experiments, and whether a-syn pathologies spread in a neural circuit–dependent manner in the mouse brain. We injected a-syn preformed fibrils (PFFs), which are seeds for the propagation of a-syn deposits, either before or after callosotomy, to disconnect bilateral hemispheric connections. In mice that underwent callosotomy before the injection, the propagation of a-syn pathology to the contralateral hemisphere was clearly reduced. In contrast, mice that underwent callosotomy 24 h after a-syn PFFs injection showed a-syn pathology similar to that seen in mice without callosotomy. These results suggest that a-syn seeds are rapidly disseminated through neuronal circuits immediately after seed injection, in a prion-like seeding experiment in vivo, although it is believed that clinical a-syn pathologies take years to spread throughout the brain. In addition, we found that botulinum toxin B blocked the transsynaptic transmission of a-syn seeds by specifically inactivating the synaptic vesicle fusion machinery. This study offers a novel concept regarding a-syn propagation, based on the Braak hypothesis, and also cautions that experimental transmission systems may be examining a unique type of transmission, which differs from the clinical disease state.

Keywords: Rapid dissemination, A-syn, Propagation, Callosotomy

Introduction

Parkinson's disease (PD) is one of the most common neurodegenerative disorders. The primary manifestations of PD consist of movement disturbances, such as bradykinesia, tremor, and rigidity [14], while the main cellular pathological features include neuronal degeneration along with inclusions called Lewy bodies (LBs), and neuronal loss in the substantia nigra (SN) [4]. The protein alpha-synuclein (a-syn), a major component of LBs and Lewy neurites, is deposited in a phosphorylated form. These a-syn deposits are also observed in dementia with Lewy body and in multiple system atrophy [15]. However,

the reason for the a-syn deposits to result in distinct disease phenotypes [16, 35] remains unclear.

Studies on PD brains reveal that a-syn pathologies spread to the brainstem from the olfactory bulb and the enteric vagus nerve during the first several years of the disease. As the disease progresses, the pathology spreads to other brain areas, over the course of 5–10 years [4, 5, 18]. Therefore, the intracerebral growth of a-syn pathologies is considered to be the underlying mechanism for disease progression, and the localization and abundance of a-syn deposits tend to correlate with the clinical symptoms. Consequently, a deeper understanding regarding the spread of a-syn deposits is needed, in order to clarify the mechanisms underlying disease progression. In recent years, both in vitro and in vivo studies have indicated that pathological a-syn spreads to adjacent cells and anatomically connected areas of the brain.

* Correspondence: nhattori@juntendo.ac.jp; nnukina@mail.doshisha.ac.jp
[1]Department of Neurology, Juntendo University Graduate School of Medicine, 2-1-1 Hongo, Bunkyo-ku, Tokyo 113-8421, Japan
Full list of author information is available at the end of the article

In addition, this spreading has been reported to occur in a prion-like manner, upon the injection of recombinant a-syn including monomers, oligomers, fibrils or insoluble a-syn derived from diseased brain, or spinal cord homogenates into the brain of a-syn overexpressing/wild-type rodents [17, 19, 25, 26, 28, 29, 33, 35, 40–42] or primate [37, 44] and also into the intestine wall of the stomach [19]. Another report has proposed the hypothesis that these seeds induce the conversion of endogenous a-syn to the abnormal form of a-syn and its deposition, although this has not been demonstrated in vivo [32].

This observation suggests that the synaptic connections between neurons may be involved in the spread of a-syn pathologies. However, this possibility needs to be investigated experimentally. Therefore, in this study, we used a neural disconnection approach in the mouse brain, in which either callosotomy or botulinum toxin B (BoNT/B) injection was performed before and after a-syn seeds injection to examine transmission speed, and the specific neural circuits through which a-syn pathologies spread. Although it is believed that clinical a-syn pathologies take years to spread throughout the brain, this study showed that seeds exhibit rapid dissemination throughout the brain via neural networks, within 24 h. This offers a novel concept to add to the existing discussion of disease progression in the brain, and also cautions that artificial experimental transmission systems may be examining a unique type of transmission, which differs from the clinical disease state.

To avoid confusion, we use the term "transmission" to refer to the intercellular transport of seeds or the cellular incorporation of exogenous seeds, and the term "propagation" to refer to the increase in misfolded a-syn induced by the seeds.

Materials and methods

Antibodies

The antibodies used in the study are listed in Additional file 1: Table S1.

Preparation of recombinant a-syn

His-tagged a-syn was expressed and purified using and Ni affinity resin. In the last step of the purification protocol, the His tag was eliminated. As a result, the a-syn protein used in this experiment had no tag attached. We removed the tag because it might affect propagation and aggregation. Both, human and mouse a-syn were used in the study. The *Escherichia coli* strain BL21 (DE3) was transformed with the expression vector pET15b, encoding wild type (WT) human or mouse a-syn. The expression of His-tagged a-syn proteins was induced by the addition of 0.5 mM isopropyl β-d-thiogalactoside at 37 °C for 3 h. Cells were lysed by ultrasonication in PBS containing 2%

Triton X-100, centrifuged at 20,000×g for 30 min. The supernatant thus obtained was loaded on a Ni Sepharose 6 Fast Flow column (1 mL, GE Healthcare). a-Syn was eluted with a buffer containing 50 mM Tris-HCl, 100 mM NaCl, and 250 mM imidazole, at pH 8.0. The eluted samples were concentrated by centrifugation at 3000×g for 15 min using Vivaspin Turbo (5 K MW) tubes (15 mL) with buffer containing 50 mM Tris-HCl and 100 mM NaCl, pH 8.0. Proteins were treated with thrombin (GE Healthcare) to remove the N-terminal His-tag.

Fibril formation

Purified a-syn monomers (100 μM, 150 μl) were incubated at 37 °C in a shaking incubator at 1200 rpm, in 50 mM Tris–HCl containing 100 mM NaCl (pH 8.0), for 5 days. Measurements at OD 600 (or other wavelengths) were used to check turbidity. After 5 days a-syn pre-formed fibrils (PFFs) were pelleted by spinning at 50,000×g for 20 min and suspended in PBS.

Animals

C57BL/6J mice were obtained from CLEA Japan, Inc. All breeding, housing, and experimental procedures were performed according to the guidelines for Animal Care of Juntendo University and approved by the Juntendo University Animal Care and Use Committee. Only male mice were used for this study.

Seeds injection

We sonicated a-syn PFFs before the intracerebral injection (using Bioruptor UC100-D2, TOS; 20 pulses; each pulse consisting of a 20-s 'ON' period and a 20-s 'OFF' period). Mice ranging between 2 to 3 months of age were anesthetized using an isoflurane/oxygen/nitrogen mixture and were unilaterally injected with 5 μg/2.5 μl of recombinant mouse or human a-syn PFFs into the right striatum (A-P: 0.2 mm; M-L + 2.3 mm; D-V: − 2.6 mm, from bregma) using a 10 μL Hamilton syringe at a rate of 0.1 μl per min. Control animals received sterile PBS. Mice were anesthetized with an isoflurane/oxygen/nitrogen mixture and killed by decapitation at various pre-determined time points (1 week, 0.75, 1.5, 3, and 6 months). For histological studies, mice were perfused with PBS followed by 4% paraformaldehyde (PFA) in PBS followed by overnight incubation of the tissue post-fixation, in either neutral buffered formalin (Fisher Scientific) or 70% ethanol before undergoing processing and embedding in paraffin.

Callosotomy

We used a surgical stitching needle (straight, 17-mm long), the tip of which was filed down with sandpaper. An incision was made from bregma, extending 3 mm anteriorly and 4 mm posteriorly, cutting in a continuous line perpendicular to the cerebral ventricle, with the needle at a depth of 3 mm. All incisions were made 0.4 mm to the left of bregma. The corpus callosum was severed either 1 day before or 1 day after the a-syn PFFs injection, and dissection was performed 1.5 months later.

Botulinum toxin B (BoNT/B) injection

BoNT/B was used in this study. NerBloc (rimabotulinumtoxin B) 2500 units/500 μL solution was purchased from Eisai. In total, 10 units/2 μL of BoNT/B was administered to the left striatum of each mouse, according to the stereotaxic surgical procedure described above (A-P: 0.2 mm, M-L: – 2.3 mm, D-V: – 2.6 mm from the bregma). BoNT/B was administered either 3 days prior to or 1 day after a-syn PFFs injection.

Tissue preparation

Mice were perfused with PBS, followed by 4% PFA in PBS. To prepare paraffin sections, brains were post-fixed, dehydrated, and embedded in paraffin wax. Sections of 5-μm thickness were cut with an HM430 sliding microtome (Leica).

Immunohistochemistry

Autoclaved paraffin sections were incubated with blocking solution containing 5% skim milk in TBST (20 mM Tris-HCl, pH 8.0, 150 mM NaCl, 0.05% Tween 20) for 1 h. Sections were incubated with the primary antibodies in TBST overnight at 4 °C, followed by the secondary antibodies. For diaminobenzidine (DAB) staining, sections were quenched with 3% H_2O_2/methanol for 30 min before blocking and incubated with the VECTASTAIN Elite ABC Kit reagent (Vector Laboratories) for 30 min after secondary antibody incubation. Color development ensued using 3,3′-diaminobenzidine/H_2O_2. For the immunofluorescent study, sections were incubated with appropriate fluorescent secondary antibodies conjugated with Alexa-Fluor 488 or 594 (Invitrogen). After washing, sections were mounted to coverslips with VECTASHIELD Mounting Medium (Vector Laboratories).

For human samples, formalin-fixed autopsied brains (midbrains) of two separate PD patients were provided by the neuropathologic library of Juntendo Neurology. Sections of 6-μm thickness were cut with an HM430 sliding microtome (Leica).

For human samples, before mounting with VECTA-SHIELD Mounting Medium, potential lipofuscin autofluorescence in the tissue sections was quenched using the TrueBlack Lipofuscin Autofluorescence Quencher (Biotium).

The Images were taken with a BIOREVO BZ-9000 and BZ-X700 (Keyence), TCS SP5 confocal microscope (Leica), and an inverted laser scanning confocal microscope (Zeiss LSM 880, Carl Zeiss), using a 63× oil immersion objective and the ZEN Software (Carl Zeiss). Care was taken to capture approximately similar regions in each comparative sample. For counting phosphorylated a-syn (p-syn) inclusions, whole-brain sections were imaged with a Keyence microscope (BZ-9000) using bright field capture. Multiple fields were captured using a 10× objective and stitched together using the Keyence Merge function. The p-syn - deposits per area were quantified using the BZ-9000 Generation II Analyzer (Keyence) Single Extraction function of the Hybrid Cell Count software, based on hue (details are described in Additional file 1: Figure S11).

Statistics

Sample sizes were determined on the basis of pilot experiments and previous data from similar experiments. To examine whether the samples had the same variances, we first analyzed them with an F-test. Data are presented as mean ± SEM. In Fig. 2b-f, 3d-f, 4c-d, the quantitative comparison of p-syn positive inclusions between the a-syn PFFs administered side (ips) and the contralateral side (contra) was analyzed using a paired t-test. In Fig. 2, the mixed effect model with contrast-based test was carried out to evaluate the significance of trends in time related response using the linear contrast. In Fig. 4b, analysis of covariance (ANCOVA) was conducted by adjusting for the area factor (ips, contra) to examine the time related response. For Fig. 5, we used an unpaired Student's t-test with Bonferroni correction ($^*p < 0.05$, $^{**}p < 0.01$, $^{***}p < 0.001$ and $^{****}p < 0.0001$). A p-value of < 0.05 was considered statistically significant.

Results

a-Syn PFF seeds are transported in both retrograde and anterograde directions

To elucidate whether the a-syn pathology spreads through neural circuits in the brain, recombinant mouse a-syn PFFs (Additional file 1: Figure S1) were injected as "seeds" into the right dorsal striatum of C57BL/6J mice. Immunohistological methods were then used to examine in detail the expansion of a-syn pathology in the mouse brains 6 months later. Cytoplasmic inclusions and neuritic inclusions (threads) were identified as phosphorylated a-syn (p-syn) accumulations using anti-phospho-alpha-synuclein antibody (anti-p-syn #64). These pathological accumulations were observed in the medium spiny neurons (MSNs) of the striatum, identified as DARPP-32-positive neurons (Fig. 1a). In addition, pathological p-syn accumulations were observed in the tyrosine hydroxylase (TH)-positive neurons of the substantia nigra pars compacta (SNpc), which project their axons into the striatum (Fig. 1b-c). Orthogonal projection studies identified an anti-p-syn#64-positive deposit (green) inside the DARPP-32-positive neuron or the TH-positive neuron (red) (Fig. 1a and Additional file 1: Figure S2), suggesting the presence of p-syn uptake in these cells. Thread-like deposits were detected not only in

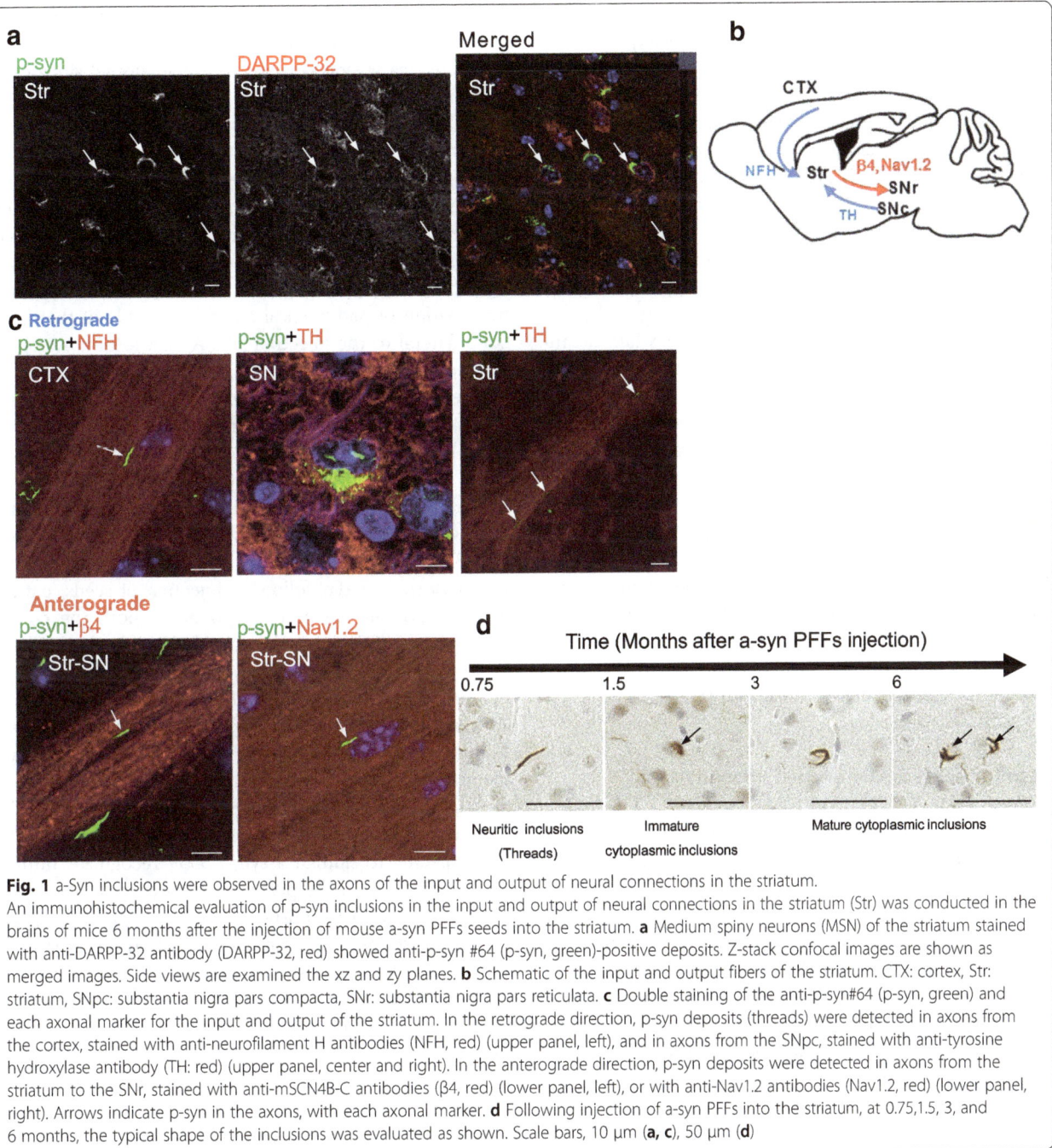

Fig. 1 a-Syn inclusions were observed in the axons of the input and output of neural connections in the striatum. An immunohistochemical evaluation of p-syn inclusions in the input and output of neural connections in the striatum (Str) was conducted in the brains of mice 6 months after the injection of mouse a-syn PFFs seeds into the striatum. **a** Medium spiny neurons (MSN) of the striatum stained with anti-DARPP-32 antibody (DARPP-32, red) showed anti-p-syn #64 (p-syn, green)-positive deposits. Z-stack confocal images are shown as merged images. Side views are examined the xz and zy planes. **b** Schematic of the input and output fibers of the striatum. CTX: cortex, Str: striatum, SNpc: substantia nigra pars compacta, SNr: substantia nigra pars reticulata. **c** Double staining of the anti-p-syn#64 (p-syn, green) and each axonal marker for the input and output of the striatum. In the retrograde direction, p-syn deposits (threads) were detected in axons from the cortex, stained with anti-neurofilament H antibodies (NFH, red) (upper panel, left), and in axons from the SNpc, stained with anti-tyrosine hydroxylase antibody (TH: red) (upper panel, center and right). In the anterograde direction, p-syn deposits were detected in axons from the striatum to the SNr, stained with anti-mSCN4B-C antibodies (β4, red) (lower panel, left), or with anti-Nav1.2 antibodies (Nav1.2, red) (lower panel, right). Arrows indicate p-syn in the axons, with each axonal marker. **d** Following injection of a-syn PFFs into the striatum, at 0.75,1.5, 3, and 6 months, the typical shape of the inclusions was evaluated as shown. Scale bars, 10 μm (**a, c**), 50 μm (**d**)

TH-positive axons but also in sodium channel β4 subunit (β4)-positive [30] or sodium channel, voltage-gated, type II (Nav1.2)-positive axons, which project to the globus pallidus or substantia nigra pars reticulata (SNr) from the striatum, as well as in the neurofilament H-positive axons that project to the striatum from the cortex (Fig. 1b-c). Images from the orthogonal projection demonstrate the localization of p-syn in axonal projections. Additionally, the anti-p-syn#64-positive deposits (green) located in apposition to each axonal marker (red). These results strongly suggest that p-syn forms aggregated or was transported in those axons.

Next, to evaluate how the size of a-syn deposits changed over time, we performed a chronological analysis at 0.75, 1.5, 3, and 6 months following injection with mouse a-syn PFFs. The a-syn deposits propagated gradually following injection, and they developed from thread-like or faint cytoplasm deposits, at 0.75 months, to concentrated, perinuclear tangle-like inclusions (hereafter called cytoplasmic inclusions) at 3 to 6 months (Fig. 1d). The formation and distribution of these inclusions following injection with a-syn seeds are displayed chronologically in histograms (Additional file 1: Figure S3). There was a tendency for the aggregates to be larger and more numerous in the a-syn PFFs-injected (ipsilateral) side compared with those in the contralateral side, which consisted of many smaller-sized inclusions, such as threads. However, the largest inclusions on each side of the brain were almost the same size (Additional file 1: Figure S3). It is possible that a-syn deposits gradually increase in size (propagate) at each transmitted (disseminated) site. In contrast to the injection of a-syn seeds, no pathological a-syn inclusions were found at any sites at any point in time, when the injection consisted of phosphate-buffered saline (PBS) alone, as a negative control (Additional file 1: Figure S4).

Double staining with glial cell markers and anti-p-syn#64 were conducted to investigate whether there was an uptake of a-syn seeds by other cell types, in addition to neurons (Additional file 1: Figure S5). The localization of p-syn (green) within iba-1 (red) positive cells was also observed, although this occurred infrequently. This too was confirmed through orthogonal projection. Although infrequent, double staining with antibodies against the oligodendrocyte marker GST-pi and p-syn revealed p-syn deposits in some oligodendrocytes of the white matter. In contrast, anti-GFAP staining showed that astrocytes did not have any p-syn inclusions.

a-Syn PFF seeds are transmitted through neural connections

The distribution of a-syn inclusions at 6 months post-injection is illustrated in Fig. 2a. Accumulation of a-syn was seen in regions with both direct and indirect connections to the injected striatum (Fig. 2a).Time-dependent propagation of pathological a-syn was detected between 0.75 and 6 months (Fig. 2b-f, Additional file 1: Figure S6). The mixed effect model with contrast-based testing was carried out to evaluate the significance of trends in time related to response using the linear contrast. Significant trends in time related to response were observed in striatum, cortex, substantia nigra (SN) and entorhinal cortex (EC), and the amygdala (Amyg). The accumulation of pathological a-syn spread from the injected site to the ipsilateral cortex, contralateral cortex (Fig. 2c), contralateral striatum (Fig. 2b), ipsilateral and contralateral Amyg (Fig. 2f), and ipsilateral SN (Fig. 2d); with the contralateral striatum and contralateral SN demonstrating delayed accumulation. In addition, despite the lack of a direct fiber connection to the striatum, accumulation of pathological a-syn was also detected in the EC (Fig. 2e), which has direct connections to the Amyg and cortex. On the side contralateral to the injection, propagation of a syn deposits was detected in a time-dependent manner, between 0.75 and 6 months. In the striatum (Fig. 2b), SN (Fig. 2d), and Amyg (Fig. 2f), the total

area of pathological a-syn accumulation tended to be small, in the side contralateral to the injection. These regions are connected via several synapses from the injected side of the striatum.

Callosotomy inhibited propagation of a-syn deposits in the contralateral side

Further, to examine whether transmission of a-syn seeds occurred through specific neural circuits, we investigated the impact of disrupting neural circuits (by callosotomy) (Additional file 1: Figure S7) on the transmission and propagation of pathological a-syn in the side of the brain contralateral to the injection site. A callosotomy was performed either 1 day before or 1 day after the injection of mouse a-syn PFFs into the right striatum (Fig. 3b-c and e-f). Compared to the mice in which mouse a-syn PFFs were injected without callosotomy (Fig. 3a, d), mice that received callosotomy before the injection showed a clear reduction in the transmission and propagation of pathological a-syn to the contralateral side (Fig. 3b, e). In contrast, in the mice in which callosotomy was performed 1 day following injection of seeds, pathological a-syn propagation was found in both the cortex and striatum of the contralateral side (Fig. 3c, f).

Extrinsic seeds first moved to the contralateral side within 24 h and then gradually propagated to form aggregates

To detect exogenous a-syn seeds directly and differentiate them from a-syn deposits produced from the endogenous protein, human a-syn PFFs were injected as seeds into the right dorsal striatum and detected with LB509, an antibody specific to human a-syn. LB509 recognizes human a-syn, regardless of the presence or absence of phosphorylation. In contrast, anti-p-syn antibody (phospho S129, Abcam), also used in this experiment, recognizes both mouse and human phosphorylated a-syn. Therefore, p-syn deposits were determined to be mouse-derived when they were recognized by this anti-p-syn antibody (phospho S129) but not by LB509 (Fig. 4a, Additional file 1: Figure S8). Our results indicate that the exogenous human a-syn PFFs were detected only by LB509 at 3 and 6 weeks (0.75 and 1.5 months), at which times no staining with the anti-p-syn antibody was detected (phospho S129) (Fig. 4a). Sections of SN from autopsied brains of patients with PD were double stained with two antibodies, LB509 and phospho S129. Stained Lewy bodies were detected by both LB509 and phospho S129 and were colocalized. (Additional file 1: Figure S8). Mouse-derived pathological p-syn accumulations were observed gradually following the seed injection (Fig. 4a-b). Human a-syn seed accumulations were found in the same areas where inclusions were observed after mouse a-syn PFFs were injected, but these visible human a-syn inclusions disappeared after 12 weeks (Fig. 4b). From 3 weeks after injection, pathological

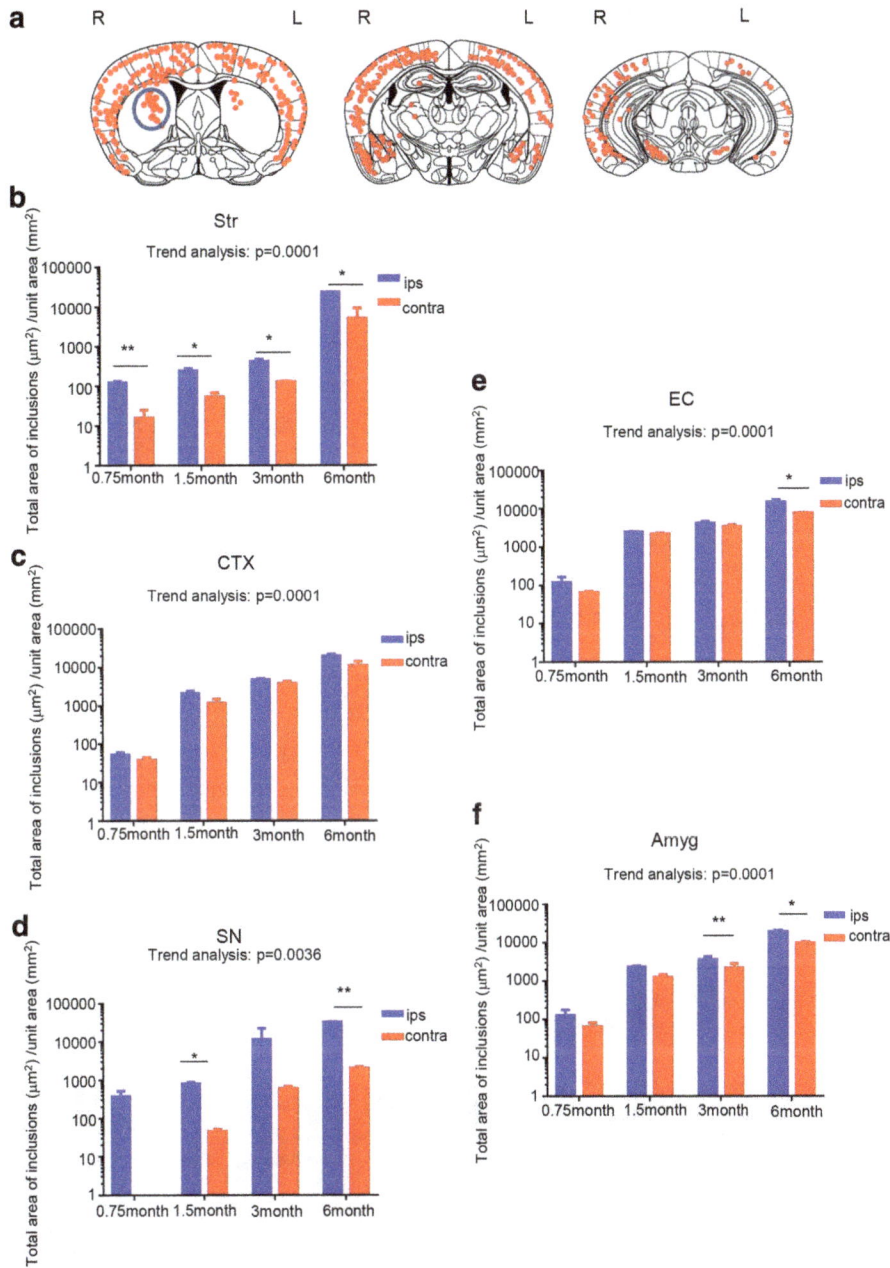

Fig. 2 P-syn inclusions were found in neural systems directly or indirectly connected with the striatum where a-syn seeds were injected. **a** Distribution of p-syn pathology in a-syn PFFs-injected mouse brain 6 months after injection. Red dots indicate neuritic inclusions (threads) or cytoplasmic inclusions. Blue circles indicate the injection site in the striatum. L = left hemisphere of the brain; R = right hemisphere. (**b-f**) Total area of the p-syn-positive inclusions (deposits) quantified chronologically at 0.75, 1.5, 3, and 6 months for each region (Str, CTX, SN, EC, and Amyg) of the brain. Horizontal axis: Time following a-syn PFFs injection; vertical axis: Total area of p-syn-positive inclusions (μm^2) per unit area (mm^2). **b** Str (0.75 month $p = 0.0062$, 1.5 month $p = 0.031$, 3 month $p = 0.0413$, 6 month $p = 0.0117$), **c** CTX, **d** SN (1.5 month $p = 0.0122$, 6 month $p = 0.0013$), **e** EC (6 month $p = 0.0235$), and **f** Amyg 3 month $p = 0.0025$, 6 month $p = 0.0189$. Mixed effect model with contrast-based testing: Fig. 2b $p < 0.0001$, Fig. 2c $p < 0.0001$, Fig. 2d $p < 0.0001$, Fig. 2e $p < 0.0001$, Fig. 2f $p < 0.0001$. Data is represented as mean area per region ± SEM, $n = 5$ mice per group. Paired t-test and the mixed effect model with contrast-based test was carried out to evaluate the significance of trends in time related response using the linear contrast; *$p < 0.05$, **$p < 0.01$. Str, striatum; CTX, cortex; SN, substantia nigra; EC, entorhinal cortex; Amyg, amygdala

mouse p-syn deposits were detected and increased subsequently in the areas where human a-syn seeds spread (Fig. 4b). ANCOVA was conducted to examine time related response, and significant differences were observed in the number of a-syn inclusions in striatum, cortex, SN, EC, and Amyg (Fig. 4b). Further, we examined the effects of callosotomy on the transmission of human a-syn PFF seeds and the

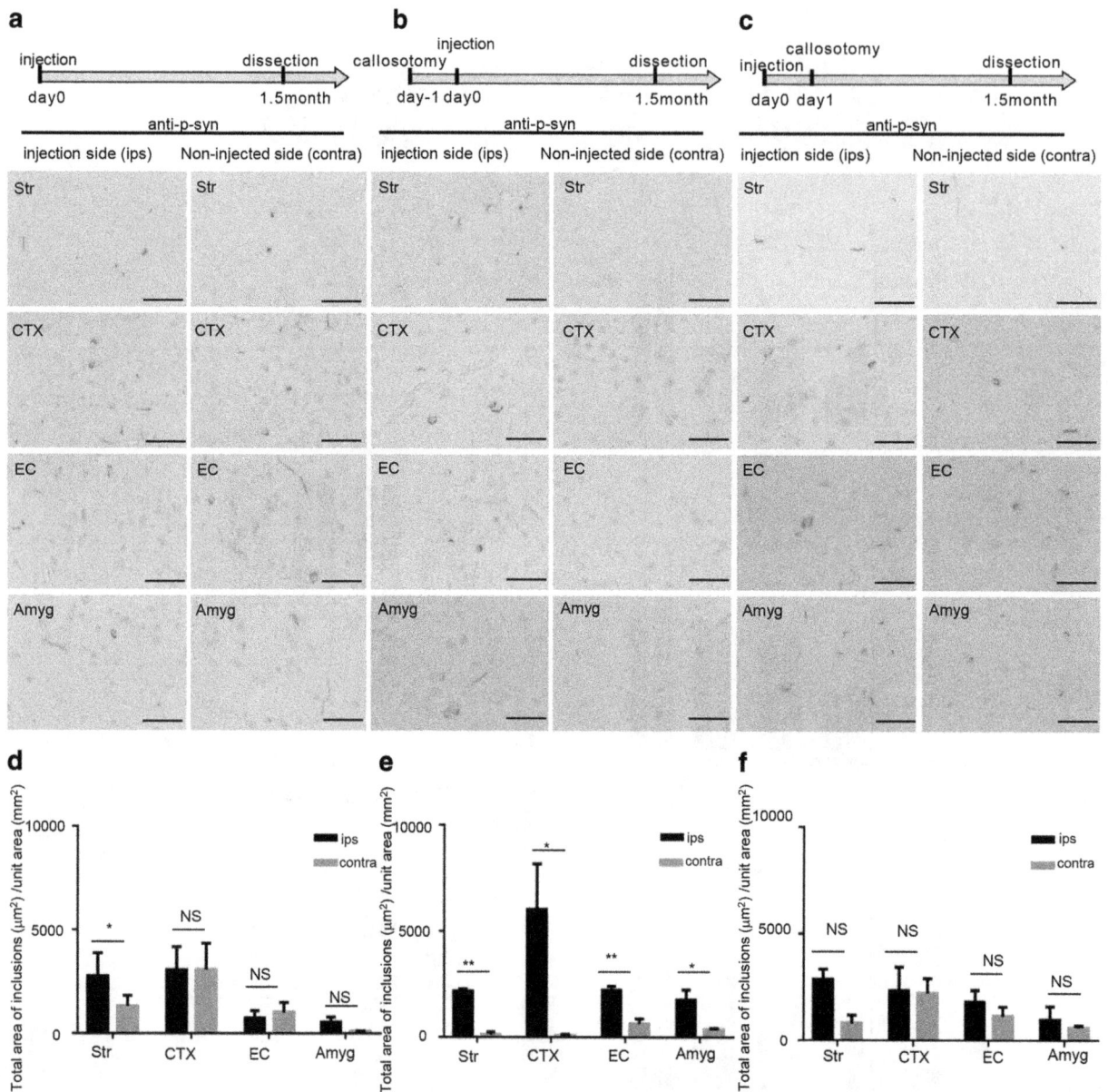

Fig. 3 The propagation of a-syn deposits in the contralateral hemisphere was reduced after callosotomy. Callosotomy was conducted 1 day before or 1 day after injection with mouse a-syn PFFs. As a control, a-syn PFFs were injected into mice without callosotomy. (**a-c**)Schematic representation of the experimental protocol and p-syn deposits detected with anti-p-syn#64. Scale bars, 50 μm. (**a, d**) Injection with a-syn PFFs only (no callosotomy) (Str $p = 0.0171$). (**b, e**) Callosotomy 1 day before injection with a-syn PFFs (Str $p = 0.0098$, CTX $p = 0.0205$, EC $p = 0.0025$, Amyg $p = 0.0476$). (**c, f**) Callosotomy 1 day after injection with a-syn PFFs. (**d-f**) The total area of p-syn-positive inclusions (deposits) was quantified for each region (Str, CTX, EC, Amyg) of the brain. Horizontal axis: Brain region; Vertical axis: Total area of p-syn-positive inclusions (μm²) per unit area (mm²). Data is represented as mean area per region ± SEM, $n = 5$ mice per group, paired t-test; *$p < 0.05$; **$p < 0.01$. Str: striatum, CTX: cortex, EC: entorhinal cortex, Amyg: amygdala

propagation of mouse a-syn deposits. Callosotomy of the mouse brains was conducted 1 day before or 1 day after injection with human a-syn PFFs, and dissection was performed 3 weeks afterward. When the callosotomy was performed prior to injection of human a-syn seeds, significantly less human a-syn deposits were found in the striatum, cortex, and EC on the contralateral side, and the

accumulation of mouse pathological p-syn was significantly reduced in these areas, as well (Fig. 4c). In contrast, when the callosotomy was performed after human a-syn seeds were injected, human a-syn seeds were found to have transmitted and formed visible inclusions in the contralateral hemisphere, and the accumulation of mouse pathological p-syn was also detected (Fig .4d).

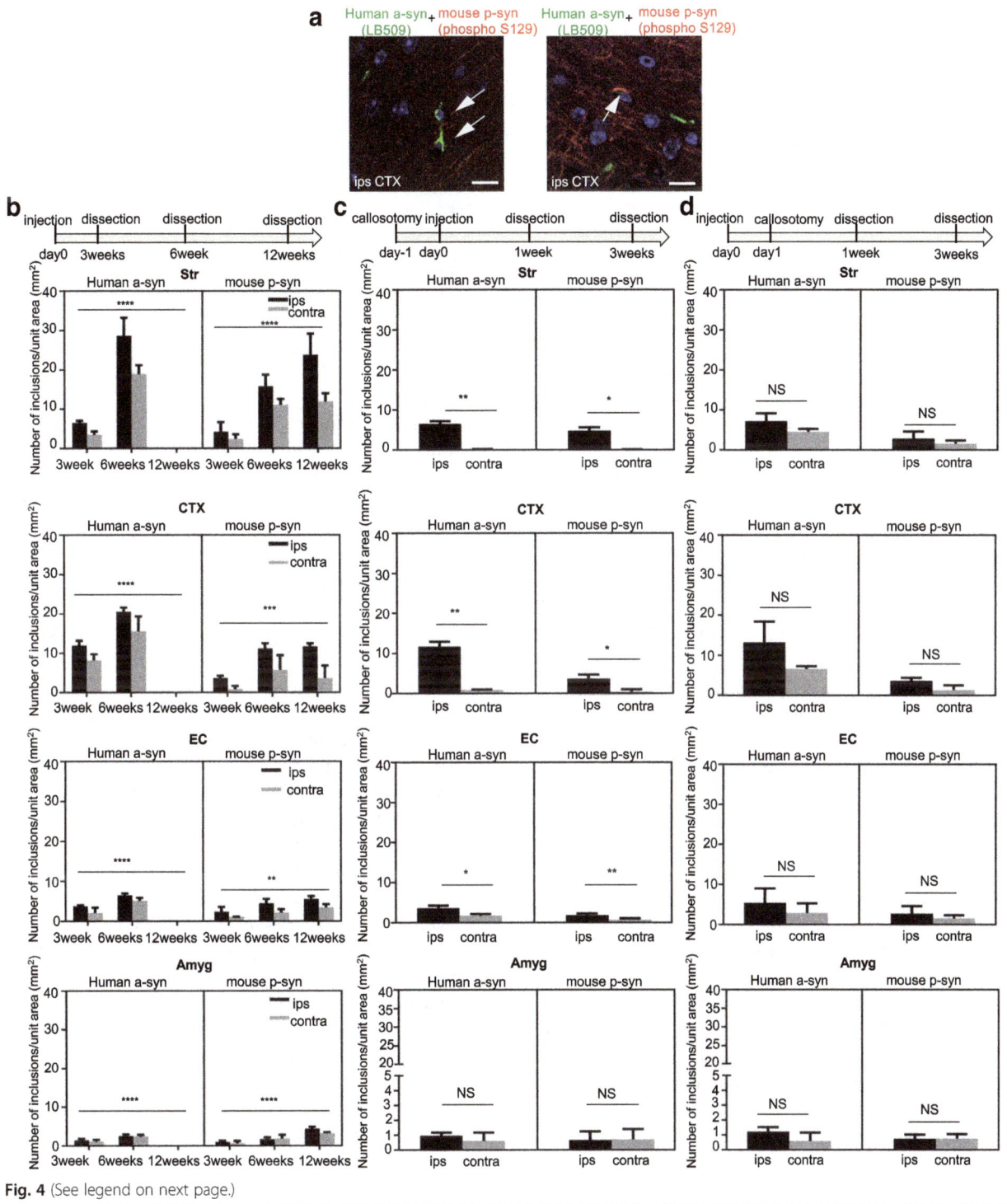

Fig. 4 (See legend on next page.)

(See figure on previous page.)

Fig. 4 Extrinsic a-syn seeds were transmitted to the contralateral side within 24 h. **a** Mouse brains were stained with human a-syn-specific antibody LB509 (green) and anti-p-syn antibody (phospho S129) (red). Scale bars, 10 μm. **b** The number of human a-syn (left panels) and mouse a-syn (right panels) inclusions after human a-syn PFFs injection was quantified chronologically in each region of the brain: Str (Human a-syn $p < 0.0001$, mouse p-syn $p < 0.0001$), CTX (Human a-syn $p < 0.0001$, mouse p-syn $p = 0.0008$), EC (Human a-syn $p < 0.0001$, mouse p-syn $p = 0.0014$), and Amyg (Human a-syn $p < 0.0001$, mouse p-syn $p < 0.0001$). Data is represented as mean number of a-syn inclusions per region ± SEM, $n = 5$ mice per group, analysis of covariance (ANCOVA) was conducted to adjust area factor (ips, contra) to examine time related response. **c** Callosotomy 1 day before injection with human a-syn PFFs. **d** Callosotomy 1 day after injection with human a-syn PFFs. (**c, d**) The number of human a-syn (left panels) and mouse p-syn (right panels) inclusions (deposits) was quantified chronologically in each region (Str Human a-syn $p = 0.0024$, mouse p-syn $p = 0.0114$, CTX Human a-syn $p = 0.0040$, mouse p-syn $p = 0.0484$, EC Human a-syn $p = 0.0216$, mouse p-syn $p = 0.0015$, Amyg) of the brain. Horizontal axis: Time after human a-syn PFFs injection; Vertical axis: Number of a-syn inclusions/unit area (mm^2). Data are the mean number of a-syn inclusions per region ± SEM, $n = 5$ mice per group, paired t-test for mouse and human a-syn at 3 weeks in CTX, Str, EC and Amyg for **c** and **d**. *$p < 0.05$,**$p < 0.01$,***$p < 0.001$, ****$p < 0.0001$. Str: striatum, CTX: cortex, EC: entorhinal cortex, Amyg: amygdala

Inhibition of synaptic vesicle fusion blocks the transmission of a-syn seeds

Thus far, our results appear to support the hypothesis that a-syn seeds are transmitted via synapses, and that synaptic machinery may be involved in neuron-to-neuron transmission. We used botulinum toxin (BoNT) to determine whether the transmission of a-syn seeds was dependent upon synaptic vesicle fusion. BoNT is a sequence-specific endoprotease with precise specificity for its molecular targets, and there are no known off-target interactions. BoNT degrades unique structural factors in the synapse vesicle docking and fusion complex SNARE, which is necessary for the release of neurotransmitters that catalyze membrane fusion. We specifically used BoNT/B, which degrades and deactivates VAMP-2 [19, 26].

BoNT/B was injected into the left (contralateral to the seeds injection site) dorsal striatum, either 3 days prior to, or 1 day after, injection with mouse a-syn PFFs. We evaluated the propagation of p-syn deposits 1.5 months later by immunohistochemistry. Physiological saline was used as a control for the BoNT/B injection. Pathological p-syn deposits in axons (threads) and intracellular p-syn deposits (cytoplasmic inclusions) were quantified separately. When BoNT/B was injected 3 days before the mouse a-syn PFFs injection, we observed that the pathological p-syn accumulation significantly declined in the striatum, Amyg, and EC of the BoNT/B-injected side, compared with control (Fig. 5a,b and Additional file 1: Figure S9). In particular, in the striatum and Amyg, thread-like p-syn deposits decreased (Fig. 5a). A marked reduction in the cytoplasmic inclusions was also observed in striatum and Amyg, as well as EC, which is connected to Amyg (Fig. 5b). In contrast, when BoNT/B was injected 1 day after injection of a-syn seeds, no reduction in a-syn accumulation was observed, similar to what was seen in the control group, injected with physiological saline (Fig. 5c, d). Thus, transmission of a-syn seeds was blocked by BoNT/B, thus our results further confirm that a-syn seeds transmission occurs via synaptic connections.

Discussion

Accumulating evidence indicates that misfolded protein pathologies can spread throughout the nervous system in a prion-like fashion [2, 17]. It appears that neuronal connections are more important than physical distance for the propagation of a-syn deposits among brain regions. The hypothesis that synaptic transmission of a-syn seeds is responsible for the stepwise expansion of Lewy lesions has been proposed.

In the previous reports, this hypothesis has been discussed from a neuropathological point of view, which stipulated that a-syn accumulation only occurs in the regions where anatomical neural connections exist [4, 17, 19, 25, 28, 29, 33, 40, 41, 49]. Holmqvist et al. have reported that a-syn propagated to the brain stem through the vagus nerve from the intestinal tract [19]. Rey et al. reported that monomers and oligomers of human a-syn injected into the olfactory bulb of mice were transported along the axonal pathways within a few hours [40]. Furthermore, Peelaerts et al. observed that dopaminergic neurons take in all types of a-syn including oligomers, fibrils and ribbons to complete the trans-synaptic transportation [35].In this study, we used callosotomy, a different experimental method from the previous reports, to investigate whether a-syn seeds are specifically transmitted across neural connections, and we experimentally demonstrated the speed of a-syn transmission.

First, in order to confirm the direction of a-syn seeds axonal transport and propagation, we analyzed the accumulation of p-syn in the input and output fibers of the striatum, into which the a-syn seeds were injected. We confirmed that injected a-syn seeds were incorporated into the MSNs of the striatum, to which the a-syn PFFs were administered, and showed the formation of p-syn inclusion bodies. In the neurofilament H-positive axons projecting from the cortex into the striatum, TH-positive axons projecting from neurons in the SNpc, as well as β4- or Nav 1.2-positive fibers projecting from the striatum to the globus pallidus and SNr, thread-like inclusion

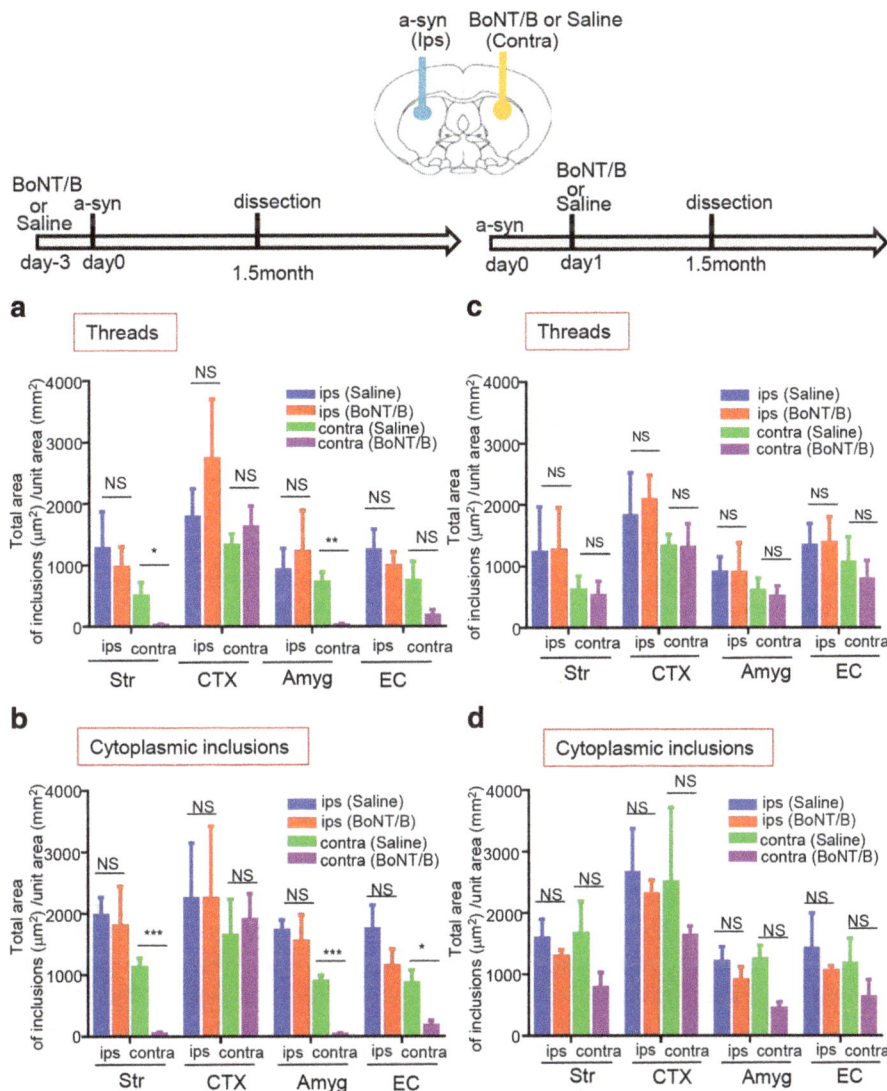

Fig. 5 BoNT/B injection into the contralateral side of the seeds injection reduced the propagation of a-syn in the connected areas. Top: Schematic view of the injection sites and the experimental procedures. Injection with BoNT/B to the contralateral side of the seeds injection was conducted 3 days before or 1 day after injection with mouse a-syn PFFs. As a control, physiological saline was administered instead of BoNT/B 3 days before or 1 day after injection of mouse a-syn PFFs. The mice were dissected 1.5 months later. (a, b) Injection with saline or BoNT/B 3 days before injection with mouse a-syn PFFs. a: Threads (Str $p = 0.0468$, Amyg $p = 0.0025$) b: Cytoplasmic inclusions (Str $p = 0.0002$, Amyg $p = 0.0002$, EC $p = 0.0101$). (c, d) Injection with saline or BoNT/B 1 day after injection with mouse a-syn PFFs. (a–d) The total area of p-syn-positive inclusions (deposits) was quantified for each region (Str, CTX, EC, Amyg) of the brain. Ips: mouse a-syn PFFs injection side, contra: the contralateral side to the mouse a-syn PFFs injection side. Horizontal axis: Brain region; Vertical axis: Total area of p-syn-positive inclusions (μm^2)/unit area (mm^2). The p-syn-positive were divided into neuritic inclusions (threads) and cytoplasmic inclusions, and quantified separately. $n = 5$ mice per group, unpaired t-test with Student's correction and Bonferroni correction (significance level $0.05/2 = 0.025$); Data are the mean area per region ± SEM; $*p < 0.05$, $**p < 0.01$, $***p < 0.001$. Str: striatum, CTX: cortex, Amyg: amygdala, EC: entorhinal cortex

bodies were detected by anti-p-syn antibody. These results strongly suggest that bidirectional (anterograde and retrograde) transport of seeds occurs in axons from the striatal MSNs, or axons projecting into striatum (Fig. 1a-c).

In our experiments, there were no p-syn inclusions observed inside astrocytes in any of the images. Loria et al. demonstrated that astrocytes degrade a-syn immediately after uptake [23]. Thus it may have been difficult to detect astrocytic p-syn inclusions in the images, obtained at a single time point. In addition, the ability of neurons to degrade a-syn may be lower than that of astrocytes. This presumably indicates that a-syn tends to be accumulated by neurons.

We analyzed the propagation of pathological a-syn over time after the injection of a-syn PFFs into the right striatum. The results showed that accumulation of pathological a-syn tended to increase over time. We observed spreading in the contralateral striatum and in regions connected to the striatum through multiple synapses, such as the contralateral striatum and SN, although the amount of spreading decreased. These data suggest that the transmission of a-syn amounts depended on connectivity. Paumier et al. reported a reduction of the a-syn pathology in SNpc within 180 days after administration of the a-syn fibrils, based on the observation of neuron degeneration [33]. Similarly, Rey et al. observed that the density of the pathology as a whole in the brain tends to decrease over the longer term after administration of the a-syn PFFs [39]. In the present study, brains of mice were analyzed over a period ranging from 0.75 months to 6 months after administration of a-syn PFFs, the p-syn positive deposits in the SN increased within 6 months. The difference could likely be attributed to factors such as the adjustment of synthetic recombinant a-syn. However further longer-term observation is warranted to assess this hypothesis.

Moreover, analysis of the areas and quantities of individual p-syn deposits over time revealed the size of each p-syn deposit to be larger on ipsilateral side as compared to the contralateral side. However, the maximum size of the deposits was equivalent on both sides (Additional file 1: Figure S3). These results suggest that the injected a-syn PFFs initially spread to each area as seeds and formed inclusions over time by recruiting endogenous a-syn. P-syn accumulation in the ipsilateral cortex is the most frequent, and transmission to the striatum and contralateral SN to the site of a-syn PFFs administration tended to be less frequent. This is presumably because the transmission of seeds via multiple synapses is required to reach the striatum and SN on the contralateral side, and the number of seeds declines during transmission.

We further confirmed that a-syn seeds are transmitted through neural circuits using callosotomy (Fig. 3). We designed an experiment using callosotomy to determine whether nerve fiber disconnection inhibits a-syn propagation, in a neural circuit-dependent manner. When callosotomy disconnected the contralateral side from the injected side before the injection of a-syn seeds, the transmission and propagation of pathological a-syn to the contralateral side substantially decreased. This is likely because the delivery of the a-syn seeds to the contralateral side was blocked by severing the axons of the corpus callosum. From this result, we confirmed that the seeds were transported along the path of the nerves. Some propagation of p-syn deposits in the limbic system (EC and Amyg), including routes other than the corpus callosum, such as hippocampal traffic and the anterior commissure, also seem likely to be involved [8], however, the decreased p-syn deposits in these regions

after callosotomy suggest that the transmission through the striatum may affect the results through the striatum-Amyg and Amyg-EC connection. In contrast, when the callosotomy was performed 24 h after injection of the a-syn seeds, p-syn accumulated in the contralateral side in a similar fashion as in the control (without callosotomy). This result suggests that exogenous seed migration occurs within a 24-h period.

We also examined the dynamics of the seeds transmission itself. Human a-syn PFFs can be differentiated from mouse a-syn PFFs by the human a-syn-specific antibody LB509 (Fig. 4a). Exogenous human a-syn PFFs injected into the right striatum spread to the contralateral side, in the cortex, striatum, Amyg, and EC, forming visible aggregates (inclusions) 3 weeks (0.75 months) after injection. However, 12 weeks after seed administration, the exogenous human a-syn deposits were no longer detected. Meanwhile, endogenous mouse a-syn inclusions began to appear (Fig. 4b). These results suggest that exogenous human seeds interact with each other and bind other human seeds more rapidly than they convert endogenous mouse a-syn to the misfolded form, due to conformational and species-specific sequence differences (Additional file 1: Figure S10).

The administration of human a-syn PFFs resulted in a slower and reduced formation of a-syn inclusions compared with the administration of mouse a-syn PFFs. This observation has been previously reported [41]. As suggested in previous studies, the species barrier may be the reason for this effect [6]. This observation was also noted by Rey et al. [41]. Further, Luk et al. proposed that the seeding efficiency on a molecular level is determined by the sequence homology of the a-syn PFF seeds and the soluble a-syn monomer, and the result of the present study which showed delayed propagation ability when human a-syn PFFs was administered to mice is also consistent with this proposal [24]. In the present study, the human a-syn deposit itself was undetectable 3 months after seeds administration. We suppose that the majority of exogenous seeds were degraded when the human a-syn deposits disappeared. The later disappearance of human a-syn deposits was also confirmed by the previous studies [2, 3, 24, 29, 39, 41]. Rey et al. stated [39] that this elimination could be due to the degeneration of cells itself, or degradation caused by the autophagy/lysosomal, ubiquitin-proteasome systems [48], or phagocytosis by microglia [7] or astrocytes [23].

Interestingly, the exogenous seeds were not phosphorylated, while the endogenous a-syn aggregates were phosphorylated, suggesting that the exogenous seeds are not phosphorylated inside the cell and can recruit and convert endogenous p-syn more easily than the non-phosphorylated form. Sections of SN from autopsied brains of patients with Parkinson's disease were double stained with two antibodies, LB509 and phospho S129. Stained Lewy bodies were detected by both LB509 and phospho S129 and were colocalized. Thus, it was inferred that these antibodies did not compete for their epitopes, and this confirmed that the human a-syn PFFs was not phosphorylated. We also examined the spread of the seeds themselves and their speed using callosotomy with the administration of human a-syn PFFs (Fig. 4c, d). When the callosotomy was performed prior to the administration of human a-syn PFFs, transmission to the contralateral side decreased and the emergence of mouse p-syn deposits also decreased. When the callosotomy was conducted 1 day after the injection of human a-syn PFFs, transmission of human a-syn to the contralateral side was observed, and the emergence of mouse p-syn was also observed. From these results, we confirmed that the spread of the exogenous seeds occurs within 24 h. This rapid dissemination/transmission of a-syn phenomenon is very surprising and raises several questions. In clinical cases of PD and dementia with Lewy bodies (DLB)/PD with dementia (PDD), a-syn pathologies spread slowly over a period of 5–10 years [4, 5, 18]. Incidentally, in reports of Lewy body pathology in fetal SN transplants, which provide important evidence for a-syn transmission, it is estimated that Lewy bodies cannot be positively detected until more than 10 years after transplantation [21, 22]. There are several possible explanations for the difference in progression from around 24 h to over 10 years, between experimental transmission systems and the clinic. First, it is plausible that administering artificial protein aggregates to the experimental transmission systems creates a unique situation which does not necessarily reflect the clinical disease. Alternatively, it could be that the seeds themselves, which form the initial explosive trigger for the transmission and aggregation of the pathological protein, can spread within 24 h, while it takes more time for the exogenous seeds to recruit endogenous proteins by altering their conformation. This could represent a novel pathological concept in the disease progression of synucleinopathies. Indeed, since the transmission experiments involve injecting a large dose of seed proteins directly into the brain, they could be viewed as a way to capture the clinical pathological condition in a shorter period of time. Meanwhile, prion disease has been shown to spread extremely quickly after onset, both experimentally and clinically [27]. This difference could arise from the fact that prion disease causes changes in the cell membrane [36] which lead to a rapid worsening of disease, while synuclein causes changes within the cytoplasm [20, 45, 47] which may lead to slower progression.

In recent years, the propagation of pathological a-syn to anatomically adjacent neurons or cells has been observed in other studies as well, further supporting the trans-neuronal and trans-synaptic transportation of a-syn seeds [4, 9, 19, 28, 33, 35, 40, 41]. However, a study using cultured primary neurons reported that the transmission of pathological a-syn may not necessarily occur via synapses. Indeed, the transmission between axons and soma has been observed during the early culture phase (1 to 4 days), prior to the formation of synapses [11]. There are additional studies that report mechanisms other than synaptic transmission, such as transport via nanotubes [1], exocytosis or exosomes, or by receptor-mediated endocytosis [10, 17, 38]. However, our results strongly suggest that a synaptic mechanism underlies the trans-neuronal transmission of a-syn seeds in-vivo. Understanding the pathways involved in the pathological propagation of proteins is an important step for developing therapeutic interventions. The results of the present study using callosotomy suggest that the rapid dissemination of seeds through synapses does indeed occur. Finally, we used BoNT/B to investigate whether the transmission of seeds was inhibited by the cessation of synaptic release (Fig. 5). BoNT blocks synaptic vesicle fusion in the presynaptic terminal by breaking down and inactivating SNARE proteins in a highly specific manner (VAMP-2 by BoNT/B). BoNT has been shown to block vesicle exocytosis, but not endocytosis [31]. The role of VAMP-2 in the presynaptic SNARE complex that mediates vesicle fusion is widely accepted [46]. In our present study, BoNT/B injected into the striatum inhibited the exocytosis of a-syn seeds from the synapses of axons entering the striatum from the cortex. Transmission and propagation of pathological a-syn in the contralateral striatum and Amyg were inhibited. As a result, we observed that BoNT/B treatment reduced accumulation of p-syn in an area in which the seeds transmission should occur, confirming the presence of trans-synaptic transmission using an in vivo model, for the first time. Previously, it was reported that BoNT inhibited the spread of huntingtin protein in primary cultures, but the actual substances used were β-bungarotoxin [34], at least as far as the product numbers suggest. Thus, ours is the first study to definitively demonstrate trans-synaptic transmission of a pathological protein using BoNT in vivo. In recent years, the association of inflammation with PD or other diseases has been discussed. A study reported that inflammation alters neuronal functions, leading to an increase in cell death [43] and another study reported that inflammatory environments enhance a-syn spreading [13].

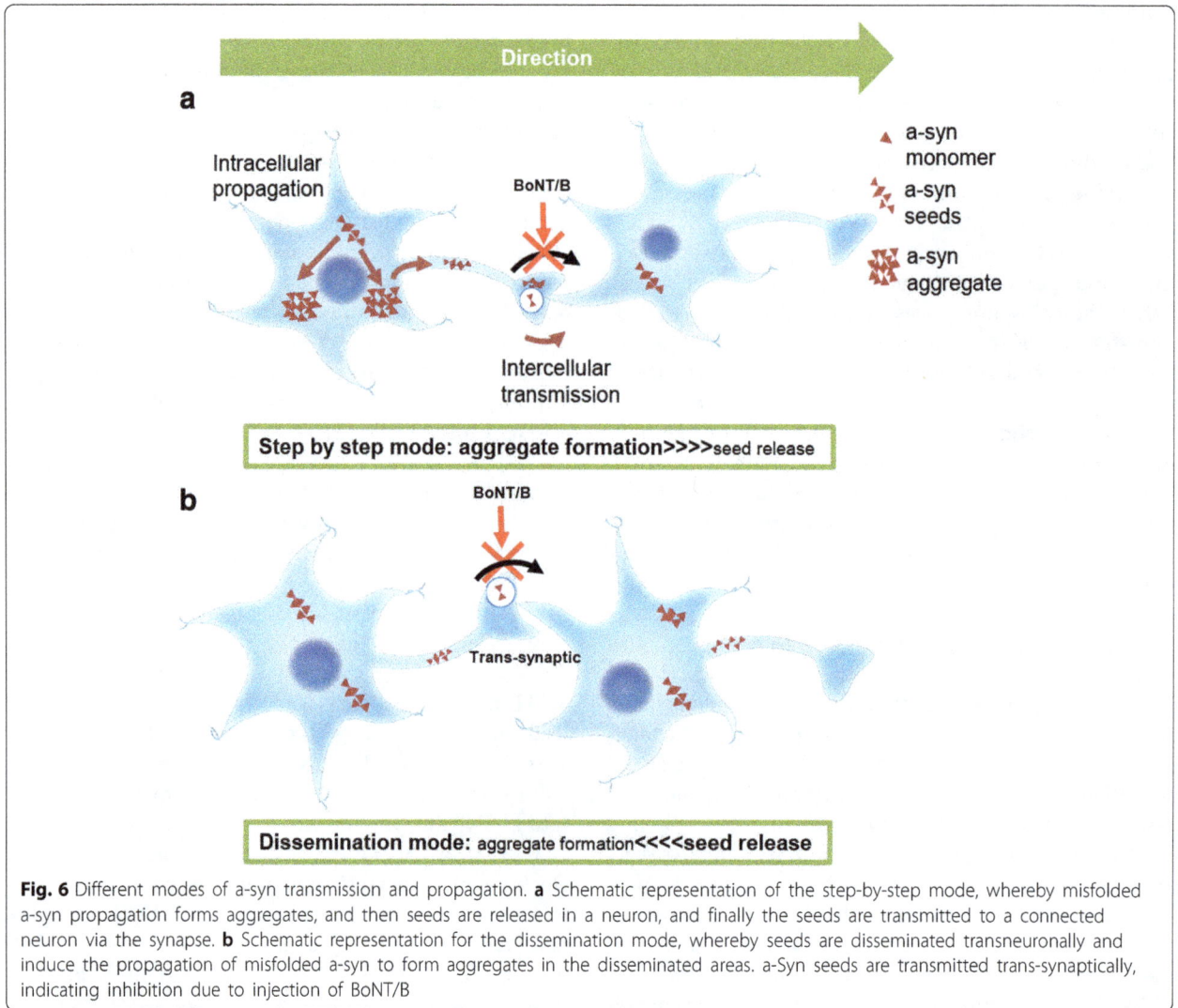

Fig. 6 Different modes of a-syn transmission and propagation. **a** Schematic representation of the step-by-step mode, whereby misfolded a-syn propagation forms aggregates, and then seeds are released in a neuron, and finally the seeds are transmitted to a connected neuron via the synapse. **b** Schematic representation for the dissemination mode, whereby seeds are disseminated transneuronally and induce the propagation of misfolded a-syn to form aggregates in the disseminated areas. a-Syn seeds are transmitted trans-synaptically, indicating inhibition due to injection of BoNT/B

The possibility that inflammation was caused by a surgical procedure such as callosotomy and injection of BoNT cannot be denied. Thus in this study, we performed callosotomy or injection of BoNT before or after administration of a-syn PFFs. When we performed callosotomy or injection of BoNT before a-syn PFFs administration, the spreading of a-syn inclusions decreased. However, when the administration of a-syn PFFs was performed after callosotomy or injection of BoNT, spreading of a-syn inclusions occurred equally as that with a-syn PFFs administration alone. Therefore, we concluded that inflammation had little effect in this study. Combined with the results of the experiments using callosotomy, we confirmed the rapid transmission and dissemination of a-syn seeds through circuit and synapses. Our findings provide empirical support for a dissemination mode (Fig. 6b) of a-syn propagation, where a-syn seeds are disseminated and then induced to

form aggregates, and not a step-by-step mode (Fig. 6a) where each neuron forms inclusions and releases seeds. Typical PD shows only limited affected regions and usually has a slowly progressive course. However, the distribution and rapid dissemination of a-syn seeds observed in this study seems to represent a different point in the recognition of PD, beyond its usual disease course. The dissemination mode may be a mechanism underlying the pathology of dementia with Lewy body disease, in which larger regions are affected in the cortex, including in the rapidly progressive phenotype [12]. Further studies will be necessary to elucidate this regulatory mechanism and to develop therapeutic strategies for synucleinopathies.

Conclusion

In the current study, even when a callosotomy was performed 24 h after seeds injection, a-syn was observed to have propagated to the contralateral hemisphere of the brain, indicating that seeds dissemination throughout the brain occurs very rapidly, within 24 h of injection. This is a new concept that differs from traditional notions of pathological progression; that is, aggregates are gradually formed from preceding, widely transmitted seeds. Moreover, the synaptic transmission of seeds was confirmed using BoNT in vivo.

Abbreviations

Amyg: Amygdala; ANCOVA: Analysis of covariance; a-syn: Alpha-synuclein; BoNT: Botulinum toxin; BoNT/B: Botulinum toxin B; CTX: Cortex; DAB: Diaminobenzidine; DLB: PD and dementia with Lewy bodies; EC: Entorhinal cortex; LBs: Lewy bodies; MSNs: Medium spiny neurons; Nav1.2: Sodium channel, voltage-gated, type II; PBS: Phosphate-buffered saline; PD: Parkinson's disease; PDD: PD with dementia; PFFs: Pre-formed fibrils; p-syn : Phosphorylated a-syn; SN: Substantia nigra; SNpc: Substantia nigra pars compacta; SNr: Substantia nigra pars reticulata; Str : Striatum; TH: Tyrosine hydroxylase; WT: Wild type; β4: Sodium channel β4 subunit

Acknowledgements

This research is supported by the Strategic Research Program for Brain Sciences from Japan Agency for Medical Research and Development, AMED under Grant Number JP18dm0107140 to N.N., from the Ministry of Education, Culture, Sports, Science and Technology (MEXT) of Japan to N.N. (17H01564), T.H.(25461290), by a Grant-in-Aid for Research on Measures for Ataxic Diseases to N.N, and by Grants-in Aid from the Research Committee of CNS Degenerative Disease, Research on Policy Planning and Evaluation for Rare and Intractable Diseases, Health, Labour and Welfare Sciences Research Grants to N.H. from the Ministry of Health, Labour and Welfare,Japan. We thank Itsuko Yamamoto for mice maintenance and thank Akiko Sumi for Immunostaining for human samples.

Authors' contributions

AO and MK mainly performed the experiments, YF, HM, SY, TS, MT, TF and TY provided the constructs and others for these experiments and prepared the PFFs, AO, MK, TH, HN and NN designed the experiments and AO, YF,TY and NN wrote the manuscript. SN performed the statistical analysis. All authors read and approved the final manuscript.

Competing interests

The authors declared that they have no competing interest.

Author details

[1]Department of Neurology, Juntendo University Graduate School of Medicine, 2-1-1 Hongo, Bunkyo-ku, Tokyo 113-8421, Japan. [2]Institute for Environmental and Gender-specific Medicine, Juntendo University Graduate School of Medicine, 2-1-1 Tomioka, Urayasu-shi, Chiba 279-0021, Japan. [3]Department of Neurology Juntendo University Koshigaya Hospital, 560 Fukuroyama, Koshigaya city, Saitama 343-0032, Japan. [4]Medical Technology Innovation Center, Clinical Research and Trial Center, Juntendo University Graduate School of Medicine, Tokyo, Japan. [5]Laboratory of Structural Neuropathology, Doshisha University Graduate School of Brain Science, 1-3 Tatara Miyakodani, Kyotanabe-shi, Kyoto 610-0394, Japan. [6]Laboratory for Mechanistic Chemistry of Biomolecules, Department of Chemistry, Keio University, 3-14-1 Hiyoshi, Kohoku, Yokohama 223-8522, Japan. [7]Laboratory for Molecular Mechanisms of Brain Development, RIKEN Center for Brain Science, 2-1 Hirosawa, Wako, Saitama 351-0198, Japan.

References

1. Abounit S, Bousset L, Loria F, Zhu S, de Chaumont F, Pieri L et al (2016) Tunneling nanotubes spread fibrillar alpha-synuclein by intercellular trafficking of lysosomes. EMBO J 35:2120–2138. https://doi.org/10.15252/embj.201593411
2. Aguzzi A, Rajendran L (2009) The transcellular spread of cytosolic amyloids, prions, and prionoids. Neuron 64:783–790. https://doi.org/10.1016/j.neuron.2009.12.016
3. Aulic S, Le TT, Moda F, Abounit S, Corvaglia S, Casalis L et al (2014) Defined alpha-synuclein prion-like molecular assemblies spreading in cell culture. BMC neuroscience 15:69. https://doi.org/10.1186/1471-2202-15-69
4. Braak H, Del Tredici K, Rub U, de Vos RA, Jansen Steur EN, Braak E (2003) Staging of brain pathology related to sporadic Parkinson's disease. Neurobiol Aging 24:197–211
5. Braak H, Muller CM, Rub U, Ackermann H, Bratzke H, de Vos RA et al (2006) Pathology associated with sporadic Parkinson's disease--where does it end? J Neural Transm Suppl:89–97
6. Bruce M, Chree A, McConnell I, Foster J, Pearson G, Fraser H (1994) Transmission of bovine spongiform encephalopathy and scrapie to mice: strain variation and the species barrier. Philos Trans R Soc Lond Ser B Biol Sci 343:405–411. https://doi.org/10.1098/rstb.1994.0036
7. Bruck D, Wenning GK, Stefanova N, Fellner L (2016) Glia and alpha-synuclein in neurodegeneration: a complex interaction. Neurobiol Dis 85:262–274. https://doi.org/10.1016/j.nbd.2015.03.003
8. Cho YT, Ernst M, Fudge JL (2013) Cortico-amygdala-striatal circuits are organized as hierarchical subsystems through the primate amygdala. J Neurosci 33:14017–14030. https://doi.org/10.1523/JNEUROSCI.0170-13.2013
9. Danzer KM, Ruf WP, Putcha P, Joyner D, Hashimoto T, Glabe C et al (2011) Heat-shock protein 70 modulates toxic extracellular alpha-synuclein oligomers and rescues trans-synaptic toxicity. FASEB J 25:326–36. https://doi.org/10.1096/fj.10-164624
10. Emmanouilidou E, Melachroinou K, Roumeliotis T, Garbis SD, Ntzouni M, Margaritis LH et al (2010) Cell-produced alpha-synuclein is secreted in a calcium-dependent manner by exosomes and impacts neuronal survival. J Neurosci 30:6838–6851. https://doi.org/10.1523/jneurosci.5699-09.2010
11. Freundt EC, Maynard N, Clancy EK, Roy S, Bousset L, Sourigues Y et al (2012) Neuron-to-neuron transmission of alpha-synuclein fibrils through axonal Transport. Ann Neurol 72:517–524. https://doi.org/10.1002/ana.23747
12. Gaig C, Valldeoriola F, Gelpi E, Ezquerra M, Llufriu S, Buongiorno M et al (2011) Rapidly progressive diffuse Lewy body disease. Mov Disord 26:1316–323. https://doi.org/10.1002/mds.23506
13. Gao HM, Zhang F, Zhou H, Kam W, Wilson B, Hong JS (2011) Neuroinflammation and alpha-synuclein dysfunction potentiate each other, driving chronic progression of neurodegeneration in a mouse model of Parkinson's disease. Environ Health Perspect 119:807–814. https://doi.org/10.1289/ehp.1003013
14. Gibb WR, Lees AJ (1988) The relevance of the Lewy body to the pathogenesis of idiopathic Parkinson's disease. J Neurol Neurosurg Psychiatry 51:745–752
15. Goedert M, Clavaguera F, Tolnay M (2010) The propagation of prion-like protein inclusions in neurodegenerative diseases. Trends Neurosci 33:317–325. https://doi.org/10.1016/j.tins.2010.04.003
16. Guo JL, Covell DJ, Daniels JP, Iba M, Stieber A, Zhang B et al (2013) Distinct alpha-synuclein strains differentially promote tau inclusions in neurons. Cell 154:103–117. https://doi.org/10.1016/j.cell.2013.05.057
17. Guo JL, Lee VM (2014) Cell-to-cell transmission of pathogenic proteins in neurodegenerative diseases. Nat Med 20:130–138. https://doi.org/10.1038/nm.3457
18. Hawkes CH, Del Tredici K, Braak H (2010) A timeline for Parkinson's disease. Parkinsonism Relat Disord 16:79–84. https://doi.org/10.1016/j.parkreldis.2009.08.007
19. Holmqvist S, Chutna O, Bousset L, Aldrin-Kirk P, Li W, Bjorklund T et al (2014) Direct evidence of Parkinson pathology spread from the gastrointestinal tract to the brain in rats. Acta Neuropathol 128:805–820. https://doi.org/10.1007/s00401-014-1343-6
20. Iwai A, Masliah E, Yoshimoto M, Ge N, Flanagan L, de Silva HA et al (1995) The precursor protein of non-a beta component of Alzheimer's disease amyloid is a presynaptic protein of the central nervous system. Neuron 14:467–475
21. Kordower JH, Chu Y, Hauser RA, Freeman TB, Olanow CW (2008) Lewy body-like pathology in long-term embryonic nigral transplants in Parkinson's disease. Nat Med 14:504–506. https://doi.org/10.1038/nm1747

22. Li JY, Englund E, Holton JL, Soulet D, Hagell P, Lees AJ et al (2008) Lewy bodies in grafted neurons in subjects with Parkinson's disease suggest host-to-graft disease propagation. Nat med 14:501–03. https://doi.org/10.1038/nm1746

23. Loria F, Vargas JY, Bousset L, Syan S, Salles A, Melki R et al (2017) alpha-Synuclein transfer between neurons and astrocytes indicates that astrocytes play a role in degradation rather than in spreading. Acta Neuropathol 134:789–808. https://doi.org/10.1007/s00401-017-1746-2

24. Luk KC, Covell DJ, Kehm VM, Zhang B, Song IY, Byrne MD et al (2016) Molecular and Biological Compatibility with Host Alpha-Synuclein Influences Fibril Pathogenicity. Cell Rep 16:3373–3387. https://doi.org/10.1016/j.celrep.2016.08.053

25. Luk KC, Kehm V, Carroll J, Zhang B, O'Brien P, Trojanowski JQ et al (2012) Pathological alpha-synuclein transmission initiates Parkinson-like neurodegeneration in nontransgenic mice. Science 338:949–953. https://doi.org/10.1126/science.1227157

26. Mao X, Ou MT, Karuppagounder SS, Kam TI, Yin X, Xiong Y et al (2016) Pathological alpha-synuclein transmission initiated by binding lymphocyte-activation gene 3. Science 353: Doi https://doi.org/10.1126/science.aah3374

27. Masters CL, Harris JO, Gajdusek DC, Gibbs CJ Jr, Bernoulli C, Asher DM (1979) Creutzfeldt-Jakob disease: patterns of worldwide occurrence and the significance of familial and sporadic clustering. Ann Neurol 5:177–188. https://doi.org/10.1002/ana.410050212

28. Masuda-Suzukake M, Nonaka T, Hosokawa M, Kubo M, Shimozawa A, Akiyama H et al (2014) Pathological alpha-synuclein propagates through neural networks. Acta neuropathol commun 2: 88 https://doi.org/10.1186/s40478-014-0088-8 10.1186/preaccept-1296467154135944

29. Masuda-Suzukake M, Nonaka T, Hosokawa M, Oikawa T, Arai T, Akiyama H et al (2013) Prion-like spreading of pathological alpha-synuclein in brain. Brain 136:1128–138. https://doi.org/10.1093/brain/awt037

30. Miyazaki H, Oyama F, Inoue R, Aosaki T, Abe T, Kiyonari H et al (2014) Singular localization of sodium channel beta4 subunit in unmyelinated fibres and its role in the striatum. Nat commun 5:5525. https://doi.org/10.1038/ncomms6525

31. Neale EA, Bowers LM, Jia M, Bateman KE, Williamson LC (1999) Botulinum neurotoxin a blocks synaptic vesicle exocytosis but not endocytosis at the nerve terminal. J Cell Biol 147:1249–1260

32. Olanow CW, Prusiner SB (2009) Is Parkinson's disease a prion disorder? Proc Natl Acad Sci U S A 106:12571–12572. https://doi.org/10.1073/pnas.0906759106

33. Paumier KL, Luk KC, Manfredsson FP, Kanaan NM, Lipton JW, Collier TJ et al (2015) Intrastriatal injection of pre-formed mouse alpha-synuclein fibrils into rats triggers alpha-synuclein pathology and bilateral nigrostriatal degeneration. Neurobiol Dis 82:185–199. https://doi.org/10.1016/j.nbd.2015.06.003

34. Pecho-Vrieseling E, Rieker C, Fuchs S, Bleckmann D, Esposito MS, Botta P et al (2014) Transneuronal propagation of mutant huntingtin contributes to non-cell autonomous pathology in neurons. Nat Neurosci 17:1064–1072. https://doi.org/10.1038/nn.3761

35. Peelaerts W, Bousset L, Van der Perren A, Moskalyuk A, Pulizzi R, Giugliano M et al (2015) alpha-Synuclein strains cause distinct synucleinopathies after local and systemic administration. Nature 522:340–344. https://doi.org/10.1038/nature14547

36. Prusiner SB (1998) Prions. Proc Natl Acad Sci U S A 95:13363–13383

37. Recasens A, Dehay B, Bove J, Carballo-Carbajal I, Dovero S, Perez-Villalba A et al (2014) Lewy body extracts from Parkinson disease brains trigger alpha-synuclein pathology and neurodegeneration in mice and monkeys. Ann Neurol 75:351–362. https://doi.org/10.1002/ana.24066

38. Ren PH, Lauckner JE, Kachirskaia I, Heuser JE, Melki R, Kopito RR (2009) Cytoplasmic penetration and persistent infection of mammalian cells by polyglutamine aggregates. Nat Cell Biol 11:219–225. https://doi.org/10.1038/ncb1830

39. Rey NL, George S, Steiner JA, Madaj Z, Luk KC, Trojanowski JQ et al (2018) Spread of aggregates after olfactory bulb injection of alpha-synuclein fibrils is associated with early neuronal loss and is reduced long term. Acta Neuropathol 135:65–83. https://doi.org/10.1007/s00401-017-1792-9

40. Rey NL, Petit GH, Bousset L, Melki R, Brundin P (2013) Transfer of human alpha-synuclein from the olfactory bulb to interconnected brain regions in mice. Acta Neuropathol 126:555–573. https://doi.org/10.1007/s00401-013-1160-3

41. Rey NL, Steiner JA, Maroof N, Luk KC, Madaj Z, Trojanowski JQ et al (2016) Widespread transneuronal propagation of alpha-synucleinopathy triggered in olfactory bulb mimics prodromal Parkinson's disease. J Exp Med 213:1759–1778. https://doi.org/10.1084/jem.20160368

42. Sacino AN, Ayers JI, Brooks MM, Chakrabarty P, Hudson VJ 3rd, Howard JK et al (2016) Non-prion-type transmission in A53T alpha-synuclein transgenic mice: a normal component of spinal homogenates from naive non-transgenic mice induces robust alpha-synuclein pathology. Acta Neuropathol 131:151–154. https://doi.org/10.1007/s00401-015-1505-1

43. Sanchez-Guajardo V, Tentillier N, Romero-Ramos M (2015) The relation between alpha-synuclein and microglia in Parkinson's disease: recent developments. Neuroscience 302:47–58. https://doi.org/10.1016/j.neuroscience.2015.02.008

44. Shimozawa A, Ono M, Takahara D, Tarutani A, Imura S, Masuda-Suzukake M et al (2017) of the input and output of neural connectionsbrain. Acta neuropathol commun 5:12. https://doi.org/10.1186/s40478-017-0413-0

45. Spillantini MG, Schmidt ML, Lee VM, Trojanowski JQ, Jakes R, Goedert M (1997) Alpha-synuclein in Lewy bodies. Nature 388:839–840. https://doi.org/10.1038/42166

46. Sudhof TC, Rizo J (2011) Synaptic vesicle exocytosis. Cold Spring Harb Perspect Biol 3. https://doi.org/10.1101/cshperspect.a005637

47. Wakabayashi K, Tanji K, Mori F, Takahashi H (2007) The Lewy body in Parkinson's disease: molecules implicated in the formation and degradation of alpha-synuclein aggregates. Neuropathology : official journal of the Japanese Society of Neuropathology 27:494–506

48. Xilouri M, Brekk OR, Stefanis L (2013) Alpha-Synuclein and protein degradation systems: a reciprocal relationship. Mol Neurobiol 47:537–551. https://doi.org/10.1007/s12035-012-8341-2

49. Zhou J, Gennatas ED, Kramer JH, Miller BL, Seeley WW (2012) Predicting regional neurodegeneration from the healthy brain functional connectome. Neuron 73:1216–1227. https://doi.org/10.1016/j.neuron.2012.03.004

7

Transcriptomic and epigenetic profiling of 'diffuse midline gliomas, H3 K27M-mutant' discriminate two subgroups based on the type of histone H3 mutated and not supratentorial or infratentorial location

David Castel[1,2*], Cathy Philippe[1,12], Thomas Kergrohen[1,2], Martin Sill[3,4], Jane Merlevede[1], Emilie Barret[1], Stéphanie Puget[5], Christian Sainte-Rose[5], Christof M. Kramm[6], Chris Jones[7], Pascale Varlet[8], Stefan M. Pfister[3,4,9], Jacques Grill[1,2], David T. W. Jones[3,10] and Marie-Anne Debily[1,11,13*] (ID)

Abstract

Diffuse midline glioma (DMG), H3 K27M-mutant, is a new entity in the updated WHO classification grouping together diffuse intrinsic pontine gliomas and infiltrating glial neoplasms of the midline harboring the same canonical mutation at the Lysine 27 of the histones H3 tail.

Two hundred and fifteen patients younger than 18 years old with centrally-reviewed pediatric high-grade gliomas (pHGG) were included in this study. Comprehensive transcriptomic ($n = 140$) and methylation ($n = 80$) profiling was performed depending on the material available, in order to assess the biological uniqueness of this new entity compared to other midline and hemispheric pHGG.

Tumor classification based on gene expression (GE) data highlighted the similarity of K27M DMG independently of their location along the midline. T-distributed Stochastic Neighbor Embedding (tSNE) analysis of methylation profiling confirms the discrimination of DMG from other well defined supratentorial tumor subgroups. Patients with diffuse intrinsic pontine gliomas (DIPG) and thalamic DMG exhibited a similarly poor prognosis (11.1 and 10.8 months median overall survival, respectively). Interestingly, H3.1-K27M and H3.3-K27M primary tumor samples could be distinguished based both on their GE and DNA methylation profiles, suggesting that they might arise from a different precursor or from a different epigenetic reorganization.

These differences in DNA methylation profiles were conserved in glioma stem-like cell culture models of DIPG which mimicked their corresponding primary tumor. ChIP-seq profiling of H3K27me3 in these models indicate that H3.3-K27M mutated DIPG stem cells exhibit higher levels of H3K27 trimethylation which are correlated with fewer genes expressed by RNAseq. When considering the global distribution of the H3K27me3 mark, we observed that intergenic regions were more trimethylated in the H3.3-K27M mutated cells compared to the H3.1-K27M mutated ones.

H3 K27M-mutant DMG represent a homogenous group of neoplasms compared to other pediatric gliomas that could be further separated based on the type of histone H3 variant mutated and their respective

(Continued on next page)

* Correspondence: david.castel@gustaveroussy.fr; marie-anne.debily@gustaveroussy.fr
[1]UMR8203,Vectorologie et Nouvelles Thérapies Anticancéreuses, CNRS, Gustave Roussy, Univ. Paris-Sud, Université Paris-Saclay, 94805 Villejuif, France
Full list of author information is available at the end of the article

(Continued from previous page)

epigenetic landscapes. As these characteristics drive different phenotypes, these findings may have important implication for the design of future trials in these specific types of neoplasms.

Keywords: Pediatric high-grade glioma, Diffuse midline glioma, H3 K27M-mutant, Diffuse intrinsic pontine glioma, Epigenetics, DNA methylation profiling, Gene expression profiling, H3K27me3 landscape, Glioma stem cell,

Introduction

Diffuse intrinsic pontine glioma and malignant midline gliomas have the worst prognosis of all types of malignant tumors in children and adolescents [3, 4, 10]. The nosological shift in the 2016 WHO classification now based on both phenotype and genotype has redefined the family tree of diffuse gliomas [17]. Glial tumors are now grouped according to their driver mutation, e.g. *IDH1* mutation, and their astrocytic or oligodendroglial phenotypes which are often associated with additional specific genetic alterations such as *ATRX* mutations or 1p/19q co-deletion, respectively. The discovery of recurrent mutations in the histone H3 genes in pediatric high-grade glioma has definitively separated these gliomas from the ones seen in adults [21, 26]. While G34R/V mutations in the *H3F3A* gene are exclusively found in the hemispheres, K27M/I mutations in several histone H3 variants genes are specific to midline tumors [23]. The 2016 release of the WHO classification has therefore created a new entity to describe these latter tumors as diffuse midline glioma, H3K27M mutant, irrespective of their specific location along the midline.

In pediatric brain tumors, location has however long been seen as a master driver of oncogenesis that could reflect their different cells of origin [8, 9]. Whether the oncogenic driver mutation is overriding location as a crucial determinant of oncogenesis is therefore to be examined since biologic identity of all these tumors would call for a common therapeutic framework. There is however no reported data showing at once a similar biology and outcome of diffuse midline gliomas (DMG) irrespective of their location in the presence of a histone H3-K27M mutation.

Moreover, we have shown two distinct forms of diffuse intrinsic pontine gliomas according to the type of histone H3 gene mutated, *H3F3A versus HIST1H3B*, with respect to differentiation markers, oncogenic programs, response to therapy and evolution [1, 2]. These mutations are mutually exclusive either because their effect is redundant [16] leading to a global loss of H3K27me3 repressive mark, or because they cannot transform the same cell, suggesting the idea of distinct cells of origin.

The purpose of this work was therefore to better characterize a large series of pediatric midline high grade gliomas from the (epi)genomic, transcriptomic and anatomic point of view in order to identify the respective influences of these parameters on their biology described by their gene expression, methylome, and clinical behaviour.

Moreover, we compared the H3-K27me3 landscape between the two main subgroups of DIPG, H3.1-K27M and H3.3-K27M, in patient deriving cellular models.

Materials & methods
Central pathology review

High-grade glioma cases were reviewed centrally to confirm the diagnosis according to the 2007 WHO classification and its 2016 update as previously described [10, 20].

Specific immunostainings were performed to detect nuclear expression of the trimethylation mark at position K27 of the histone 3 tail (1:1000, polyclonal rabbit antibody, Diagenode, Belgium) as well as nuclear expression of the K27M form of histone H3 (1:1000, polyclonal rabbit antibody, Millipore, CA).

Derivation and culture of glioma stem-like cells (GSCs)

GSCs were derived from DIPG tumors at diagnosis as previously described [19]. Briefly, tumor cells were mechanically dissociated from biopsies within 24 h of surgery, and further cultured as an adherent monolayer in laminin-coated flask (Sigma) in neural stem cells medium consisting of NeuroCult NS-A proliferation medium (Stemcell technologies) supplemented with heparin (2 µg/mL, Stemcell technologies), human-basic FGF (20 ng/ml, Peprotech), human-EGF (20 ng/ml, Peprotech), PDGF-AA (10 ng/ml, Peprotech), and PDGF-BB (10 ng/ml, Perprotech). Medium was renewed every other day, and passaging performed when cells reached 80% confluence using Accutase (Thermo).

Case selection for overall survival analysis and gene expression profiling by microarray

Frozen tissue samples were obtained from 119 pediatric patients with brain tumors of WHO grade III and IV (all locations, below 18 years old). The samples were collected at Necker Hospital (Paris, France). Complete follow-up information was available for 82.5% of patients ($n = 99$). Histone H3 gene mutational status was determined by Sanger sequencing for *H3F3A*, *HIST1H3B/C* and *HIST2H3C* [2]. The distribution of samples in the distinct genotype subgroups and location are detailed in Table 1.

Table 1 Contingency table of samples used for microarray gene expression profiling and overall survival analysis

Tumor location	Histone H3 mutational status				Total number of samples
	H3.3-G34R	H3.1-K27M	H3.3-K27M	H3.1 & H3.3-WT	
Cortex	6	0	0	35	41
Pons	0	13	26	6	45
Non-thalamic midline	0	0	2	12	14
Thalamic midline	0	0	12	7	19

One hundred and nineteen high-grade glioma samples were divided in four groups according to their location either in the pontine (DIPG), cortical or thalamic area of the brain as well as the non-thalamic midline, i.e. spinal cord, cerebellum or peduncle tumors classified as 'non-thalamic midlines'

Case and sample selections for methylation analysis

Eighty primary tumor samples were selected for methylome analysis: 22 among the DIPG patient cohort collected in Necker Hospital; 15 from the HERBY trial [10], all the remaining samples were collected by the Heidelberg group. The distribution of samples in the distinct genotype subgroups and their location are detailed in Table 2.

Gene expression profiling was also conducted by either microarray or RNA sequencing for 5 of these tumors. Eight glioma stem-like cell (GSC) cultures derived from patient biopsies at diagnosis and matching primary tumors were analyzed similarly [19].

Methylation profiling

DNA was extracted from tumors and genome-wide DNA methylation analysis was performed using either the Illumina HumanMethylation450 BeadChip (450 k) or EPIC arrays. DNA methylation analysis was performed with custom approaches as previously described [12, 23]. DNA methylation profiles from 50 K27M pHGG were compared to defined supratentorial tumor subgroups, i.e. G34R-H3.3 mutated ($n = 10$), *MYCN* ($n = 10$) and *PDGFRA*/pedRTK1 ($n = 10$) subgroup tumors. For t-SNE analysis (t-Distributed Stochastic Neighbor Embedding, Rtsne package version 0.11), 428,230 uniquely mapping autosomal probes in common between the 450 k and EPIC arrays were used. The input for the t-SNE calculation is 1-Pearson correlation, weighted by variance. Clustering analyses were performed using the beta values of the top 10,000 most variably methylated probes by standard deviation. Methylation probes in the heatmap representation were reordered by unsupervised hierarchical clustering using Pearson correlation distance and median linkage.

Microarray gene expression profiling

Gene expression analysis was conducted on an Agilent platform as previously described [2] but using RUV4 correction of batch effects [7] implemented in the R package ruv. GE data from DIPG were collected from one of our previous study [2] and microarray analysis was performed for 75 additional pHGG tumors located outside the brainstem. PCA, k-means and t-SNE analysis were performed using the same parameters as for RNA-seq data on the probes associated with the highest standard deviation. One hundred and twenty genes accounting for 0.79% of the entire probeset were selected.

RNA-seq gene expression profiling

RNA-seq was performed on 21 primary tumor samples. Libraries were prepared using the TruSeq stranded mRNA sample preparation kit according to the supplier recommendations and paired-end sequencing was conducted on Illumina NextSeq500 to generate a mean of 150 million reads of 75 base pairs by sample. Trimmed reads were then mapped using tophat2 (v2.1.0) and bowtie2 (v2.2.5) first to the reference transcriptome, then to the reference genome for the remaining reads. Genes with a row sum of raw counts over the studied samples equal to or below 10 were filtered out to remove non-expressed genes. We handled outliers as default using minReplicatesForReplace = 7 in DESeq() function used to estimate size factors, dispersion and model coefficients. Distances between samples were computed by using '1-Pearson correlation coefficient' as the distance measure. PCA and t-SNE analysis were performed on the 250 genes associated with the highest variance to keep the same proportion of genes selected with the microarray analysis. All samples were projected on the two first principal components computed with rlog transformation of the counts of the 120 genes with the highest standard deviation. Using

Table 2 Contingency table of samples used for methylation profiling

Tumor location	Histone H3 mutational status				*PDGFRA* subgroup	*MYCN* subgroup	Total number of samples
	H3.3-G34R	H3.1-K27M	H3.3-K27M	H3.2-K27M			
Cortex	10	0	0	0	10	10	30
Pons	0	12	19	1	0	0	32
Thalamic midline	0	1	17	0	0	0	18

Eighty high grade gliomas were analyzed by 450 k and EPIC Illumina bead arrays. Tumor location and histone H3 mutations or *PDGFRA* and *MYCN* molecular subgroups were considered for sample stratification

Rtsne package (v 0.11), we applied t-SNE on the same data matrix with the Pearson correlation as a distance and the following parameters: theta = 0, perplexity = min(floor((ncol(rlog_VariableGenes)-1)/3), 30), check_-duplicates = FALSE, pca = FALSE, max_iter = 10,000, verbose = TRUE, is_distance = TRUE.

RNA-seq was also performed on 6 distinct GSC models using TruSeq stranded total RNA sample preparation kit according to the supplier recommendations (Illumina) and then processed similarly as primary tumors.

Histone ChIP-sequencing and data processing

ChIP-seq of H3K27me3 epigenetic modification was performed in 6 GSC models at Active Motif according to proprietary methods. The 75-nt sequence reads were generated on a Illumina NextSeq 500 platform, mapped using BWA algorithm and peak calling was performed using SICER1.1 algorithm [27] with cutoff FDR 1e-10 and gap parameter of 600 bp. False positive ChIP-seq peaks were removed as defined within the ENCODE blacklist [5]. Overlapping intervals between the different samples were merged, and the average number of normalized reads in the different samples were calculated for these 16,977 genomic intervals defined as 'bound regions'. These bound regions were separated for further analysis in overlapping or not overlapping gene loci using Genecode annotation (gencode.v19.chr_patch_-hapl_scaff_annotation.gtf). PCA for all samples were generated after scaling to unit variance using the PCA function from the FactoMineR package (v1.41) and plotted using Factoextra (v1.0.5).

Merging of the 3 biological replicates of H3.1- or H3.3-K27M subgroups was performed using bigWigMerge tool (UCSC kent utils, http://hgdownload.soe.ucsc.edu/admin/exe/macOSX.x86_64/). Heatmaps of H3K27me3 ChIPseq enrichment across genomic loci were calculated using deepTools version 1.5.11. ComputeMatrix was used with regions of either +/− 5 kb or +/− 10 kb around the center of the genomic intervals for 'bound regions' or TSS for differentially expressed genes, respectively. Heatmaps were plotted with or without k-means ($k = 5$) and their average profiles of ChIP-Seq enrichment in the same − 10/+ 10 kb genomic intervals were also generated for each k-means group. The bigWig files (all signal) were annotated with chipSeeker package using UCSC hg19 known gene annotation and visualized by peakAnno and Vennpie.

Survival curve comparisons

The distribution of overall survival (OS) was calculated according to the Kaplan-Meier method and all survival function estimate comparisons were performed in PRISM software using a log-rank test. OS was calculated from the date of histo-radiological diagnosis until death of patient from disease or last contact for patients who were still alive.

Results

Histone H3 K27M midline pHGG and K27M DIPG display similar gene expression profiles and survival but differ significantly from other high-grade gliomas

We conducted microarray gene expression profiling of the single center cohort from Necker Enfants Malades hospital of 119 pHGG with histone H3 genotype previously determined either by Whole Genome Sequencing [25] or targeted Sanger sequencing [2] (Table 1 and Additional file 1: Table S1). In total, 131 distinct gene expression microarrays were hybridized as 12 samples were analyzed twice to control for potential batch effects. The 12 duplicated samples were located in close proximity on PCA plot when projected on the 2 first principal components, confirming the appropriate removal of a batch effect in our dataset (*data not shown*). Then, we selected a set of genes associated with the highest standard deviation for subsequent tumor classification analysis ($n = 120$). Gene Ontology over-representation analysis showed an enrichment of genes involved in brain development (Bonferroni adjusted *p*-value 8.29e-09) and morphogenesis (adjusted *p*-value 2.67e-07); many homeobox genes belong to this later set of genes reflecting probably the differences in tumor location.

Principal component analysis (PCA) was performed to highlight the principal sources of variation among pHGG tumors (Additional file 2: Table S2: weight in principal components 1 and 2 associated to each gene). The DIPG group appeared rather homogenous as all samples clustered together in the PCA plot, separated from the tumors originating from thalamic or cortical areas of the brain which were more scattered (Fig. 1a). Considering the mutational status of histone H3 genes, the results clearly showed that H3-K27M tumors, whichever their pontine or thalamic location, could be separated from the wild-type and G34R/V tumors on the first principal component (Fig. 1b). Indeed, all H3-K27M mutated thalamic and spinal tumors were close to DIPG samples, whereas histone H3 wild-type thalamic tumors are distributed on the right side of the plot among histone H3 wild-type non-thalamic midline and cortical tumors. Interestingly, 5 DIPG without any mutation in *H3F3A*, *HIST1H3B/C* and *HIST2H3A/C* were located within the K27M DIPG subgroup. These tumors all showed H3K27-trimethylation loss by immunohistochemistry (Additional file 3: Figure S1A). Unsupervised K-means analysis was performed on the same dataset (using $k = 2$ which showed the best BIC value) and led to a similar conclusion as the k-mean group 1 corresponded to H3-K27M and H3-wild type samples presenting H3K27-trimethylation loss whereas k-mean group 2

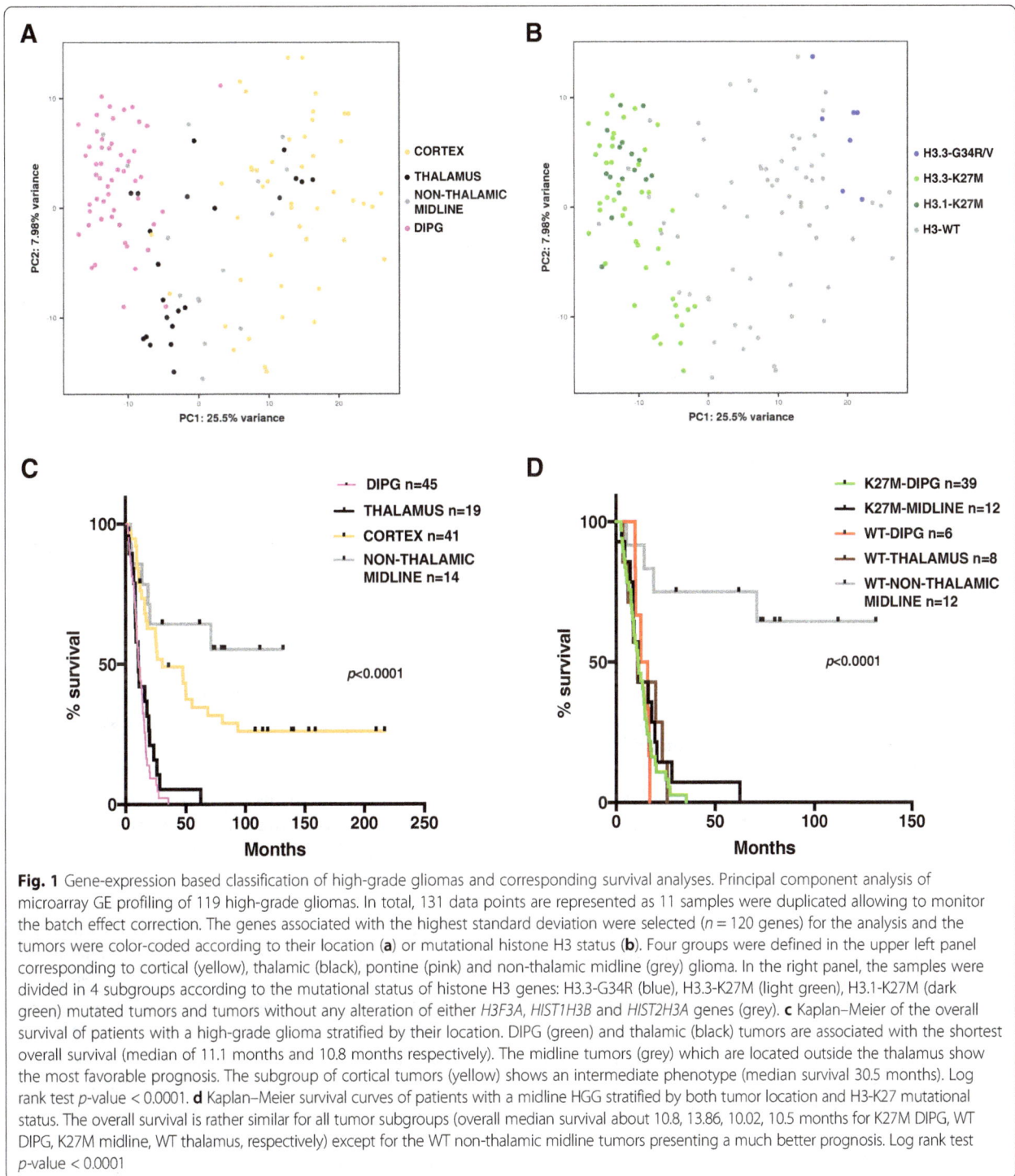

Fig. 1 Gene-expression based classification of high-grade gliomas and corresponding survival analyses. Principal component analysis of microarray GE profiling of 119 high-grade gliomas. In total, 131 data points are represented as 11 samples were duplicated allowing to monitor the batch effect correction. The genes associated with the highest standard deviation were selected ($n = 120$ genes) for the analysis and the tumors were color-coded according to their location (**a**) or mutational histone H3 status (**b**). Four groups were defined in the upper left panel corresponding to cortical (yellow), thalamic (black), pontine (pink) and non-thalamic midline (grey) glioma. In the right panel, the samples were divided in 4 subgroups according to the mutational status of histone H3 genes: H3.3-G34R (blue), H3.3-K27M (light green), H3.1-K27M (dark green) mutated tumors and tumors without any alteration of either *H3F3A*, *HIST1H3B* and *HIST2H3A* genes (grey). **c** Kaplan–Meier of the overall survival of patients with a high-grade glioma stratified by their location. DIPG (green) and thalamic (black) tumors are associated with the shortest overall survival (median of 11.1 months and 10.8 months respectively). The midline tumors (grey) which are located outside the thalamus show the most favorable prognosis. The subgroup of cortical tumors (yellow) shows an intermediate phenotype (median survival 30.5 months). Log rank test *p*-value < 0.0001. **d** Kaplan–Meier survival curves of patients with a midline HGG stratified by both tumor location and H3-K27 mutational status. The overall survival is rather similar for all tumor subgroups (overall median survival about 10.8, 13.86, 10.02, 10.5 months for K27M DIPG, WT DIPG, K27M midline, WT thalamus, respectively) except for the WT non-thalamic midline tumors presenting a much better prognosis. Log rank test *p*-value < 0.0001

contained all other pHGG tumors (Additional file 3: Figure S1B). Additionally, this GE dataset was analyzed in parallel with another dimension reduction and visualization technique for high-dimensional data, t-SNE, as it was shown to be more robust than PCA with respect to outliers. Moreover, t-SNE has also been frequently used for pediatric brain tumor classification based on DNA methylation profiles [23]. This analysis of GE profiles led to similar observations, re-iterating the similarity of H3-K27M thalamic midline and DIPG (Additional file 3: Figure S1C-D). Histone H3-G34R/V samples were tightly clustered together in particular in this analysis, thus reflecting a strong similarity in their gene expression profiles.

In agreement with these observations, a huge number of differentially expressed genes were identified between H3-K27M and H3-wild-type tumors as well as between H3-K27M and H3-G34R tumors (adjusted p-value < 0.01) in comparison with the other contrasts (Additional file 3: Figure S1E and Additional file 4: Table S3). In contrast, only 14 genes were significantly modulated between H3-G34R and H3-WT tumors which were not discriminated by PC1 (Fig. 1b). Gene ontology analysis showed an important enrichment of modulated genes associated with neurogenesis (4.37e-12 – 1.41e-11) and neuron differentiation (3e-07 - 4.87e-13) signaling pathways in both contrasts (H3-K27M vs. H3-WT and H3-K27M vs. H3-G34R) , as well as an upregulation of genes involved in ion transmembrane transport (1.6e-04) and apoptotic processes (5.9e-18) and an downregulation of genes linked to cell cycle (8.3e-11) and gliogenesis (6.87e-10) in the case of the comparison between H3-wild-type and H3-K27M tumors. Also, geneset enrichment analysis (GSEA) identified the ontology GO_oligodendrocyte_differentiation (Enrichment Score 0.70) enriched in upregulated genes in H3-K27M tumors and GO_Cerebral_cortex_neuron_differentiation (Enrichment Score – 0.79) enriched in genes upregulated in H3-G34R. Some of these biological processes were previously identified as significantly enriched in differentially expressed genes when comparing H3.1- and H3.3-K27M tumors [2].

We next conducted a survival analysis on this cohort ($n = 119$) using only location information and then both location and H3 mutation status for patient stratification (Fig. 1c and d). DIPG and thalamic tumors were associated with similar poor prognosis, i.e. 11.1 and 10.8 months median OS, respectively. Non-thalamic midline tumors exhibited the best prognosis (median OS not reached), whereas tumors arising in the cortex presented an intermediate outcome with a median survival around 30.5 months (p-value < 0.0001, Fig. 1c). Focusing on Kaplan-Meier estimates for midline tumors, our data clearly indicate that H3-WT non-thalamic midline have a significantly higher overall survival, whereas the other midline malignant gliomas (mostly thalamic), with or without alteration of histone H3 genes, display equivalent poor survival (p-value < 0.0001, Fig. 1d).

Methylation profiling separates *HIST1H3B* and *H3F3A* K27M tumors

Previous studies have shown that genome-wide DNA methylation data can provide a robust classification of pediatric brain tumors into clinically meaningful epigenetic subgroups mostly characterized by recurrent genetic alterations [14, 15, 22]. Consequently, we compared the methylation profiles of K27M-mutated diffuse midline gliomas (including DIPG) to G34R-mutated tumors and well-characterized supratentorial tumors without mutation in

histone H3 genes, i.e. *MYCN* and *PDGFRA* tumor subgroups (Fig. 2a, Table 2) [15]. Eighty primary tumor samples were used in this analysis and t-SNE visualization of the DNA methylation data was conducted. We confirmed that H3-G34R, *PDGFRA* and *MYCN* subgroups constitute 3 distinct homogenous entities, as they defined three distinct clusters. All H3-K27M samples were located on the opposite side of the 2D representation, reflecting important differences in the methylome compared to these three well-defined pHGG subgroups. This observation was thus concordant with our results on GE profiling by microarray.

In addition, the same methylation profiling splits H3-K27M samples in two subgroups that corresponded to either H3.1 or H3.3 mutated tumors. The obvious separation of these tumors in an analysis containing other very distinct biological entities clearly indicated the significant difference between them. Also, the unique H3.2-K27M sample appeared closer to H3.1-K27M than H3.3-K27M samples (Fig. 2a).

The same classification by t-SNE was repeated for the subset of H3-K27M mutated midline gliomas. First, t-SNE analysis did not reveal a segregation of these samples according to their location, as all DIPG and thalamic midline were scattered in the 2D plot (Fig. 2b). Conversely, when considering samples based on the mutated histone H3 gene, the t-SNE analysis clearly highlighted two non-overlapping subgroups corresponding to H3.1/H3.2-K27M and H3.3-K27M classes (Fig. 2c). This observation indicates that H3.3-K27M DIPG are closer to other midline H3.3-K27M HGG than to H3.1-K27M DIPG. The histone H3 variant affected by the K27M substitution thus has a stronger correlation with the modulation of DNA methylation profile than the tumor location across the midline.

An additional analysis was performed on a subset of 21 primary DIPG tumors and 8 glioma stem-like cells (GSCs) deriving from these same biopsies. The sample classification by unsupervised hierarchical clustering confirmed the previous result, with two main clusters corresponding to H3.3-K27M and H3.1/2-K27M samples (Fig. 3a). Additionally, we observed that the majority of the GSCs clustered with their corresponding primary tumors indicating the close similarity of their methylome profile. This consequently underlined that GSC population remained very similar to their primary counterpart with respect to DNA methylation, reflecting the variation in DNA methylation observed between the two subgroups of H3.1 and H3.3 mutated tumors.

RNA-seq profiling also discriminates *HIST1H3B/C* and *H3F3A* K27M mutated gliomas

DNA methylation is a relatively stable component of the epigenome involved in the establishment and maintenance of distinct gene expression patterns. Consequently,

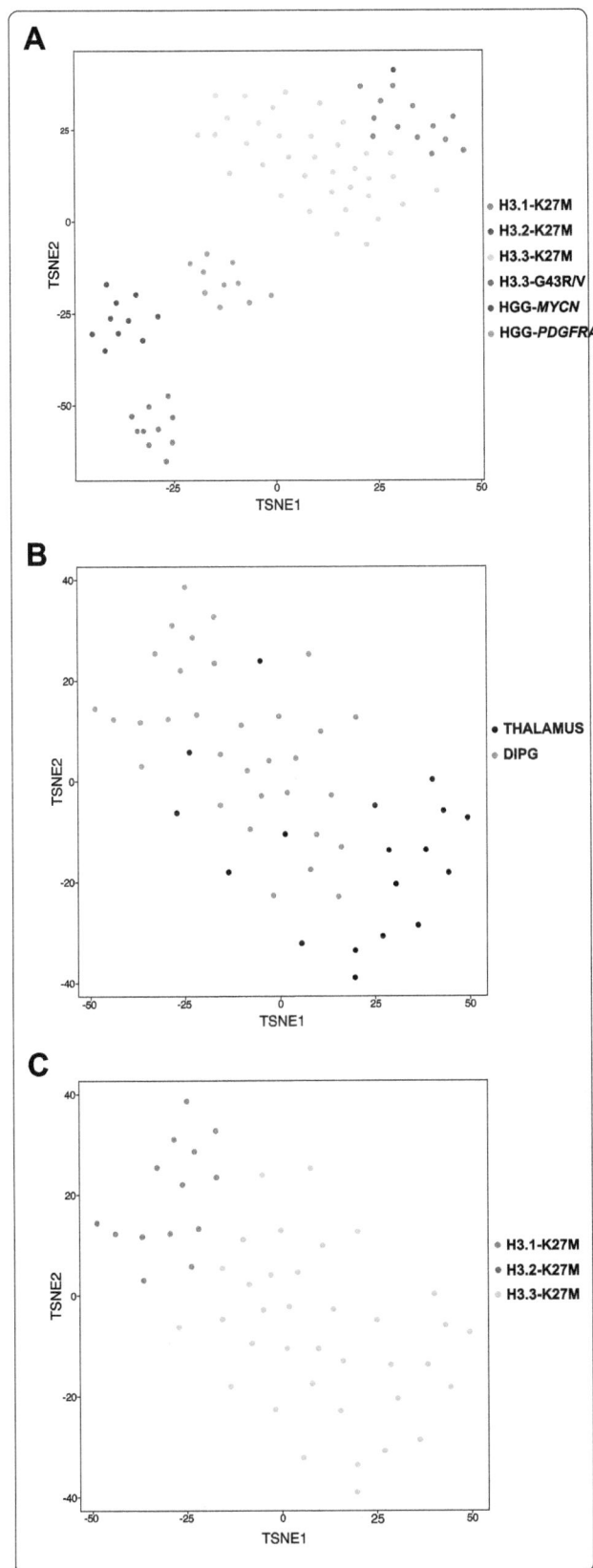

Fig. 2 Classification of high-grade gliomas based on genome-wide DNA methylation profiles. **a** t-SNE analysis of the methylation profiles of 80 pediatric high-grade gliomas using the topmost differentially methylated probes across the sample set (s.d. > 0.25). Midline tumors are color-coded according to the histone H3 gene mutated: dark green for H3.1-K27M (*n* = 13), purple for H3.2-K27M (*n* = 1) and light green for H3.3-K27M tumors (*n* = 36). Others H3-WT high-grade glioma are also presented: H3.3-G34R mutated tumors (*n* = 10, blue), *PDGFRA* (*n* = 10, orange) and *MYCN* (*n* = 10, brown) amplified tumors. **b-c** Analysis of methylation patterns of 50 pediatric H3-K27M midline tumors by t-SNE indicates that H3.1-K27M and H3.3-K27M tumors are clearly distinct from each other. Dimensionality reduction and visualization of methylome data was performed by t-SNE after selection of the probes with the greatest variance (*n* = 10,000; See Methods). Samples were color-coded according to their location (**b**), the histone H3 gene mutated (**c**). t-SNE show two main clusters corresponding to H3.1/H3.2-K27M and H3.3-K27M subgrouping

we decided to evaluate if the different DNA methylation profiles were associated with distinct transcriptome profiles. PCA analysis of GE measurements by microarrays did not clearly discriminate H3.1 and H3.3 mutated tumor samples (Fig. 1b). Indeed, even if H3.1-K27M DIPG were closer to each other in the 2-dimensional PCA plot, they are surrounded by H3.3-K27M samples. However, as microarray data were generated in several batches, we could not exclude that this could obscure the dataset, despite the use of a batch correction method. Therefore, we took advantage of a RNA-seq study of 21 new H3-K27M DIPGs samples which appeared more suitable as it provides an exhaustive measurement of transcriptome in contrast to microarray analysis. Grouping of tumors based on their RNA-seq expression profiles in either t-SNE or PCA classifications confirmed the discrimination of H3.1-K27M from H3.3-K27M tumors observed in our DNA methylation study (Fig. 3b and Additional file 5: Figure S2).

H3.1- and H3.3-K27M mutations are associated with different genomic distribution of the H3K27me3 epigenetic mark

To complement the description of the epigenetic landscape of DIPGs, we decided to assess the direct epigenetic consequences of the K27M mutation in H3.1-K27M and H3.3-K27M tumors, i.e. the loss and redistribution of the trimethylation mark at position K27. We thus took advantage of 6 GSC models of different genotypes as an expandable source of material and interrogated the genome-wide distribution of this mark with ChIP-seq. We conducted a PCA analysis on all genomic regions showing enrichment for this mark and could again separate the samples based on the type of mutated histone (Fig. 3c). This implied that despite the similar biochemical impact of both H3.1-K27M and H3.3-K27M mutated histones on PRC2, interferences of the two

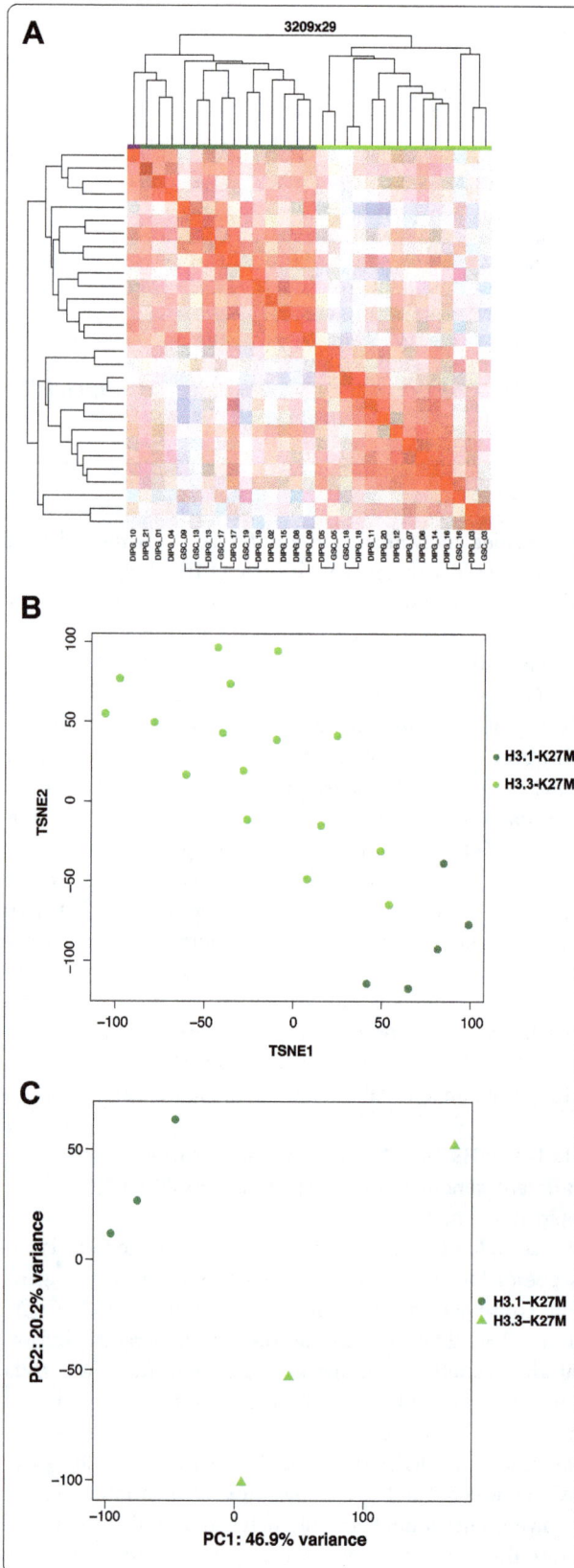

Fig. 3 Subclassification of DIPG based on RNA-seq, methylome and H3K27me3 epigenetic profiles. **a** Heatmap and hierarchical clustering of the Pearson correlation matrix of 19 DIPG and 8 matched GSC cultures (H3.3-K27M and H3.1-K27M in light and dark green respectively) across 3209 probes used for DNA methylation measurements. **b** t-SNE analysis of RNA-seq data in DIPG. RNA sequencing of 21 DIPG samples was performed and the genes associated with the highest standard deviation ($n = 250$) were selected to conduct t-SNE analysis. The tumors were color-coded according to histone H3 mutated, i.e. H3.3-K27M in light green and H3.1-K27M in dark green. **c** Principal component analysis of 3 H3.1- and 3 H3.3-K27M GSC models of DIPG based on H3K27me3 epigenetic mark profiling ($n = 16,977$ genomic intervals)

different mutated histones H3 on PRC2 is not similarly distributed in the genome and this may induce meaningful changes in the epigenetic landscapes of these DIPGs.

The average signal of all H3K27me3 peak regions was equivalent in H3.1- and H3.3-K27M tumors (Additional file 6: Figure S3A, top). We plotted the ChIP-seq signal of the union of H3K27me3 peaks identified from all the GSC samples and did not observed a specificity of the genomic regions presenting a H3K27me3 deposition between H3.1 and H3.3 K27M subgroups but rather a difference in the level of the signal enrichment (Additional file 6: Figure S3A, bottom). However, the genome distribution of H3K27me3 showed an enrichment of peaks in distal intergenic regions in H3.3-K27M GSC and in contrast in intronic and at a lesser extent exonic regions in H3.1-K27M cells (Fig. 4a).

Subsequently, we divided the active genomic loci presenting H3K27me3 deposition according to their location. Overall, the global signal was significantly higher in regions overlapping genes *versus* intergenic regions (Additional file 6: Figure S3B-C). The heatmap displayed that the majority of regions overlapping genes presented a lower level of H3K27me3 in H3.1-K27M samples (Additional file 6: Figure S3C). This observation was concordant with a higher number of expressed genes in H3.1, which are moreover associated with higher expression levels (Additional file 6: Figure S3D).

The clustering of genomic intervals by k-means highlighted the existence of distinct subgroups of loci, smaller gene clusters with a significantly higher level of H3K27me3 in H3.1-mutated cells (C1, C2 and C3 for genic and C1' and C3' for intergenic loci, Fig. 4b and c respectively). Consequently, the vast majority of loci were enriched in K27me3 in H3.3-mutated cells.

Thereafter, we focused on the differentially expressed genes identified by RNA-seq between the 2 subgroups (adj *p*-value< 0.01). The results showed that upregulated genes in H3.1-K27M are associated with a lower average signal of H3K27me3 and *vice et versa* for downregulated genes (Fig. 5a). The ChIP-seq read coverage are shown for two representative genes, *OLIG2* and *SLFN11*, even

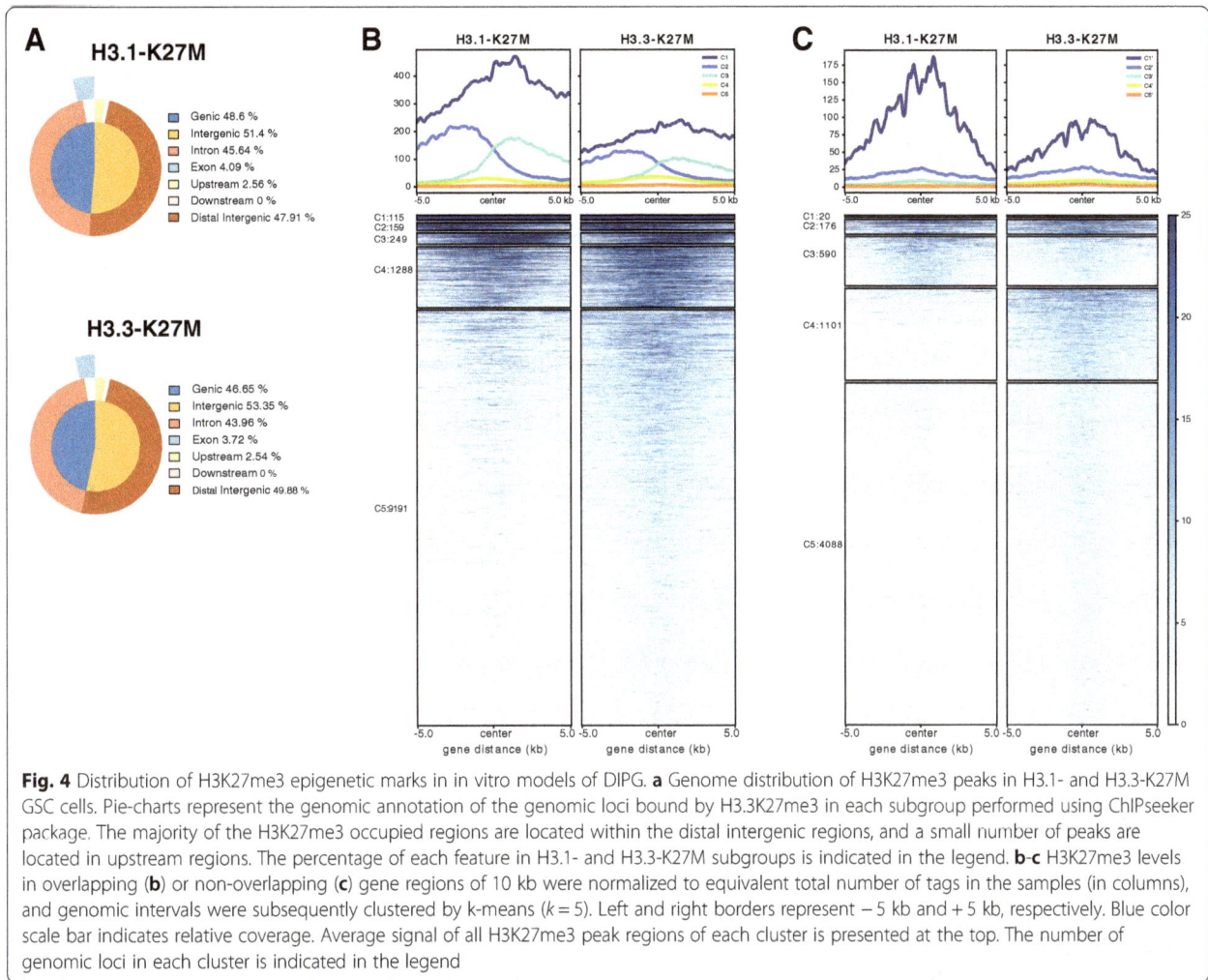

Fig. 4 Distribution of H3K27me3 epigenetic marks in in vitro models of DIPG. **a** Genome distribution of H3K27me3 peaks in H3.1- and H3.3-K27M GSC cells. Pie-charts represent the genomic annotation of the genomic loci bound by H3.3K27me3 in each subgroup performed using ChIPseeker package. The majority of the H3K27me3 occupied regions are located within the distal intergenic regions, and a small number of peaks are located in upstream regions. The percentage of each feature in H3.1- and H3.3-K27M subgroups is indicated in the legend. **b-c** H3K27me3 levels in overlapping (**b**) or non-overlapping (**c**) gene regions of 10 kb were normalized to equivalent total number of tags in the samples (in columns), and genomic intervals were subsequently clustered by k-means (k = 5). Left and right borders represent − 5 kb and + 5 kb, respectively. Blue color scale bar indicates relative coverage. Average signal of all H3K27me3 peak regions of each cluster is presented at the top. The number of genomic loci in each cluster is indicated in the legend

if distinct localization of H3K27me3 is observed between both, located mainly upstream and downstream of transcribed region for *SLFN11* and overlapping gene body for *OLIG2* (Fig. 5b and c). However, gene expression modulations between H3.1- and H3.3-mutated tumors was not restricted to changes in H3K27me3 deposition at the close vicinity of the gene body as shown for *HOXD8* which is upregulated and associated with an increased H3K27me3 deposition in H3.1-K27M tumors (Fig. 5d).

Discussion and conclusions

The recent update of the WHO classification aggregated DIPG and infiltrating glial neoplasms of the midline presenting a H3-K27M substitution as a new entity: diffuse midline glioma (DMG) H3 K27M-mutant. But this implied that the histone H3-K27M would be a stronger driver of oncogenesis than location. We used a pHGG cohort at diagnosis to evaluate the similarity of these H3-K27M mutated tumors at both DNA methylation and gene expression levels and compared them to other

pHGG tumor subgroups in order to support or question the new update of the WHO classification [23].

Tumor classification based on microarray gene expression profiling revealed that K27M mutated tumors, either thalamic or pontine, can be discriminated from all others. Consequently, the molecular subtype appears to influence more the gene expression profile than the infratentorial *vs.* supratentorial location of the tumor in the brain. Alternatively, location may not be considered at the structural level (i.e. brainstem *vs.* thalamus) but rather at the embryological level (midline *vs.* hemispheres) thus unifying midline tumors. Accordingly, survival analyses highlighted a similarly poor prognosis for DIPG and thalamic tumors, either mutated or not for histone H3. The bad outcome of all midline gliomas with K27M mutations was also observed by Karreman et al. [13]. Taken together these data support the rationale to define the same treatment paradigms for both midline K27M tumors and DIPG.

The stratification based on DNA methylation profiling of our pHGG population also supports the similarity

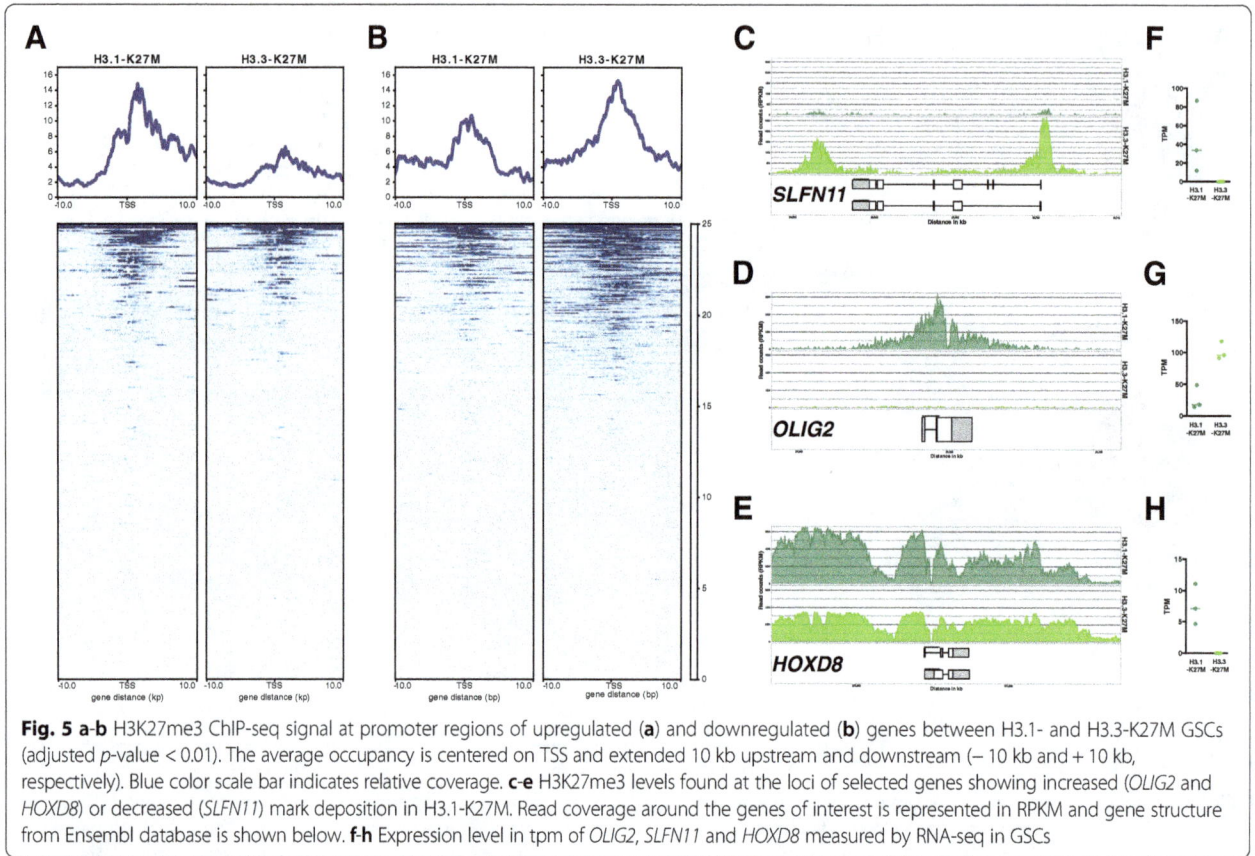

Fig. 5 a-b H3K27me3 ChIP-seq signal at promoter regions of upregulated (**a**) and downregulated (**b**) genes between H3.1- and H3.3-K27M GSCs (adjusted *p*-value < 0.01). The average occupancy is centered on TSS and extended 10 kb upstream and downstream (− 10 kb and + 10 kb, respectively). Blue color scale bar indicates relative coverage. **c-e** H3K27me3 levels found at the loci of selected genes showing increased (*OLIG2* and *HOXD8*) or decreased (*SLFN11*) mark deposition in H3.1-K27M. Read coverage around the genes of interest is represented in RPKM and gene structure from Ensembl database is shown below. **f-h** Expression level in tpm of *OLIG2*, *SLFN11* and *HOXD8* measured by RNA-seq in GSCs

between thalamic and pontine H3-K27M tumors. Our results are concordant with previous reports concerning the discrimination of G34R/V and K27M mutated tumors depending on DNA methylation [18, 23]. Moreover, t-SNE analysis highlighted a clear distinction of H3-K27M tumors from all other pHGG subtypes. Indeed, G34 mutated tumors, *PDGFRA* and *MYCN* subtypes represent three homogenous groups distinct from K27M tumors.

The DIPG median survival was similar to the large retrospective pHGG cohort recently analyzed by Mac-Kay and collaborators [18]. However, midline and hemispheric tumors were associated with longer median survival in our cohort, 18 *versus* 13.5 months and 30.5 *versus* 18 months, respectively. Survival analyses also pointed out a significantly better outcome of histone H3 wild-type non-thalamic midline tumors, which likely reflects that they may be less diffusely growing gliomas and could therefore be more amenable to surgical resection, or that they exhibit a behavior of low-grade gliomas.

Finally, in the gene expression analysis some diffuse midline gliomas without any H3-K27M mutation are grouped with the H3K27M tumors. Interestingly, they all exhibit a loss of the H3K27me3 mark as well. Thus,

defining the entity by the H3K27M mutation only may therefore be too restrictive. Further studies are needed to sort this issue, especially since diffuse pontine and thalamic malignant gliomas have a poor prognosis irrespective of the presence of an H3K27M mutation or not as also recently shown in the HERBY trial (Mackay et al., Cancer Cell 2018).

Interestingly, our methylation profiling data showed a subclassification of DMG, H3 K27M-mutant into two subgroups according to the histone gene affected by the K27M substitution, i.e. *H3F3A* or *HIST1H3B/C*. The sole H3.2-K27M sample clustered together with H3.1-K27M tumors, as expected given that they are both canonical histone H3 with identical role in the cell [24]. Yet, the similarity of H3.1 and H3.2 mutated tumors should be confirmed with additional H3.2 mutated samples from other cohorts, as only two were reported in the literature [2, 18]. Histone H3.1 and H3.3-K27M tumors were also discriminated by RNAseq transcriptome profiling, supporting their intrinsic divergence. This could support the recently reported superiority of RNAseq over expression microarrays for tumor classification purposes [28]. MacKay *and coll.* did not report this distinction between H3.1 and H3.3 mutated tumors using DNA methylation profiling. This difference might result from a 10 times smaller proportion of H3.1 mutated samples analyzed (8 out of 441 samples) hiding out the variability brought by these tumors in their huge dataset. In addition, we used a 7 times larger set of probes (10,000 instead of 1381) that might have captured more variations in the overall pHGG DNA methylation landscape.

It is assumed -and was recently demonstrated by Hoadley et al., that DNA methylation can reflect the epigenetic memory of cancer cell-of-origin [11]. Indeed, DNA methylation is inherited through successive division and is shown to be not only tumor-type specific, but can also reflect the cell type and differentiation state of the transformed cells [6]. The clear separation by DNA methylation profiling of H3.1-K27M from H3.3-K27M tumors may support that these tumors would arise from distinct cells of origin or at distinct differentiation steps in the lineage. This strongly corroborates our previous results showing that DIPG can be divided in two main H3.1-K27M and H3.3-K27M tumor subgroups, associated with distinct histological and molecular phenotypes, age of onset and location along the midline, H3.1-K27M mutation being almost exclusively seen in the brainstem while H3.3-K27M mutation are distributed everywhere along the midline [2]. Also, the conservation of DNA methylation discrepancies in GSCs confirm they are intrinsic characteristic of the tumor cells as opposed to the peri-tumor stroma. Furthermore, we demonstrate that despite the same global biochemical consequence of the H3K27M driver mutation, significant differences exist in the H3K27me3 landscape relying on the type of histone H3 variant affected (i.e. H3.1 or H3.3) as shown by PCA.

As a whole, the distribution of the H3K27me3 marks along the genome is different, both at the quantitative and qualitative levels. Average level of trimethylation at K27 is similar in both subtypes since only a small number of loci are highly enriched in H3K27me3 in H3.1 K27M mutated tumors, whereas the majority of the regions presenting this epigenetic mark are associated with a higher signal in H3.3-K27M. These H3K27me3 variations among the two subgroups are associated with the modulations of gene expression, many more genes being repressed in H3.3-K27M tumors. Qualitatively, K-means clustering of the distribution of this mark identified 5 clusters of genic regions and 5 clusters of intergenic regions differentially trimethylated at position K27 in the two subgroups of DIPG. We show that among differentially expressed genes, levels of H3K27me3 are anti-correlated with gene expression in general. However, gene expression could not be strictly explained by the levels of H3K27me3 in all cases leaving the possibility of additional levels of regulation for gene expression in DIPG.

Overall, we provide molecular and clinical evidence in favor of the unification of all midline K27M mutated tumors that was proposed in the 2016 WHO CNS classification based on their common driver mutation. As such, these gliomas need to be considered as a unique entity in future clinical trials. Further analyses on the biology of H3.3 and H3.1 mutated diffuse gliomas are required to explain the distinction we have reported so far; this could allow testing specific precision medicine approaches in these two subgroups of diffuse midline gliomas.

Additional files

Additional file 1: Table S1. Summary of the 215 pHGG samples analyzed by either gene expression microarray, RNA-seq or methylation array. (XLSX 9 kb)

Additional file 2: Table S2. PCA weights in gene expression analysis of pHGG. Table containing the weights of the 2 first principal components of each of the 120 genes used for the analysis of gene expression of the pHGG by PCA (Fig. 1). (XLSX 14 kb)

Additional file 3: Figure S1. A. Principal component analysis of microarray GE profiling of 119 high grade gliomas as presented in Fig. 1b colored by mutational histone H3 status. Five pontine WT tumors that also harbor a H3K27 trimethylation loss by IHC are highlighted with red arrowheads. B- The gene expression data of the 120 genes associated with the highest standard deviation ($n = 120$ genes) were used for k-means analysis ($k = 2$) and the results represented in the same PCA as in panel A. The samples were color-coded according to k-means results, symbols reflect the histone H3 mutational status and their location are indicated in the plot. C-D. t-SNE analysis of the GE profiles of 119 pediatric high-grade gliomas using the genes associated with the highest standard deviation ($n = 120$ genes). The tumors were color-coded according to their location (A) or mutational histone H3 status (B) as described in Fig. 1. E- Overlapping of the gene lists resulting from differential analysis between: H3-K27M and wild-type tumors, H3-K27M and G34R tumors, H3-G34R and wild-type tumors, H3.1 K27M and H3.3-K27M tumors (adjusted p-value< 0.01). (PDF 224 kb)

Additional file 4: Table S3. Lists of differentially expressed genes in microarrays data from H3-K27M vs. H3-WT, H3-G34R vs. H3-K27M, H3-G34R vs. H3-WT comparisons (adj p-value< 0.01). (XLSX 174 kb)

Additional file 5: Figure S2. Principal component analysis of the GE profile of 21 DIPG using the gene associated with the highest standard deviation ($n = 250$ genes, H3.1-K27M DIPG in dark green and H3.3-K27M DIPG in light green). (PDF 54 kb)

Additional file 6: Figure S3. A-C. Metaplots showing average signal accumulation in reads of all the regions bound by H3K27me3 in at least one sample (A, $n = 16,979$) or H3K27me3 occupied regions with or without overlapping genes (B, $n = 11,003$ and C, $n = 5976$ respectively) in both H3.1- and H3.3-K27M GSC cells. Each plot is centered on the summit of the average occupancy and extended 10 kb upstream and downstream (− 10 kb and + 10 kb, respectively). Below the metaplots, heatmaps illustrating average H3K27me3 levels in the 20 kb genomic intervals centered on the summit of the peak in each subgroup are presented. D. Violin plot displaying transcript expression level of RNA-seq data in tpm in H3.1- and H3.3-K27M subgroups. Boxplots represent the 5th,25th,75th and 95th percentiles and the median of the transcript distribution, The distributions were divided in 4 categories: non expressed genes (< 0.1 tpm), low expressed genes (from 0.1 to 1 tpm), intermediate (from 1 to 10 tpm) and highly expressed genes (> 10 tpm). (PDF 2819 kb)

Acknowledgements

DC, CP, TK, JM, EB, JG, MAD acknowledge financial support from Etoile de Martin and Carrefour through the campaign "Les Boucles du Coeur", DC from Cancéropôle Île-de-France "Émergence 2018", and SP from Association pour la Recherche en Neurochirurgie Pédiatrique. CJ acknowledges NHS funding to the NIHR Biomedical Research Centre at The Royal Marsden Hospital and the ICR.

Authors' contributions

SP, CSR, KK, CJ and JG collected the patient cohort. DC, CP, TK, EB, JM, MS, CJ, DJ and MAD collected genomic data and performed bioinformatics analyses. DC, CP, TK, JG, DJ and MAD analyzed and interpreted the results. PV performed central pathology review. DC, JG and MAD wrote the manuscript. All authors read and approved the final manuscript.

Competing interests

The authors declare that they have no competing interests.

Author details

[1]UMR8203,Vectorologie et Nouvelles Thérapies Anticancéreuses, CNRS, Gustave Roussy, Univ. Paris-Sud, Université Paris-Saclay, 94805 Villejuif, France. [2]Département de Cancérologie de l'Enfant et de l'Adolescent, Institut de Cancérologie Gustave Roussy, Université Paris-Sud, Université Paris-Saclay, 114 rue Édouard Vaillant, 94805 Villejuif Cedex, France. [3]Hopp Children's Cancer Center at the NCT Heidelberg (KiTZ), Heidelberg, Germany. [4]Division of Pediatric Neurooncology (B062), German Cancer Research Center (DKFZ) and German Cancer Consortium (DKTK), Im Neuenheimer Feld 280, 69120 Heidelberg, Germany. [5]Department of Pediatric Neurosurgery, Hôpital Necker-Enfants Malades, Université Paris V Descartes, Sorbonne Paris Cité, Paris, France. [6]Division of Pediatric Hematology and Oncology, University Medical Center Goettingen, Goettingen, Germany. [7]Divisions of Molecular Pathology and Cancer Therapeutics, The Institute of Cancer Research, Sutton, Surrey, UK. [8]Department of Neuropathology, Hôpital Sainte-Anne, Université Paris V Descartes, Sorbonne Paris Cité, Paris, France. [9]Department of Pediatric Hematology and Oncology, Heidelberg University Hospital, Heidelberg, Germany. [10]Pediatric Glioma Research Group, German Cancer Research Center (DKFZ) and German Cancer Consortium (DKTK), Im Neuenheimer Feld 280, 69120 Heidelberg, Germany. [11]Université Evry, Université Paris-Saclay, 91057 Evry Cedex, France. [12]NeuroSpin/UNATI, CEA, Université Paris-Saclay, Gif-sur-Yvette, France. [13]Univ. Evry, Université Paris-Saclay, 91057 Evry Cedex, France.

References

1. Castel D, Grill J, Debily M-A (2016) Histone H3 genotyping refines clinico-radiological diagnostic and prognostic criteria in DIPG. Acta Neuropathol 131:795–796. https://doi.org/10.1007/s00401-016-1568-7
2. Castel D, Philippe C, Calmon R, Le Dret L, Truffaux N, Boddaert N, Pagès M, Taylor KR, Saulnier P, Lacroix L, Mackay A, Jones C, Sainte-Rose C, Blauwblomme T, Andreiuolo F, Puget S, Grill J, Varlet P, Debily M-A (2015) Histone H3F3A and HIST1H3B K27M mutations define two subgroups of diffuse intrinsic pontine gliomas with different prognosis and phenotypes. Acta Neuropathol 130:815–827. https://doi.org/10.1007/s00401-015-1478-0
3. Cohen KJ, Jabado N, Grill J (2017) Diffuse intrinsic pontine gliomas-current management and new biologic insights. Is there a glimmer of hope? Neuro-Oncology 19:1025–1034. https://doi.org/10.1093/neuonc/nox021
4. Eisenstat DD, Pollack IF, Demers A, Sapp MV, Lambert P, Weisfeld-Adams JD, Burger PC, Gilles F, Davis RL, Packer R, Boyett JM, Finlay JL (2015) Impact of tumor location and pathological discordance on survival of children with midline high-grade gliomas treated on Children's Cancer Group high-grade glioma study CCG-945. J Neuro-Oncol 121:573–581. https://doi.org/10.1007/s11060-014-1669-x
5. ENCODE Project Consortium, Bernstein BE, Birney E, Dunham I, Green ED, Gunter C, Snyder M (2012) An integrated encyclopedia of DNA elements in the human genome. Nature 489:57–74. https://doi.org/10.1038/nature11247
6. Fernandez AF, Assenov Y, Martin-Subero JI, Balint B, Siebert R, Taniguchi H, Yamamoto H, Hidalgo M, Tan A-C, Galm O, Ferrer I, Sanchez-Cespedes M, Villanueva A, Carmona J, Sanchez-Mut JV, Berdasco M, Moreno V, Capella G, Monk D, Ballestar E, Ropero S, Martinez R, Sanchez-Carbayo M, Prosper F, Agirre X, Fraga MF, Graña O, Perez-Jurado L, Mora J, Puig S, Prat J, Badimon L, Puca AA, Meltzer SJ, Lengauer T, Bridgewater J, Bock C, Esteller M (2012) A DNA methylation fingerprint of 1628 human samples. Genome Res 22:407–419. https://doi.org/10.1101/gr.119867.110
7. Gagnon-Bartsch JA, Jacob L, Speed TP (2013) Removing unwanted variation from high dimensional data with negative controls. https://statistics.berkeley.edu/sites/default/files/tech-reports/ruv.pdf

8. Gibson P, Tong Y, Robinson G, Thompson MC, Currle DS, Eden C, Kranenburg TA, Hogg T, Poppleton H, Martin J, Finkelstein D, Pounds S, Weiss A, Patay Z, Scoggins M, Ogg R, Pei Y, Yang Z-J, Brun S, Lee Y, Zindy F, Lindsey JC, Taketo MM, Boop FA, Sanford RA, Gajjar A, Clifford SC, Roussel MF, McKinnon PJ, Gutmann DH, Ellison DW, Wechsler-Reya R, Gilbertson RJ (2010) Subtypes of medulloblastoma have distinct developmental origins. Nature 468:1095–1099
9. Gilbertson RJ, Gutmann DH (2007) Tumorigenesis in the brain: location, location, location. Cancer Res 67:5579–5582. https://doi.org/10.1158/0008-5472.CAN-07-0760
10. Grill J, Massimino M, Bouffet E, Azizi AA, McCowage G, Cañete A, Saran F, Le Deley M-C, Varlet P, Morgan PS, Jaspan T, Jones C, Giangaspero F, Smith H, Garcia J, Elze MC, Rousseau RF, Abrey L, Hargrave D, Vassal G (2018) Phase II, open-label, randomized, multicenter trial (HERBY) of bevacizumab in pediatric patients with newly diagnosed high-grade glioma. J Clin Oncol 36: 951–958. https://doi.org/10.1200/JCO.2017.76.0611
11. Hoadley KA, Yau C, Hinoue T, Wolf DM, Lazar AJ, Drill E, Shen R, Taylor AM, Cherniack AD, Thorsson V, Akbani R, Bowlby R, Wong CK, Wiznerowicz M, Sanchez-Vega F, Robertson AG, Schneider BG, Lawrence MS, Noushmehr H, Malta TM, Network CGA, Stuart JM, Benz CC, Laird PW (2018) Cell-of-origin patterns dominate the molecular classification of 10,000 tumors from 33 types of cancer. Cell 173:291–304.e6. https://doi.org/10.1016/j.cell.2018.03.022
12. Hovestadt V, Remke M, Kool M, Pietsch T, Northcott PA, Fischer R, Cavalli FMG, Ramaswamy V, Zapatka M, Reifenberger G, Rutkowski S, Schick M, Bewerunge-Hudler M, Korshunov A, Lichter P, Taylor MD, Pfister SM, Jones DTW (2013) Robust molecular subgrouping and copy-number profiling of medulloblastoma from small amounts of archival tumour material using high-density DNA methylation arrays. Acta Neuropathol 125:913–916. https://doi.org/10.1007/s00401-013-1126-5
13. Karremann M, Gielen GH, Hoffmann M, Wiese M, Colditz N, Warmuth-Metz M, Bison B, Claviez A, van Vuurden DG, von Bueren AO, Gessi M, Kühnle I, Hans VH, Benesch M, Sturm D, Kortmann R-D, Waha A, Pietsch T, Kramm CM (2018) Diffuse high-grade gliomas with H3 K27M mutations carry a dismal prognosis independent of tumor location. Neuro-Oncology 20:123–131. https://doi.org/10.1093/neuonc/nox149
14. Korshunov A, Ryzhova M, Hovestadt V, Bender S, Sturm D, Capper D, Meyer J, Schrimpf D, Kool M, Northcott PA, Zheludkova O, Milde T, Witt O, Kulozik AE, Reifenberger G, Jabado N, Perry A, Lichter P, von Deimling A, Pfister SM, Jones DTW (2015) Integrated analysis of pediatric glioblastoma reveals a subset of biologically favorable tumors with associated molecular prognostic markers. Acta Neuropathol 129: 669–678. https://doi.org/10.1007/s00401-015-1405-4
15. Korshunov A, Schrimpf D, Ryzhova M, Sturm D, Chavez L, Hovestadt V, Sharma T, Habel A, Burford A, Jones C, Zheludkova O, Kumirova E, Kramm CM, Golanov A, Capper D, von Deimling A, Pfister SM, Jones DTW (2017) H3-/IDH-wild type pediatric glioblastoma is comprised of molecularly and prognostically distinct subtypes with associated oncogenic drivers. Acta Neuropathol. https://doi.org/10.1007/s00401-017-1710-1
16. Lewis PW, Müller MM, Koletsky MS, Cordero F, Lin S, Banaszynski LA, Garcia BA, Muir TW, Becher OJ, Allis CD (2013) Inhibition of PRC2 activity by a gain-of-function H3 mutation found in pediatric glioblastoma. Science 340:857–861. https://doi.org/10.1126/science.1232245
17. Louis DN, Perry A, Reifenberger G, von Deimling A, Figarella-Branger D, Cavenee WK, Ohgaki H, Wiestler OD, Kleihues P, Ellison DW (2016) The 2016 World Health Organization classification of tumors of the central nervous system: a summary. Acta Neuropathol 131:803–820. https://doi.org/10.1007/s00401-016-1545-1
18. Mackay A, Burford A, Carvalho D, Izquierdo E, Fazal-Salom J, Taylor KR, Bjerke L, Clarke M, Vinci M, Nandhabalan M, Temelso S, Popov S, Molinari V, Raman P, Waanders AJ, Han HJ, Gupta S, Marshall L, Zacharoulis S, Vaidya S, Mandeville HC, Bridges LR, Martin AJ, Al-Sarraj S, Chandler C, Ng H-K, Li X, Mu K, Trabelsi S, Brahim DH-B, Kisljakov AN, Konovalov DM, Moore AS, Carcaboso AM, Sunol M, de Torres C, Cruz O, Mora J, Shats LI, Stavale JN, Bidinotto LT, Reis RM, Entz-Werle N, Farrell M, Cryan J, Crimmins D, Caird J, Pears J, Monje M, Debily M-A, Castel D, Grill J, Hawkins C, Nikbakht H, Jabado N, Baker SJ, Pfister SM, Jones DTW, Fouladi M, von Bueren AO, Baudis M, Resnick A, Jones C (2017) Integrated molecular meta-analysis of 1,000 pediatric high-grade and diffuse intrinsic pontine glioma. Cancer Cell 32:520–537.e5. https://doi.org/10.1016/j.ccell.2017.08.017
19. Plessier A, Le Dret L, Varlet P, Beccaria K, Lacombe J, Mériaux S, Geffroy F, Fiette L, Flamant P, Chrétien F, Blauwblomme T, Puget S, Grill J, Debily M-A,

Castel D (2017) New in vivo avatars of diffuse intrinsic pontine gliomas (DIPG) from stereotactic biopsies performed at diagnosis. Oncotarget 8: 52543–52559. https://doi.org/10.18632/oncotarget.15002

20. Puget S, Boddaert N, Veillard A-S, Garnett M, Miquel C, Andreiuolo F, Sainte-Rose C, Roujeau T, DiRocco F, Bourgeois M, Zerah M, Doz F, Grill J, Varlet P (2011) Neuropathological and neuroradiological spectrum of pediatric malignant gliomas: correlation with outcome. Neurosurgery 69:215–224. https://doi.org/10.1227/NEU.0b013e3182134340

21. Schwartzentruber J, Korshunov A, Liu X-Y, Jones DTW, Pfaff E, Jacob K, Sturm D, Fontebasso AM, Quang D-AK, Tönjes M, Hovestadt V, Albrecht S, Kool M, Nantel A, Konermann C, Lindroth A, Jäger N, Rausch T, Ryzhova M, Korbel JO, Hielscher T, Hauser P, Garami M, Klekner A, Bognar L, Ebinger M, Schuhmann MU, Scheurlen W, Pekrun A, Frühwald MC, Roggendorf W, Kramm C, Dürken M, Atkinson J, Lepage P, Montpetit A, Zakrzewska M, Zakrzewski K, Liberski PP, Dong Z, Siegel P, Kulozik AE, Zapatka M, Guha A, Malkin D, Felsberg J, Reifenberger G, von Deimling A, Ichimura K, Collins VP, Witt H, Milde T, Witt O, Zhang C, Castelo-Branco P, Lichter P, Faury D, Tabori U, Plass C, Majewski J, Pfister SM, Jabado N (2012) Driver mutations in histone H3.3 and chromatin remodelling genes in paediatric glioblastoma. Nature 482:226–231. https://doi.org/10.1038/nature10833

22. Sturm D, Orr BA, Toprak UH, Hovestadt V, Jones DTW, Capper D, Sill M, Buchhalter I, Northcott PA, Leis I, Ryzhova M, Koelsche C, Pfaff E, Allen SJ, Balasubramanian G, Worst BC, Pajtler KW, Brabetz S, Johann PD, Sahm F, Reimand J, Mackay A, Carvalho DM, Remke M, Phillips JJ, Perry A, Cowdrey C, Drissi R, Fouladi M, Giangaspero F, Łastowska M, Grajkowska W, Scheurlen W, Pietsch T, Hagel C, Gojo J, Lötsch D, Berger W, Slavc I, Haberler C, Jouvet A, Holm S, Hofer S, Prinz M, Keohane C, Fried I, Mawrin C, Scheie D, Mobley BC, Schniederjan MJ, Santi M, Buccoliero AM, Dahiya S, Kramm CM, von Bueren AO, von Hoff K, Rutkowski S, Herold-Mende C, Frühwald MC, Milde T, Hasselblatt M, Wesseling P, Rößler J, Schüller U, Ebinger M, Schittenhelm J, Frank S, Grobholz R, Vajtai I, Hans V, Schneppenheim R, Zitterbart K, Collins VP, Aronica E, Varlet P, Puget S, Dufour C, Grill J, Figarella-Branger D, Wolter M, Schuhmann MU, Shalaby T, Grotzer M, van Meter T, Monoranu C-M, Felsberg J, Reifenberger G, Snuderl M, Forrester LA, Koster J, Versteeg R, Volckmann R, van Sluis P, Wolf S, Mikkelsen T, Gajjar A, Aldape K, Moore AS, Taylor MD, Jones C, Jabado N, Karajannis MA, Eils R, Schlesner M, Lichter P, von Deimling A, Pfister SM, Ellison DW, Korshunov A, Kool M (2016) New brain tumor entities emerge from molecular classification of CNS-PNETs. Cell 164:1060–1072. https://doi.org/10.1016/j.cell.2016.01.015

23. Sturm D, Witt H, Hovestadt V, Khuong-Quang D-A, Jones DTW, Konermann C, Pfaff E, Tönjes M, Sill M, Bender S, Kool M, Zapatka M, Becker N, Zucknick M, Hielscher T, Liu X-Y, Fontebasso AM, Ryzhova M, Albrecht S, Jacob K, Wolter M, Ebinger M, Schuhmann MU, van Meter T, Frühwald MC, Hauch H, Pekrun A, Radlwimmer B, Niehues T, von Komorowski G, Dürken M, Kulozik AE, Madden J, Donson A, Foreman NK, Drissi R, Fouladi M, Scheurlen W, von Deimling A, Monoranu C, Roggendorf W, Herold-Mende C, Unterberg A, Kramm CM, Felsberg J, Hartmann C, Wiestler B, Wick W, Milde T, Witt O, Lindroth AM, Schwartzentruber J, Faury D, Fleming A, Zakrzewska M, Liberski PP, Zakrzewski K, Hauser P, Garami M, Klekner A, Bognar L, Morrissy S, Cavalli F, Taylor MD, van Sluis P, Koster J, Versteeg R, Volckmann R, Mikkelsen T, Aldape K, Reifenberger G, Collins VP, Majewski J, Korshunov A, Lichter P, Plass C, Jabado N, Pfister SM (2012) Hotspot mutations in H3F3A and IDH1 define distinct epigenetic and biological subgroups of glioblastoma. Cancer Cell 22:425–437. https://doi.org/10.1016/j.ccr.2012.08.024

24. Szenker E, Ray-Gallet D, Almouzni G (2011) The double face of the histone variant H3.3. Cell Res 21:421–434. https://doi.org/10.1038/cr.2011.14

25. Taylor KR, Mackay A, Truffaux N, Butterfield YS, Morozova O, Philippe C, Castel D, Grasso CS, Vinci M, Carvalho D, Carcaboso AM, de Torres C, Cruz O, Mora J, Entz-Werle N, Ingram WJ, Monje M, Hargrave D, Bullock AN, Puget S, Yip S, Jones C, Grill J (2014) Recurrent activating ACVR1 mutations in diffuse intrinsic pontine glioma. Nat Genet 46:457–461. https://doi.org/10.1038/ng.2925

26. Wu G, Broniscer A, McEachron TA, Lu C, Paugh BS, Becksfort J, Qu C, Ding L, Huether R, Parker M, Zhang J, Gajjar A, Dyer MA, Mullighan CG, Gilbertson RJ, Mardis ER, Wilson RK, Downing JR, Ellison DW, Zhang J, Baker SJ (2012) Somatic histone H3 alterations in pediatric diffuse intrinsic pontine gliomas and non-brainstem glioblastomas. Nat Genet 44:251–253. https://doi.org/10.1038/ng.1102

27. Zang C, Schones DE, Zeng C, Cui K, Zhao K, Peng W (2009) A clustering approach for identification of enriched domains from histone modification ChIP-Seq data. Bioinformatics 25:1952–1958. https://doi.org/10.1093/bioinformatics/btp340

28. Zhang W, Yu Y, Hertwig F, Thierry-Mieg J, Zhang W, Thierry-Mieg D, Wang J, Furlanello C, Devanarayan V, Cheng J, Deng Y, Hero B, Hong H, Jia M, Li L, Lin SM, Nikolsky Y, Oberthuer A, Qing T, Su Z, Volland R, Wang C, Wang MD, Ai J, Albanese D, Asgharzadeh S, Avigad S, Bao W, Bessarabova M, Brilliant MH, Brors B, Chierici M, Chu T-M, Zhang J, Grundy RG, He MM, Hebbring S, Kaufman HL, Lababidi S, Lancashire LJ, Li Y, Lu XX, Luo H, Ma X, Ning B, Noguera R, Peifer M, Phan JH, Roels F, Rosswog C, Shao S, Shen J, Theissen J, Tonini GP, Vandesompele J, Wu P-Y, Xiao W, Xu J, Xu W, Xuan J, Yang Y, Ye Z, Dong Z, Zhang KK, Yin Y, Zhao C, Zheng Y, Wolfinger RD, Shi T, Malkas LH, Berthold F, Wang J, Tong W, Shi L, Peng Z, Fischer M (2015) Comparison of RNA-seq and microarray-based models for clinical endpoint prediction. Genome Biol 16:133. https://doi.org/10.1186/s13059-015-0694-1

8

Detection of tau in Gerstmann-Sträussler-Scheinker disease (*PRNP* F198S) by [18F]Flortaucipir PET

Shannon L. Risacher[1,2*], Martin R. Farlow[2,3], Daniel R. Bateman[2,4], Francine Epperson[2,5], Eileen F. Tallman[1,2], Rose Richardson[2,5], Jill R. Murrell[2,5], Frederick W. Unverzagt[2,4], Liana G. Apostolova[1,2,3,6], Jose M. Bonnin[3,5], Bernardino Ghetti[2,3,4,5,6*] and Andrew J. Saykin[1,2,6*]

Abstract

This study aimed to determine the pattern of [18F]flortaucipir uptake in individuals affected by Gerstmann-Sträussler-Scheinker disease (GSS) associated with the *PRNP* F198S mutation. The aims were to: 1) determine the pattern of [18F]flortaucipir uptake in two GSS patients; 2) compare tau distribution by [18F]flortaucipir PET imaging among three groups: two GSS patients, two early onset Alzheimer's disease patients (EOAD), two cognitively normal older adults (CN); 3) validate the PET imaging by comparing the pattern of [18F]flortaucipir uptake, in vivo, with that of tau neuropathology, *post-mortem*. Scans were processed to generate standardized uptake value ratio (SUVR) images. Regional [18F]flortaucipir SUVR was extracted and compared between GSS patients, EOADs, and CNs. Neuropathology and tau immunohistochemistry were carried out *post-mortem* on a GSS patient who died 9 months after the [18F]flortaucipir scan. The GSS patients were at different stages of disease progression. Patient A was mildly to moderately affected, suffering from cognitive, psychiatric, and ataxia symptoms. Patient B was moderately to severely affected, suffering from ataxia and parkinsonism accompanied by psychiatric and cognitive symptoms. The [18F]flortaucipir scans showed uptake in frontal, cingulate, and insular cortices, as well as in the striatum and thalamus. Uptake was greater in Patient B than in Patient A. Both GSS patients showed greater uptake in the striatum and thalamus than the EOADs and greater uptake in all evaluated regions than the CNs. Thioflavin S fluorescence and immunohistochemistry revealed that the anatomical distribution of tau pathology is consistent with that of [18F]flortaucipir uptake. In GSS patients, the neuroanatomical localization of pathologic tau, as detected by [18F]flortaucipir, suggests correlation with the psychiatric, motor, and cognitive symptoms. The topography of uptake in *PRNP* F198S GSS is strikingly different from that seen in AD. Further studies of the sensitivity, specificity, and anatomical patterns of tau PET in diseases with tau pathology are warranted.

Keywords: Positron emission tomography (PET), [18F]flortaucipir/AV-1451/T-807, Gerstmann-Sträussler-Scheinker disease (GSS), Tau, Prion protein (PrP), *PRNP* F198S mutation

Introduction

Gerstmann-Sträussler-Scheinker disease (GSS) [9] is a rare dominantly inherited prion protein (PrP) amyloidosis. GSS patients, from a large kindred, have been extensively studied in three generations [13]; they carry a

TTC to TCC DNA change at codon 198 of the prion protein gene (*PRNP*) resulting in a phenylalanine to serine substitution (F198S) in the prion protein [6, 7, 11, 12, 14, 16, 35]. Neuropathologic examinations in these patients have shown that the extracellular PrP amyloid coexists with a severe intraneuronal tau pathology, characterized by deposits of hyperphosphorylated tau and neurofibrillary tangles (NFT) in the cerebral gray matter, but not in the cerebellum [10, 11, 14]. Clinically, *PRNP* F198S mutation carriers present with cerebellar ataxia and dysarthria, with later bradykinesia and

* Correspondence: srisache@iupui.edu; bghetti@iupui.edu; asaykin@iu.edu
[1]Department of Radiology and Imaging Sciences, Indiana University School of Medicine, 355 West 16th Street, Suite 4100, Indianapolis, IN 46202, USA
[2]Indiana Alzheimer Disease Center, Indiana University School of Medicine, Indianapolis, IN, USA
Full list of author information is available at the end of the article

rigidity. These neurologic symptoms may be preceded by psychiatric manifestations including drug dependence, depression, and/or psychosis [7]. As the disease progresses, memory impairment and cognitive dysfunction become severe [35].

In the brain of individuals carrying the *PRNP* F198S mutation, PrP amyloid deposits occur in the form of multicentric plaques and diffuse deposits throughout the cerebral cortex, subcortical nuclei, cerebellum, and brainstem [10, 12]. Neuropathologically, the pattern of distribution of PrP amyloid differs substantially from that of the amyloid β (Aβ) peptide, which is the major component of the plaques in the dominantly inherited and sporadic forms of Alzheimer's disease (AD). Limited neuropathologic data from non-symptomatic *PRNP* F198S carriers suggest that extracellular PrP amyloid deposits precede the development of tau pathology [11]. Deposition of tau occurs in the form of tau-immunoreactive intracytoplasmic deposits in neurons, NFT, and neuropil threads [10, 12]. By transmission electron microscopy and Western blot analysis, the neurofibrillary tangles in GSS associated with the *PRNP* F198S mutation are similar to those seen in AD [33]. Tau deposition occurs in close proximity to the PrP amyloid deposits, and thus, the pattern of tau pathology in the cerebrum mirrors that of PrP amyloid. As a consequence, both tau spread and topography in this prion disease differ substantially from those observed in AD and other neurodegenerative diseases with tau pathology.

Neuroimaging studies of patients with GSS have employed structural magnetic resonance imagin (MRI), positron emission tomography (PET), and single photon emission computerized tomography (SPECT). To date, only a few studies have evaluated neuroimaging measures in *PRNP* F198S GSS patients. Vitali et al. (2011) studied changes on fluid-attenuated inversion recovery (FLAIR) and diffusion-weighted imaging (DWI) in patients with GSS, including two who carried the *PRNP* F198S mutation and demonstrated hyperintense signal in *PRNP* F198S individuals in limbic, neocortical, and subcortical regions [36]. Kepe et al. (2010) evaluated alterations in GSS patients, including two symptomatic and two asymptomatic *PRNP* F198S GSS patients from the Indiana kindred, on 2-(1-(6-[(2-[fluorine-18]fluoroethyl)(methyl)amino]-2-naphthyl)-ethylidene)malononitrile ([18F]FDDNP) PET, [18F]fluorodeoxyglucose (FDG) PET, and structural MRI [19] images. In that report, the symptomatic *PRNP* F198S GSS patients and one asymptomatic carrier had increased [18F]FDDNP binding in the basal ganglia, thalamus, cerebral cortex, and cerebellum. Reduced metabolism and mild atrophy were also seen in similar regions in symptomatic *PRNP* F198S patients. Recently, another study demonstrated that [11C]PiB, which is selective for Aβ deposition, showed

no specific signal in asymptomatic and symptomatic individuals carrying the *PRNP* P102L mutation or the *PRNP* F198S mutation [4]. Currently, no ligand is available to specifically demonstrate PrP amyloid deposition by PET.

In this study, we sought to: 1) determine the pattern of [18F]flortaucipir uptake in *PRNP* F198S GSS patients; 2) compare the tau distribution on [18F]flortaucipir PET among the following three groups: *PRNP* F198S GSS affected individuals, sporadic early onset AD patients (EOAD), cognitively normal older adults (CN); and, 3) compare the pattern of [18F]flortaucipir uptake, in vivo, with that of tau neuropathology, *post-mortem*. Based on the neuropathological similarity of the tau NFT in *PRNP* F198S GSS and AD [33], we hypothesized that [18F]flortaucipir, a recently developed PET tracer that is specifically sensitive to tau NFTs [2, 37], would permit in vivo detection of tau deposits in *PRNP* F198S GSS patients. In the present study, we report, for the first time, data showing [18F]flortaucipir uptake in two symptomatic GSS individuals carrying the F198S *PRNP* mutation and compare the uptake patterns in these individuals with patterns observed in cognitively normal older adults (CN) and in patients with EOAD. The [18F]flortaucipir PET results are also validated by the neuropathologic demonstration of PrP amyloid and tau deposits in one of the two GSS patients, who died 9 months after the [18F]flortaucipir PET scan.

Materials and methods
Clinical assessment

All participants were evaluated in the context of annual research visits to the Indiana Alzheimer Disease Center (IADC). The clinical assessments included neurological examinations, structured informant interviews for symptoms and function, and neuropsychological assessments. Diagnoses were made by consensus panel using research criteria. Assessments were compliant with National Alzheimer's Coordinating Center (NACC) procedures at the time of the visits including: demographics, health histories, medications, family histories, Clinical Dementia Rating (CDR), Functional Assessment Scale (FAS), Geriatric Depression Scale (GDS), and Neuropsychiatric Interview Questionnaire (NPI-Q). At the time of the [18F]flortaucipir PET scans, cognitive testing with the UDS3 measures included: Montreal Cognitive Assessment (MoCA), Craft Stories immediate and delayed recall, Benson Complex Figure copy and delayed recall, the Multilingual Naming Test (MINT), Animal fluency, Vegetable fluency, Phonemic fluency (letters F and L), Trail Making Test Parts A and B (TMT-A and TMT-B), and Number Span forward and backward. The Rey Auditory Verbal Learning Test (RAVLT) and Digit Symbol Substitution Test were also given to all participants. Written informed consent was obtained from all participants in accordance with the Declaration of Helsinki and the Belmont Report. All procedures were approved by the Indiana University School of Medicine Institutional Review Board.

Genetics

DNA was extracted from fresh blood samples of patients A and B and the open-reading frame of the Prion Protein gene (PRNP) was analyzed by direct sequencing. The same procedure was used to study DNA extracted from the brain tissue of patient B and several previously deceased family members [16].

Structural MRI

A T1-weighted magnetization-prepared rapid gradient-echo (MPRAGE) structural MRI sequence was acquired at the time of the [18F]flortaucipir PET scan on a 3 Tesla Siemens Prisma scanner for both patients. Automatic parcellation with Freesurfer version 5.1 (https://surfer.nmr.mgh.harvard.edu/fswiki/FreeSurferWiki) was completed to create subject-specific regions of interest (ROIs) to use for extraction of mean [18F]flortaucipir standardized uptake value ratio (SUVR; see [18F]Flortaucipir section) from target regions. MPRAGE scans were also segmented in Statistical Parametric Mapping 8 (SPM8) to generate subject-specific spatial normalization parameters for use in PET scan processing.

[18F]Flortaucipir PET

Both patients were studied with [18F]flortaucipir PET within two months of the nearest clinical visit (mean age in the sixth decade). They were injected intravenously with approximately 10 mCi of [18F]flortaucipir and after a 75-min uptake period were scanned for 30 min on a Siemens mCT (six 5-min frames). Scans were reconstructed according to the Alzheimer's Disease Neuroimaging Initiative (ADNI)-2 protocol (http://adni.loni.usc.edu/wp-content/uploads/2015/02/01_DOD-ADNI_Tau-Addendum-Protocol_23Oct2014.pdf). Standard processing, including spatial alignment for motion and normalization to Montreal Neurologic Institute (MNI) space using parameters from the MRI segmentation, was completed in SPM8. Mean static images from 80 to 100 min post-injection were generated by averaging the appropriate frames and smoothed with an 8 mm full-width half maximum (FWHM) Gaussian kernel. Finally, [18F]flortaucipir SUVR images were generated by intensity normalizing by mean cerebellar crus uptake. The [18F]flortaucipir PET scans were qualitatively visualized using MRIcron (http://www.mccauslandcenter.sc.edu/mricro/mricron/). Mean [18F]flortaucipir SUVR values were extracted from subject-specific ROIs, including the caudate nucleus, putamen, pallidum, thalamus, insula, anterior cingulate gyrus, posterior cingulate gyrus, overall lobar regions (frontal, parietal, temporal, and occipital), the overall cingulate cortex, the sensory-motor cortices, and the global cortex.

[18F]Flortaucipir PET scans from two CN (mean age of approximately 67.5 years) and two Aβ-positive EOAD patients (mean age of approximately 61 years; mean age of onset of approximately 59 years) were used as comparisons. The patients were selected to match the PRNP F198S GSS patients by sex and, as closely as possible, by age and global cognition on the MoCA. All scans were processed as described above. Scans were visualized using MRIcron and mean SUVR was extracted from Freesurfer-generated subject-specific ROIs for the regions described above. For display purposes (Fig. 4), mean SUVR values were calculated for the target ROIs in both CN individuals and both EOAD patients as comparisons to the PRNP F198S GSS patients.

Neuropathology

Patient B expired 9 months after the [18F]flortaucipir PET scan. The brain, harvested at Indiana University School of Medicine, was hemisected along the mid-sagittal plane. The left hemibrain was fixed in formalin. Following fixation in a 10% formalin solution, the left cerebral and cerebellar hemispheres, as well as the left half of the brainstem, were sliced and tissue samples were selected. In order to compare neuropathology with tau PET imaging, six hemispheric coronal slabs were selected that included areas of the frontal, insular, temporal, parietal, and occipital lobes. These were submitted in their entirety for histology and immunohistochemistry. In addition, blocks of the following CNS areas were also submitted: superior frontal gyrus, middle frontal gyrus, anterior cingulate gyrus, superior temporal gyrus, middle temporal gyrus, hippocampus at two levels, entorhinal cortex, precentral cortex, postcentral cortex, inferior parietal lobule, posterior cingulate gyrus and precuneus, calcarine cortex, caudate nucleus, putamen, globus pallidus, amygdala, claustrum, thalamus, subthalamic nucleus, cerebellar vermis, cerebellar cortex and dentate nucleus, midbrain, pons, medulla, and spinal cord at cervical, thoracic, lumbar, and sacral levels. The areas submited were representative of the following Brodmann Areas: 1, 2, 3, 4, 5, 6, 7, 8, 9, 11, 12, 17, 18, 19, 20, 21, 22, 23, 24, 27, 28, 31, 32, 36, 37, 38, 44, 47. The right hemibrain was sliced, frozen, and stored at − 70 °C for structural, biochemical and molecular genetic studies of PrP and tau and for the analysis of the seeding properties of PrP and tau in PRNP F198S GSS.

Brain tissue samples from the left hemibrain were dehydrated in graded alcohols, cleared in xylene, and embedded in paraffin. Eight-micrometer-thick sections from multiple brain areas were stained using the histological and immunohistochemical methods described below. Hematoxylin and eosin (H&E) and Luxol fast blue-hematoxylin & eosin (LFB-H&E) were used to survey gray and white matters for neuronal loss, gliosis, vascular pathology, and other possible pathologic lesions.

The Thioflavin S method was used to visualize amyloid deposits and neurofibrillary tangles. Prussian blue stain enhanced by DAB (Prussian Blue-DAB) visualized the ferric iron deposits in the tissue. Neurodegenerative pathology was further analyzed using antibodies raised against PrP (3F4, 1:800, Dr. Richard Kacsak, Staten-Island, New York, USA), tau (AT8, 1:300, Thermo Fisher Scientific, Waltham, MA, USA; PHF-1, 1:10, gift of Dr. P. Davies); 3-repeat tau (3R, 1:3000, Millipore, Billerica Massachusetts, USA), 4-repeat tau (4R, 1:100, Millipore, Billerica Massachusetts, USA), anti-phospho-TDP-43 (1:1000, Cosmo Biologicals, Carlsbad, CA, USA), α-synuclein (ASy119–137, 1:300, Dr. P. Piccardo, Dr. B. Ghetti) and amyloid β (Aβ 21F12, 1:1000, Janssen Research & Development, South San Francisco, CA, USA). AT8 recognizes tau phosphorylated at serine 202 and threonine 205, while PHF-1 recognizes tau phosphorylated at serine 396 and serine 404. The signal from polyclonal or monoclonal antibodies was visualized using avidin-biotin, with goat anti-rabbit immunoglobulin or goat anti-mouse as the secondary antibody as required, followed by horseradish peroxidase-conjugated streptavidin and the chromogen diaminobenzidine. Immunohistochemical sections were counterstained with hematoxylin.

Results

Case histories

Patient A

Patient A had a family history of GSS and completed 15 IADC clinical yearly assessments before the tau PET scan. The subject was right-handed, had a few years of college education, and was first examined neurologically in their fourth decade. At the first twelve annual visits, clinical, neurologic, and neuropsychological assessments were within normal limits in all respects. During this time period, Patient A was found to have the *PRNP* F198S mutation. In the sixth decade, Patient A developed mild depression and the patient's informant reported the onset of a gradually progressive memory impairment accompanied by a change in personality, characterized by sadness and withdrawal developing over an 18-month period. The NPI-Q also indicated mild apathy and irritability. Otherwise, the neurological and neuropsychological exams were unremarkable and the patient was determined to be cognitively normal. Approximately 1 year later, the patient's informant reported mild worsening of the psychiatric symptoms, including mild depression, irritability, and changes in motor behaviors. Neurologically and cognitively, however, the patient was considered normal except for a mild decline in psychomotor speed that remained within the normal range for the patient's age. The neurological examination on the next visit, approximately 1 year later,was again unremarkable but the supplemental CDR for the behavioral, comportment, and personality domains now indicated mild impairment (a 0.5 rating). NPI-Q revealed progression of symptoms, including mild changes in motor behaviors and mild ataxia, moderate depressive and anxiety symptoms, and altered nighttime behaviors and appetite. The neuropsychological battery indicated mild decline in psychomotor speed and complex sequencing, but these were still within the normal range. Normal cognition was again the consensus diagnosis.

The [18F]flortaucipir PET and the structural MRI scans were completed at the sixteenth clinical assessment. The informant reported a continued decline in memory, progressive changes in personality, as well as slowly progressive decline in language. At the neurological examination, gait abnormalities, slowness, and falls were observed. Results of the neuropsychological examination are shown in Table 1. The global CDR was 0.5, indicating mild global impairment, with mild impairment (a 0.5 rating) in the memory domain and mild-to-moderate impairment (a 1.0 rating) in the judgement and problem-solving domain. The FAS indicated difficulty understanding books and TV shows, difficulty remembering appointments and medications, and need for assistance with finances. The NPI-Q again showed mild depressive symptoms, changes in motor behavior, and changes in appetite. The neuropsychological assessment revealed a decline in global cognitive status, moderate impairment in complex sequential tracking and psychomotor speed, moderate impairment in manual motor skills, and mild impairment in new learning and memory. Self-reported mood was within normal limits on the GDS. The consensus diagnosis at this visit was mild cognitive impairment due to GSS. One year following the tau PET scan (the 17th clinical assessment), Patient A showed progression of neurologic, psychiatric, and cognitive symptoms; the informant reported continued gradually progressive decline in memory, language, judgment, reasoning, and attention. The consensus diagnosis at that time was mild dementia due to GSS.

Patient B

Patient B had a family history of GSS, was first assessed at the IADC in the sixth decade, and was found to have the *PRNP* F198S mutation. At time of the examination, the informant reported a one-year history of gradually progressive memory difficulties and a language disorder, as well as a six-month history of difficulties with judgment and reasoning, accompanied by changes in personality characterized by irritability, withdrawal, sadness, socially inappropriate behavior, and agitation. On neurological examination, there was slight tremor, bradykinesia, and ataxic gait. The global CDR was 0.5, indicating mild global impairment, with mild impairment (a 0.5 rating) in the memory, orientation, judgement and problem-solving, community affairs, and home and hobbies domains, and

Table 1 Neuropsychological performance of participants at the time of the [^{18}F]flortaucipir scan

	GSS Participants		Early-Onset Alzheimer's		Cognitive Normals	
	Patient A	Patient B	Patient #1	Patient #2	#1	#2
MoCA	22	18	18	17	29	26
CDR Global	0.5	1	0.5	0.5	0	0
CDR Sum of Boxes	1.5	7	3	3.5	0	0
Digit Span Forward	10	5	10	8	9	9
Digit Span Backward	8	5	10	6	12	10
Trail Making Test A	49	76	53	35	23	20
Trail Making Test B	129	300	209	159	61	38
WAIS Digit Symbol	36	20	40	27	68	82
Animal Fluency	15	8	13	21	24	23
Vegetable Fluency	9	11	11	3	18	13
Letter Fluency	25	11	36	26	36	25
MINT	31	28	27	30	32	24
RAVLT Immediate	41	22	27	22	56	51
RAVLT Delayed	7	3	0	0	11	8
Craft Stories Immediate	9	5	6	5	18	15
Craft Stories Delayed	10	4	2	0	17	16
Benson Figure Copy	16	10	14	17	15	15
Benson Figure Recall	10	8	2	0	12	13
GDS	4	4	2	2	1	0
FAS	7	13	14	17	1	0
NPI-Q	3	10	7	9	1	2
Finger Tapping – Dom	39	24	48	58	39	42
Finger Tapping – ND	33	25	36	52	43	40

CDR Clinical Dementia Rating scale, *Dom* dominant hand, *FAS* Functional Assessment Scale, *GDS* Geriatric Depression Scale, *GSS* Gerstmann-Sträussler-Scheinker disease, *MINT* Multi-lingual Naming Test, *MoCA* Montreal Cognitive Assessment, *ND* non-dominant hand, *NPI-Q*Neuropsychiatric Inventory Questionnaire, *RAVLT* Rey Auditory Verbal Learning Test, *WAIS* Wechsler Adult Intelligence Scale

moderate impairment (a 1.0 rating) in the behavior, comportment, and personality domains of the supplemental CDR. The NPI-Q indicated the presence of agitation, depression, anxiety, disinhibition, irritability, nighttime behaviors, and problems with appetite, with severity scores predominantly in the mild range. The FAS indicated mild impairment in daily functioning, including shopping, playing games, using and turning off the stove, meal preparation, keeping track of current events, remembering dates, and traveling out of the neighborhood. The neuropsychological battery revealed mild impairments in efficiency of new learning, verbal fluency, response inhibition, complex sequential tracking, and manual motor speed. The Mini-Mental State Examination score was 26/30. The GDS was within normal limits. The consensus diagnosis was mild dementia due to GSS.

At the follow-up IADC assessment approximately 1 year later, the informant reported continued loss of memory, language, judgment, and reasoning, as well as continued deterioration in personality, including the

appearance of delusions. On neurological examination, there was evidence of parkinsonism and slowness, with frequent falls and gait disturbance. Results of the neuropsychological examination are shown in Table 1. The global CDR had worsened to 1.0, indicating mild impairment, with very mild impairment (a 0.5 rating) in memory and orientation domains, mild to moderate impairment (a 1.0 rating) in judgement and problem-solving, community affairs, and personal care domains, and severe impairment (a 3.0 rating) in the home and hobbies domain. The NPI-Q now included delusions in addition to the problems noted on the previous visit, with most symptoms rated as moderate in severity. The FAS total score had worsened to 13, with need for assistance in shopping, simple meal preparation and cooking, and traveling. The second neuropsychological examination revealed mild to moderate declines in new learning, memory, executive cognitive function, psychomotor speed, and manual motor skills. The MoCA score was 18/30 (equivalent to a MMSE score of

24/30 [34]) and GDS was within normal limits. The consensus diagnosis was dementia due to GSS. The [^{18}F]flortaucipir PET and the structural MRI scans were completed at this visit.

Patient B died while at hospice care 9 months after the completion of the [^{18}F]flortaucipir PET scan from progression of the GSS dementia.

Early-onset AD patient #1

EOAD patient #1 was found to be amyloid positive on a [^{18}F]florbetapir PET scan and showed medial temporal and global atrophy on the structural MRI. At the time of the [^{18}F]flortaucipir PET scan, EOAD patient #1 was aged in the seventh decade and had a global CDR of 0.5, indicating mild impairment, with mild impairment (a 0.5 rating) in the orientation and judgment and problem-solving domains and mild to moderate impairment (a 1.0 rating) in the memory and home and hobbies domains, but normal functioning (a 0.0 rating) in the behavioral, comportment, and personality domains of the supplemental CDR. The informant reported a four-year history of gradually progressive memory problems, a 1 year history of gradually progressive problems with judgment and reasoning, and a 3–4 month history of gradually progressive problems with attention and concentration. There were no neurological abnormalities. Results of the neuropsychological examination are shown in Table 1. The NPI-Q revealed depression and anxiety at a moderate level and agitation, irritability, and abnormal nighttime behaviors at a mild level of severity. The FAS total score was 14, indicating mild difficulties with finances, shopping, meal preparation, remembering appointments, pastimes, current events, and travel outside of the neighborhood. The neuropsychological battery revealed moderate impairments in global cognitive status, complex sequential tracking, and psychomotor speed, and severe impairment in new learning and memory. The consensus diagnosis was dementia due to AD [25].

Early-onset AD patient #2

EOAD patient #2 was found to be amyloid positive on a [^{18}F]florbetapir PET scan and showed medial temporal and global atrophy on the structural MRI. At the time of the [^{18}F]flortaucipir PET scan, EOAD patient #2 was aged in the sixth decade and had a global CDR of 0.5, indicating mild impairment, with mild impairment (a 0.5 rating) in the judgment and problem-solving domain and mild to moderate impairment (a 1.0 rating) in the memory, orientation, and home and hobbies domains, and mild impairment (a 0.5 rating) the behavioral, comportment, and personality domains of the supplemental CDR. The informant reported a three-year history of gradually progressive memory loss and a two-year history of gradually progressive difficulty with judgment, reasoning, and

attention. There were no abnormal neurological manifestations. Results of the neuropsychological examination are shown in Table 1. The NPI-Q reflected mild problems with delusions, depression, indifference, disinhibition, irritability, abnormal nighttime behaviors, and problems with eating. The FAS total score was 17, indicating a substantial impairment and dependency in many activities of daily living. The neuropsychological battery revealed moderate impairment in global cognitive status and severe impairment in new learning and memory. There were moderate impairments in complex sequential tracking. The consensus diagnosis was mild dementia due to AD.

Cognitively Normal individuals

At the time of their [^{18}F]flortaucipir PET scans, both CN individuals had global CDRs and Sum of Boxes scores of 0.0, with no informant-rated impairments or depression. On examination, there were no neurological or neuropsychological abnormalities and consensus diagnoses were normal cognition. Results of the neuropsychological examination are shown in Table 1.

Genetics

There was a single nucleotide (T to C) substitution in codon 198 of one allele of Patient A's and Patient B's *PRNP* genes. This change results in a serine for phenylalanine amino acid change (F198S). For patient A, the first base of *PRNP* codon 129 was heterozygous guanine/adenine (G/A), coding for valine/methionine (GTG/ATG). For patient B, the first base of *PRNP* codon 129 was homozygous guanine (G), coding for valine (GTG).

[^{18}F]Flortaucipir PET scans in *PRNP* F198S GSS patients

The [^{11}C]PiB PET scans showed no specific uptake in the Patients A and B, as previously reported ([4]; Additional file 1: Figure S1). In contrast, the [^{18}F]flortaucipir PET scans showed significant uptake in multiple regions in both GSS patients (Figs. 1, 2, and 4). As compared with Patient A (Fig. 1), Patient B (Fig. 2) showed a more severe clinical presentation and a wider spread of [^{18}F]flortaucipir uptake. GSS Patient A also showed evidence of tracer uptake in regions (Fig. 1) that were not seen in Patient B, including the primary sensory cortex and the left temporal cortex. This [^{18}F]flortaucipir uptake was determined to be within cortical tissue and did not correspond to any lesion observable on MRI. On visual inspection, both individuals showed uptake in the basal ganglia, cingulate gyrus, insular cortex, and thalamus.

Comparison of [^{18}F]Flortaucipir between GSS patients, Alzheimer's patients, and cognitively normal individuals

Selected [^{18}F]flortaucipir sections of the two GSS patients, two EOAD patients, and two CN older adults are

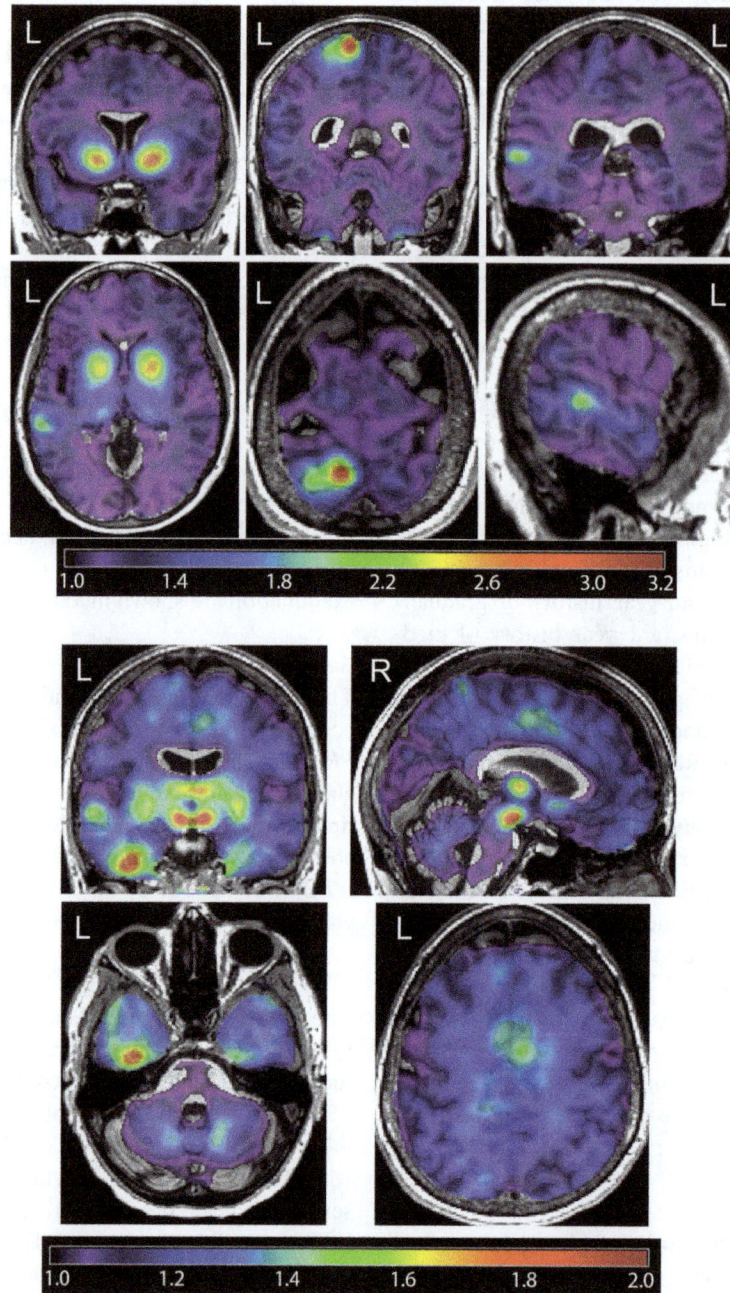

Fig. 1 [^{18}F]Flortaucipir PET in Patient A – Mildly to Moderately Impaired *PRNP* F198S GSS Patient. [^{18}F]Flortaucipir scans from a mildly to moderately impaired GSS *PRNP* F198S mutation carrier (Patient **a**) show specific binding of the tracer in the basal ganglia, thalamus, insular cortex, postcentral gyrus, and inferior temporal lobe. At a lower threshold (lower panels), additional binding is seen in the medial temporal lobe and cingulate gyrus.

shown in Fig. 3. Qualitatively, dramatically higher [^{18}F]flortaucipir uptake was observed in the basal ganglia of Patient A (Fig. 3a) and Patient B (Fig. 3b) relatively to the EOAD (Fig. 3c, d) and CN (Fig. 3e, f) individuals. Less dramatic, but still notable, increased uptake in the thalamus was observed in both GSS patients relative to the EOAD and CN individuals. Further, greater uptake in the cingulate gyrus, bilaterally, and in the insula, anteriorly, was observed in GSS Patient B relatively to both CN individuals. Alternatively, the EOAD patients showed much higher temporal, parietal, and frontal lobes [^{18}F]flortaucipir uptake than the GSS patients and the CN individuals.

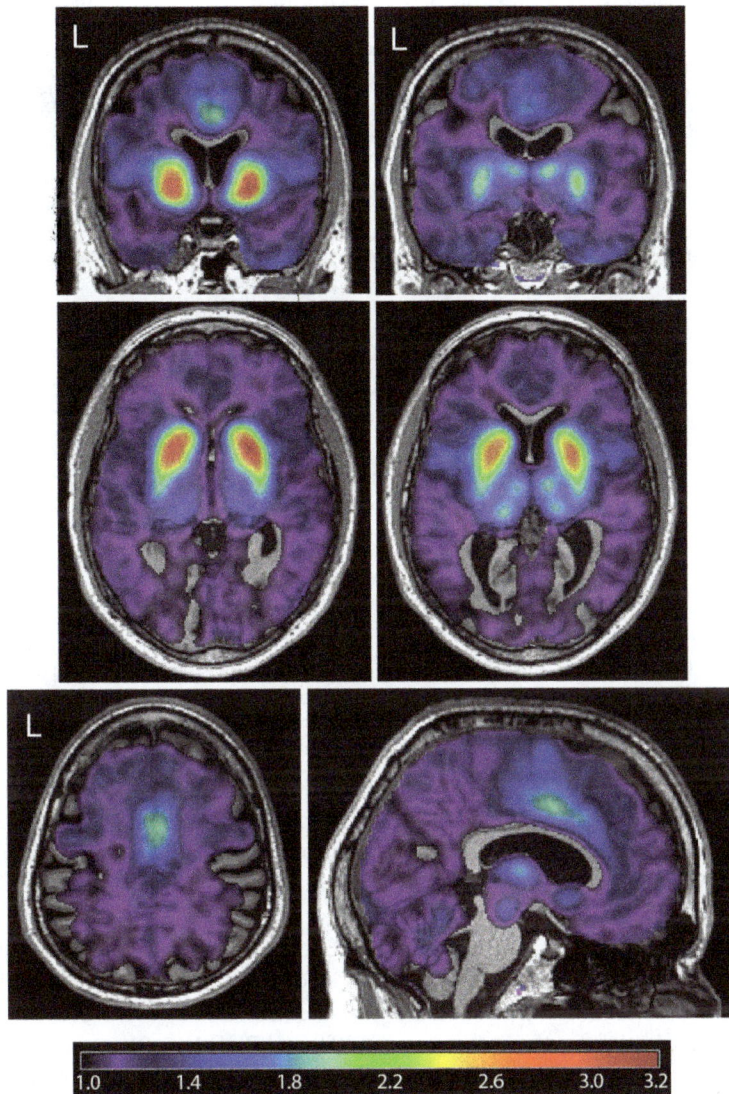

Fig. 2 [¹⁸F]Flortaucipir PET in Patient B – Moderately to Severely Impaired *PRNP* F198S GSS Patient. [¹⁸F]Flortaucipir scans from a moderately to severely impaired GSS *PRNP* F198S mutation carrier (Patient **b**) show specific binding of the tracer in the basal ganglia, thalamus, cingulate gyrus, frontal lobe, and insula/claustrum

Quantitative analysis confirmed much of the qualitative observation of increased [¹⁸F]flortaucipir uptake in GSS patients. Both GSS patients showed increased mean [¹⁸F]flortaucipir SUVR in subcortical areas, including the striatum and thalamus (Fig. 4a & b; Additional file 2: Table S1). These areas were increased relative to both the EOAD and CN individuals. Cortical areas such as insula, anterior cingulate, posterior cingulate, and, globally, in the cortical grey matter (Fig. 4c-f; Additional file 2: Table S1) also showed increased mean [¹⁸F]flortaucipir SUVR in the GSS patients relative to the CN individuals. However, the EOAD patients showed considerably greater mean [¹⁸F]flortaucipir SUVR in the majority of

cortical regions than either the CN individuals or GSS patients.

Neuropathology

The fresh brain of Patient B weighed 1452.5 g. There was no appreciable atrophy of the cerebral hemispheres and no focal lesions or atheromatous changes were noted on external examination. The left cerebral hemisphere was cut into twenty-seven coronal slices. The cerebellar cortex and the dentate nucleus appeared atrophic. The substantia nigra and the locus coeruleus were moderately to severely depigmented. The inferior olivary nuclei were atrophic.

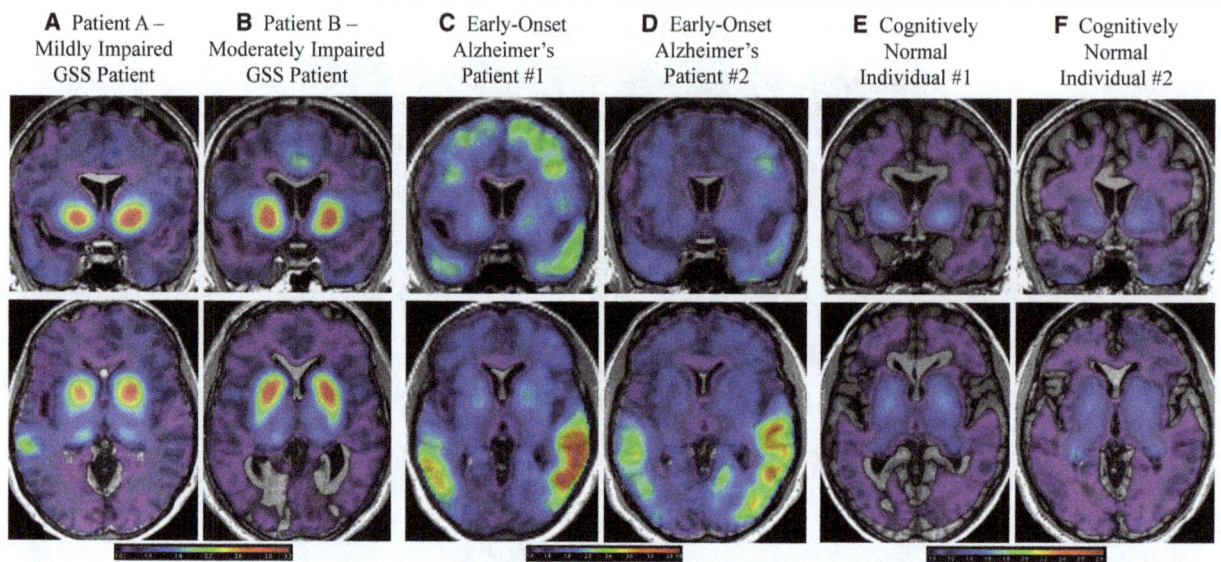

Fig. 3 Qualitative Comparison of [^{18}F]Flortaucipir PET in *PRNP* F198S GSS Patients Relative to Early-Onset Alzheimer's Patients and Cognitively Normal Older Adults. Comparisons of selected [^{18}F]flortaucipir sections of the two GSS patients with two early-onset Alzheimer's disease (EOAD) patients and two cognitively normal older adults (CN) are shown. Higher [^{18}F]flortaucipir uptake is observed in the basal ganglia of the *PRNP* F198S GSS patients (**a, b**) relative to the EOAD patients (**c, d**) and CN individuals (**e, f**). In the *PRNP* F198S GSS patients, there is also increased uptake in the thalamus relative to the EOAD patients and CN individuals. Greater uptake in the cingulate gyrus bilaterally is observed in *PRNP* F198S GSS Patient B (**b**) relative to EOAD Patient #2 (**d**) and both CN individuals (**e, f**). There is slightly increased uptake in the anterior insula bilaterally for *PRNP* F198S GSS Patient B (**b**) relative to EOAD Patient #2 (**d**) and both CN individuals (**e,f**)

Serial coronal sections, stained with LFB-H&E, revealed mild and global cerebral atrophy, neuronal loss and gliosis in the gray matter, as well as a diffuse loss of myelin stain in the deep white matter of the frontal, temporal, and parietal lobes (Fig. 5, 1st **column**).

In Thioflavin S-stained sections of cerebrum and cerebellum, diffuse plaques and plaques with multicentric cores were numerous (Fig. 6a). The diffuse deposits were not fluorescent, but appeared brighter than the surrounding neuropil; the cores of the plaque were fluorescent and, therefore, have the tinctorial properties of amyloid. In the Thioflavin S preparations of the cerebrum, but not in preparations of the cerebellum, NFTs were seen within neuronal perikarya and in neurites that surround the amyloid cores.

Serial sections, adjacent to those stained with Thioflavin S, were immunostained for PrP and revealed that both diffuse plaques and plaques with amyloid core were decorated by PrP antibodies (Fig. 6b). By PrP immunohistochemistry, labeling of the gray matter structures of the cerebral hemisphere and of the cerebellum was observed. PrP immunopositive diffuse and multicentric cored plaques were extensively distributed in the neuropil. No intracellular PrP inclusions were present. Within the gray matter of the cerebral hemisphere, the most severe PrP immunolabeling was seen in the superior, middle, and inferior frontal gyri, the cingulate gyrus, the pre- and post-central gyri, the superior, middle and inferior temporal gyri, the fusiform gyrus, the entorhinal cortex, the parahippocampal gyrus, as well as the upper portion of the insular cortex, the caudate nucleus, putamen, and thalamus (Fig. 5, 3rd **column**; Additional file 1: Figure S1).

Serial sections, adjacent to those stained with Thioflavin S and to those immunolabeled for PrP were immunostained for tau. Decorated by the monoclonal antibodies AT8 and PHF-1 were not just the NFTs, but also multiple structures, including cytoplasm of neuronal perikarya, dentritic processes, neuropil threads, and neurites surrounding cores of plaques (Fig. 6c & d). In fact, using AT8 and PHF-1, the pattern of hyperphosphorylated tau immunohistochemical labeling mirrored that of PrP throughout the cerebral cortex and the subcortical nuclei except in the thalamus, where PrP immunoreactivity was much stronger than tau immunoreactivity (Fig. 5, 4th **column**; Fig. 7; Additional file 1: Figure S1). Tau deposits were most numerous in the superior, middle and inferior frontal gyri, inferior temporal, fusiform, and cingulate gyri, as well as in the insular, parahippocampal, and entorhinal cortices, caudate nucleus, and putamen (Fig. 5, 4th **column**; Fig. 7). Patient B showed a large number of NFT (Fig. 6d, Fig. 7). Tau deposits were not present in the cerebellar cortex.

In comparing tau immunolabeled tissue preparations with those stained with Thioflavin S, it was evident that profiles labeled with AT8 or PHF-1 were more numerous

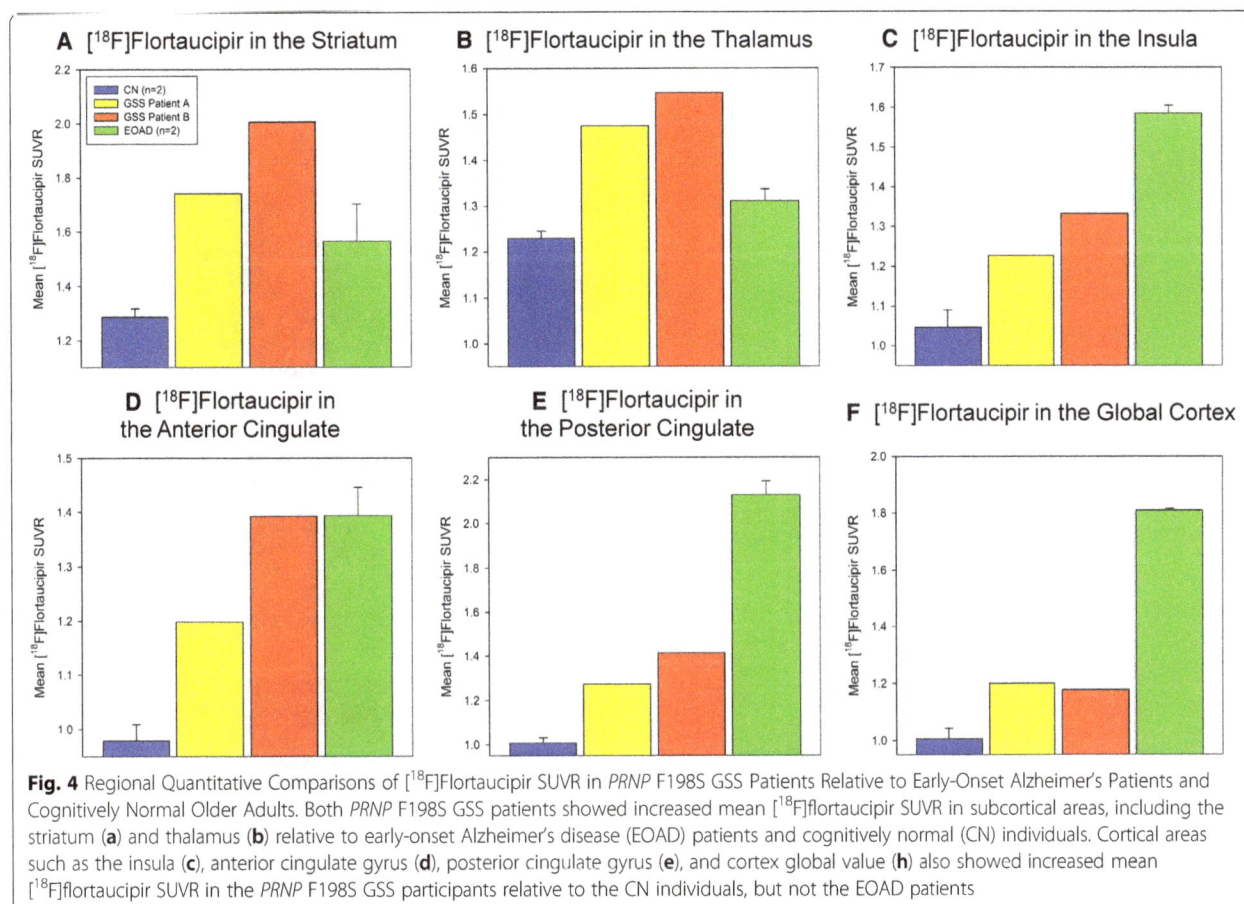

Fig. 4 Regional Quantitative Comparisons of [^{18}F]Flortaucipir SUVR in *PRNP* F198S GSS Patients Relative to Early-Onset Alzheimer's Patients and Cognitively Normal Older Adults. Both *PRNP* F198S GSS patients showed increased mean [^{18}F]flortaucipir SUVR in subcortical areas, including the striatum (**a**) and thalamus (**b**) relative to early-onset Alzheimer's disease (EOAD) patients and cognitively normal (CN) individuals. Cortical areas such as the insula (**c**), anterior cingulate gyrus (**d**), posterior cingulate gyrus (**e**), and cortex global value (**h**) also showed increased mean [^{18}F]flortaucipir SUVR in the *PRNP* F198S GSS participants relative to the CN individuals, but not the EOAD patients

than the fluorescent profiles seen in Thioflavin S preparations (Fig. 6). However, it was also evident that AT8 appeared to label a larger number of profiles than PHF-1 (Fig. 6; Fig. 7). These findings suggest that while Thioflavin S detects exclusively the filament cores of tau NFTs, AT8 and PHF-1 label the NFTs, as well as portions of the tau fuzzy coat, hyperphosporylated tau, and possibly tau in various states of aggregation.

In AD, tau inclusions are immunopositive for 3R and 4R tau [8]. Similarly, the tau aggregates in the GSS patient were immunolabeled by monoclonal antibodies to 3R and to 4R tau; however, the 4R antibody appeared to give a stronger labeling than the 3R (Fig. 8).

Immunohistochemistry for Aβ revealed neither diffuse nor cored plaques. Immunohistochemical preparations using antibodies to TDP-43 and α-synuclein did not show intracellular inclusions in neurons or glia.

Similar to what was observed previously in GSS F198S affected individuals [11], ferric iron deposits in the brain of Patient B were most abundant in the globus pallidus and the substantia nigra (Fig. 9a-b), however at the microscopic examination they were detected also in the caudate nucleus and putamen. Iron deposits were not detected in the thalamus (Fig. 9b).

Discussion

The PET tracer [^{18}F]flortaucipir was used to investigate the pattern of tau deposition in two GSS patients who carry the *PRNP* F198S mutation and are members of a pedigree that has been previously studied extensively from the clinical and neuropathological points of view [7, 11, 14, 35].

GSS caused by the *PRNP* F198S mutation is a PrP amyloidosis associated with severe tau deposition in all regions of the cerebrum and brainstem in which misfolded PrP amyloid is observed. On the contrary, tau does not aggregate in the cerebellum, in spite of the heavy PrP burden. DNA changes in the *PRNP* gene, including missense, nonsense, insertion, and deletion mutations, may be associated with a PrP amyloidosis that coexists with severe tau deposition [1, 10, 14, 17, 20, 26, 31]. Patients with different forms of dominantly inherited PrP amyloidosis may present with neuropsychiatric manifestations including depression, personality changes, psychosis, and hallucinations, as well as with frontotemporal dementia-like phenotypes, similar to those previously observed in some *PRNP* F198S mutation carriers [7, 21, 30]. Therefore, it is notable that the two GSS *PRNP* F198S carriers reported in the present

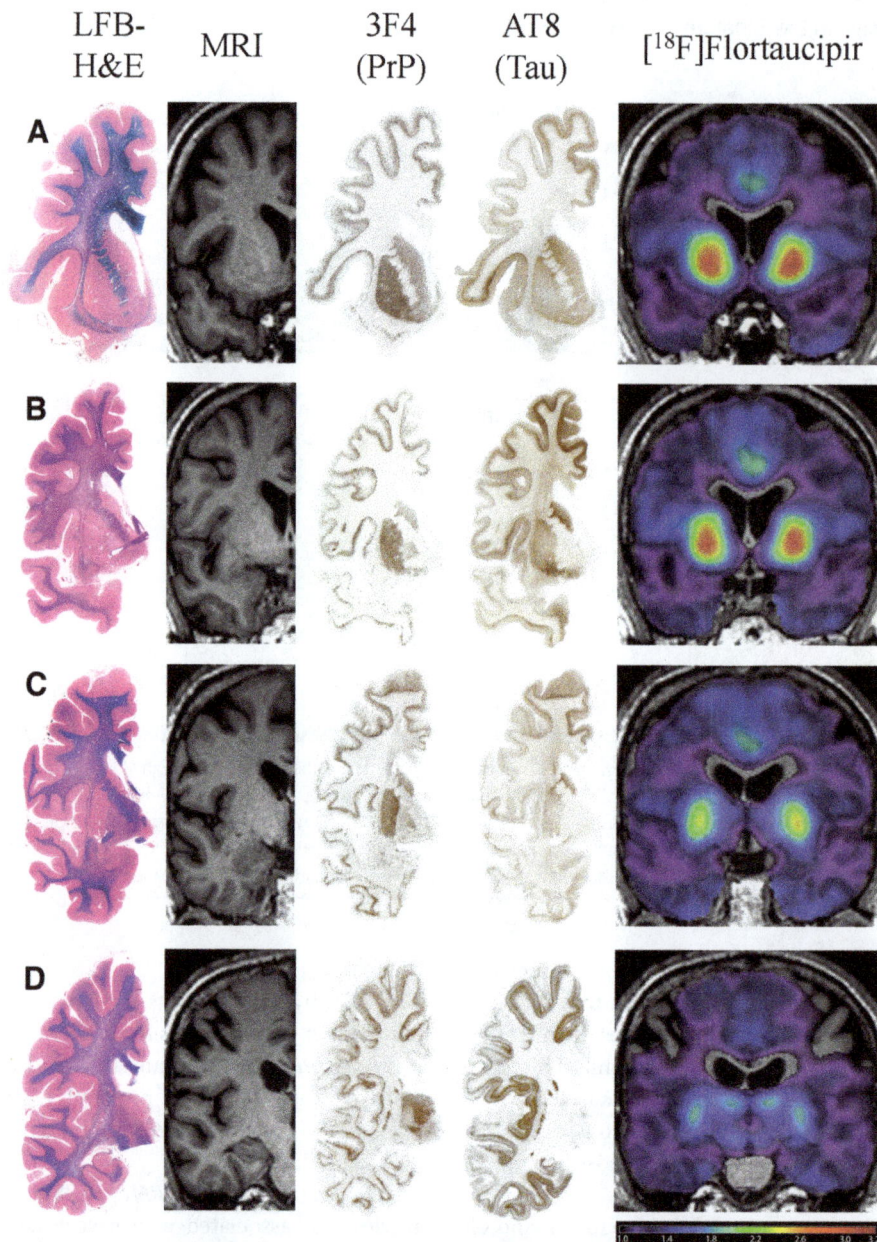

Fig. 5 Neuropathologic Analysis of the Moderately to Severely Impaired GSS Patient B. Good correspondence between the [^{18}F]flortaucipir SUVR (5th column) and AT8 immunolabeling of tau (4th column) was observed across multiple regions, including the basal ganglia and cingulate gyrus (**a-c**), as well as the frontal (**a-d**) and insular cortices (**b,c,d**). These areas also feature considerable structural atrophy on MRI (1st column) and LFB-H&E stain (2nd column), as well as PrP amyloid deposition on 3F4 (3rd column). The only region of non-correspondence occurred in the thalamus (**d**), where [^{18}F]flortaucipir PET (5th column) showed increased uptake but no AT8 immunolabeling of tau (4th column) was observed; PrP deposition was observed in the thalamus (3rd column). LFB-H&E = luxol fast blue with hematoxylin & eosin; MRI = magnetic resonance imaging; PrP = prion protein

study had neurological signs that were preceded by psychiatric symptoms.

This study reveals for the first time that there is a considerable uptake of [^{18}F]flortaucipir in various brain regions of both GSS patients with the *PRNP* F198S mutation. Specifically, [^{18}F]flortaucipir uptake is evident in the anterior and posterior cingulate gyri, insular

cortex, caudate nucleus, nucleus accumbens, putamen, globus pallidus, thalamus, and entorhinal cortex. Furthermore, in comparing the more affected individual with the less affected one, the uptake in the former was greater than that in the latter in the majority of the regions mentioned above. This suggests that a correlation between clinical severity and [^{18}F]flortaucipir uptake

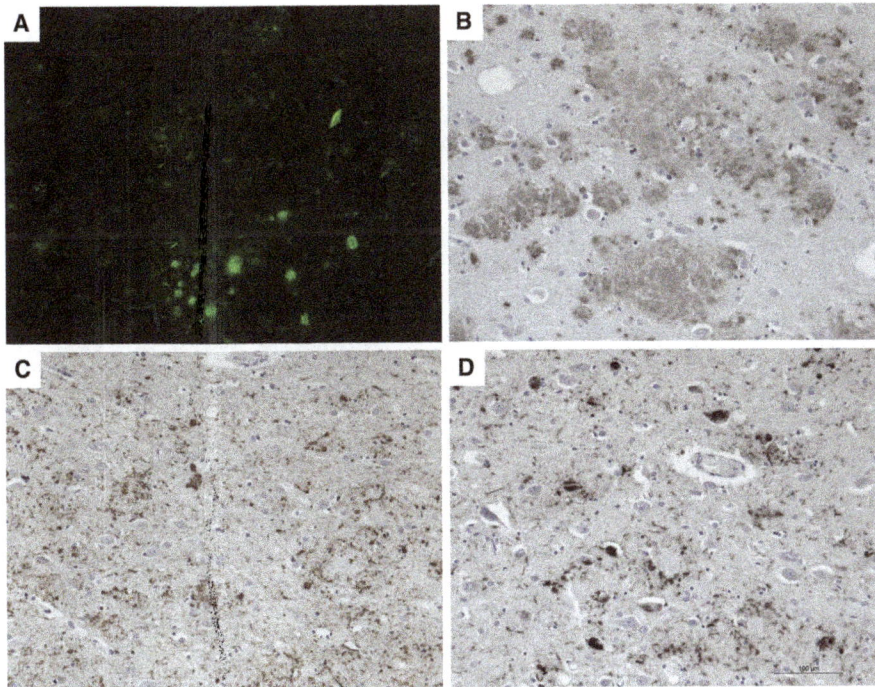

Fig. 6 PrP and Tau in the Frontal Lobe of the Moderately to Severely Impaired GSS Patient B. PrP amyloid plaques and neurofibrillary tangles (NFTs) were observed using Thioflavin S in the frontal lobe (**a**). Significant immunolabeling of PrP amyloid (**b**; 3F4) and tau (**c**; AT8; **d**; PHF-1) was also observed

may exist and that greater [18F]flortaucipir uptake may correlate with a higher burden of aggregated tau.

Similar to what occurs in AD, the NFT present in symptomatic *PRNP* F198S mutation carriers are made of 3R and 4R tau; however, the anatomical pattern of [18F]flortaucipir PET uptake differs considerably from that seen in early- and late-onset AD [5, 18, 28, 29, 32]. In AD, tau pathology as visualized by [18F]flortaucipir PET, appears to be distributed over widespread brain areas in the amnestic, non-amnestic, behavioral, corticobasal, and posterior cortical atrophy variants of the disease [29]. Further, tau PET patterns have been shown to reflect the variability of clinical syndromes and topography of pathologic regions [29]. Many of the anatomical regions found to have high [18F]flortaucipir uptake in *PRNP* F198S GSS patients belong to the salience network, as well as to the reward system [27]. Reduction in the function of these networks has been associated with numerous neuropsychiatric disorders, drug dependence, and psychosis. Taken together, our findings and those reported in the literature suggest that in GSS patients carrying the *PRNP* F198S allele the behavioral, psychiatric, and neurological symptoms, as well the dementia that develops in the late stage, result from the interaction of misfolded PrP amyloid and tau. The spreading of tau throughout the entire cerebral cortex and subcortical nuclei contributes to the progression and severity of the

psychiatric, neurologic, and cognitive dysfunctions [7, 11, 12, 14].

The neuropathologic results observed in Patient B support the concept that [18F]flortaucipir uptake likely reflects the anatomical localization of misfolded tau and NFT that are distributed in the cerebral gray structures. In fact, there is a definite topographic correspondence between [18F]flortaucipir uptake and the extent of fluorescent NFT in Thioflavin S preparations of cingulate gyrus, caudate nucleus, putamen, and insular cortex. Immunohistochemical preparations of adjacent serially cut sections of these anatomical regions also revealed a strong immunoreactivity to monoclonal antibodies AT8 and PHF-1 in the cingulate gyrus, caudate nucleus, putamen, and insular cortex. It is also important to note that no Aβ immunoreactivity was present in any CNS area affected by PrP or tau pathology.

A finding that needs to be emphasized and that is relevant to the mechanisms of tau spread and to the correlations between [18F]flortaucipir PET images with those obtained by neuropathologic studies is that many CNS gray matter regions demonstrated notable tau immunopositivity, but not an increased signal on PET images. This discrepancy may be due to differences in tau species in these regions, as [18F]flortaucipir is known to recognize the NFT, similarly to what Thioflavin S recognizes in histological preparations. Whether [18F]flortaucipir

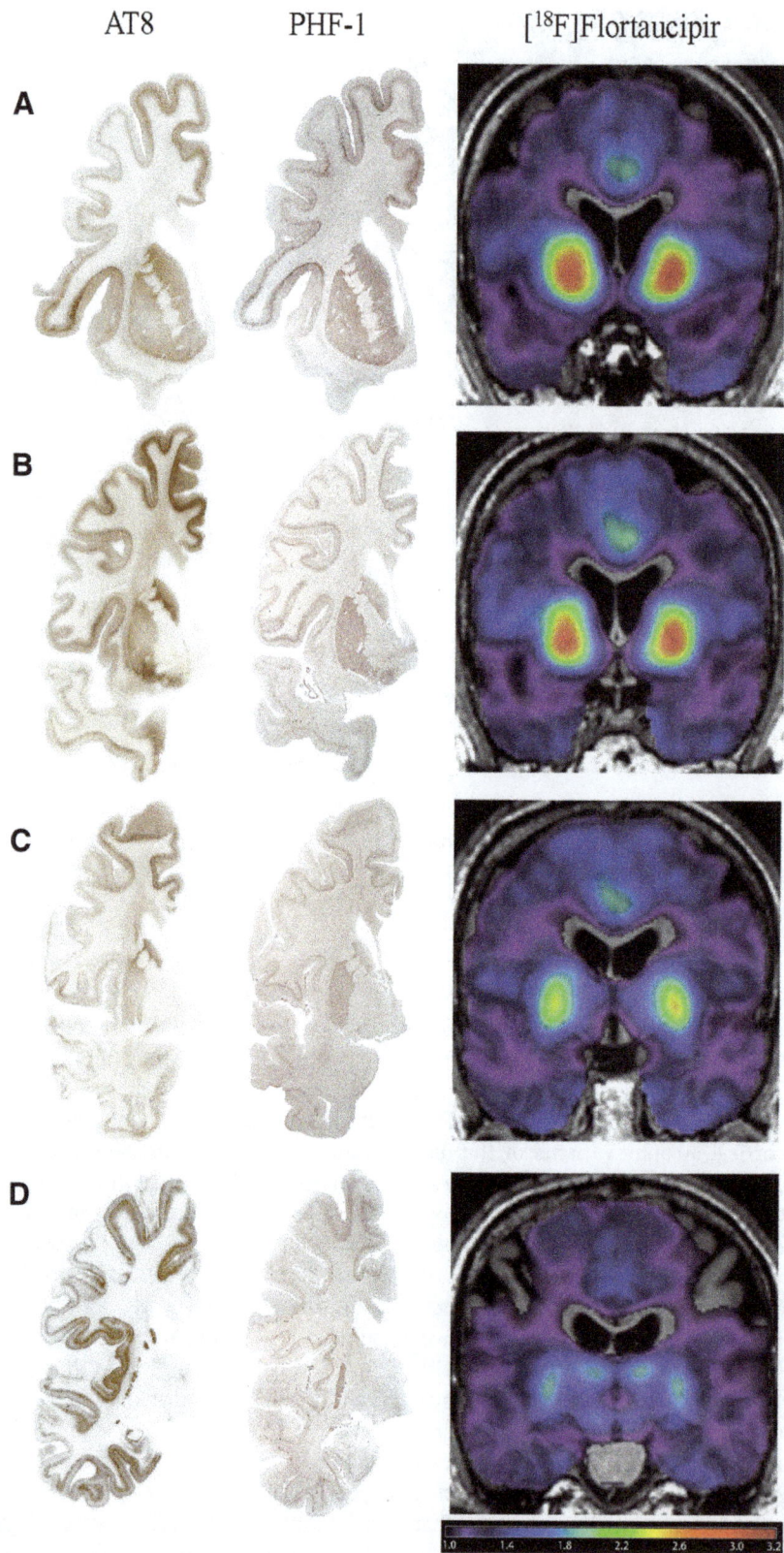

Fig. 7 (See legend on next page.)

(See figure on previous page.)
Fig. 7 Comparison of AT8 and PHF-1 Staining to [^{18}F]Flortaucipir in the Moderately to Severely Impaired GSS Patient B. Good correspondence between the [^{18}F]flortaucipir SUVR (3rd column) and both the AT8 (1st column) and PHF-1 (2nd column) immunolabeling of tau and neurofibrillary tangles, respectively, was observed across the basal ganglia and cingulate gyrus (**a-c**), as well as the frontal (**a-d**) and insular cortices (**b,c,d**). However, while the AT8 immunolabeling was more widespread throughout the cortical and subcortical regions, the PHF-1 immunolabeling was more restricted to areas that corresponded to increased [^{18}F]flortaucipir signal, with the exception of the thalamus

may detect states of tau aggregation that precede NFT formation needs further investigation. Thus, tau immunolabeled tissue preparations and those stained with Thioflavin S reveal presence of tau in different states of aggregation. AT8 or PHF-1 reveal the hyperphosphorylated tau burden, which is known to be more widespread than that represented by the fluorescent profiles detected in Thioflavin S preparations. The process of tau becoming hyperphosphorylated is not completely understood; however, this process is known to precede tangle formation. Thus, while Thioflavin S detects only the NFTs made of aggregated tau filament cores, by knowing which tau epitopes are recognized by AT8 or PHF-1, we can conclude that the labeling observed in the specific immunohistochemical preparations recognizes neurons containing not only NFT but also portions of the tau fuzzy coat. It is also possible that the inherent spatial and sensitivity limitations of PET imaging may lead to an inability to detect low levels of tau deposition in vivo. Novel tracers with greater specificity for particular tau filaments are needed [15].

Another region lacking good correspondence between PET imaging and immunohistochemistry is the thalamus, where [^{18}F]flortaucipir uptake is relatively strong in both patients, but is weak in the immunohistochemical preparation for tau in GSS Patient B. It should be noted that the thalamus and cerebellum are strongly labeled by immunohistochemistry for PrP; however, no tau immunopositivity is seen in the cerebellum and only a weak immunopositivity is detected in the thalamus. The [^{18}F]flortaucipir PET signal in the thalamus may represent "off-target" binding similarly to what has been reported in other studies with [^{18}F]flortaucipir tracer showing binding to neuromelanin-containing cells and other targets [22–24]. In view of published studies that showed high iron binding in GSS patients [11] and non-specific binding of [^{18}F]flortaucipir to iron [3], we studied neuropathologically Patient B using a method to detect iron deposits, and showed that iron deposits occur mostly in the globus pallidus and the substantia nigra, but not in the thalamus. Therefore, additional

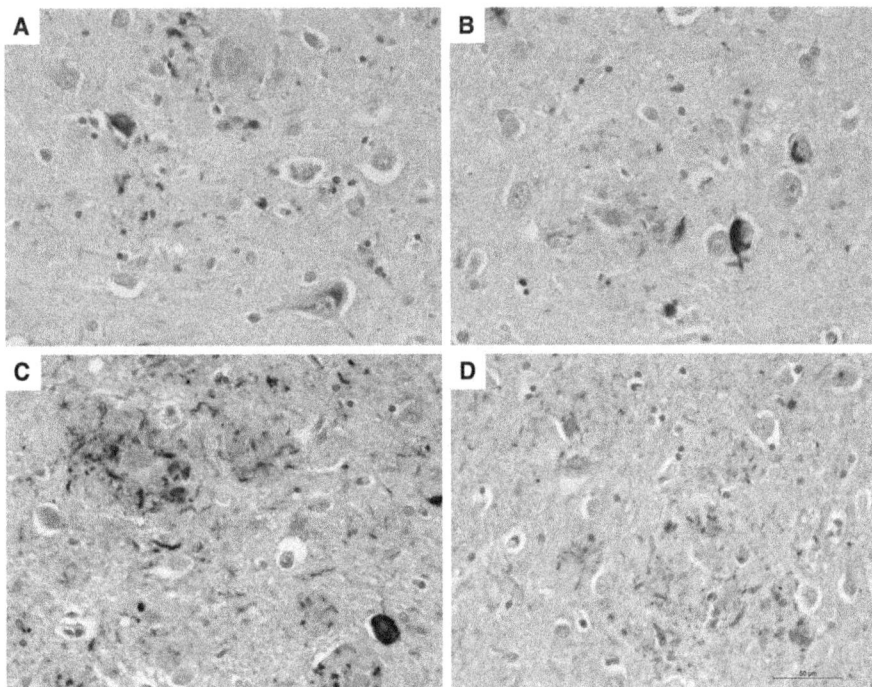

Fig. 8 3R and 4R Tau Deposition in the Frontal Lobe of the Moderately to Severely Impaired GSS Patient B. Both 3R (**a-b**) and 4R (**c-d**) tau were observed in GSS Patient B, although the 4R tau appeared to be more prevalent

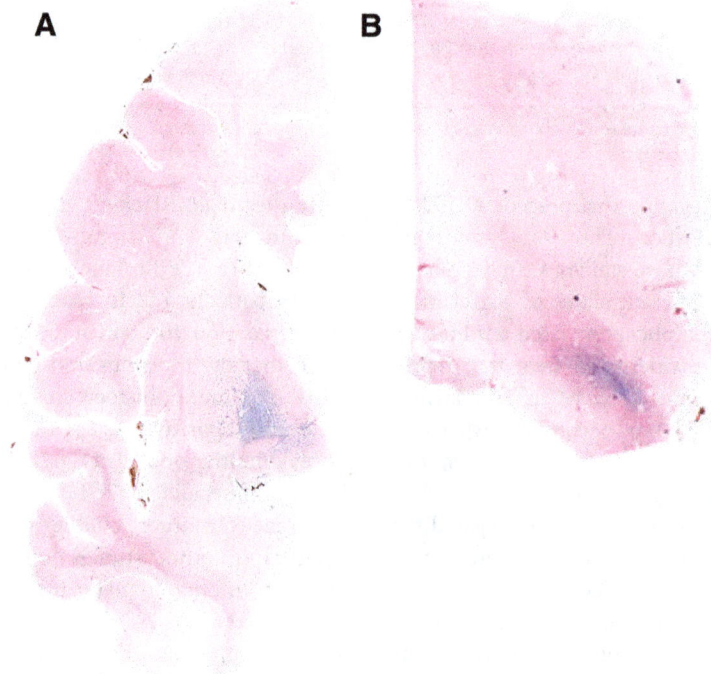

Fig. 9 Iron Deposition in the Moderately to Severely Impaired GSS Patient B. Significant iron accumulation is seen in the globus pallidum, as well as in the caudate and putamen (**a**). Iron is also observed in the substantia nigra, while minimal iron binding is observed in the thalamus (**b**)

studies will be needed to clarify the significance of the uptake of [18F]flortaucipir in the thalamus.

Overall, the present study shows for the first time that [18F]flortaucipir detects in vivo the severe neurofibrillary pathology that is a significant neuropathologic phenotype in GSS patients carrying the *PRNP* F198S mutation, which potentially has a profound impact on the pathogenesis of psychiatric and neurological symptoms of the disease [11, 12, 14]. Based on evidence obtained in two unpublished presymptomatic mutation carriers, PrP amyloid deposits are detected prior to the occurrence of tau pathology and NFT formation; however, additional in vivo evidence is needed to confirm the PrP-tau relationship and its temporal evolution [11].

In conclusion, it is shown that deposits of tau are detected in vivo by [18F]flortaucipir PET in patients who carry the *PRNP* F198S mutation and that tau accumulates with a pattern that is strikingly different from that seen in AD. The patterns of tau anatomical spread seen in GSS *PRNP* F198S and AD may reflect the mechanisms of PrP and Aβ distribution. The results of this study support the view that tau pathology, and not just PrP, contributes significantly to both the psychiatric and the motor symptoms that characterize the phenotype of GSS *PRNP* F198S and that the different clinical phenotypes of GSS *PRNP* F198S and AD correlate with the specific pattern of tau anatomical distribution seen in each disease.

Future studies, comparing in vivo longitudinal PET imaging with the *post-mortem* PrP and tau immunolabeled preparations may allow a precise assessment of the spread of the abnormally conformed proteins over time during the evolution of the *PRNP* F198S GSS disease process.

Abbreviations

3R: 3-repeat; 4R: 4-repeat; AD: Alzheimer's disease; ADNI: Alzheimer's disease neuroimaging initiative; Aβ: Amyloid β; CDR: Clinical Dementia Rating; DWI: Diffusion-weighted imaging; EOAD: Early-onset Alzheimer's disease; FAS: Functional Assessment Scale; FDDNP: [18F]2-(1-(6-[(2-[fluorine-18]fluoroethyl)(methyl)amino]-2-naphthyl)-ethylidene)malononitrile; FDG: [18F]Fluorodeoxyglucose; FLAIR: Fluid-attenuated inversion recovery; FWHM: Full-width half maximum; GDS: Geriatric Depression Scale; GSS: Gerstmann-Sträussler-Scheinker; H&E: Hematoxylin and eosin; IADC: Indiana Alzheimer Disease Center; IHC: Immunohistochemistry; LFB-H&E: Luxol fast blue with hematoxylin & eosin; MCI: Mild cognitive impairment; MINT: Multi-lingual Naming Test; MNI: Montreal Neurologic Institute; MoCA: Montreal Cognitive Assessment; MPRAGE: Magnetization-prepared rapid gradient-echo; MRS: Magnetic resonance spectroscopy; NPI-Q: Neuropsychiatric Inventory Questionnaire; PiB: [11C]Pittsburgh Compound B; PrP: Prion protein; PTSD: Post-traumatic stress disorder; RAVLT: Rey Auditory Verbal Learning Test; rsfMRI: Resting-state functional MRI; SPECT: Single photon emission computerized tomography; SPM8: Statistical Parametric Mapping 8; SUVR: Standardized uptake value ratio; TMT-A: Trail Making Test A; TMT-B: Trail Making Test B; UDS-3: Uniform Dataset 3; WAIS: Wechsler Adult Intelligence Scale

Acknowledgements

The authors thank Trina Bird, Christina Brown, Steve Brown, Madeline Cassidy, Ryan Crosbie, Su Gao, Bradley Glazier, Kala Hall, Lili Kyurkchiyska, Heather Polson, Dr. Adam Schwarz, and Wendy Territo for their contributions to this work. We would also like to thank Dr. Kimberly Quaid for her assistance and support with genetic counseling for the patients described in this manuscript and others in the Indiana Alzheimer Disease Center (IADC).

Funding

This work was supported in part by the National Institute on Aging (NIA, P30 AG010133, R01 AG19771 and K01 AG049050), the Alzheimer's Association, the Indiana University Health-Indiana University School of Medicine Strategic Research Initiative, and the Indiana Clinical and Translational Sciences Institute (CTSI) and a collaborative research grant from Eli Lilly. Precursor for the [18F]flortaucipir tracer was provided by Avid Radiopharmaceuticals, a wholly-owned subsidiary of Eli Lilly. In addition, this research was supported in part by Lilly Endowment, Inc., through its support for the Indiana University Pervasive Technology Institute and the Indiana METACyt Initiative, and, in part, upon work supported by the National Science Foundation under Grant No. CNS-0521433.

Authors' contributions

All authors contributed to the manuscript. Drs. Risacher, Ghetti, Unverzagt, and Saykin authored the majority of the text. Drs. Apostolova, Bateman, and Farlow conducted the clinical and cognitive evaluations of included participants. Drs. Ghetti and Bonnin were the primary neuropathologists. Dr. Risacher did the majority of the PET image processing and analysis. Dr. Murrell was the primary individual responsible for genotyping of the individuals. Francine Epperson and Rose Richardson were the primary technologists involved in the neuropathologic analysis. Ms. Tallman was the primary coordinator responsible for the neuroimaging studies. All authors reviewed, edited, and approved the final manuscript submission.

Competing interests

The authors declare that they have no competing interests.

Author details

[1]Department of Radiology and Imaging Sciences, Indiana University School of Medicine, 355 West 16th Street, Suite 4100, Indianapolis, IN 46202, USA. [2]Indiana Alzheimer Disease Center, Indiana University School of Medicine, Indianapolis, IN, USA. [3]Department of Neurology, Indiana University School of Medicine, Indianapolis, IN, USA. [4]Department of Psychiatry, Indiana University School of Medicine, Indianapolis, IN, USA. [5]Department of Pathology and Laboratory Medicine, Indiana University School of Medicine, Indianapolis, IN, USA. [6]Department of Medical and Molecular Genetics, Indiana University School of Medicine, Indianapolis, IN, USA.

References

1. Alzualde A, Indakoetxea B, Ferrer I, Moreno F, Barandiaran M, Gorostidi A, Estanga A, Ruiz I, Calero M, van Leeuwen FW et al (2010) A novel PRNP Y218N mutation in Gerstmann-Straussler-Scheinker disease with neurofibrillary degeneration. J Neuropathol Exp Neurol 69:789–800. https://doi.org/10.1097/NEN.0b013e3181e85737
2. Chien DT, Bahri S, Szardenings AK, Walsh JC, Mu F, Su MY, Shankle WR, Elizarov A, Kolb HC (2013) Early clinical PET imaging results with the novel PHF-tau radioligand [F-18]-T807. J Alzheimer's Dis 34:457–468. https://doi.org/10.3233/JAD-122059
3. Choi JY, Cho H, Ahn SJ, Lee JH, Ryu YH, Lee MS, Lyoo CH (2018) Off-target (18)F-AV-1451 binding in the basal ganglia correlates with age-related Iron accumulation. J Nucl Med 59:117–120. https://doi.org/10.2967/jnumed.117.195248
4. Deters KD, Risacher SL, Yoder KK, Oblak AL, Unverzagt FW, Murrell JR, Epperson F, Tallman EF, Quaid KA, Farlow MR et al (2016) [(11)C]PiB PET in Gerstmann-Straussler-Scheinker disease. Am J Nucl Med Mol Imaging 6:84–93
5. Dickerson B, Domoto-Reilly K, Daisy S, Brickhouse M, Stepanovic M, Johnson KA (2014) Imaging tau pathology In Vivo in FTLD: initial experience with [18F]T807 PET. Alzheimer's Dement 10:P131
6. Dlouhy SR, Hsiao K, Farlow MR, Foroud T, Conneally PM, Johnson P, Prusiner SB, Hodes ME, Ghetti B (1992) Linkage of the Indiana kindred of Gerstmann-Straussler-Scheinker disease to the prion protein gene. Nat Genet 1:64–67. https://doi.org/10.1038/ng0492-64
7. Farlow MR, Yee RD, Dlouhy SR, Conneally PM, Azzarelli B, Ghetti B (1989) Gerstmann-Sträussler-Scheinker disease. I. Extending the clinical spectrum. Neurology 39:1446–1452
8. Fitzpatrick AWP, Falcon B, He S, Murzin AG, Murshudov G, Garringer HJ, Crowther RA, Ghetti B, Goedert M, Scheres SHW (2017) Cryo-EM structures of tau filaments from Alzheimer's disease. Nature 547:185–190. https://doi.org/10.1038/nature23002
9. Gerstmann J, Straussler E, Scheinker I (1936) Uber eine eigenartige hereditar-familiare Erkrankung des Zentralnervensystems. Zugleich ein Beitrag zur Frage des vorzeitigen lokalen Alters. Z Neur Psychiat 154:736–762
10. Ghetti B, Bugiani O, Tagliavini F, Piccardo P (2011) Gerstmann–Sträussler–Scheinker Disease. In: Dickson DW, Weller RO (eds) Neurodegeneration: the molecular pathology of dementia and movement disorders 2 edn. Wiley-Blackwell, City, pp 364–377
11. Ghetti B, Dlouhy SR, Giaccone G, Bugiani O, Frangione B, Farlow MR, Tagliavini F (1995) Gerstmann-Straussler-Scheinker disease and the Indiana kindred. Brain Pathol 5:61–75
12. Ghetti B, Tagliavini F, Giaccone G, Bugiani O, Frangione B, Farlow MR, Dlouhy SR (1994) Familial Gerstmann-Straussler-Scheinker disease with neurofibrillary tangles. Mol Neurobiol 8:41–48. https://doi.org/10.1007/BF02778006
13. Ghetti B, Tagliavini F, Hsiao K, Dlouhy SR, Yee RD, Giaccone G, Conneally PM, Hodes ME, Bugiani O, Prusiner SB et al (1992) Indiana variant of Gerstmann-Straussler-Scheinker disease. In: Prusiner SB, Collinge J, Powell J, Anderton B (eds) Prion diseases of humans and animals. Ellis Horwood Ltd., Hemel Hempstead, Hertfordshire, UK, pp 154–167
14. Ghetti B, Tagliavini F, Masters CL, Beyreuther K, Giaccone G, Verga L, Farlow MR, Conneally PM, Dlouhy SR, Azzarelli B et al (1989) Gerstmann-Straussler-Scheinker disease. II. Neurofibrillary tangles and plaques with PrP-amyloid coexist in an affected family. Neurology 39:1453–1461
15. Goedert M, Yamaguchi Y, Mishra SK, Higuchi M, Sahara N (2018) Tau filaments and the development of positron emission tomography tracers. Front Neurol 9:70. https://doi.org/10.3389/fneur.2018.00070
16. Hsiao K, Dlouhy SR, Farlow MR, Cass C, Da Costa M, Conneally PM, Hodes ME, Ghetti B, Prusiner SB (1992) Mutant prion proteins in Gerstmann-Sträussler-Scheinker disease with neurofibrillary tangles. Nat Genet 1:68–71. https://doi.org/10.1038/ng0492-68
17. Jansen C, Parchi P, Capellari S, Vermeij AJ, Corrado P, Baas F, Strammiello R, van Gool WA, van Swieten JC, Rozemuller AJ (2010) Prion protein amyloidosis with divergent phenotype associated with two novel nonsense mutations in PRNP. Acta Neuropathol 119:189–197. https://doi.org/10.1007/s00401-009-0609-x
18. Johnson KA, Schultz A, Betensky RA, Becker JA, Sepulcre J, Rentz D, Mormino E, Chhatwal J, Amariglio R, Papp K et al (2016) Tau positron emission tomographic imaging in aging and early Alzheimer disease. Ann Neurol 79:110–119. https://doi.org/10.1002/ana.24546
19. Kepe V, Ghetti B, Farlow MR, Bresjanac M, Miller K, Huang SC, Wong KP, Murrell JR, Piccardo P, Epperson F et al (2010) PET of brain prion protein amyloid in Gerstmann-Straussler-Scheinker disease. Brain pathology 20:419–430. https://doi.org/10.1111/j.1750-3639.2009.00306.x
20. Kumar N, Boeve BF, Boot BP, Orr CF, Duffy J, Woodruff BK, Nair AK, Ellison J, Kuntz K, Kantarci K et al (2011) Clinical characterization of a kindred with a novel 12-octapeptide repeat insertion in the prion protein gene. Arch Neurol 68:1165–1170. https://doi.org/10.1001/archneurol.2011.187
21. Laplanche JL, Hachimi KH, Durieux I, Thuillet P, Defebvre L, Delasnerie-Laupretre N, Peoc'h K, Foncin JF, Destee A (1999) Prominent psychiatric features and early onset in an inherited prion disease with a new insertional mutation in the prion protein gene. Brain 122(Pt 12):2375–2386

22. Lowe VJ, Curran G, Fang P, Liesinger AM, Josephs KA, Parisi JE, Kantarci K, Boeve BF, Pandey MK, Bruinsma T et al (2016) An autoradiographic evaluation of AV-1451 tau PET in dementia. Acta Neuropathol Commun 4: 58. https://doi.org/10.1186/s40478-016-0315-6

23. Marquie M, Normandin MD, Vanderburg CR, Costantino IM, Bien EA, Rycyna LG, Klunk WE, Mathis CA, Ikonomovic MD, Debnath ML et al (2015) Validating novel tau positron emission tomography tracer [F-18]-AV-1451 (T807) on postmortem brain tissue. Ann Neurol 78:787–800. https://doi.org/10.1002/ana.24517

24. Marquie M, Verwer EE, Meltzer AC, Kim SJW, Aguero C, Gonzalez J, Makaretz SJ, Siao Tick Chong M, Ramanan P, Amaral AC et al (2017) Lessons learned about [F-18]-AV-1451 off-target binding from an autopsy-confirmed Parkinson's case. Acta Neuropathol Commun 5:75. https://doi.org/10.1186/s40478-017-0482-0

25. McKhann GM, Knopman DS, Chertkow H, Hyman BT, Jack CR Jr, Kawas CH, Klunk WE, Koroshetz WJ, Manly JJ, Mayeux R et al (2011) The diagnosis of dementia due to Alzheimer's disease: recommendations from the National Institute on Aging-Alzheimer's Association workgroups on diagnostic guidelines for Alzheimer's disease. Alzheimers Dement 7:263–269. https://doi.org/10.1016/j.jalz.2011.03.005

26. Mead S, Gandhi S, Beck J, Caine D, Gallujipali D, Carswell C, Hyare H, Joiner S, Ayling H, Lashley T et al (2013) A novel prion disease associated with diarrhea and autonomic neuropathy. N Engl J Med 369: 1904–1914. https://doi.org/10.1056/NEJMoa1214747

27. Menon V (2015) Salience network. In: Toga AW (ed) Brain mapping: an encyclopedic reference. Elsevier, City, pp 597–611

28. Ossenkoppele R, Schonhaut DR, Baker SL, O'Neil JP, Janabi M, Ghosh PM, Santos M, Miller ZA, Bettcher BM, Gorno-Tempini ML et al (2015) Tau, amyloid, and hypometabolism in a patient with posterior cortical atrophy. Ann Neurol 77:338–342. https://doi.org/10.1002/ana.24321

29. Ossenkoppele R, Schonhaut DR, Scholl M, Lockhart SN, Ayakta N, Baker SL, O'Neil JP, Janabi M, Lazaris A, Cantwell A et al (2016) Tau PET patterns mirror clinical and neuroanatomical variability in Alzheimer's disease. Brain 139:1551–1567. https://doi.org/10.1093/brain/aww027

30. Paucar M, Xiang F, Moore R, Walker R, Winnberg E, Svenningsson P (2013) Genotype-phenotype analysis in inherited prion disease with eight octapeptide repeat insertional mutation. Prion 7:501–510

31. Piccardo P, Dlouhy S, Lievens P, Young K, Bird T, Nochlin D, Dickson D, Vinters H, Zimmerman T, Mackenzie I et al (1998) Phenotypic variability of Gerstmann-Straussler-Scheinker disease is associated with prion protein heterogeneity. J Neuropathol Exp Neurol 57:979–988

32. Suhara T, Shimada H, Shinotoh H, Hirano S, Eguchi Y, Takahata K, Kimura Y, Yamada M, Ito H, Higuchi M (2014) In vivo tau PET imaging using [11C]PBB3 in Alzheimer's disease and non-Alzheimer's disease tauopathies. J Nucl Med 55:1824

33. Tagliavini F, Giaccone G, Prelli F, Verga L, Porro M, Trojanowski JQ, Farlow MR, Frangione B, Ghetti B, Bugiani O (1993) A68 is a component of paired helical filaments of Gerstmann-Straussler-Scheinker disease, Indiana kindred. Brain Res 616:325–329

34. Trzepacz PT, Hochstetler H, Wang S, Walker B, Saykin AJ, Alzheimer's Disease Neuroimaging I (2015) Relationship between the Montreal cognitive assessment and mini-mental state examination for assessment of mild cognitive impairment in older adults. BMC Geriatr 15:107. https://doi.org/10.1186/s12877-015-0103-3

35. Unverzagt FW, Farlow MR, Norton J, Dlouhy SR, Young K, Ghetti B (1997) Neuropsychological function in patients with Gerstmann-Sträussler-Scheinker disease from the Indiana kindred (F198S). J Int Neuropsychol Soc 3:169–178

36. Vitali P, Maccagnano E, Caverzasi E, Henry RG, Haman A, Torres-Chae C, Johnson DY, Miller BL, Geschwind MD (2011) Diffusion-weighted MRI hyperintensity patterns differentiate CJD from other rapid dementias. Neurology 76:1711–1719. https://doi.org/10.1212/WNL.0b013e31821a4439

37. Xia CF, Arteaga J, Chen G, Gangadharmath U, Gomez LF, Kasi D, Lam C, Liang Q, Liu C, Mocharla VP et al (2013) [(18)F]T807, a novel tau positron emission tomography imaging agent for Alzheimer's disease. Alzheimers Dement 9:666–676. https://doi.org/10.1016/j.jalz.2012.11.008

9

SETD2 mutations in primary central nervous system tumors

Angela N. Viaene[1], Mariarita Santi[1], Jason Rosenbaum[2], Marilyn M. Li[1], Lea F. Surrey[1] and MacLean P. Nasrallah[2,3]*

Abstract

Mutations in *SETD2* are found in many tumors, including central nervous system (CNS) tumors. Previous work has shown these mutations occur specifically in high grade gliomas of the cerebral hemispheres in pediatric and young adult patients. We investigated *SETD2* mutations in a cohort of approximately 640 CNS tumors via next generation sequencing; 23 mutations were detected across 19 primary CNS tumors. Mutations were found in a wide variety of tumors and locations at a broad range of allele frequencies. *SETD2* mutations were seen in both low and high grade gliomas as well as non-glial tumors, and occurred in patients greater than 55 years of age, in addition to pediatric and young adult patients. High grade gliomas at first occurrence demonstrated either frameshift/truncating mutations or point mutations at high allele frequencies, whereas recurrent high grade gliomas frequently harbored subclones with point mutations in *SETD2* at lower allele frequencies in the setting of higher mutational burdens. Comparison with the TCGA dataset demonstrated consistent findings. Finally, immunohistochemistry showed decreased staining for H3K36me3 in our cohort of *SETD2* mutant tumors compared to wildtype controls. Our data further describe the spectrum of tumors in which *SETD2* mutations are found and provide a context for interpretation of these mutations in the clinical setting.

Keywords: SETD2, Histone, Brain tumor, Glioma, Epigenetics, H3K36me3

Introduction

Histone modifying enzymes regulate gene expression and play a role in numerous genomic functions through the modification of histones and non-histone proteins [20]. The disruption of normal epigenetic mechanisms secondary to mutations in histone modifying enzymes has been implicated in tumorigenesis [2] and in chemotherapeutic resistance in cancer patients [26]. Specifically, the loss of normal histone modifying enzyme activity is thought to result in alterations in chromatin configuration, disrupting cellular transcription and predisposing a cell to cancerous development [11]. In addition, multiple epigenetic therapies are in development or undergoing testing [23].

The *SETD2* gene encodes SET domain-containing 2 (SETD2), a histone modifying enzyme responsible for all trimethylation of the lysine 36 residue on Histone 3

(H3K36me3) in humans. Decreases in H3K36me3 lead to alterations in gene regulation, increased spontaneous mutation frequency and chromosomal instability [13, 14]. Prior studies have indicated that loss of one allele of *SETD2* does not significantly decrease levels of H3K36me3 [5, 8]; however, it is important to note that biallelic inactivation of *SETD2* may not be the sole mechanism leading to the loss of H3K36me3. For example, overexpression of other proteins such as HOX Transcript Antisense RNA (HOTAIR) can decrease levels of H3K63me3 as well [14].

SETD2-inactivating mutations have been implicated in a number of tumor types (for a review, see [14]). Most frequently, *SETD2* mutations are seen in clear cell renal cell carcinoma (CCRCC) and are thought to confer a poor prognosis [16]. *SETD2* mutations have also been reported in neoplasms of the central nervous system (CNS) [1, 6, 27]. These mutations have been found to be specific to pediatric and young adult high grade gliomas located in the cerebral hemispheres, affecting 15% and 8% of pediatric and adult high grade gliomas, respectively, and not found in other gliomas [6]. In the 2016 WHO Classification of Tumors of the Central Nervous

* Correspondence: maclean.nasrallah@uphs.upenn.edu
[2]Department of Pathology and Laboratory Medicine, University of Pennsylvania Perelman School of Medicine, Philadelphia, PA, USA
[3]Hospital of the University of Pennsylvania, FO6.089 3400 Spruce St, Philadelphia PA 19104, USA
Full list of author information is available at the end of the article

System, *SETD2* mutations are listed under frequent genetic alterations in pediatric (but not adult) high-grade diffuse astrocytic tumors within the cerebral hemispheres [18].

Western blot studies have shown *SETD2*-mutant gliomas have decreased levels of H3K36me3, indicating that the mutations in these tumors are loss-of-function [6]. Similarly, immunohistochemical studies of CCRCC, chondroblastomas, and chordomas have been used to demonstrate decreased staining for H3K36me3 in tumors with *SETD2* mutations [8, 16, 19, 25]. To our knowledge, immunohistochemistry has not been used to evaluate levels of H3K36me3 in *SETD2*-mutant brain tumors.

Here we describe 19 cases of CNS tumors with mutations in *SETD2*. *SETD2* mutation allele frequency and co-occurring mutations in other genes are investigated, and results are correlated with the effects of *SETD2* mutations on epigenetic change, specifically histone methylation and acetylation as shown by immunohistochemistry for H3K36me3, H3K36ac and H3K27me3. Our findings indicate that *SETD2* mutations occur at a wide range of allele frequencies in a variety of tumors of the central nervous system and that those mutations most likely to have functional impact on the gene product are seen most often but not exclusively in pediatric and young adult high grade gliomas of the cerebral hemispheres.

Materials and methods

This study was approved by an independent institutional review board at the Hospital of the University of Pennsylvania (HUP IRB 827290). All CNS tumors with *SETD2* mutations identified on routine next generation sequencing (NGS) studies performed September 17, 2016 through June 30, 2017 at HUP and from February 1, 2016 to June 30, 2018 at CHOP are included in the current study. Fifteen tumors from HUP and four tumors from Children's Hospital of Philadelphia (CHOP) are included. Patients whose tumor showed single nucleotide polymorphisms or otherwise benign variants in *SETD2* were excluded.

Next generation sequencing

At our institutions, targeted NGS of brain tumor specimens is performed as part of routine patient care. Genomic tumor testing was performed at the Center for Personalized Diagnostics (CPD) at the University of Pennsylvania and the Division of Genomic Diagnostics (DGD) at the CHOP, both CLIA-approved laboratories. Genomic DNA from brain tumor specimens is extracted from fresh tissue, formalin-fixed paraffin-embedded tissues or frozen tissue. Tumor DNA is sequenced on an Illumina MiSeq or HiSeq, and the data are analyzed using in-house bioinformatics pipelines.

At the CPD, the Solid Tumor Sequencing panel uses a custom Agilent HaloPlex library preparation (Agilent,

Santa Clara, CA) to cover approximately 0.5 megabases, including the entire exonic (coding) sequence of 152 genes, + 10 base pairs of intronic sequence. The 152 genes sequenced on the CPD panel may be found at (https://www.pennmedicine.org/departments-and-centers/center-for-personalized-diagnostics/gene-panels). The library preparation includes unique molecular identifiers to identify duplicate reads. Specimens are sequenced on the Illumina HiSeq 2500 platform (Illumina, San Diego, CA) using multiplexed, paired end reads. Analysis and interpretation is performed using a customized bioinformatics pipeline, Halo_v1.2. All variants are annotated with reference to the hg19 Genome build. Variants are reported according to HGVS nomenclature and classified into 3 categories: Disease-Associated Variants, Variants of Uncertain Significance, and Benign. Variant allele frequency (VAF) is defined as the number of reads of a variant from the reference sequence divided by the total number of reads at that base.

The Comprehensive Solid Tumor Panel v1 at CHOP includes sequence and copy number analyses of 237 cancer genes, and 586 known fusions and many more novel fusions associated with 106 fusion gene partners. The genes included in the panel can be found at (https://www.testmenu.com/chop/Tests/785967). Fusion genes were evaluated by targeted RNA-seq using anchored multiplex PCR with custom designed primers (ArcherDx, Boulder, CO). Full exonic and select intronic/promotor sequence of 237 cancer genes were evaluated by next generation sequencing. Regions of interest were captured using SureSelect^{QTX} target enrichment technology (Agilent Technologies, Santa Clara, CA). Sequencing was performed on Illumina MiSeq or HiSeq (San Diego, CA). Sequencing data were processed using the homebrew software ConcordS v1 and NextGENe v2 NGS Analysis Software (Softgenetics, State College, PA). Variant interpretation was performed according to AMP/ASCO/CAP standards and guidelines for somatic variant interpretation and reporting [15].

Immunohistochemistry

All tumors with nonsense or frameshift mutations in *SETD2* and those with missense mutations with AF greater than 40% were used for immunohistochemical (IHC) studies. In addition, glioblastomas, anaplastic astrocytomas, pilocytic astrocytomas and meningiomas confirmed to be *SETD2*-wildtype by NGS were used as controls.

H3K36me3 (Abcam ab9050), H3K36ac (Abcam ab177179), and H3K27me3 (Cell Signaling 9733) antibodies were used to stain formalin fixed paraffin embedded slides. Staining was performed on a Bond Max automated staining system (Leica Biosystems). The Bond Refine polymer staining kit (Leica Biosystems) was used. The standard protocol was followed with the exception of the primary antibody incubation which was extended to 1 h at room temperature. The antibodies were used at 1:5 K (H3K36me3), 1:100 (H3K36ac) and 1:150 (H3K36me3) dilutions and antigen retrieval was performed with E1 (H3K36me3 & H3K36ac) or E2 (H3K27me3) (Leica Biosystems) retrieval solution for 20 min. Slides were rinsed, dehydrated through a series of ascending concentrations of ethanol and xylene, then coverslipped.

Immunohistochemistry was scored using the semiquantitative H-score system. H-scores were calculated as 3x the percentage of strongly staining nuclei +2x the percentage of moderately staining nuclei + the percentage of weakly staining nuclei (giving a range of 0 to 300). The H-scores were independently assessed by two neuropathologists board-certified by the American Board of Pathology (MPN and ANV) on de-identified slides.

TCGA

The Cancer Genome Atlas (TCGA) dataset was retrieved from cbioportal (http://www.cbioportal.org) by searching for SETD2 mutations in "CNS/Brain" tumors (headings: diffuse glioma, glioblastoma, oligodendroglioma, pilocytic astrocytoma and medulloblastoma). The search was performed 11/30/2017.

Statistical analysis

Statistical analysis was performed using SPSS version 23.0 (IBM Corp.). Statistical significance was defined as $p < .05$ and based on two-tailed tests. For the analysis of the number of co-occurring mutations in SETD2-mutant tumors, only data from the CPD were used in calculations.

Results

From September 17, 2016 through June 30, 2017, approximately 400 CNS tumors, including metastases, were sequenced at the University of Pennsylvania CPD. From February 1, 2016 to June 30, 2018 approximately 240 CNS tumors were sequenced at the DGD at CHOP. Nineteen primary brain tumors (fifteen at the University of Pennsylvania and four at CHOP) with SETD2 mutations were identified on routine NGS studies (Tables 1 and 2). Eleven tumors had nonsense or frameshift mutations (truncating mutations) in SETD2 and eight had missense mutations. The age of the patients ranged from 9 to 80 years old (mean 43 years, median 42 years), and there was no statistically significant difference ($p = 0.49$) in age between patients with nonsense or frameshift mutations and those with missense mutations (Fig. 1a); however, of high grade gliomas, recurrences often showed missense mutations, whereas frameshift and nonsense mutations were preferentially seen in de novo tumors (Tables 1 and 2). The male to female ratio of the cohort was 3:1.

Twelve of these SETD2-mutant tumors were located within the cerebral hemispheres while seven occurred outside the hemispheres (two extra-axial, one thalamic, and four posterior fossa; Fig. 1b). A broad range of tumor histologies were seen, including high grade gliomas ($n = 10$, 62.5%, with 4 of them recurrent), low grade astrocytic tumors ($n = 5$, 12.5%), atypical meningiomas ($n = 2$, 12.5%), a medulloblastoma ($n = 1$, 6.3%) and a choroid plexus papilloma ($n = 1$, 6.3%). Examples of tumor histology are show in Fig. 1d. Overall, eleven of the SETD2-mutant tumors were classified as high grade (WHO grade III or IV) and eight were low grade tumors (WHO grade I or II) (Tables 1 and 2).

In total, 23 SETD2 changes amongst the 19 tumors were detected at a wide range of VAF (range 2–51%); 4 tumors had more than one SETD2 missense mutation, 3 of which were recurrent high grade gliomas, and the fourth a medulloblastoma. No statistically significant difference ($p = 0.49$) in VAF was seen between truncating mutations and missense mutations.

The detected mutations were distributed throughout SETD2 with the majority of the high grade glioma nonsense or frameshift mutations occurring 5′ to the SET domain (VAF 4–44%) (Fig. 2a). The nonsense or frameshift mutations for the low grade gliomas occurred throughout the SETD2 gene (VAF 6–34%).

Missense mutations occurred throughout the SETD2 gene, and in gliomas, were found predominantly in recurrent high grade gliomas, including recurrent glioblastomas (Table 2). The exceptions were patients 10 and 12. For patient 10 in Table 2, diagnosed with an IDH-wildtype anaplastic astrocytoma, a p.I1398T change in SETD2 was found; however, this may represent a benign single nucleotide polymorphism as it is seen at > 0.1% frequency in the Ashkenazi Jewish population (http://gnomad.broadinstitute.org/) [12]. Patient 12, with otherwise similar characteristics, showed SETD2 p.A2242V, which we classify as a variant of uncertain significance, given that is not been identified previously. The remaining missense mutations found in SETD2 may represent changes found with the increased mutational load seen with tumor recurrence in this cohort (4.57 ± 3.40 mutations in recurrent tumors vs. 1.41 ± 1.24 mutations in primary tumors, $p < 0.01$), and known in the literature, particularly after treatment with temozolomide [3, 9]. The largest number of co-occurring mutations (11) was seen in patient 14 following chemotherapy and radiation. Of note, this patient also had two MM in SETD2. Within the adult cohort, tumors with missense mutations in SETD2 had more concurrent mutations than did those with truncations of SETD2 (5.17 ± 3.31 vs. 1.50 ± 1.35, $p < 0.05$). Mutations in EGFR were found to be the most commonly co-occurring change with SETD2 changes and were seen in 40% of the high grade gliomas in this cohort, similar to

Table 1 Demographics of patients with frameshift and nonsense (truncating) mutations in SETD2

Patient #	Age at time of resection	Gender	Location	Diagnosis	Histologic Grade	SETD2 mutation (AF)	Other disease-associated mutations (AF)[a]	Prior CNS tumor	Follow up from initial tumor resection (months)
1	60	M	Left thalamus	Glioblastoma, IDH-wildtype, WHO grade IV	IV	p.K846Ifs*4 (30%)	PTEN p.P246L (47%)	None	8[b]
2	48	F	Left temporal lobe	Glioblastoma, IDH-wildtype, WHO grade IV	IV	p.E282Rfs*9 (4%)	PIK3CA p.G1049R (6%) BRAF p.G466V (2%) NF1 p.F124?Ifs*18 (7%)	None	7[b]
3	37	M	Right frontoparietal lobe	Glioblastoma, IDH-wildtype, WHO grade IV	IV	p.F1135Sfs*22 (23%)	None	None	12[c]
4	55	M	Left frontal lobe	Anaplastic astrocytoma, IDH-wildtype, WHO grade III	III	p.R1598* (44%)	EGFR amplification	None	2[b]
5	75	M	Right frontal lobe	Recurrent/residual glioblastoma, IDH-wildtype	IV	p.W1341* (5%)	ARID1A p.? (3%) FBXW7 p.Q548* (6%) EGFR p.A289V (15%) ARID2 p.Q1215* (11%)	History of glioblastoma resected in 2012 status-post chemoradiation	61[b]
6	80	F	Right frontal lobe resection, gliomatosis cerebri pattern	Diffuse astrocytoma, IDH-wildtype, WHO grade II	II	p.E1907Rfs*4 (6%)	EGFR p.A244T (19%)	None	9[d]
7	10	M	Cerebellum, left hemisphere	Pilocytic astrocytoma, WHO grade I	I	p.R2109* (34%)	KIAA1549-BRAF fusion	None	12[b]
8	16	F	Left temporal lobe	Diffuse astrocytoma	II	p.Q1764Pfs*3 (11%)	QKI-NTRK2 fusion	None	3[b]
9	9	M	Left temporal lobe	Recurrent/residual Pilocytic Astrocytoma	I	p.Q7* (51%)	KIAA1549-BRAF fusion	History of pilocytic astrocytoma resected 2012 (x3) status-post chemotherapy	72[b]
10	17	M	Cerebellum	Pilocytic Astrocytoma	I	p.N261* (28%)	NF1 p.R2269Vfs*11	None	2[b]
11	68	F	Right temporoparietal, extra axial	Atypical meningioma, WHO grade II	II	p.E282Kfs*19 (10%)	NF2 p.L163Wfs*11 (71%)	History of grade I menginomas resected 2005 and 2006	7[a]

Mutation calls were made using transcript ID NM_014159.6

[a]Changes considered variants of uncertain significance are not listed with other disease-associated mutations

[b]No definitive tumor progression detected on surveillance imaging

[c]Surveillance imaging studies not available

[d]Tumor progression suspected on surveillance imaging

Table 2 Demographics of patients with missense mutations in SETD2

Patient #	Age at time of resection	Gender	Location	Diagnosis	Histologic Grade	SETD2 point mutation (AF)	Other disease-associated mutations (AF)[a]	Prior CNS tumor	Follow up from initial tumor resection (months)
12	32	M	Right frontal lobe	Recurrent/residual high grade glioma, IDH-mutant	IV	p.G1659D (4%) p.S1268F (3%)	IDH1 p.R132H (49%) CDKN2A p.A36Rfs*17 (72%) NOTCH1 p.? (3%) TP53 p.? (84%) EP300 p.Q2224* (2%)	History of anaplastic astrocytoma resected in 2011 and 2012 status-post resection and chemoradiation	72[c]
13	69	M	Right frontal lobe	Anaplastic astrocytoma, IDH-wildtype, WHO grade III	III	p.I1398T (49%)[b]	EGFR p.G598V (94%) EGFR amplification KMT2C p.S777Kfs*19 (24%)	None	13[d]
14	60	M	Left frontal lobe	Recurrent/residual glioblastoma, IDH-wildtype	IV	p.A2458T (32%) p.S1088F (9%)	MSH6 p.F1088Lfs*5 (9%) TET2 p.W184* (14%) EZH2 p.? (10%) PTCH1 p.Y1316Tfs*56 (6%) PTEN p.? (4%) TP53 p.H179Y (3%), p.P152L (49%), p.S127F (8%) NF1 p.? (9%), p.W2229* (6%) KDM6A p.? (9%)	History of glioblastoma resected 2013 and 2015 status-post chemoradiation	44[e]
15	64	M	Right frontal lobe	Anaplastic astrocytoma, IDH-wildtype, WHO grade III	III	p.A2242V (49%)[b]	EGFR p.A289T (32%) PTEN p.E7Rfs*17 (18%), p.R130del (7%)	None	2[c]
16	27	F	Right frontal	Recurrent/residual glioblastoma, IDH-mutant	IV	p.E1692K (7%) p.R385K (2%)	IDH1 p.R132H (38%) KMT2C p.? (3%) MEN1 p.? (2%) ARID2 p.Q1604* (2%) BRCA2 p.Q2009* (23%) TP53 p.Y220Pfs*28 (90%)	History of glioblastoma resected 2013 and 2015 status-post chemoradiation	49[f]
17	42	M	Superior saggital sinus, extra axial	Recurrent/residual atypical meningioma	III	p.G1014D (22%)	BRCA2 p.R2494* (3%)	History of atypical meningioma resected 2009 status-post radiation	96[c]
18	33	M	4th ventricle	Choroid plexus papilloma, WHO grade I	I	p.R1089Q (51%)[b]	None	None	5[c]
19	18	M	Cerebellum, left hemisphere	Medulloblastoma, nodular desmoplastic variant, SHH subgroup, WHO grade IV	IV	p.V2371L (5%) p.T1663M (6%)	ATM p.L1327* (42%) CTCF p.R448* (7%) PTCH1 p.C454* (41%) TERT p.? (57%)	None	40[d]

Mutation calls were were made using transcript ID NM_014159.6

aChanges considered variants of uncertain significance are not listed with other disease-associated mutations

bMissense mutations likely represent germline variant

cNo definitive tumor progression detected on surveillance imaging

dPatient had tumor recurrences and resections, now with no definitive progression detected on surveillance imaging

eSurveillance imaging studies not available

fTumor progression suspected on surveillance imaging

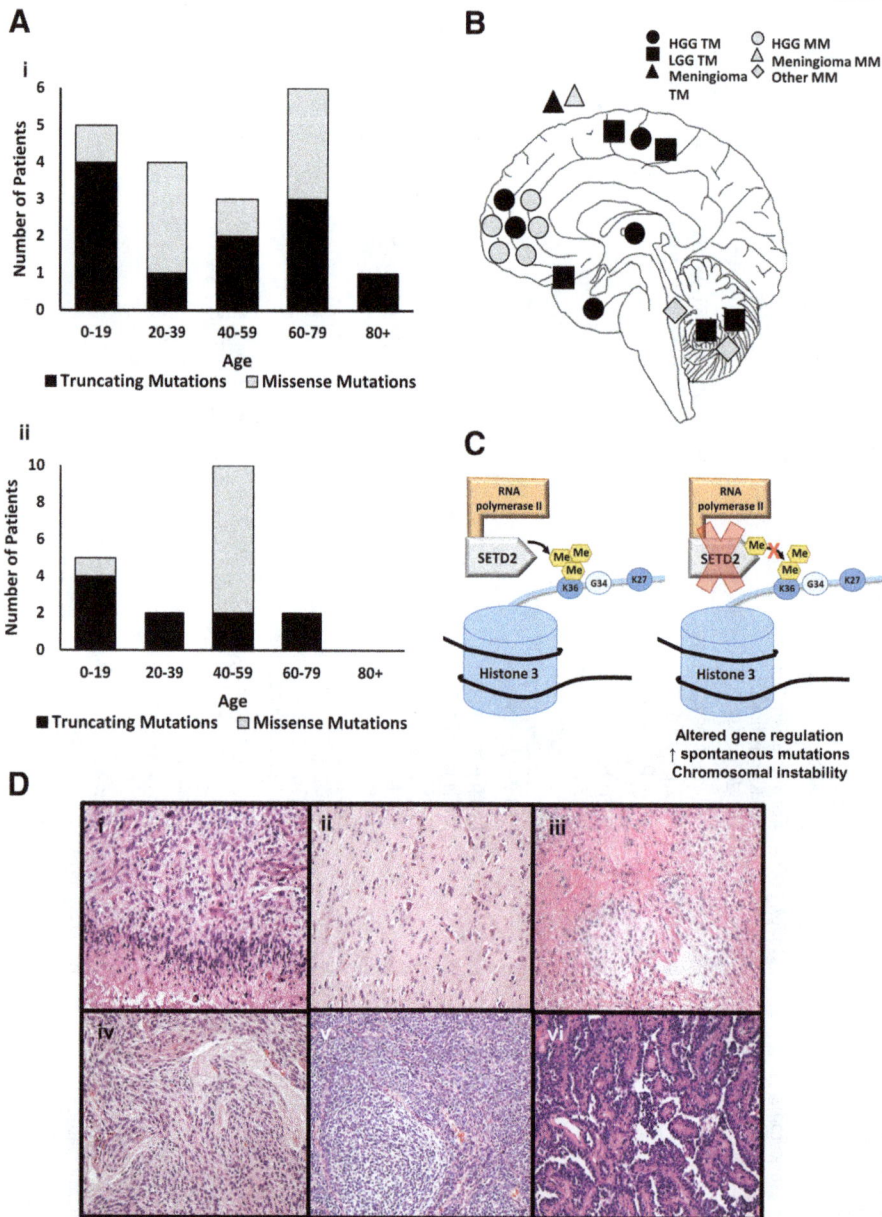

Fig. 1 Demographics, locations and histologies of *SETD2* mutant brain tumors. **a** Histograms of patient ages at time of tumor resection for the 19 cases presented in the current study (i) and from the TCGA database (ii). **b** Schematic representation of *SETD2* mutant tumor locations within the CNS. **c** A schematic illustrating the proposed epigenetic effects of *SETD2* alterations. **d** Representative histologies of *SETD2* mutant tumors: Glioblastoma (i), Diffuse astrocytoma (ii), Pilocytic astrocytoma (iii), Atypical meningioma (iv), Medulloblastoma (v), Choroid plexus papilloma (vi). All tumors stained with Hematoxylin and Eosin. All photographs taken at 200x magnification. Truncating mutations (TM), missense mutation (MM)

the frequency of EGFR mutations found in high grade gliomas overall (Fig. 2b) [1]. Pathogenic mutations in *TP53* were seen in 30% of high grade gliomas with *SETD2* changes, and IDH mutations were seen in 20%. However, *TP53* and *IDH* mutations were only seen in tumors with missense mutations in *SETD2* and not those with nonsense or frameshift mutations in *SETD2*. No mutations in *H3F3A* were seen to co-occur with *SETD2* changes.

Immunohistochemistry

Immunohistochemistry for H3K36me3, H3K36ac and H3K27me3 expression were assessed with H-scores by two neuropathologists (ANV and MPN) on *SETD2*-mutant tumors and histologic controls confirmed to be wildtype for *SETD2* by NGS. Gliomas with SETD2 mutations showed significantly lower H-scores for H3K36me3 compared to wildtype controls (140.8 ± 65.4

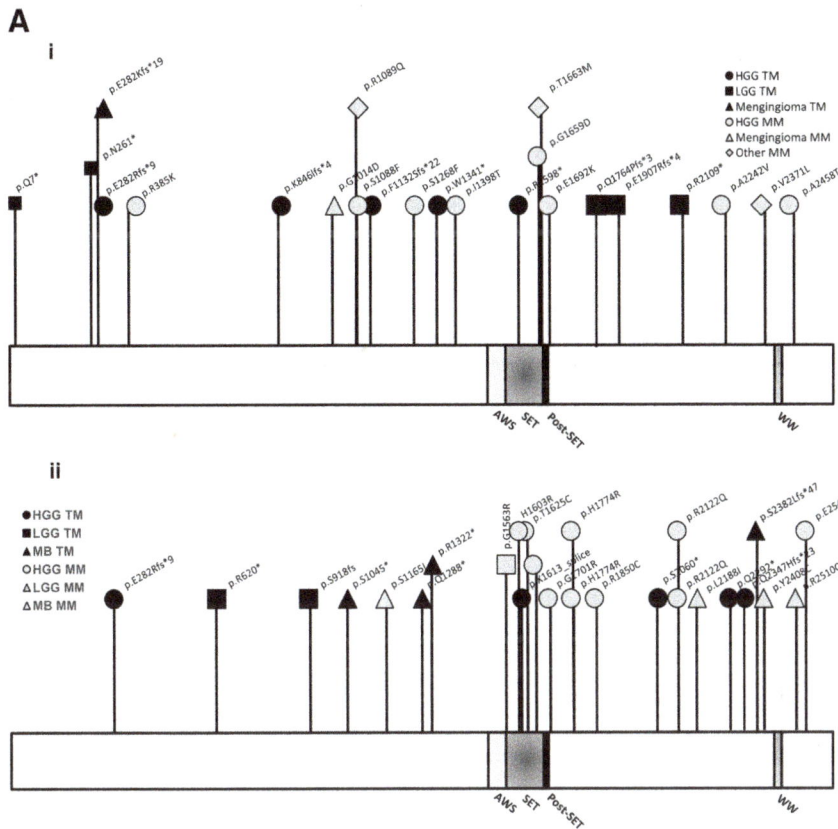

Fig. 2 Location of mutations within *SETD2* and co-occurring pathogenic mutations. **a** Schematic representation of the locations of mutations in SETD2 for the 16 cases presented in the current study (i) and the TCGA database (ii) (AWS, Associated with SET). **b** Other pathogenic mutations co-occurring in tumors with *SETD2* mutations with the percentage of tumors with each mutation is labeled within each cell. Darker shading corresponds to higher percentages. Truncating mutations (TM), missense mutation (MM)

vs. 228.8 ± 29.1, $p < 0.01$) (Fig. 3). In contrast, statistically significant differences in staining for H3K36ac and H3K27me3 between SETD2 mutants and controls were not observed (H3K36ac: 140.1 ± 35.7 vs. 160.0 ± 41.8, $p = 0.13$; H3K27me3: 206.1 ± 24.2 vs. 190.8 ± 33.5, $p = 0.23$). There was no correlation between AF and H-score for any of the immunohistochemical markers [H3K36me3: $F_{1,8} = 0.55$, $p = .48$ with an R^2 of 0.06 (Fig. 3c); H3K36ac: $F_{1,8} = 0.54$, $p = .48$ with an R^2 of 0.06; H3K27me3: $F_{1,8} = 0.46$, $p = .53$ with an R^2 of 0.08]. The concordance correlation coefficients for the three antibodies were as

follows: H3K36me3 concordance correlation coefficient of 0.88 [95% CI 0.69–0.96]; H3K36ac concordance correlation coefficient of 0.58 (95% CI 0.12–0.83); H3K27me3: concordance correlation coefficient of 0.51 (95% CI 0.16–0.75).

TCGA

The results shown here are based upon data generated by the TCGA Research Network: http://cancergenome. nih.gov/, via http://www.cbioportal.org/ [4, 7]. A total of 22 CNS tumors with *SETD2* mutations were identified across the cohorts included in the TCGA datasets, with

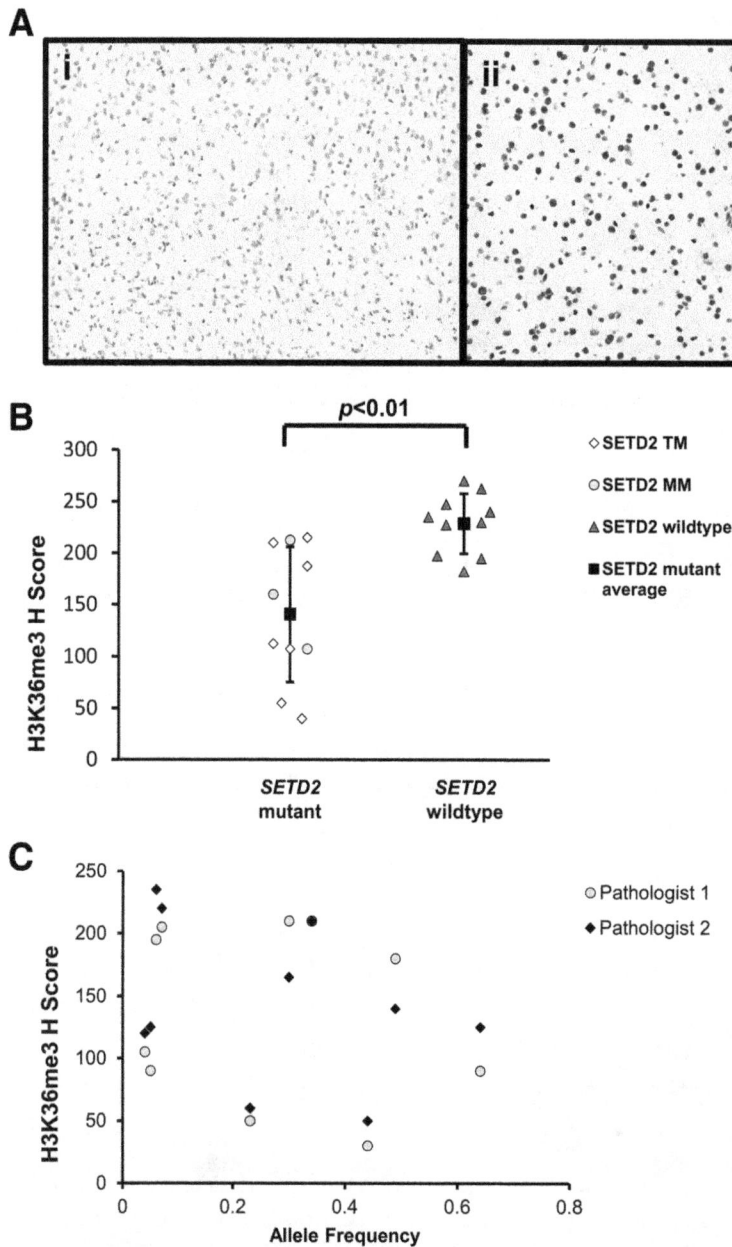

Fig. 3 Immunohistochemical staining for H3K36me3. a Examples of immunohistochemical staining for H3K36me3 in high grade gliomas with a truncating mutation in *SETD2* (i) and wildtype control (ii); both images were taken at 200x magnification. b H scores for *SETD2* mutant tumors and wildtype tumors. Averages for each group are shown as black squares and with error bars representing the standard deviation. c H scores calculated by two independent pathologists for *SETD2* mutants plotted against allele frequency. Truncating mutations (TM), missense mutation (MM)

0–14% of CNS tumors harboring a *SETD2* mutation depending on the cohort (Fig. 4). Eleven tumors had truncating mutations, ten had missense mutations and one had a splice-site mutation. The age of the patients ranged from 2 to 74 years (mean 40.1 ± 23.6 years) with a male to female ratio of 2.3:1. There was no statistically significant difference ($p = 0.22$) in age between patients with truncating mutations and those with missense mutations. *SETD2* mutations were found in high grade gliomas ($n = 14$, 63%), low grade gliomas ($n = 3$, 14%), and medulloblastomas ($n = 5$, 23%). The low grade gliomas included two pilocytic astrocytomas and an IDH-mutant, 1p/19q-codeleted, WHO grade II oligodendroglioma. Data on the location of the tumors is limited; a study of glioblastomas found that all tumors with *SETD2* mutations were located in the cerebral hemispheres [6]. However, it is likely *SETD2* mutant tumors were also present in the posterior fossa as mutations

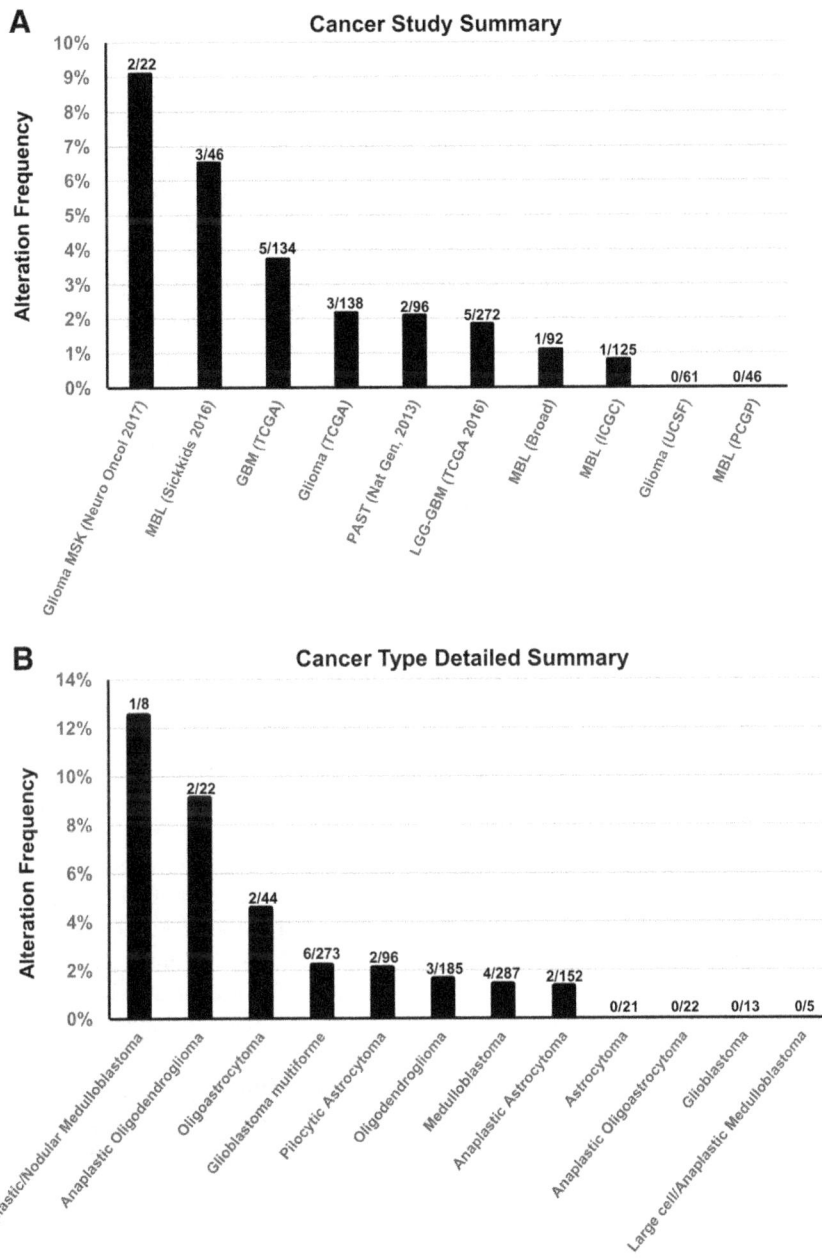

Fig. 4 *SETD2* mutations in CNS tumors retrieved from the TCGA database. **a** Frequency of *SETD2* alterations detected per study. **b** Frequency of *SETD2* alterations detected per tumor type. The number of cases with SETD2 variants over the denominator of the total number of analyzed cases for each group is indicated above the bars

were seen in 5 medulloblastomas and 2 pilocytic astrocytomas, tumors which both have a strong association with the posterior fossa. In total, 26 *SETD2* mutations were seen among the 22 tumors with one medulloblastoma having 3 *SETD2* missense mutations. For the 11 tumors for which data on AF was available, the frequency ranged from 5 to 48%. No statistically significant difference in AF was seen between truncating mutations and missense mutations ($p = 0.82$). The mutations were distributed throughout SETD2 (Fig. 2 aii). Survival data

is available on 16 patients (15 patients with gliomas and 1 patient with medulloblastoma). The average follow-up was 19.1 ± 17.3 months (range 5 to 72 months) for all tumors and 15.8 ± 11.4 months (range 5 to 45 months) for patients with high grade gliomas. Twelve patients were still living. High grade gliomas with TM had an average follow-up of 13.2 ± 10.8 months and those with MM had an average follow-up of 17.7 ± 12.3 months ($p = .52$). Four deceased patients all had high grade gliomas (two of which were recurrent) with an average survival of 16.3 ± 10.0 months (range 7 to 30 months). Two of the deceased patients had TM (survival 7 months and 30 months) and two patients had MM (survivals of 11 and 17 months).

Discussion

Epigenetic changes, such as DNA methylation and histone modifications affect the structure of chromatin, and therefore have a potentially broad impact on transcription. Epigenetic changes have been detected in a wide range of tumors, and a variety of drugs have been developed to target these changes; for a review, see [23]. Epigenetic mutations in gliomas include H3 K27 M mutations in diffuse midline gliomas and H3.3 G34R/V mutations in gliomas of the cerebral hemispheres [18]. In diffuse midline gliomas, the H3 K27 M mutation has been shown to globally reduce levels of H3K27me3 levels, altering transcription and driving tumorigenesis. Several therapies that target enzymes responsible for chromatin modifications in these gliomas have been developed; for a review, see [17]. In gliomas, mutations have also been reported in SETD2, whose protein product is an enzyme responsible for trimethylation of the lysine 36 residue on Histone 3 (H3K36me3) in humans. These mutations potentially decrease H3K36me3, which may alter gene regulation, increase spontaneous mutation frequency and lead to chromosomal instability, with theoretically targetable effects (Fig. 1c).

Our investigation of SETD2 mutations in brain tumors yields findings consistent with the previous report of SETD2 mutations in gliomas, which shows that loss-of-function SETD2 mutations occur in older children and young adults in high grade gliomas of the cerebral cortex [6]. In addition, we expand on those results to demonstrate that subclonal mutations in SETD2 are seen in a broad range of tumors and locations. Prior studies focusing on gliomas illustrate that SETD2 mutations are found nearly exclusively within the cerebral hemispheres [1, 6, 22, 27]. Similarly, in our cohort, mutations were most commonly seen in high grade gliomas within the cerebral hemispheres (12 of 19 tumors). However, our results include a broader range of CNS tumor types, and demonstrate SETD2 truncating mutations in atypical meningiomas and pilocytic astrocytomas, as well as missense mutations in a choroid plexus papilloma and a medulloblastoma. Data from the TCGA database also showed SETD2 mutations in pilocytic astrocytomas, an oligodendroglioma, and medulloblastomas. Prior studies of medulloblastomas did not detect mutations in SETD2 [10] suggesting SETD2 mutations are rare in these tumors. The medulloblastoma described in our cohort belongs to the Sonic Hedgehog genetic group, and has two point mutations in SETD2 with reported VAFs of 5% and 6%.

In contrast to previous work showing that SETD2 mutations are seen in high grade gliomas but not low grade

gliomas, we found frameshift mutations in SETD2 in two diffuse astrocytomas, WHO grade II. However, one SETD2-mutant astrocytoma in an older patient (#6) also harbors an EGFR mutation and lacks IDH changes, and so is in essence a "molecular glioblastoma," in addition to radiologically showing a gliomatosis cerebri pattern of growth. Given the previous findings that SETD2 mutations are specific to high grade gliomas, the SETD2 change in this tumor may be hypothesized to indicate or correlate with aggressive behavior. The patient experienced slow radiological progression and clinical decline over 8 months despite temozolomide therapy, and subsequently transitioned to hospice and comfort care. Along the same lines, we found truncating mutations in three pilocytic astrocytomas. Although pilocytic astrocytomas are grade I tumors, they can show anaplastic changes, and one of these three tumors did have increased mitotic activity (#7). Additionally, another pilocytic astrocytoma was a recurrent tumor with a history of three prior resections and chemotherapy (#9).

In addition, not all patients conform to the previously reported age and tumor location profile. For example, the patient diagnosed with the diffuse astrocytoma mentioned above was 80 years old at the time of diagnosis. Also, a 60-year-old patient presented with a thalamic glioblastoma, which demonstrated a frameshift mutation in SETD2 at a 30% VAF. Data from the TCGA database also showed a wide range of patient ages (2–74 years).

In our cohort, mutations were seen in a variety of regions within the SETD2 gene and at a broad range of VAF in tumors. In high grade gliomas, nonsense and frameshift mutations were mostly located 5′ to the SET domain. These findings are similar to what has been reported [6]. In contrast, in the low grade astrocytic tumors, nonsense or frameshift mutations often occurred 3′ to the SET domain, including in tumor #6. Missense mutations were found throughout SETD2. The significance of the location of mutation with respect to nonsense mediated decay of the RNA is unknown. SETD2 mutations with low VAF (defined as VAF < 10%), were seen to co-occur with an average of 3.8 ± 1.7 other mutations (range 1–6 mutations). Those tumors with higher SETD2 mutation VAF (≥10%) had an average of 1.8 ± 2.9 additional co-occurring mutations (range 0–11 mutations).

Several tumors in our cohort were recurrent/residual gliomas. Sequencing for SETD2 mutations was not performed on the prior resection specimens. However, one patient (#13) had tumor recurrence and a subsequent resection which showed the same SETD2 mutation (p.I1398T) at a similar VAF. Patients 13, 15, and 18 had MM occurring at VAF around 50%. It is possible that these mutations are germline though this cannot be confirmed as paired normal sequencing for SETD2 was not performed.

We attempted to determine whether the *SETD2* mutation resulted in a functional effect through immunohistochemical studies of epigenetic markers. If *SETD2* mutations are indeed driving tumorigenesis in some CNS tumors, the exact mechanism by which this occurs also requires further elucidation. One of the leading hypotheses suggests that loss of *SETD2* function in tumor cells decreases levels of H3K36me3, which subsequently leads to alterations in gene regulation, increased spontaneous mutation frequency and chromosomal instability (Fig. 1c) [13, 14]. Evidence also indicates that increased levels of H3K36ac are seen when the levels of H3K36me3 decrease [21]. We employed IHC for H3K36me3, H3K36ac and H3K27me3 to investigate the impact of *SETD2* mutations on histone methylation and acetylation. We hypothesized that decreased H3K36me3 staining and increased staining for H3K36ac would be present in *SETD2* mutant tumors with mutation seen at high VAF. Additionally, prior investigations have shown that cells depleted for all H3K36-directed methyltransferases have a reduction in H3K36me3 and also have elevated levels of H3K27me3 [19]. Based on these findings, we investigated whether staining for H3K27me3 is increased in *SETD2* mutant tumors.

Immunohistochemical staining for H3K36me3 showed a statistically significant decrease in staining for *SETD2* mutant gliomas compared to *SETD2* wildtype histologic controls. However, given the variability in staining and the lack of correlation with allele frequency, IHC for the detection of *SETD2* mutations is impractical in a clinical setting. Prior work in gliomas also found a significant decrease in levels of H3K36me3 in gliomas with heterozygous mutations in *SETD2* by Western Blot [6]. In contrast, studies have indicated that bi-allelic loss of *SETD2* is needed to significantly decrease levels of H3K36me3 in in vitro models and renal cell carcinoma [5, 8, 14]. For example, the most significant decreases in staining for H3K36me3 in non-CNS tumors with *SETD2* mutations were seen when both *SETD2* allelic copies were lost [8, 16, 19, 25]. Specifically, studies of clear cell renal cell carcinoma indicate that mutations occurring at higher AFs may not result in significant decreases in H3K36me3 unless both *SETD2* alleles are affected [5, 8]. Further studies are needed to assess whether this statistically significant decrease in levels of H3K36me3 in gliomas with heterozygous mutations in *SETD2* has a function impact on tumorigenesis, as well as to determine if there is loss of the alternate allele.

Immunohistochemical stains for H3K36ac and H3K27me3 did not show statistically significant differences in staining between mutants and controls, although an increase in staining for H3K27me3 were seen in *SETD2* mutants compared to controls. There was no correlation between VAF and levels of staining for any

antibodies though this may be due to the small number of tumors evaluated.

An alternative mechanistic hypothesis is that *SETD2* mutations are interacting with other mutations to drive tumorigenesis. For example, SETD2 may bind to p53 and regulate the transcription of specific genes [28]. Studies of lung adenocarcinomas found loss of H3K36me3 lead to accelerated progression of early- and late-stage tumors; however SETD2 loss alone was not sufficient to overcome the p53-regulated barrier that suppresses the formation of higher grade adenocarcinomas [24]. It is possible that *SETD2* mutations work in conjunction with other mutations such as *TP53* or mutations in growth factor pathways to promote tumorigenesis. Although one of the most frequently observed concurrently mutated genes in our cohort of high grade gliomas is *TP53*, *TP53* mutations were only seen in tumors with *SETD2* missense mutations and not in those tumors with *SETD2* nonsense or frameshift mutations. Most often, the co-occurrence of *SETD2* and *TP53* mutations was seen in recurrent gliomas, and the VAFs varied. These findings do not lend support to the hypothesis that *SETD2* mutations synergize with *TP53* mutations, and further studies are necessary.

In addition to *TP53*, the other most frequently observed genes showing mutations concurrent with *SETD2* mutation within the high grade glioma subset were *EGFR* and *PTEN*, likely due to the frequency of mutation in these genes in glioblastoma. Recurrent tumors with *SETD2* mutations had significantly more concurrent mutations than did first occurrence *SETD2*-mutant tumors. *IDH* mutations were present in a subset (18%) of diffuse gliomas with *SETD2* changes, which in this study were all *SETD2* missense mutations rather than nonsense or frameshift mutations. Concurrent mutations in *SETD2* and *H3F3A* were not seen. Both of these findings are consistent with prior investigation [6].

Data on the long-term survival for patients with *SETD2*-mutant CNS tumors is limited. Twelve of sixteen patients from the TCGA cohort were still living, and the data on follow-up does not allow any conclusions to be drawn regarding the impact of the SETD2 mutations. At the conclusion of the current study, all patients were still living. Focusing on patients with high grade gliomas, the average follow-up period from initial presentation was 18.0 ± 24.3 months (range 2 to 61 months) for truncating mutations and 36.0 ± 28.3 months (range 2 to 72 months) for missense mutations. Two tumors with *SETD2* missense mutations were positive for *IDH1* mutations; when comparing tumors with *SETD2* missense mutations, *IDH*-mutant tumors had follow-up periods of 79 and 42 months versus follow-up periods ranging from 2 to 44 months with an average follow-up of 19.7 ± 21.8 months for *IDH*-wildtype gliomas. On average, longer follow-up data was available for patients with tumors with missense mutations as several of these were identified in recurrences (4 of 5 high grade gliomas with missense mutations had recurrences available for analysis). It is important to note that the initial tumor resections of three of these tumors were not sequenced for *SETD2*, so it is uncertain if the changes were present at the time of initial presentation. However, one patient (#13) had an *IDH*-wildtype anaplastic astrocytoma recur with progression to glioblastoma; the initial frontal lobe resection and the frontal lobe recurrence demonstrated the same mutational profile, including the same *SETD2* missense mutation, whereas an intervening temporoparietal tumor resection demonstrated different mutations. EGFR p.G589 V and a copy number gain of EGFR were detected in both frontal lobe resections, and EGFR p.T263P and PTEN p.T366Hfs*50 were detected in the temporoparietal resection. In these recurrent/residual high grade gliomas with changes in *SETD2*, longer durations of follow-up were seen after initial presentation (mean of 79 and 42 months for *IDH*-mutant tumors and 52.5 ± 12.0 months for *IDH*-wildtype tumors) than is common for high grade gliomas. Further studies are required to better elucidate how nonsense or frameshift mutations and missense mutations in *SETD2* relate to prognosis.

Another question that requires further investigation is the difference between truncating mutations and missense *SETD2* mutations. Prior Western blot studies found a decrease in levels of H3K36me3 for both truncating and missense mutations [6]. As a number of different missense mutations occurring throughout the *SETD2* gene have been seen in CNS tumors, as well as in other tumor types, the role of individual missense mutations in tumorigenesis is unclear. One possibility is that a subset of missense mutations are passenger mutations that occur following glioma therapy. Three recurrent high grade gliomas (#12, 14 and 16) in our subset had multiple missense mutations in *SETD2*. In these cases, a higher mutational burden was present following chemoradiation. It is likely that the missense *SETD2* mutations seen at low VAF are not drivers of tumorigenesis in these tumors. In contrast, for the tumors with nonsense or frameshift mutations in *SETD2*, fewer concurrent PM were detected, and in one tumor (#3), the PM in *SETD2* was the only mutation detected on the NGS panel, at a VAF of 23%.

Conclusions

In summary, these findings suggest that *SETD2* mutations, although most common in high grade gliomas of the cerebral hemispheres, may be found in a variety of primary CNS tumors and locations. Immunohistochemistry shows a decrease in H3K36me3 in tumor with *SETD2* mutations, implicating epigenetic pathways in tumor biology. Additional studies are needed to investigate the role of *SETD2* mutations in tumorigenesis.

Abbreviations
CCRCC: Clear cell renal cell carcinoma; CHOP: Children's Hospital of Philadelphia; CNS: Central nervous system; CPD: Center for Personalized Diagnostics; DGD: Division of Genomic Diagnostics; H3K27me3: Trimethylation of the lysine 27 residue on Histone 3; H3K36ac: Acetylation of the lysine 36 residue on Histone 3; H3K36me3: Trimethylation of the lysine 36 residue on Histone 3; HOTAIR: HOX Transcript Antisense RNA; HUP: Hospital of the University of Pennsylvania; IHC: Immunohistochemistry; MM: Missense mutation; NGS: Next generation sequencing; SETD2: SET domain-containing 2; TCGA: The Cancer Genome Atlas; TM: Truncating mutation; VAF: Variant allele frequency

Acknowledgements
The authors thank Dr. John Wojcik for thoughtful review of this work and Daniel Martinez and the Children's Hospital of Philadelphia Pathology Core Laboratory for optimizing and performing immunohistochemistry.

Funding
Not applicable.

Authors' contributions
ANV and MPN Conceived and designed the analysis; Collected the data; Contributed data; Performed the analysis; Wrote the paper. MS Contributed data and immunohistochemical staining. LFS, MML and JR Contributed data and assisted in analysis. All authors read and approved the final manuscript.

Competing interests
The authors declare that they have no competing interests.

Author details
[1]Department of Pathology and Laboratory Medicine, Children's Hospital of Philadelphia, University of Pennsylvania Perelman School of Medicine, Philadelphia, PA, USA. [2]Department of Pathology and Laboratory Medicine, University of Pennsylvania Perelman School of Medicine, Philadelphia, PA, USA. [3]Hospital of the University of Pennsylvania, FO6.089 3400 Spruce St, Philadelphia, PA 19104, USA.

References
1. Brennan CW, Verhaak RG, McKenna A, Campos B, Noushmehr H, Salama SR, Zheng S, Chakravarty D, Sanborn JZ, Berman SH, Beroukhim R, Bernard B, Wu CJ, Genovese G, Shmulevich I, Barnholtz-Sloan J, Zou L, Vegesna R, Shukla SA, Ciriello G, Yung WK, Zhang W, Sougnez C, Mikkelsen T, Aldape K, Bigner DD, Van Meir EG, Prados M, Sloan A, Black KL, Eschbacher J, Finocchiaro G, Friedman W, Andrews DW, Guha A, Iacocca M, O'Neill BP, Foltz G, Myers J, Weisenberger DJ, Penny R, Kucherlapati R, Perou CM, Hayes DN, Gibbs R, Marra M, Mills GB, Lander E, Spellman P, Wilson R, Sander C, Weinstein J, Meyerson M, Gabriel S, Laird PW, Haussler D, Getz G, Chin L, Network TR (2013) The somatic genomic landscape of glioblastoma. Cell 155:462–477. https://doi.org/10.1016/j.cell.2013.09.034
2. Butler JS, Koutelou E, Schibler AC, Dent SY (2012) Histone-modifying enzymes: regulators of developmental decisions and drivers of human disease. Epigenomics 4:163–177. https://doi.org/10.2217/epi.12.3
3. Cancer Genome Atlas Research N (2008) Comprehensive genomic characterization defines human glioblastoma genes and core pathways. Nature 455:1061–1068. https://doi.org/10.1038/nature07385
4. Cerami E, Gao J, Dogrusoz U, Gross BE, Sumer SO, Aksoy BA, Jacobsen A, Byrne CJ, Heuer ML, Larsson E, Antipin Y, Reva B, Goldberg AP, Sander C, Schultz N (2012) The cBio cancer genomics portal: an open platform for exploring multidimensional cancer genomics data. Cancer Discov 2:401–404. https://doi.org/10.1158/2159-8290.CD-12-0095
5. Duns G, van den Berg E, van Duivenbode I, Osinga J, Hollema H, Hofstra RM, Kok K (2010) Histone methyltransferase gene SETD2 is a novel tumor

suppressor gene in clear cell renal cell carcinoma. Cancer Res 70:4287–4291. https://doi.org/10.1158/0008-5472.CAN-10-0120

6. Fontebasso AM, Schwartzentruber J, Khuong-Quang DA, Liu XY, Sturm D, Korshunov A, Jones DT, Witt H, Kool M, Albrecht S, Fleming A, Hadjadj D, Busche S, Lepage P, Montpetit A, Staffa A, Gerges N, Zakrzewska M, Zakrzewski K, Liberski PP, Hauser P, Garami M, Klekner A, Bognar L, Zadeh G, Faury D, Pfister SM, Jabado N, Majewski J (2013) Mutations in SETD2 and genes affecting histone H3K36 methylation target hemispheric high-grade gliomas. Acta Neuropathol 125:659–669. https://doi.org/10.1007/s00401-013-1095-8

7. Gao J, Aksoy BA, Dogrusoz U, Dresdner G, Gross B, Sumer SO, Sun Y, Jacobsen A, Sinha R, Larsson E, Cerami E, Sander C, Schultz N (2013) Integrative analysis of complex cancer genomics and clinical profiles using the cBioPortal. Sci Signal 6:pl1. https://doi.org/10.1126/scisignal.2004088

8. Ho TH, Park IY, Zhao H, Tong P, Champion MD, Yan H, Monzon FA, Hoang A, Tamboli P, Parker AS, Joseph RW, Qiao W, Dykema K, Tannir NM, Castle EP, Nunez-Nateras R, Teh BT, Wang J, Walker CL, Hung MC, Jonasch E (2016) High-resolution profiling of histone h3 lysine 36 trimethylation in metastatic renal cell carcinoma. Oncogene 35:1565–1574. https://doi.org/10.1038/onc.2015.221

9. Hunter C, Smith R, Cahill DP, Stephens P, Stevens C, Teague J, Greenman C, Edkins S, Bignell G, Davies H, O'Meara S, Parker A, Avis T, Barthorpe S, Brackenbury L, Buck G, Butler A, Clements J, Cole J, Dicks E, Forbes S, Gorton M, Gray K, Halliday K, Harrison R, Hills K, Hinton J, Jenkinson A, Jones D, Kosmidou V, Laman R, Lugg R, Menzies A, Perry J, Petty R, Raine K, Richardson D, Shepherd R, Small A, Solomon H, Tofts C, Varian J, West S, Widaa S, Yates A, Easton DF, Riggins G, Roy JE, Levine KK, Mueller W, Batchelor TT, Louis DN, Stratton MR, Futreal PA, Wooster R (2006) A hypermutation phenotype and somatic MSH6 mutations in recurrent human malignant gliomas after alkylator chemotherapy. Cancer Res 66: 3987–3991. https://doi.org/10.1158/0008-5472.CAN-06-0127

10. Jones DT, Jager N, Kool M, Zichner T, Hutter B, Sultan M, Cho YJ, Pugh TJ, Hovestadt V, Stutz AM, Rausch T, Warnatz HJ, Ryzhova M, Bender S, Sturm D, Pleier S, Cin H, Pfaff E, Sieber L, Wittmann A, Remke M, Witt H, Hutter S, Tzaridis T, Weischenfeldt J, Raeder B, Avci M, Amstislavskiy V, Zapatka M, Weber UD, Wang Q, Lasitschka B, Bartholomae CC, Schmidt M, von Kalle C, Ast V, Lawerenz C, Eils J, Kabbe R, Benes V, van Sluis P, Koster J, Volckmann R, Shih D, Betts MJ, Russell RB, Coco S, Tonini GP, Schuller U, Hans V, Graf N, Kim YJ, Monoranu C, Roggendorf W, Unterberg A, Herold-Mende C, Milde T, Kulozik AE, von Deimling A, Witt O, Maass E, Rossler J, Ebinger M, Schuhmann MU, Fruhwald MC, Hasselblatt M, Jabado N, Rutkowski S, von Bueren AO, Williamson D, Clifford SC, McCabe MG, Collins VP, Wolf S, Wiemann S, Lehrach H, Brors B, Scheurlen W, Felsberg J, Reifenberger G, Northcott PA, Taylor MD, Meyerson M, Pomeroy SL, Yaspo ML, Korbel JO, Korshunov A, Eils R, Pfister SM, Lichter P (2012) Dissecting the genomic complexity underlying medulloblastoma. Nature 488:100–105. https://doi.org/10.1038/nature11284

11. la Rosa AH, Acker M, Swain S, Manoharan M (2015) The role of epigenetics in kidney malignancies. Cent Eur J Urol 68:157–164. https://doi.org/10.5173/ceju.2015.453

12. Lek M, Karczewski KJ, Minikel EV, Samocha KE, Banks E, Fennell T, O'Donnell-Luria AH, Ware JS, Hill AJ, Cummings BB, Tukiainen T, Birnbaum DP, Kosmicki JA, Duncan LE, Estrada K, Zhao F, Zou J, Pierce-Hoffman E, Berghout J, Cooper DN, Deflaux N, DePristo M, Do R, Flannick J, Fromer M, Gauthier L, Goldstein J, Gupta N, Howrigan D, Kiezun A, Kurki MI, Moonshine AL, Natarajan P, Orozco L, Peloso GM, Poplin R, Rivas MA, Ruano-Rubio V, Rose SA, Ruderfer DM, Shakir K, Stenson PD, Stevens C, Thomas BP, Tiao G, Tusie-Luna MT, Weisburd B, Won HH, Yu D, Altshuler DM, Ardissino D, Boehnke M, Danesh J, Donnelly S, Elosua R, Florez JC, Gabriel SB, Getz G, Glatt SJ, Hultman CM, Kathiresan S, Laakso M, McCarroll S, McCarthy MI, McGovern D, McPherson R, Neale BM, Palotie A, Purcell SM, Saleheen D, Scharf JM, Sklar P, Sullivan PF, Tuomilehto J, Tsuang MT, Watkins HC, Wilson JG, Daly MJ, MacArthur DG, Exome Aggregation C (2016) Analysis of protein-coding genetic variation in 60,706 humans. Nature 536:285–291. https://doi.org/10.1038/nature19057

13. Li F, Mao G, Tong D, Huang J, Gu L, Yang W, Li GM (2013) The histone mark H3K36me3 regulates human DNA mismatch repair through its interaction with MutSalpha. Cell 153:590–600. https://doi.org/10.1016/j.cell.2013.03.025

14. Li J, Duns G, Westers H, Sijmons R, van den Berg A, Kok K (2016) SETD2: an epigenetic modifier with tumor suppressor functionality. Oncotarget 7: 50719–50734. https://doi.org/10.18632/oncotarget.9368

15. Li MM, Datto M, Duncavage EJ, Kulkarni S, Lindeman NI, Roy S, Tsimberidou AM, Vnencak-Jones CL, Wolff DJ, Younes A, Nikiforova MN (2017) Standards and guidelines for the interpretation and reporting of sequence variants in Cancer: A Joint Consensus Recommendation of the Association for Molecular Pathology, American Society of Clinical Oncology, and College of American Pathologists. J Mol Diagn 19:4–23. https://doi.org/10.1016/j.jmoldx.2016.10.002

16. Liu W, Fu Q, An H, Chang Y, Zhang W, Zhu Y, Xu L, Xu J (2015) Decreased expression of SETD2 predicts unfavorable prognosis in patients with nonmetastatic clear-cell renal cell carcinoma. Medicine (Baltimore) 94:e2004. https://doi.org/10.1097/MD.0000000000002004

17. Long W, Yi Y, Chen S, Cao Q, Zhao W, Liu Q (2017) Potential new therapies for pediatric diffuse intrinsic pontine glioma. Front Pharmacol 8:495. https://doi.org/10.3389/fphar.2017.00495

18. Louis DN, Perry A, Reifenberger G, von Deimling A, Figarella-Branger D, Cavenee WK, Ohgaki H, Wiestler OD, Kleihues P, Ellison DW (2016) The 2016 World Health Organization classification of tumors of the central nervous system: a summary. Acta Neuropathol 131:803–820. https://doi.org/10.1007/s00401-016-1545-1

19. Lu C, Jain SU, Hoelper D, Bechet D, Molden RC, Ran L, Murphy D, Venneti S, Hameed M, Pawel BR, Wunder JS, Dickson BC, Lundgren SM, Jani KS, De Jay N, Papillon-Cavanagh S, Andrulis IL, Sawyer SL, Grynspan D, Turcotte RE, Nadaf J, Fahiminiyah S, Muir TW, Majewski J, Thompson CB, Chi P, Garcia BA, Allis CD, Jabado N, Lewis PW (2016) Histone H3K36 mutations promote sarcomagenesis through altered histone methylation landscape. Science 352:844–849. https://doi.org/10.1126/science.aac7272

20. Marmorstein R, Trievel RC (2009) Histone modifying enzymes: structures, mechanisms, and specificities. Biochim Biophys Acta 1789:58–68. https://doi.org/10.1016/j.bbagrm.2008.07.009

21. Pai CC, Deegan RS, Subramanian L, Gal C, Sarkar S, Blaikley EJ, Walker C, Hulme L, Bernhard E, Codlin S, Bahler J, Allshire R, Whitehall S, Humphrey TC (2014) A histone H3K36 chromatin switch coordinates DNA double-strand break repair pathway choice. Nat Commun 5:4091. https://doi.org/10.1038/ncomms5091

22. Suzuki H, Aoki K, Chiba K, Sato Y, Shiozawa Y, Shiraishi Y, Shimamura T, Niida A, Motomura K, Ohka F, Yamamoto T, Tanahashi K, Ranjit M, Wakabayashi T, Yoshizato T, Kataoka K, Yoshida K, Nagata Y, Sato-Otsubo A, Tanaka H, Sanada M, Kondo Y, Nakamura H, Mizoguchi M, Abe T, Muragaki Y, Watanabe R, Ito I, Miyano S, Natsume A, Ogawa S (2015) Mutational landscape and clonal architecture in grade II and III gliomas. Nat Genet 47: 458–468. https://doi.org/10.1038/ng.3273

23. Toh TB, Lim JJ, Chow EK (2017) Epigenetics in cancer stem cells. Mol Cancer 16:29. https://doi.org/10.1186/s12943-017-0596-9

24. Walter DM, Venancio OS, Buza EL, Tobias JW, Deshpande C, Gudiel AA, Kim-Kiselak C, Cicchini M, Yates TJ, Feldser DM (2017) Systematic in vivo inactivation of chromatin-regulating enzymes identifies Setd2 as a potent tumor suppressor in lung adenocarcinoma. Cancer Res 77:1719–1729. https://doi.org/10.1158/0008-5472.CAN-16-2159

25. Wang L, Zehir A, Nafa K, Zhou N, Berger MF, Casanova J, Sadowska J, Lu C, Allis CD, Gounder M, Chandhanayingyong C, Ladanyi M, Boland PJ, Hameed M (2016) Genomic aberrations frequently alter chromatin regulatory genes in chordoma. Genes Chromosomes Cancer 55:591–600. https://doi.org/10.1002/gcc.22362

26. Wilting RH, Dannenberg JH (2012) Epigenetic mechanisms in tumorigenesis, tumor cell heterogeneity and drug resistance. Drug Resist Updat 15:21–38. https://doi.org/10.1016/j.drup.2012.01.008

27. Wu G, Diaz AK, Paugh BS, Rankin SL, Ju B, Li Y, Zhu X, Qu C, Chen X, Zhang J, Easton J, Edmonson M, Ma X, Lu C, Nagahawatte P, Hedlund E, Rusch M, Pounds S, Lin T, Onar-Thomas A, Huether R, Kriwacki R, Parker M, Gupta P, Becksfort J, Wei L, Mulder HL, Boggs K, Vadodaria B, Yergeau D, Russell JC, Ochoa K, Fulton RS, Fulton LL, Jones C, Boop FA, Broniscer A, Wetmore C, Gajjar A, Ding L, Mardis ER, Wilson RK, Taylor MR, Downing JR, Ellison DW, Zhang J, Baker SJ (2014) The genomic landscape of diffuse intrinsic pontine glioma and pediatric non-brainstem high-grade glioma. Nat Genet 46:444–450. https://doi.org/10.1038/ng.2938

28. Xie P, Tian C, An L, Nie J, Lu K, Xing G, Zhang L, He F (2008) Histone methyltransferase protein SETD2 interacts with p53 and selectively regulates its downstream genes. Cell Signal 20:1671–1678. https://doi.org/10.1016/j.cellsig.2008.05.012

10

Neurodegeneration in SCA14 is associated with increased PKCγ kinase activity, mislocalization and aggregation

Maggie M. K. Wong[1], Stephanie D. Hoekstra[1], Jane Vowles[2], Lauren M. Watson[1], Geraint Fuller[3], Andrea H. Németh[4,5], Sally A. Cowley[2], Olaf Ansorge[4], Kevin Talbot[4] and Esther B. E. Becker[1]* [iD]

Abstract

Spinocerebellar ataxia type 14 (SCA14) is a subtype of the autosomal dominant cerebellar ataxias that is characterized by slowly progressive cerebellar dysfunction and neurodegeneration. SCA14 is caused by mutations in the *PRKCG* gene, encoding protein kinase C gamma (PKCγ). Despite the identification of 40 distinct disease-causing mutations in *PRKCG*, the pathological mechanisms underlying SCA14 remain poorly understood. Here we report the molecular neuropathology of SCA14 in post-mortem cerebellum and in human patient-derived induced pluripotent stem cells (iPSCs) carrying two distinct SCA14 mutations in the C1 domain of PKCγ, H36R and H101Q. We show that endogenous expression of these mutations results in the cytoplasmic mislocalization and aggregation of PKCγ in both patient iPSCs and cerebellum. PKCγ aggregates were not efficiently targeted for degradation. Moreover, mutant PKCγ was found to be hyper-activated, resulting in increased substrate phosphorylation. Together, our findings demonstrate that a combination of both, loss-of-function and gain-of-function mechanisms are likely to underlie the pathogenesis of SCA14, caused by mutations in the C1 domain of PKCγ. Importantly, SCA14 patient iPSCs were found to accurately recapitulate pathological features observed in post-mortem SCA14 cerebellum, underscoring their potential as relevant disease models and their promise as future drug discovery tools.

Keywords: Ataxia, Stem cells, Purkinje cells, Neurodegeneration, Cerebellum, Protein kinase C gamma

Introduction

Spinocerebellar ataxia type 14 (SCA14) (OMIM 605361) most commonly represents with slowly progressive, relatively pure cerebellar ataxia characterized by gait disturbance, incoordination, mild dysarthria and nystagmus, with complex phenotypes such as myoclonus described in over a third of cases [9, 12]. Brain MRI in SCA14 patients shows mild to severe cerebellar atrophy [9, 12], and loss of Purkinje cells has been described at post-mortem [7].

SCA14 is caused by mutations in the *PRKCG* gene encoding the conventional protein kinase C gamma (PKCγ), which is particularly abundant in the Purkinje cells of the cerebellum [26]. To date, 40 mutations have been reported to cause SCA14 (Fig. 1a). Most of these mutations cluster in the regulatory C1 and C2 domains of PKCγ that respond to second messengers and control the activation and membrane translocation of PKCγ. Binding of calcium to the C2 domain initiates the activation of PKCγ and induces the rapid translocation of PKCγ from the cytoplasm to the plasma membrane, where it interacts with phospholipids. PKCγ is further allosterically activated by the binding of diacylglycerol (DAG) to the C1 domain, resulting in the release of a pseudo-inhibitory substrate that occupies the catalytic domain, and an open and active confirmation of PKCγ that allows phosphorylation of target substrates [2, 8].

The C1 domain is composed of two structurally and functionally similar cysteine-rich subdomains, C1A and C1B, of which the latter is preferentially affected by SCA14 mutations (Fig. 1a). Despite the wealth of mutations identified in PKCγ, the pathologic mechanisms underlying

* Correspondence: esther.becker@dpag.ox.ac.uk
[1]Department of Physiology, Anatomy and Genetics, University of Oxford, Sherrington Road, Oxford OX1 3PT, UK
Full list of author information is available at the end of the article

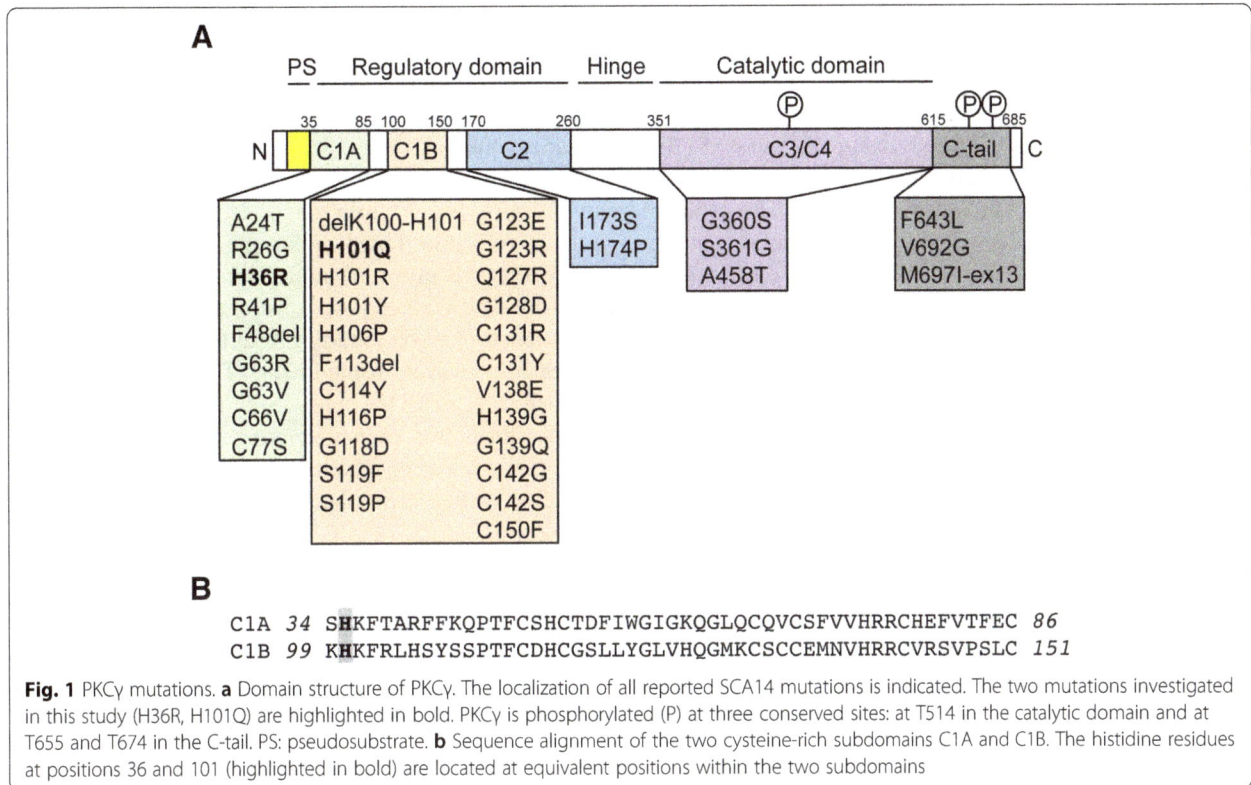

Fig. 1 PKCγ mutations. **a** Domain structure of PKCγ. The localization of all reported SCA14 mutations is indicated. The two mutations investigated in this study (H36R, H101Q) are highlighted in bold. PKCγ is phosphorylated (P) at three conserved sites: at T514 in the catalytic domain and at T655 and T674 in the C-tail. PS: pseudosubstrate. **b** Sequence alignment of the two cysteine-rich subdomains C1A and C1B. The histidine residues at positions 36 and 101 (highlighted in bold) are located at equivalent positions within the two subdomains

SCA14 remain unclear. Homozygous *Prkcg* knockout animals display only mild ataxia and show no loss of Purkinje cells [10, 22]. Therefore, the SCA14 phenotype is thought to result from a gain-of-function mechanism rather than haploinsufficiency. However, overexpression studies in cell lines and animals have yielded conflicting cellular disease mechanisms including increased kinase function [1, 43], impaired kinase function [42], protein aggregation [36] and impaired ubiquitin proteasome degradation [38], as well as aggregation-independent pathologies [37]. Thus, there is a need for authentic SCA14 models to better understand the underlying disease mechanisms.

Here, we have investigated the consequences of physiological expression of two SCA14 mutations in the C1 domain, H36R and H101Q, in both patient-derived induced pluripotent stem cells (iPSCs) and in SCA14 (H101Q) post-mortem cerebellum. We demonstrate that SCA14 patient iPSCs, in which PKCγ is expressed at levels more likely to be relevant to normal physiology compared with previous in vitro models, recapitulate pathological features observed in post-mortem SCA14 cerebellum. We found that the SCA14 mutations result in a decrease of PKCγ at the plasma membrane upon activation, but increased PKCγ aggregates in the cytoplasm of both patient iPSCs and Purkinje cells. We also observed lysosomal and autophagy impairment in SCA14 iPSCs and cerebellar tissue. PKCγ phosphorylation and downstream signaling were

increased in the SCA14 iPSCs and cerebellum. Together, our findings suggest that SCA14 pathology is likely to be caused by the combination of a loss-of-function of PKCγ at the plasma membrane and a gain-of-function of hyper-activated and mislocalized PKCγ.

Materials and methods

Generation and maintenance of iPSC lines

iPSC lines were derived from four SCA14 patients, two carrying an H36R and two carrying the H101Q mutation (Additional file 1: Figure S2). Reprogramming of donor fibroblasts to iPSCs was performed as described in the Additional file 1, and full characterization is provided in Additional file 1: Figure S2. iPSC lines from two age- and sex-matched healthy donors were used as controls (Additional file 1: Figure S2) and have been fully described elsewhere [16, 18]. iPSCs were maintained in feeder-free conditions on hESC-qualified Matrigel (Corning), in supplemented mTeSR (Stem Cell Technologies). Cells were passaged 1:3 every 4–5 days, using 0.5 mM EDTA (Invitrogen) [5]. For inhibitor experiments, iPSCs were treated with 400 nM phorbol-12-myristate-13-acetate (PMA; R&D Systems) or 200 nM phorbol-12, 13-dibutyrate (PDBu) in PBS before harvesting.

Quantitative real-time PCR

Total RNA from iPSCs and cerebellar tissue was prepared using the RNeasy Mini Kit (Qiagen). RNA from human fetal cerebellar tissue was purchased (AMS Biotechnology (Europe) Ltd., Abingdon, UK). RNA was reverse transcribed to cDNA using the High-Capacity RNA-to-cDNA Kit (Applied Biosystems). Quantitative real-time PCR was performed using the Fast SYBR Green Master Mix (Applied Biosystems) on a StepOne Plus qPCR machine (Applied Biosystems). The relative *PRKCG* levels were quantified and normalized against the housekeeping gene β-actin with reference to a negative control, using standard DDCt techniques. Primers are listed in Additional file 1: Table S1.

Biochemical assays

Frozen tissue of human cerebellum was sampled from the inferior aspect, immediately lateral to the cerebellar tonsils (that is, adjacent to the areas with relative preservation of Purkinje cells on histology). Sampling sites were consistent between SCA14 and control cerebellum.

For the preparation of protein extracts, iPSCs were washed once with PBS and then lysed in cold Pierce® RIPA buffer [25 mM Tris-HCl pH = 7.6, 150 mM NaCl, 1% NP-40, 1% sodium deoxycholate, 0.1% sodium dodecyl sulphate (SDS)] (Thermo Fisher Scientific), supplemented with Complete Protease Inhibitor Cocktail (Roche) and PhosSTOP Phosphatase Inhibitor Cocktail (Roche). Protein lysates were incubated on ice for 10 min and subsequently centrifuged at 14,000 g for 20 min at 4 °C. Snap-frozen human cerebellar tissue was homogenized in cold RIPA buffer, followed by 30-s sonication. The cerebellar lysate was incubated on ice for 10 min before centrifugation at 14,000 g for 30 min at 4 °C. 50 μg of protein extracts were analyzed by SDS-PAGE and immunoblotting.

For the preparation of (in)soluble fractions, snap-frozen cerebellar tissue was homogenized in cold lysis buffer [1% Triton X-100, 20 mM Tris, pH = 7.5, 5 mM ethylene glycol-bis(β-aminoethyl ether)-N,N,N′,N′-tetraacetic acid (EGTA), 150 mM NaCl, Complete Protease Inhibitor Cocktail, PhosSTOP Phosphatase Inhibitor Cocktail], followed by a 10-min incubation on ice and centrifugation at 14,000 g for 30 min at 4 °C. The supernatant was collected as Triton-soluble fraction. The pellet was re-suspended in cold Pierce® RIPA buffer (Triton-insoluble fraction) and sonicated for 10–20 s. Equal volumes of soluble and insoluble fractions were loaded for SDS-PAGE and analyzed by immunoblotting.

A list of primary and secondary antibodies can be found in Additional file 1: Table S2. Antibody binding was detected by enhanced chemoluminescence (ECL, GE Healthcare). The intensity of bands was quantified using ImageJ software (NIH). Data were normalized to Actin levels and respective control bands and analyzed using GraphPad Prism 7 (GraphPad Software, Inc.). All data are represented as the mean of three independent experiments ±SEM. Statistical significance was assessed by ANOVA with Bonferroni's post-hoc test, with $p < 0.05$ considered statistically significant.

Immunostaining

iPSCs were fixed in 4% paraformaldehyde at room temperature for 20 min or in ice-cold methanol at -20 °C for 15 min. Fixed cells were washed three times with PBS for 5 min and subjected to immunostaining as previously described [44]. A list of primary and secondary antibodies can be found in Additional file 1: Table S2. Images were analysed using ImageJ. The size of aggregates was measured using the ImageJ Cell Counter plugin. The area of signals was measured using Threshold and Area Measurement. The co-localization of labelled proteins was quantified using Just Another Colocalization Plugin (JACoP) [6].

Immunohistochemistry of human cerebellar sections was performed as follows. 5-μm sections were cut from formalin-fixed paraffin-embedded blocks from the vermis, paravermis and lateral neocerebellum, including dentate nucleus. The index case was matched to two control cases. All three cases were assessed for PKCγ reactivity outside the cerebellum and screened for age-related neurodegenerative pathology. De-identified sections were de-waxed through xylene, and rehydrated through decreasing concentrations of alcohol before being pre-treated for 30 min in 10% concentrated (30%) H_2O_2 and distilled water to block endogenous peroxidase. Heat-induced epitope-retrieval was performed using autoclave boiling at 121 °C for 10 min. Sections were then rinsed with Tris-buffered saline and blocked with normal goat serum (1:10 in TBS-T) for 30 min. Primary antibodies (Additional file 1: Table S2) were incubated overnight at 4 °C and visualized using the Dako Envision+ kit and HRP-DAB signal (Agilent). Positive and negative controls were used for each antibody. No staining was seen when the primary antibody was omitted. Sections were viewed and photographed with an Olympus BX43 microscope and Olympus cellSense software.

Results

Cerebellar pathology in SCA14

Given the multitude of, often conflicting, phenotypes reported in the literature that might be caused by mutations in PKCγ in heterologous models, we set out to investigate the pathological changes in SCA14 in patient-derived cells and post-mortem cerebellum. We focused on two different SCA14 mutations, H36R and H101Q. Both of these mutations are located at equivalent positions in the C1A and C1B subdomains of the regulatory domain of PKCγ (Fig. 1) [32] and are implicated in zinc coordination and phorbol ester binding [11].

Affected individuals had slowly progressive adult onset ataxia typical of SCA14, with moderate gait ataxia, mild dysarthria, titubation and relatively mild nystagmus. The H101Q family had pure ataxia, without additional features described in other pedigrees such as myoclonus and seizures. MRI showed moderate to severe generalized atrophy of the cerebellum (Fig. 2a). One individual from the SCA14 H101Q family underwent autopsy when he died of 'natural causes' at the age of 90 years (Additional file 1: Figure S1). Brain tissue was examined according to standard protocols for neurodegenerative disease, which included screening for Alzheimer disease, Lewy body disease and TDP-43 proteinopathy. We found Braak II/III neurofibrillary Alzheimer type pathology and mild cerebrovascular disease. No Lewy body

or TDP-43 proteinopathy was identified. We used a sequestosome1/p62 antibody as a highly sensitive screening tool for generic protein aggregates. We did not find any neuropathology that could not be explained by Alzheimer-related changes.

To identify Purkinje cells, tissue sections were immunolabelled with an antibody against the calcium-binding protein Calbindin D-28 k. We observed severe loss (estimated to be 80%) of Purkinje cells in all lobules of the neocerebellum, associated with Bergmann gliosis. However, Purkinje cells in the cerebellar tonsils and adjacent flocculonodular lobe were relatively preserved (Fig. 2b). Neurons of the deep cerebellar nuclei, pons

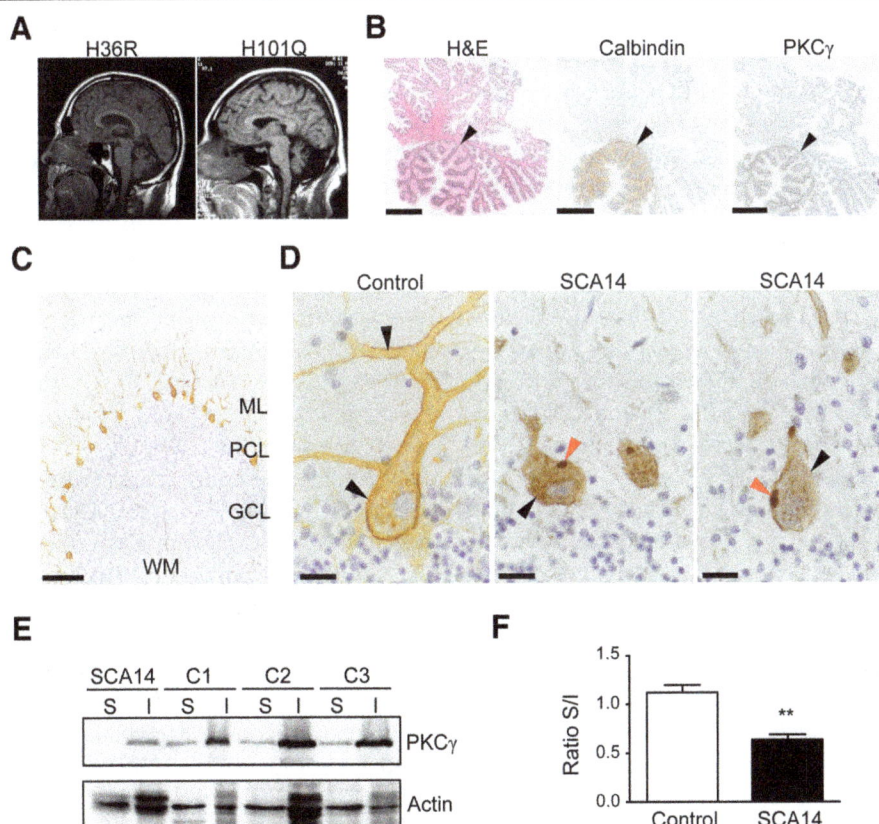

Fig. 2 Cerebellar pathology in SCA14. a Brain MRI imaging of SCA14 patients carrying the H36R and H101Q mutations, respectively, shows marked cerebellar atrophy. b Neurodegeneration of SCA14 cerebellum. There is severe loss of Purkinje cells from the lateral neocerebellum. Purkinje cells in the tonsil (and flocconodular lobe) are relatively preserved (black arrowheads). Brain sections were stained with hematoxylin and eosin (H&E) (left panel), and with antibodies against Calbindin-28 k (centre) and PKCγ (right panel). Scale bar: 5 mm. c Normal PKCγ pattern from an age-matched control cerebellum. ML: molecular layer, PCL: Purkinje cell layer, GCL: granule cell layer, WM: white matter. Scale bar: 200 μm. d PKCγ staining of control (left) and SCA14 cerebellum (centre and right panels). In control cerebellum, PKCγ showed distinct expression at the plasma membrane, both around the soma and primary and secondary dendrites (black arrowheads), with minor granular staining in the perinuclear cytoplasm. In SCA14 cerebellum, homogeneous circumferential plasmalemma localization was lost (black arrowheads) and large cytoplasmic PKCγ aggregates were found, some apparently still linked to fragments of plasma membrane (red arrowheads). Scale bar: 20 μm. e, f Enrichment of mutant PKCγ in the Triton-X-100-insoluble fraction in SCA14 cerebellum compared to controls. Cerebellar tissue lysates were separated into Triton-X-100-soluble (S) and -insoluble (I) fractions. Equal volumes of soluble and insoluble fractions were loaded for SDS-PAGE and analyzed by immunoblotting for PKCγ. (e). Actin: loading control. The intensity of the bands was quantified and the level of PKCγ was normalized against the loading control. The ratio of normalized PKCγ present in the soluble versus insoluble fractions (Ratio S/I) is shown ($n = 3$, **$p < 0.01$, unpaired students' t-test). (f). S: Triton-X-100-soluble fraction, I: Triton-X-100-insoluble fraction

and inferior olive were not obviously depleted. Thus, we conclude that SCA14 seems to be a pure Purkinje cell neuronopathy, predominantly affecting the lateral parts of the cerebellar hemispheres (neocerebellum). This is consistent with the highly restricted expression pattern of PKCγ in human control cerebellum (Fig. 2c). No other cerebellar cell type expressed PKCγ. The remaining Purkinje cells displayed variable degrees of dendritic and somatic atrophy compared to control tissue (Fig. 2d). In age-matched control autopsy material, PKCγ was localized to the plasma membrane and cytoplasmic puncta in the soma and primary dendrite of Purkinje cells (Fig. 2d). This staining pattern is consistent with the localization of PKCγ in rodent Purkinje cells [26, 39]. In contrast, PKCγ staining at the plasma membrane was lost in SCA14 Purkinje cells and associated with large cytoplasmic aggregates in the soma, sometimes preserving a link to the plasma membrane (Fig. 2d). Loss of PKCγ staining was particularly pronounced in the dendrites. PKCγ aggregates were unique to Purkinje cells. Compared to Purkinje cells, only minimal expression of PKCγ is seen in any other part of the adult human brain. In our hands, the only extracerebellar region with faint expression in age-matched controls corresponded to the CA1-CA4 sectors of the hippocampus. However, unlike in the cerebellum, staining revealed only diffuse neuropil positivity, and no distinct membrane, soma, dendrite or axonal neuronal expression (data not shown). The SCA14 index case showed no aggregates or other morphological PKCγ abnormalities in the hippocampal formation compared with controls. We conclude from our immunohistochemical studies that cytoplasmic and membrane expression of PKCγ in adult cerebellar Purkinje cells is several orders of magnitude higher than in any other cell type of the human brain. We postulate that this underpins selective vulnerability and thus clinical presentation, and that loss of PKCγ cell membrane binding, cytoplasmic aggregation and Purkinje cell death represent the morphological substrate of the SCA14 H101Q mutation in human brain.

Many neurodegenerative diseases are characterized by the formation of disease-specific inclusions including Parkinson's Disease, Huntington's Disease and the polyglutamine SCAs [25, 35]. Inclusion bodies are generated by aggregation of misfolded proteins and often become detergent-insoluble. To formally confirm the insolubility of the PKCγ aggregates in SCA14 cerebellum, we carried out biochemical fractionation of cerebellar tissue into Triton X-100-soluble and -insoluble fractions. PKCγ was found in both soluble and insoluble fractions in control cerebellum (Fig. 2e). In contrast, PKCγ in SCA14 cerebellum was found almost exclusively in the insoluble fraction (Fig. 2e, f). Together, these findings suggest that in SCA14 Purkinje cells, PKCγ is mislocalized and aggregated in detergent-insoluble inclusions.

Generation of SCA14 human iPSCs
To better understand the pathological mechanisms that cause SCA14, we generated human iPSC lines from fibroblasts obtained from two patients carrying the H36R mutation and from two patients with the H101Q mutation (Additional file 1: Figure S1 & S2, Suppl. Methods). At least two iPSC clones were generated from each patient. Age- and sex-matched control iPSC lines, reprogrammed using Sendai reprogramming viruses in the same laboratory, generated through the Oxford Parkinson's Disease Centre, have been published previously [16, 18]. All iPSC lines displayed embryonic stem cell-like morphology and expressed the pluripotency-associated proteins Tra-1-60 and Nanog (Additional file 1: Figure S2B & D). Clearance of viral transgenes was confirmed by qRT-PCR (Additional file 1: Figure S2C). Genome integrity was confirmed by Illumina SNP arrays (Additional file 1: Figure S2E). *PRKCG* genotypes were confirmed in all quality-checked iPSC lines by Sanger sequencing (Additional file 1: Figure S2F).

SCA14 mutations cause PKCγ aggregation in human iPSCs
Although PKCγ is generally known to be a neuron-specific kinase, we identified robust expression of *PRKCG* RNA in both control and patient iPSCs human iPSCs (Fig. 3a, b), consistent with previous reports [24]. This prompted us to investigate the cellular phenotypes of iPSCs expressing mutant PKCγ. Similar to our observations in post-mortem cerebellar tissue, wildtype PKCγ was present in small cytoplasmic puncta, which partially co-localized with the cis-Golgi marker GM130, early endosomal marker EEA1 and recycling endosomal marker RAB11 (data not shown). In contrast, mutant PKCγ formed large aggregates in the cytoplasm (Fig. 3c, d), with little co-localization with Golgi and endosomal markers (data not shown). This staining pattern was observed for both SCA14 mutations, H36R and H101Q.

Prolonged activation of PKC results in its accumulation in the detergent-insoluble fraction, where it is subjected to dephosphorylation and degradation [2, 15, 33]. To address whether activation of mutant PKCγ further enhanced its aggregation, we treated control and SCA14 iPSCs with 400 nM of phorbol 12-myristate 13-acetate (PMA), a potent PKC activator. Stimulation with PMA led to a more significant increase in the size of aggregates in SCA14 patient cells compared to controls (Fig. 3e). DMSO vehicle control did not affect PKCγ aggregation (Additional file 1: Figure S3). Together, these results indicate that the SCA14 H36R and H101Q mutations cause the aggregation of PKCγ in the cytoplasm of iPSCs, which is further enhanced following PKCγ activation.

Reduced membrane targeting of mutant PKCγ
The C1 domain mediates binding of PKCγ to DAG and phospholipids at the plasma membrane [8]. As both

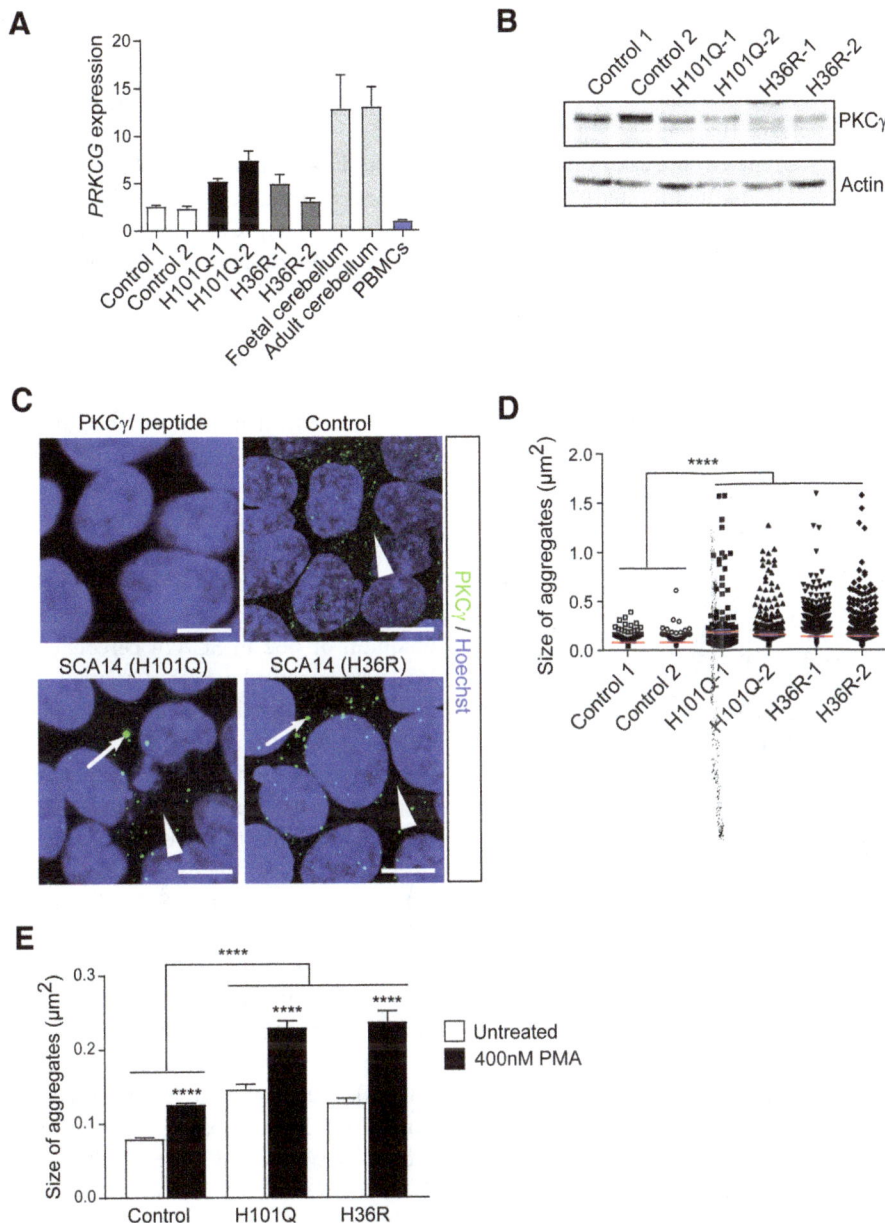

Fig. 3 Mutant PKCγ forms cytoplasmic aggregates in iPSCs. **a** *PRKCG* mRNA expression in control and patient iPSC lines. RNA extracted from fetal and adult human cerebellum was included as positive controls. *PRKCG* is not expressed in peripheral blood mononuclear cells (PBMCs) according to data from GTEx, BioGPS, and CGAP SAGE, and thus, RNA extracted from PBMCs was used as negative control. *PRKCG* gene expression levels were normalized to housekeeping gene β-actin, and are shown relative to negative control. **b** PKCγ protein expression in control and patient iPSC lines. Actin: loading control. **c** Immunostaining of iPSC lines for PKCγ. Specificity of the anti-PKCγ antibody was confirmed by peptide absorption assay (top left panel). Small punctate staining of PKCγ (white solid arrowheads) was observed in the cytoplasm of control iPSCs and SCA14 iPSCs, while large cytoplasmic aggregates (white arrows) were only present in SCA14 iPSCs. Cell nuclei are visualized by Hoechst staining. Scale bar: 10 μm. **d** PKCγ formed significantly larger aggregates in SCA14 iPSCs compared to control iPSCs (n = 3, ****p < 0.0001, ANOVA followed by Bonferroni's post-hoc test). **e** Treatment with 400 nM PMA, a potent PKCγ activator, both wildtype and mutant PKCγ aggregates increased in size. Compared to control, PKCγ formed significantly larger aggregates in SCA14 iPSCs following PMA treatment (n = 3, ****p < 0.0001, two-way ANOVA followed by Bonferroni's post-hoc test)

SCA14 mutations investigated in this study are located in the C1 domain, we next determined whether SCA14 mutants would be impaired in their membrane targeting. Interestingly, as described above, PKCγ immunostaining at the plasma membrane of Purkinje cells was markedly reduced in SCA14 post-mortem cerebellar tissue (Fig. 2d). To test whether membrane translocation of PKCγ was affected in patient iPSCs, cells were treated with 400 nM

PMA to activate PKCγ. In control iPSCs, PKCγ co-localization with sodium potassium ATPase at the plasma membrane increased after 5 min of PMA treatment, and after 15 min of PMA treatment, PKCγ was found again in the cytoplasm (Fig. 4a, b). In contrast, mutant PKCγ remained aggregated in the cytoplasm and did not translocate to the plasma membrane in response to PMA treatment (Fig. 4a, b). Similar results were obtained following treatment with phorbol 12,13-dibutyrate

(PDBu), an alternative PKCγ-activating phorbol ester (Additional file 1: Figure S4A). Together, these findings indicate that mutant PKCγ is impaired in its ability to translocate to, or be retained at, the plasma membrane.

Impaired degradation of SCA14 PKCγ aggregates

We next investigated the cellular responses to mutant and aggregated PKCγ. Cells operate two major protein degradation machineries: the ubiquitin proteasome system (UPS) and autophagy [14]. Impairment of both the UPS and autophagy have been associated with neurodegenerative disorders [14, 31]. This is further supported by the accumulation of intraneuronal aggregates of misfolded proteins in many neurodegenerative disorders [25, 31, 35]. Most of these aggregates are visible with light microscopy with immunohistochemistry against the disease-defining protein species (e.g. alpha-synuclein, C-terminal huntingtin) and components of the ubiquitin proteasome or macroautophagy systems. Interestingly, we did not find co-localization of the PKCγ aggregates with antibodies to ubiquitin or p62 in SCA14 cerebellum (data not shown). We next assessed whether mutant PKCγ aggregates in iPSCs were tagged with ubiquitin in an attempt by the cells to clear the aggregates. Control and patient iPSCs were immunostained with antibodies against PKCγ or ubiquitin in the presence or absence of PMA or PDBu. No ubiquitin-positive PKCγ aggregates were identified (Additional file 1: Figure S4), consistent with the results obtained in post-mortem SCA14 cerebellum.

The absence of PKCγ ubiquitination led us to investigate whether mutant PKCγ aggregates might be degraded through a different cellular pathway. We first looked at the formation of autophagosomes using immunostaining microtubule-associated protein 1 light chain 3 (LC3), a central protein in the autophagy pathway. In control iPSCs, we observed a significant increase in the overlap between PKCγ and LC3 following activation by PMA or PDBu (Fig. 5a, b; Additional file 1: Figure S4). In contrast, there was already a significant overlap between SCA14 PKCγ and LC3 in unstimulated iPSCs (Fig. 5a, b). This overlap did not increase upon further PKCγ activation by PMA or PDBu (Fig. 5a, b; Additional file 1: Figure S4), despite the increased formation of PKCγ aggregates observed (Fig. 3e). Overall, autophagosome levels did not significantly change in the presence of mutant PKCγ aggregates or upon PKCγ activation (Fig. 5c, d). These results indicate that aggregated mutant PKCγ is not cleared efficiently by the autophagosome in SCA14 iPSCs.

Aggregated proteins that are engulfed by autophagosomes are subsequently degraded through the fusion with lysosomes [31]. Alternatively, aggregated proteins can also be degraded by lysosomes through autophagosome-independent pathways [14]. We found that a small

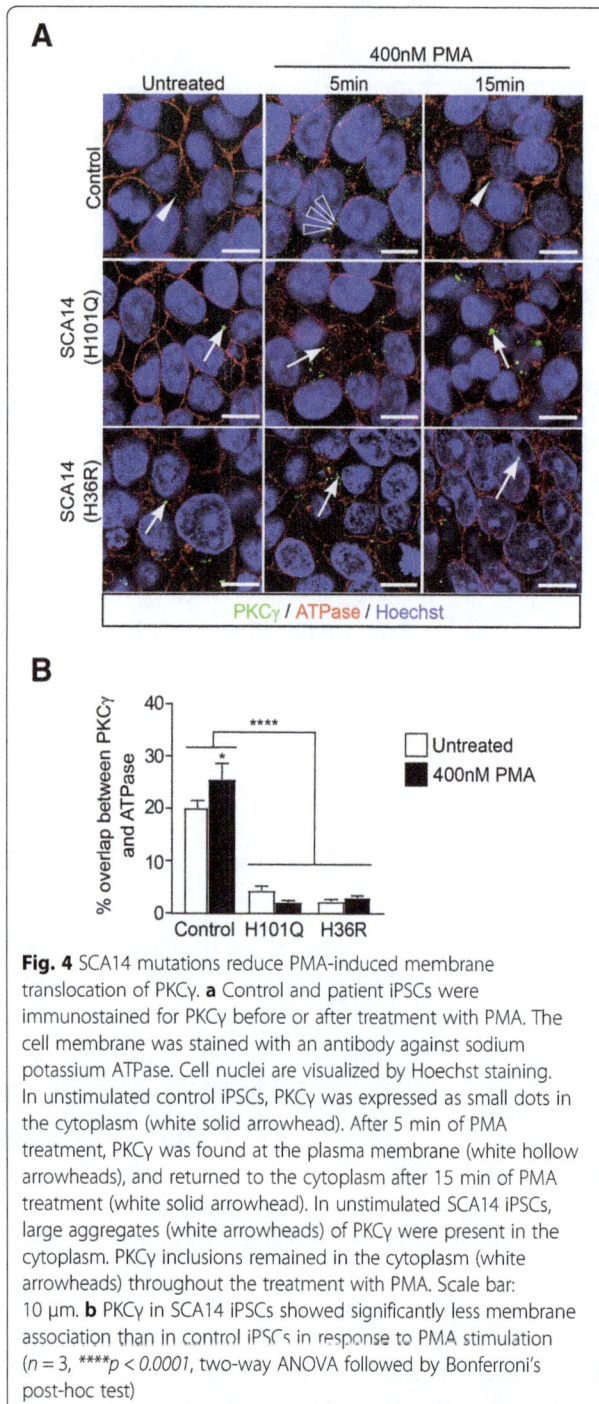

Fig. 4 SCA14 mutations reduce PMA-induced membrane translocation of PKCγ. **a** Control and patient iPSCs were immunostained for PKCγ before or after treatment with PMA. The cell membrane was stained with an antibody against sodium potassium ATPase. Cell nuclei are visualized by Hoechst staining. In unstimulated control iPSCs, PKCγ was expressed as small dots in the cytoplasm (white solid arrowhead). After 5 min of PMA treatment, PKCγ was found at the plasma membrane (white hollow arrowheads), and returned to the cytoplasm after 15 min of PMA treatment (white solid arrowhead). In unstimulated SCA14 iPSCs, large aggregates (white arrowheads) of PKCγ were present in the cytoplasm. PKCγ inclusions remained in the cytoplasm (white arrowheads) throughout the treatment with PMA. Scale bar: 10 μm. **b** PKCγ in SCA14 iPSCs showed significantly less membrane association than in control iPSCs in response to PMA stimulation ($n = 3$, ****$p < 0.0001$, two-way ANOVA followed by Bonferroni's post-hoc test)

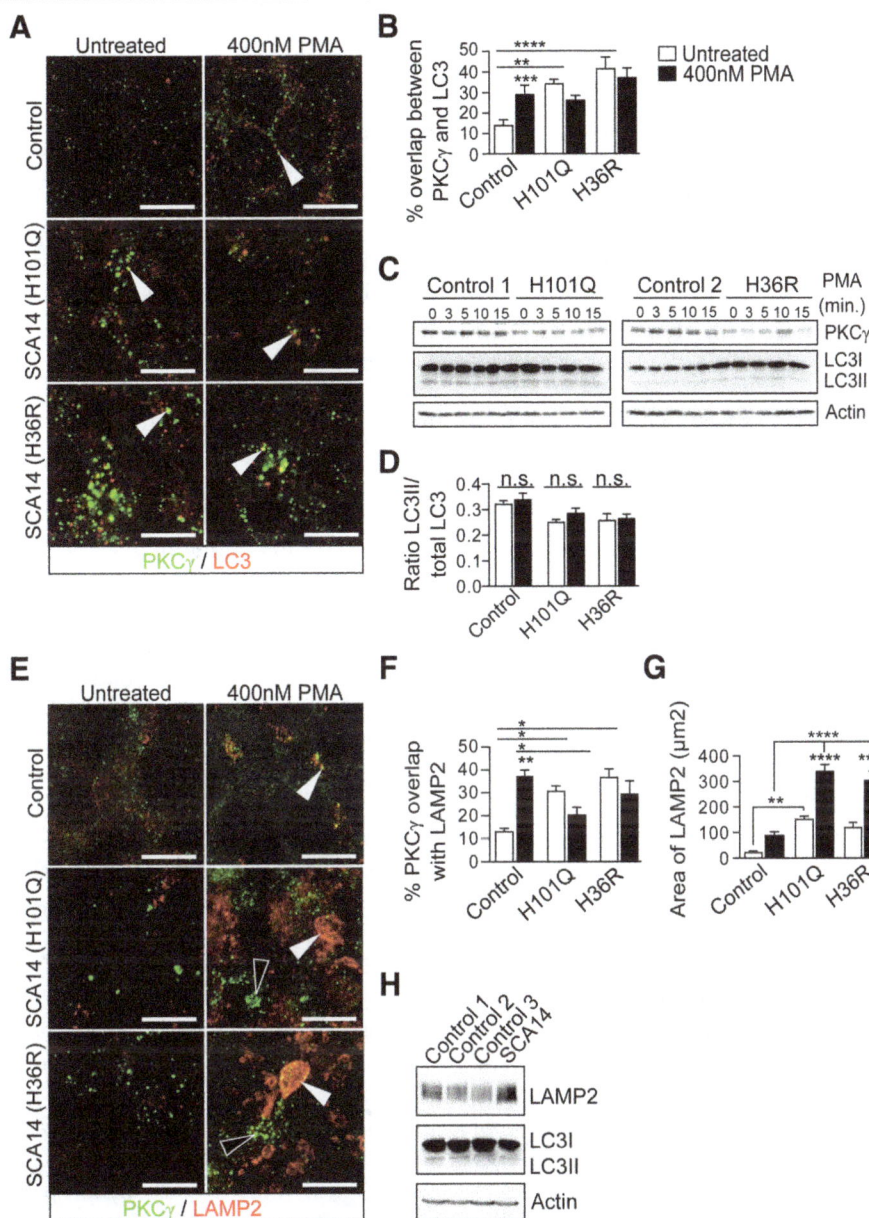

Fig. 5 Impaired degradation of SCA14 PKCγ aggregates. **a**, **b** Control and patient iPSCs were immunostained for PKCγ and the autophagosomal marker LC3 before or after treatment with PMA for 15 min. In control iPSCs, PKCγ co-localization with LC3 (white solid arrowheads) increased upon treatment with PMA. In untreated SCA14 iPSCs, there was already a significant overlap with LC3 (white solid arrowheads), which did not further increase upon PKCγ activation ($n = 3$, $**p < 0.01$, $***p < 0.001$, $****p < 0.0001$, two-way ANOVA followed by Bonferroni's post-hoc test). **c** Lysates of iPSCs were subjected to immunoblotting for PKCγ and LC3. LC3I represents free cytosolic cleaved LC3. LC3II represents LC3 that is anchored to the autophagosome membrane and indicates autophagosome load. **d** Ratio of LC3II/total LC3 levels remained constant in control and SCA14 iPSCs following PMA treatment. **e**, **f** Control and patient iPSCs were immunostained for PKCγ and the lysosomal marker LAMP2 before or after treatment with PMA for 15 min. In control iPSCs, co-localization of PKCγ with LAMP2 increased upon activation (white solid arrowheads). In SCA14 iPSCs, by contrast, lysosomes fused together into larger vesicles enclosing PKCγ aggregates (white arrowheads) in the presence of PMA. However, the majority of PKCγ aggregates did not co-localize with LAMP2-postive lysosomes (white hollow arrowheads) ($n = 3$, $*p < 0.05$, $**p < 0.001$, two-way ANOVA followed by Bonferroni's post-hoc test). **g** The area of LAMP2 signal, representing the formation of lysosomes, significantly increased in both control and SCA14 iPSCs following PMA treatment. The lysosomal area was significantly larger in SCA14 iPSCs compared to control iPSCs ($n = 3$, $**p < 0.01$, $****p < 0.0001$, two-way ANOVA followed by Bonferroni's post-hoc test). **h** Cerebellar lysates were subjected to immunoblotting for LAMP2 and LC3. LC3I represents free cytosolic cleaved LC3. LC3II represents LC3 that is anchored to the autophagosome membrane and indicates autophagosome load

proportion of wildtype PKCγ co-localized with the lyso-somal marker LAMP2 (lysosome-associated membrane protein 2) in the absence of PMA treatment (Fig. 5e, f). Following PKCγ activation in control iPSCs, both the lysosomal area, and the co-localization of PKCγ and LAMP2 significantly increased (Fig. 5f, g; Additional file 1: Figure S4). In SCA14 iPSCs, a significant enlargement of the lysosomal compartment and co-localization of PKCγ with LAMP2 was already observed prior to PMA treat-ment. (Fig. 5e-g). Upon PMA treatment, lysosomes fused together and formed very large vesicles (Fig. 5e, g; Additional file 1: Figure S4). Some PKCγ aggregates were found to be enclosed within these large lysosomes. How-ever, the majority of mutant PKCγ did not co-localize with LAMP2 (Fig. 5e, f). Moreover, compared to control iPSCs, less PKCγ was found to co-localize with LAMP2 following activation in SCA14 iPSCs (Fig. 5f). Together, these results suggest that despite lysosomal enlargement, aggre-gated mutant PKCγ is not efficiently targeted by lysosomes and thus accumulates as cytosolic aggregates in SCA14 iPSCs. Interestingly, increased expression of LAMP2 but no change in LC3 levels were also found in SCA14 cerebel-lum (Fig. 5h) indicating that the findings in SCA14 iPSCs reflect cerebellar pathology.

Increased PKCγ kinase activity in SCA14 patient cells

Phosphorylation is known to play an important role in regulating PKCγ, rendering PKCγ in a catalytically compe-tent conformation, and protecting it from degradation [2]. PKCγ phosphorylation occurs sequentially at three con-served residues: phosphoinositide-dependent kinase 1 (PDK1) phosphorylates PKCγ within the activation loop (T514), and autophosphorylation occurs within the turn motif (T655) and the hydrophobic motif (T674) at the C-terminal tail (Fig. 1a). Having identified that mutant PKCγ is not efficiently cleared in SCA14 patient cells, we next determined whether its phosphorylation status might be altered compared to wildtype PKCγ, which might affect its stability and kinase activity. Although overall PKCγ expression was lower in SCA14 iPSCs than control cells (Figs. 4b & 6a), PKCγ was highly phosphorylated at T514 and T674 in SCA14 iPSCs as determined by immunoblot-ting with phospho-specific antibodies (Fig. 6a, b). We also analyzed the phosphorylation status of PKCγ in SCA14 (H101Q) cerebellar tissue. Less PKCγ protein was present in SCA14 cerebellum compared to controls (Fig. 6c). We noted a similar reduction in Calbindin protein levels, consistent with the loss of Purkinje cells in the SCA14 cerebellum that was observed histopathologically (Fig. 2b). Despite the reduction in total PKCγ protein level, there was no reduction in phosphorylation levels of the PKCγ activa-tion loop (Fig. 6c). Quantification of the phosphoT514-PKCγ levels in three independent experiments showed that net phosphorylation of PKCγ was significantly increased in

SCA14 cerebellum compared to control tissue (Fig. 6d). Together with previous results, these findings indicate that the SCA14 mutations H36R and H101Q promote the aber-rant maturation of PKCγ into a catalytically competent and stable conformation.

Phosphorylated PKCγ increases its affinity for Ca²⁺ and promotes substrate binding [2, 8]. We therefore next asked whether the SCA14 mutations affect downstream PKCγ signaling and assessed the phosphorylation status of several PKCγ substrates. First, we employed a pan-phospho-PKC substrate antibody that recognizes cel-lular proteins (Ser-)phosphorylated at PKC consensus mo-tifs. PKC substrate phosphorylation was consistently higher in iPSCs derived from SCA14 patients than in controls (Fig. 6a). Moreover, we detected a robust increase in PKC substrate phosphorylation in the SCA14 cerebel-lum compared to controls (Fig. 6e). We also assessed the phosphorylation status of a well-known PKC target in the brain, myristoylated alanine-rich C-kinase substrate (MARCKS). Using a phospho-specific antibody, we de-tected elevated phospho-MARCKS levels in the SCA14 cerebellum compared to controls (Fig. 6e). Together, these findings suggest that the SCA14 mutations H36R and H101Q cause increased kinase activity of PKCγ in both patient iPSCs and cerebellum.

Discussion

In this study, we provide novel insights into the patho-genesis of SCA14. We present a unique in vitro model using human patient-derived iPSCs carrying two distinct SCA14 mutations in the C1 domain of PKCγ, H36R and H101Q, respectively, that recapitulate key pathological findings observed in SCA14 cerebellum. Our findings indicate that SCA14 is likely to be caused by three inter-connected pathogenic mechanisms (Fig. 7): (i) SCA14 mutations in the C1 domain enhance the aggregation of PKCγ, aided by insufficient protein degradation, (ii) a reduction of mutant PKCγ at the plasma membrane is likely to decrease its interaction with target substrates, and (iii) extended cytoplasmic retention of hyper-active PKCγ results in aberrant phosphorylation of substrates in the cytoplasm.

This study sheds light on the important question of how PKCγ harboring mutations in the C1 domain causes SCA14 pathology. Mutations in other domains of PKCγ might cause disease through other or additional mecha-nisms. Indeed, other PKCγ mutations in overexpression studies have been reported to drive a plethora of cellular phenotypes, which often contradict each other [1, 43]. This is the first study that investigates the consequences of more physiological levels of expression of two distinct SCA14 mutations in relevant human models, iPSCs and post-mortem cerebellar tissue. Only one postmortem brain of a SCA14 patient with a H101Y mutation has

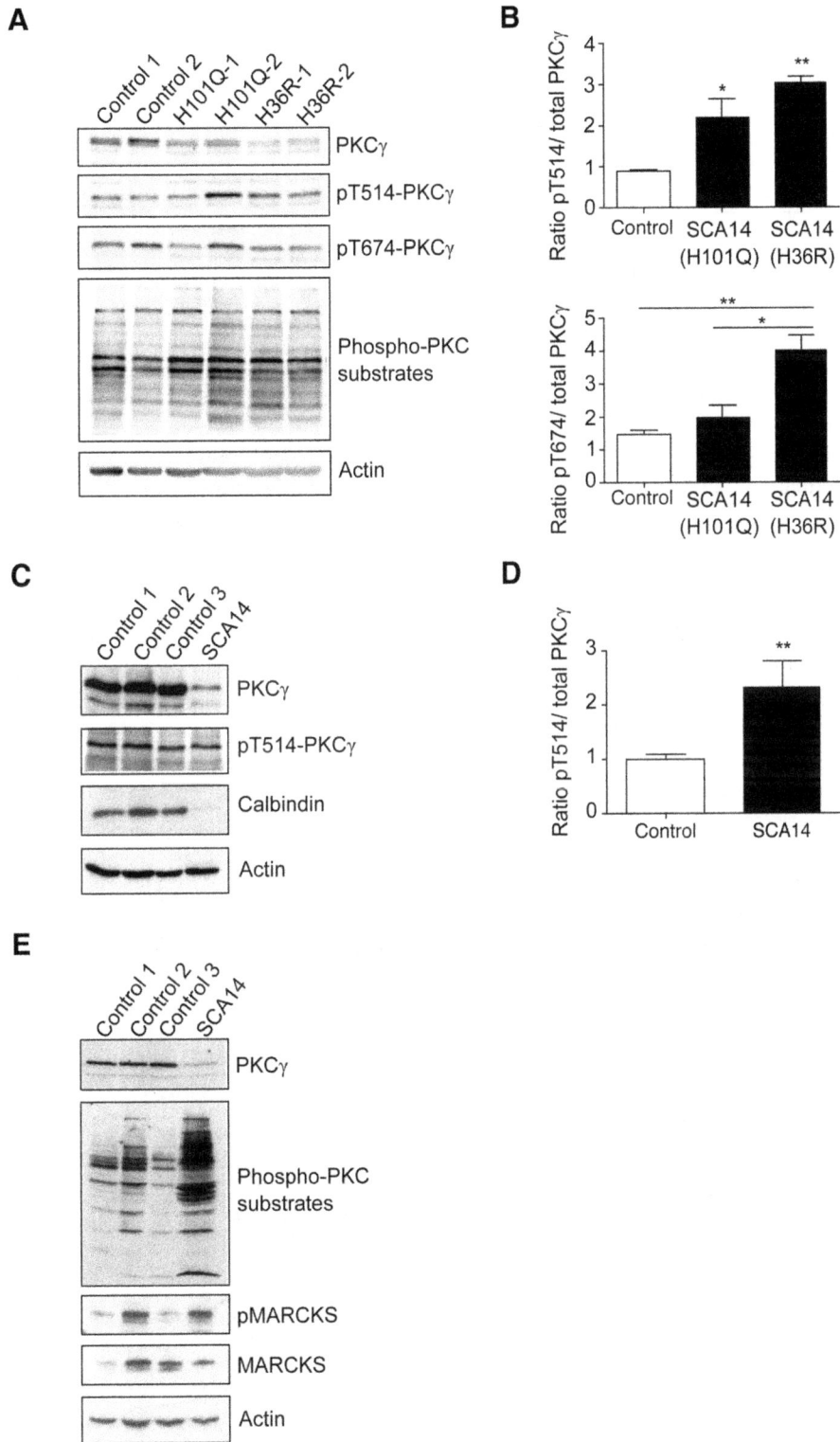

A

Control 1, Control 2, H101Q-1, H101Q-2, H36R-1, H36R-2

PKCγ
pT514-PKCγ
pT674-PKCγ
Phospho-PKC substrates
Actin

B

Ratio pT514/ total PKCγ

Control — SCA14 (H101Q) * — SCA14 (H36R) **

Ratio pT674/ total PKCγ

Control — SCA14 (H101Q) — SCA14 (H36R)

C

Control 1, Control 2, Control 3, SCA14

PKCγ
pT514-PKCγ
Calbindin
Actin

D

Ratio pT514/ total PKCγ

Control — SCA14 **

E

Control 1, Control 2, Control 3, SCA14

PKCγ
Phospho-PKC substrates
pMARCKS
MARCKS
Actin

Fig. 6 (See legend on next page.)

(See figure on previous page.)
Fig. 6 Increased PKC kinase activity in SCA14 patient cells. **a** Lysates of iPSCs were subjected to immunoblotting for PKCγ, T514- and T674-phosphorylated PKCγ and phospho-PKC substrates. Actin was used as loading control. **b** Quantification of PKCγ phosphorylation at T514 (upper panel) and T674 (lower panel) versus total PKCγ. Phosphorylation was significantly increased in SCA14 iPSCs compared to controls ($n = 3$, *$p < 0.05$, **$p < 0.01$, ANOVA followed by Bonferroni's post-hoc test). **c** Lysates from post-mortem cerebellum were subjected to immunoblotting for PKCγ, T514-phosphorylated PKCγ, Calbindin and Actin. **d** Quantification of PKCγ phosphorylation at T514 versus total PKCγ. T514 phosphorylation was significantly increased in SCA14 (H101Q) cerebellum compared to controls ($n = 3$, **$p < 0.01$, unpaired students' t-test). **e** Cerebellar lysates were subjected to immunoblotting for PKCγ, phospho-PKC substrates, phosphorylated (p) MARCKS, MARCKS and Actin

been reported previously [11]. Other than the loss of Purkinje cells, little pathology was observed, likely due to the insufficient quality of the post-mortem material. Remaining Purkinje cells were shown to display markedly reduced immunoreactivity for PKCγ without any visible protein aggregation (16). In contrast, our results suggest that aggregation of PKCγ is central to SCA14 pathology. Both mutations investigated in this study cause aggregation of PKCγ in the cytoplasm in both iPSCs and in Purkinje cells of SCA14 (H101Q) cerebellum, but not in other brain regions (which show only minimal PKCγ expression in adult human brain). The aggregation of misfolded proteins is a central feature in many neurodegenerative disorders. Owing to their post-mitotic nature, neurons are particularly vulnerable to misfolded proteins as they cannot dilute toxic substances by division [14]. Moreover, in many neurodegenerative disorders components of the protein degradation machinery are impaired, a phenomenon that is further worsened as neurons age. Interestingly, we found that mutant aggregated PKCγ did not co-localize with ubiquitin. Dephosphorylation of PKC is a prerequisite of the subsequent ubiquitination and

degradation via a proteasome pathway [28]. Given the hyper-phosphorylated state of mutant PKCγ, our results raise the possibility that mutant PKCγ might be resistant to ubiquitination and subsequent proteasomal or autophagic degradation, which is in contrast to a previous study employing transient overexpression of mutant PKCγ [46]. This discrepancy might be explained by the massive overexpression of mutant PKCγ that could trigger a cellular response that is different from that under physiological circumstances. We found that there was a significant overlap between PKCγ and LC3 in unstimulated SCA14 iPSCs, consistent with the idea that mutant PKCγ is already in an active and aggregated conformation [21, 42]. However, this overlap did not further increase following phorbol ester activation, despite the significant increase in aggregation size. This is consistent with the observation that autophagosomes mostly degrade non-aggregated or small aggregated proteins, but not large inclusions [31]. The enhanced formation of lysosomes in SCA14 iPSCs and cerebellum suggests that mutant PKCγ might enter the lysosomal pathway via alternative routes. Dephosphorylation- and ubiquitination-independent downregulation through lipid raft-mediated endocytic and lysosomal

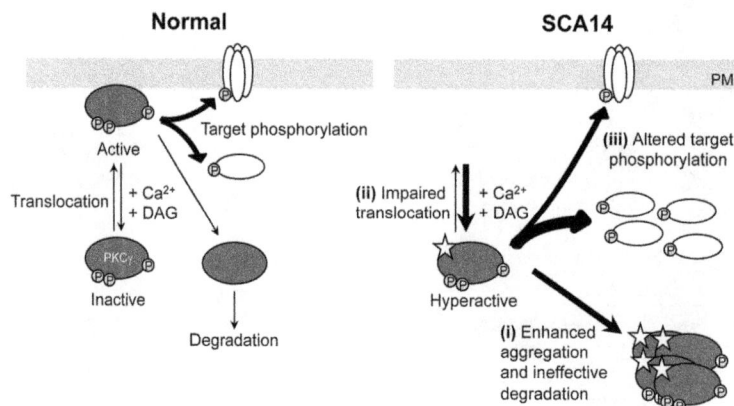

Fig. 7 Model of the functional effect of PKCγ mutations. Normally (left panel), mature wildtype PKCγ resides in the cytosol in an autoinhibited conformation. Binding of diacylglycerol (DAG) and calcium ions (Ca^{2+}) activates and promotes the translocation of PKCγ to the plasma membrane (PM), where active PKCγ phosphorylates its membrane substrates. PKCγ returns to an autoinhibited conformation (inactive) following the decay of its second messengers. The membrane-bound conformation of PKCγ is sensitive to dephosphorylation. Prolonged activation of PKCγ leads to its dephosphorylation by phosphatases. The dephosphorylated PKCγ can be tagged by ubiquitin and subsequently degraded. In contrast, in SCA14, PKCγ with mutated C1 domain adapts an open conformation and is hyper-active in the cytoplasm. (I) Highly phosphorylated mutant PKCγ forms aggregates, which accumulate in the cytoplasm due to inefficient degradation. (ii) Mutant PKCγ fails to translocation to the plasma membrane and remains in the cytoplasm. (iii) This might lead to altered phosphorylation of its substrates at the membrane and in the cytoplasm

pathways has been described for PKCα [27, 29]. Although endosomal sequestration of mutant PKCγ has been observed in vitro [17], this could not be confirmed in our study suggesting the existence of alternative mechanisms such as chaperone-mediated autophagy via LAMP2A [14].

In our study, we found reduced staining of mutant PKCγ at the Purkinje cell membrane in SCA14 cerebellum. This is consistent with previous studies that have suggested altered translocation of mutant PKCγ to the plasma membrane following activation in heterologous cell lines [1, 42] and primary Purkinje cells [39]. PKC has long been implicated in the regulation of neurotransmission and synaptic plasticity by phosphorylating membrane receptors and ion channels [8]. Mutant PKCγ might affect membrane excitability in Purkinje cells either indirectly through altering the membrane kinetics of PKCα [39] or directly via phosphorylation of critical receptors. Specific physiological targets of PKCγ remain largely unknown, and their identification might provide important clues about the selective vulnerability of Purkinje cells in SCA14. One possible membrane-associated substrate of PKCγ might be the C3-type transient receptor potential (TRPC3) channel, which is highly expressed in Purkinje cells [19]. In Purkinje cells, TRPC3 is activated downstream of mGluR1 signaling, resulting in calcium influx [19]. Interestingly, PKCγ, which is also activated downstream of mGluR1 [23], has been shown to negatively regulate calcium entry via phosphorylation of TRPC3 [40, 41]. Moreover, transiently overexpressed PKCγ mutants failed to phosphorylate TRPC3 despite their high catalytic activity [1]. Thus, a failure of mutated PKCγ to phosphorylate and inhibit TRPC3 might lead to excessive calcium influx upon TRPC3 activation and might thereby contribute to Purkinje cell dysfunction and cell death. Abnormal TRPC3 signaling is likely to be a common pathological mechanisms in different subtypes of ataxia [4, 30], suggesting a pathological role for PKCγ beyond SCA14. Indeed, *Trpc3* and *Prkcg* were recently identified as hub genes in gene networks misregulated in mouse models of SCA1 [20] and SCA2 [34].

Together, these findings suggest that SCA14 pathogenesis might be partially explained by a loss-of-function of PKCγ at the cell membrane. However, the absence of SCA14-related phenotypes in *Prkcg* knockout mice suggests that the disease cannot be fully explained by a reduction of PKCγ function. Interestingly, we found an increase in PKC substrate phosphorylation in SCA14 cerebellum and iPSCs. Increased kinase activity of mutant PKCγ has also been reported in in vitro studies [1, 3, 43], supporting and support the hypothesis that mutations in the C1 domain facilitate the ligand-induced 'open' and signaling competent conformation of PKCγ. Recently, increased PKC kinase activity has been shown to be neuroprotective in mouse models of SCA1 and SCA2 [13]. The identities of the phosphorylated PKC targets in these conditions compared to SCA14 remain to be elucidated. Similarly, it will be important to test whether the same aberrantly phosphorylated targets are found in both SCA14 cerebellum and iPSCs. Moreover, it is conceivable that PKC isoforms other than PKCγ contribute to the observed increased PKC substrate phosphorylation. Human stem cells express both canonical and non-canonical PKC isoforms [24] and Purkinje cells have been shown to express PKCα, PKCγ, PKCδ and PKCε [45].

Conclusions

Our study is the first to describe the functional neuropathology of SCA14 in post-mortem cerebellum as well as in human iPSCs derived from patients with SCA14 mutations. Unexpectedly, PKCγ aggregation, mislocalization and increased kinase activity that we observed in SCA14 cerebellum were reproduced in SCA14 iPSCs. Purkinje cells are particularly vulnerable in SCA14, likely due to their high expression of PKCγ and its specific targets that regulate the calcium homeostasis and the unique physiological properties of these neurons. While the latter cannot be modelled in undifferentiated stem cells, the fact that patient iPSCs express PKCγ and recapitulate key pathological findings observed in SCA14 cerebellum underscores their potential as relevant tools for disease modeling and drug discovery, in addition to future studies in which SCA14 iPSCs will be differentiated to Purkinje cells.

Abbreviations

DAG: Diacylglycerol; iPSCs: Induced pluripotent stem cells; LAMP2: Lysosome-associated membrane protein 2; LC3: Microtubule-associated protein 1 light chain 3; MARCKS: Myristoylated alanine-rich C-kinase substrate; PDBu: Phorbol 12, 13-dibutyrate; PKCγ: Protein kinase C gamma; PMA: Phorbol 12-myristate 13-acetate; SCA14: Spinocerebellar ataxia type 14; UPS: Ubiquitin proteasome system

Acknowledgments

We are immensely grateful to all patients for their participation. We acknowledge the Oxford Parkinson's Disease Center (OPDC) study for the original generation of iPSC lines from control donors, funded by the Monument Trust Discovery Award from Parkinson's UK, a charity registered in England and Wales (2581970) and in Scotland (SC037554), with the support of the National Institute for Health Research (NIHR) Oxford Biomedical Research Center based at Oxford University Hospitals NHS Trust and University of Oxford, and the NIHR Comprehensive Local Research Network. Human peripheral blood mononuclear cells (PBMCs) were a generous gift from Professor Quentin Sattentau, University of Oxford. We thank the High-Throughput Genomics Group at the Wellcome Trust Centre for Human Genetics, Oxford (Funded by Wellcome Trust grant reference 090532/Z/09/Z and MRC Hub grant G0900747 91070) for the generation of Illumina genotyping and transcriptome data for characterization of iPSC lines. We also acknowledge the Oxford Brain Bank, supported by the UK Medical Research Council and Alzheimer's Brain Bank UK.

Funding

Supported by the Royal Society (E.B.E.B.), Ataxia UK (E.B.E.B.), the European Union's Horizon 2020 research and innovation program (under the Marie Skłodowska-Curie grant agreement no. 699978) (L.M.W.), the John Fell OUP Fund (E.B.E.B., L.M.W.) and the Monument Trust Discovery Award from Parkinson's UK (J.V.) and the Oxford NIHR Biomedical Research Centre (O.A.). This publication reflects the views only of the authors, and the European Commission cannot be held responsible for any use, which may be made of the information contained therein. The Wellcome Trust (WTISSF121302) and The Oxford Martin School (LC0910–004) provide financial support to the James Martin Stem Cell Facility (S.A.C.). The funding bodies had no role in the design of the study and collection, analysis, and interpretation of data and in writing the manuscript.

Authors' contributions

MMKW carried out iPSC reprogramming and all functional experiments in iPSCs, designed and interpreted experiments, and was a major contributor in writing the manuscript. SDH, JV, LMW and SAC were involved in iPSC reprogramming. GF and AHN identified and diagnosed SCA14(H36R) patients. OA carried out neuropathology experiments and interpreted the patient histopathology. KT identified and diagnosed SCA14(H101Q) patients, interpreted findings and helped writing the manuscript. EBEB performed biochemical experiments on SCA14 cerebellum, designed and interpreted experiments and wrote the manuscript. All authors read and approved the final manuscript.

Competing interests

The authors declare that they have no competing interests.

Author details

[1]Department of Physiology, Anatomy and Genetics, University of Oxford, Sherrington Road, Oxford OX1 3PT, UK. [2]Sir William Dunn School of Pathology, University of Oxford, South Parks Road, Oxford OX1 3RE, UK. [3]Gloucestershire Hospitals, NHS Foundation Trust, Cheltenham General Hospital, Sandford Road, Cheltenham GL53 7AN, UK. [4]Nuffield Department of Clinical Neurosciences, University of Oxford, Level 6, West Wing, John Radcliffe Hospital, Oxford OX3 9DU, UK. [5]Oxford Centre for Genomic Medicine, ACE Building, Oxford University Hospitals NHS Trust, Nuffield Orthopaedic Centre, Windmill Road, Oxford OX3 7HE, UK.

References

1. Adachi N, Kobayashi T, Takahashi H, Kawasaki T, Shirai Y, Ueyama T, Matsuda T, Seki T, Sakai N, Saito N (2008) Enzymological analysis of mutant protein kinase Cγ causing spinocerebellar ataxia type 14 and dysfunction in Ca2+ homeostasis. J Biol Chem 283:19854–19863. https://doi.org/10.1074/jbc.M801492200

2. Antal CE, Newton AC (2014) Tuning the signalling output of protein kinase C. Biochem Soc Trans 42:1477–1483. https://doi.org/10.1042/BST20140172

3. Asai H, Hirano M, Shimada K, Kiriyama T, Furiya Y, Ikeda M, Iwamoto T, Mori T, Nishinaka K, Konishi N, Udaka F, Ueno S (2009) Protein kinase C gamma, a protein causative for dominant ataxia, negatively regulates nuclear import of recessive-ataxia-related aprataxin. Hum Mol Genet 18:3533–3543. https://doi.org/10.1093/hmg/ddp298

4. Becker EBE (2017) From mice to men: TRPC3 in cerebellar Ataxia. Cerebellum 16:877–879. https://doi.org/10.1007/s12311-015-0663-y

5. Beers J, Gulbranson DR, George N, Siniscalchi LI, Jones J, Thomson JA, Chen G (2012) Passaging and colony expansion of human pluripotent stem cells by enzyme-free dissociation in chemically defined culture conditions. Nat Protoc 7:2029–2040. https://doi.org/10.1038/nprot.2012.130

6. Bolte S, Cordelières FP (2006) A guided tour into subcellular colocalization analysis in light microscopy. J Microsc 224:213–232. https://doi.org/10.1111/j.1365-2818.2006.01706.x

7. Brkanac Z, Bylenok L, Fernandez M, Matsushita M, Lipe H, Wolff J, Nochlin D, Raskind WH, Bird TD (2002) A new dominant spinocerebellar ataxia linked to chromosome 19q13.4-qter. Arch Neurol 59:1291–1295

8. Callender JA, Newton AC (2017) Conventional protein kinase C in the brain: 40 years later. Neuronal Signal 1:NS20160005–NS20160010. https://doi.org/10.1042/NS20160005

9. Chelban V, Wiethoff S, Fabian-Jessing BK, Haridy NA, Khan A, Efthymiou S, Becker EBE, O'Connor E, Hersheson J, Newland K, Hojland AT, Gregersen PA, Lindquist SG, Petersen MB, Nielsen JE, Nielsen M, Wood NW, Giunti P, Houlden H (2018) Genotype-phenotype correlations, dystonia and disease progression in spinocerebellar ataxia type 14. Mov Disord. https://doi.org/10.1002/mds.27334

10. Chen C, Kano M, Abeliovich A, Chen L, Bao S, Kim JJ, Hashimoto K, Thompson RF, Tonegawa S (1995) Impaired motor coordination correlates with persistent multiple climbing fiber innervation in PKC gamma mutant mice. Cell 83:1233–1242

11. Chen D-H, Brkanac Z, Verlinde CLMJ, Tan X-J, Bylenok L, Nochlin D, Matsushita M, Lipe H, Wolff J, Fernandez M, Cimino PJ, Bird TD, Raskind WH (2003) Missense mutations in the regulatory domain of PKC gamma: a new mechanism for dominant nonepisodic cerebellar ataxia. Am J Hum Genet 72:839–849

12. Chen D-H, Raskind WH, Bird TD (2012) Spinocerebellar ataxia type 14. Handb Clin Neurol 103:555–559. https://doi.org/10.1016/B978-0-444-51892-7.00036-X

13. Chopra R, Wasserman AH, Pulst SM, De Zeeuw CI, Shakkottai VG (2018) Protein kinase C activity is a protective modifier of Purkinje neuron degeneration in cerebellar ataxia. Hum Mol Genet 27:1396–1410. https://doi.org/10.1093/hmg/ddy050

14. Ciechanover A, Kwon YT (2017) Protein quality control by molecular chaperones in Neurodegeneration. Front Neurosci 11:185. https://doi.org/10.3389/fnins.2017.00185

15. Curnutte JT, Erickson RW, Ding J, Badwey JA (1994) Reciprocal interactions between protein kinase C and components of the NADPH oxidase complex may regulate superoxide production by neutrophils stimulated with a phorbol ester. J Biol Chem 269:10813–10819

16. Dafinca R, Scaber J, Ababneh N, Lalic T, Weir G, Christian H, Vowles J, Douglas AGL, Fletcher-Jones A, Browne C, Nakanishi M, Turner MR, Wade-Martins R, Cowley SA, Talbot K (2016) C9orf72 Hexanucleotide expansions are associated with altered endoplasmic reticulum calcium homeostasis and stress granule formation in induced pluripotent stem cell-derived neurons from patients with amyotrophic lateral sclerosis and Frontotemporal dementia. Stem Cells 34:2063–2078. https://doi.org/10.1002/stem.2388

17. Doran G, Davies KE, Talbot K (2008) Activation of mutant protein kinase Cgamma leads to aberrant sequestration and impairment of its cellular function. Biochem Biophys Res Commun 372:447–453. https://doi.org/10.1016/j.bbrc.2008.05.072

18. Handel AE, Chintawar S, Lalic T, Whiteley E, Vowles J, Giustacchini A, Argoud K, Sopp P, Nakanishi M, Bowden R, Cowley S, Newey S, Akerman C, Ponting CP, Cader MZ (2016) Assessing similarity to primary tissue and cortical layer identity in induced pluripotent stem cell-derived cortical neurons through single-cell transcriptomics. Hum Mol Genet 25:989–1000. https://doi.org/10.1093/hmg/ddv637

19. Hartmann J, Dragicevic E, Adelsberger H, Henning HA, Sumser M, Abramowitz J, Blum R, Dietrich A, Freichel M, Flockerzi V, Birnbaumer L, Konnerth A (2008) TRPC3 channels are required for synaptic transmission and motor coordination. Neuron 59:392–398. https://doi.org/10.1016/j.neuron.2008.06.009

20. Ingram M, Wozniak EAL, Duvick L, Yang R, Bergmann P, Carson R, O'Callaghan B, Zoghbi HY, Henzler C, Orr HT (2016) Cerebellar Transcriptome profiles of ATXN1 transgenic mice reveal SCA1 disease progression and protection pathways. Neuron 89:1194–1207. https://doi.org/10.1016/j.neuron.2016.02.011

21. Jezierska J, Goedhart J, Kampinga HH, Reits EA, Verbeek DS (2013) SCA14 mutation V138E leads to partly unfolded PKCγ associated with an exposed C-terminus, altered kinetics, phosphorylation and enhanced insolubilization. J Neurochem 128:741–751. https://doi.org/10.1111/jnc.12491

22. Kano M, Hashimoto K, Chen C, Abeliovich A, Aiba A, Kurihara H, Watanabe M, Inoue Y, Tonegawa S (1995) Impaired synapse elimination during cerebellar development in PKCγ mutant mice. Cell 83:1223–1231. https://doi.org/10.1016/0092-8674(95)90147-7

23. Kano M, Watanabe T (2017) Type-1 metabotropic glutamate receptor signaling in cerebellar Purkinje cells in health and disease. F1000Res 6:416. https://doi.org/10.12688/f1000research.10485.1

24. Kinehara M, Kawamura S, Tateyama D, Suga M, Matsumura H, Mimura S, Hirayama N, Hirata M, Uchio-Yamada K, Kohara A, Yanagihara K, Furue MK (2013) Protein kinase C regulates human pluripotent stem cell self-renewal. PLoS One 8:e54122–e54113. https://doi.org/10.1371/journal.pone.0054122

25. Koeppen AH (2005) The pathogenesis of spinocerebellar ataxia. Cerebellum 4:62–73. https://doi.org/10.1080/14734220510007950

26. Kose A, Saito N, Ito H, Kikkawa U, Nishizuka Y, Tanaka C (1988) Electron microscopic localization of type I protein kinase C in rat Purkinje cells. J Neurosci 8:4262–4268

27. Leontieva OV, Black JD (2004) Identification of two distinct pathways of protein kinase Calpha down-regulation in intestinal epithelial cells. J Biol Chem 279:5788–5801. https://doi.org/10.1074/jbc.M308375200

28. Lu Z, Liu D, Hornia A, Devonish W, Pagano M, Foster DA (1998) Activation of protein kinase C triggers its ubiquitination and degradation. Mol Cell Biol 18:839–845

29. Lum MA, Pundt KE, Paluch BE, Black AR, Black JD (2013) Agonist-induced down-regulation of endogenous protein kinase c α through an endolysosomal mechanism. J Biol Chem 288:13093–13109. https://doi.org/10.1074/jbc.M112.437061

30. Meera P, Pulst SM, Otis TS (2016) Cellular and circuit mechanisms underlying spinocerebellar ataxias. J Physiol 594:4653–4660. https://doi.org/10.1113/JP271897

31. Menzies FM, Fleming A, Caricasole A, Bento CF, Andrews SP, Ashkenazi A, Füllgrabe J, Jackson A, Jimenez Sanchez M, Karabiyik C, Licitra F, Lopez Ramirez A, Pavel M, Puri C, Renna M, Ricketts T, Schlotawa L, Vicinanza M, Won H, Zhu Y, Skidmore J, Rubinsztein DC (2017) Autophagy and Neurodegeneration: pathogenic mechanisms and therapeutic opportunities. Neuron 93:1015–1034. https://doi.org/10.1016/j.neuron.2017.01.022

32. Németh AH, Kwasniewska AC, Lise S, Parolin Schnekenberg R, EBE B, Bera KD, Shanks ME, Gregory L, Buck D, Zameel Cader M, Talbot K, de Silva R, Fletcher N, Hastings R, Jayawant S, Morrison PJ, Worth P, Taylor M, Tolmie J, O'Regan M, Ataxia Consortium UK, Valentine R, Packham E, Evans J, Seller A, Ragoussis J (2013) Next generation sequencing for molecular diagnosis of neurological disorders using ataxias as a model. Brain 136:3106–3118. https://doi.org/10.1093/brain/awt236

33. Nixon JB, McPhail LC (1999) Protein kinase C (PKC) isoforms translocate to triton-insoluble fractions in stimulated human neutrophils: correlation of conventional PKC with activation of NADPH oxidase. J Immunol 163:4574–4582

34. Pflieger LT, Dansithong W, Paul S, Scoles DR, Figueroa KP, Meera P, Otis TS, Facelli JC, Pulst SM (2017) Gene co-expression network analysis for identifying modules and functionally enriched pathways in SCA2. Hum Mol Genet 14:269–212. https://doi.org/10.1093/hmg/ddx191

35. Ross CA, Poirier MA (2005) Opinion: what is the role of protein aggregation in neurodegeneration? Nat Rev MolCell Bio 6:891–898. https://doi.org/10.1038/nrm1742

36. Seki T, Adachi N, Ono Y, Mochizuki H, Hiramoto K, Amano T, Matsubayashi H, Matsumoto M, Kawakami H, Saito N, Sakai N (2005) Mutant protein kinase Cgamma found in spinocerebellar ataxia type 14 is susceptible to aggregation and causes cell death. J Biol Chem 280:29096–29106. https://doi.org/10.1074/jbc.M501716200

37. Seki T, Shimahara T, Yamamoto K, Abe N, Amano T, Adachi N, Takahashi H, Kashiwagi K, Saito N, Sakai N (2009) Mutant gammaPKC found in spinocerebellar ataxia type 14 induces aggregate-independent

38. Seki T, Takahashi H, Adachi N, Abe N, Shimahara T, Saito N, Sakai N (2007) Aggregate formation of mutant protein kinase C gamma found in spinocerebellar ataxia type 14 impairs ubiquitin-proteasome system and induces endoplasmic reticulum stress. Eur J Neurosci 26:3126–3140. https://doi.org/10.1111/j.1460-9568.2007.05933.x

maldevelopment of dendrites in primary cultured Purkinje cells. Neurobiol Dis 33:260–273. https://doi.org/10.1016/j.nbd.2008.10.013

39. Shuvaev AN, Horiuchi H, Seki T, Goenawan H, Irie T, Iizuka A, Sakai N, Hirai H (2011) Mutant PKCγ in spinocerebellar ataxia type 14 disrupts synapse elimination and long-term depression in Purkinje cells in vivo. J Neurosci 31:14324–14334. https://doi.org/10.1523/JNEUROSCI.5530-10.2011

40. Trebak M, Hempel N, Wedel BJ, Smyth JT, Bird GSJ, Putney JW (2005) Negative regulation of TRPC3 channels by protein kinase C-mediated phosphorylation of serine 712. Mol Pharmacol 67:558–563. https://doi.org/10.1124/mol.104.007252

41. Venkatachalam K (2003) Regulation of canonical transient receptor potential (TRPC) channel function by diacylglycerol and protein kinase C. J Biol Chem 278:29031–29040. https://doi.org/10.1074/jbc.M302751200

42. Verbeek DS, Goedhart J, Bruinsma L, Sinke RJ, Reits EA (2008) PKC gamma mutations in spinocerebellar ataxia type 14 affect C1 domain accessibility and kinase activity leading to aberrant MAPK signaling. J Cell Sci 121:2339–2349. https://doi.org/10.1242/jcs.027698

43. Verbeek DS, Knight MA, Harmison GG, Fischbeck KH, Howell BW (2005) Protein kinase C gamma mutations in spinocerebellar ataxia 14 increase kinase activity and alter membrane targeting. Brain 128:436–442. https://doi.org/10.1093/brain/awh378

44. Watson LM, Wong MMK, Vowles J, Cowley SA, Becker EBE (2018) A simplified method for generating Purkinje cells from human-induced pluripotent stem cells. Cerebellum 17:419–427. https://doi.org/10.1007/s12311-017-0913-2

45. Wetsel WC, Khan WA, Merchenthaler I, Rivera H, Halpern AE, Phung HM, Negro-Vilar A, Hannun YA (1992) Tissue and cellular distribution of the extended family of protein kinase C isoenzymes. J Cell Biol 117:121–133. https://doi.org/10.1083/jcb.117.1.121

46. Yamamoto K, Seki T, Adachi N, Takahashi T, Tanaka S, Hide I, Saito N, Sakai N (2010) Mutant protein kinase C gamma that causes spinocerebellar ataxia type 14 (SCA14) is selectively degraded by autophagy. Genes Cells 15:425–438. https://doi.org/10.1111/j.1365-2443.2010.01395.x

11

Unique microglia recovery population revealed by single-cell RNAseq following neurodegeneration

Tuan Leng Tay[1,2,3*†], Sagar[4†], Jana Dautzenberg[1], Dominic Grün[4*] and Marco Prinz[1,5*]

Abstract

Microglia are brain immune cells that constantly survey their environment to maintain homeostasis. Enhanced microglial reactivity and proliferation are typical hallmarks of neurodegenerative diseases. Whether specific disease-linked microglial subsets exist during the entire course of neurodegeneration, including the recovery phase, is currently unclear. Taking a single-cell RNA-sequencing approach in a susceptibility gene-free model of nerve injury, we identified a microglial subpopulation that upon acute neurodegeneration shares a conserved gene regulatory profile compared to previously reported chronic and destructive neurodegeneration transgenic mouse models. Our data also revealed rapid shifts in gene regulation that defined microglial subsets at peak and resolution of neurodegeneration. Finally, our discovery of a unique transient microglial subpopulation at the onset of recovery may provide novel targets for modulating microglia-mediated restoration of brain health.

Keywords: Microglia, Recovery, Neurodegeneration, Single-cell RNA analysis

Introduction

Microglia are tissue-resident macrophages of the central nervous system (CNS) that act as the first line of defense upon disruption of CNS homeostasis. In contrast to the lattice-like organization of sparsely (< 0.5%) renewing microglial cells in the adult brain [3, 26, 27, 35, 43], heightened microglial reactivity and microgliosis are hallmarks of all neurodegenerative diseases regardless of severity, as exemplified in local neuronal damage and widespread neurodegeneration [10, 13, 32, 37, 43].

While adult microglia originate solely from the primitive yolk sac erythromyeloid progenitors without contribution from the peripheral hematopoietic stem cells [1, 11, 12, 22, 33], gene expression and single-cell transcriptomic studies [14, 29] suggest that total CNS parenchymal microglia are not functionally homogeneous. The relative contributions to neuroprotection and neurodegeneration by microglia in neurodegenerative diseases such as Alzheimer's disease (AD), amyotrophic lateral sclerosis and multiple sclerosis remain contentious [38, 39]. Notably, we recently demonstrated that immediate activation and proliferation of microglial cells within one to two weeks of neuronal injury was not detrimental to the CNS but appeared vital to the timely recovery of tissue homeostasis and neural functions [43]. Bulk RNA-sequencing (RNAseq) analyses of microglial cells of the facial nucleus (FN) from the unilateral facial nerve axotomy (FNX) model of acute neurodegeneration showed lesion-dependent gene regulation, while compensatory alterations observed in the contralateral FN were attributed to other CNS cell types [43]. Recent reports based on single-cell analysis of microglial transcriptomes attributed specific cellular states to neurodegenerative diseases recapitulated in AD-like mouse models with chronic or severe CNS damage [21, 30]. Although these important studies highlighted the appearance of novel disease-associated microglial subtypes, they did not address the existence of distinct microglial populations during recovery due to the chronic and destructive characteristics of the transgenic mouse models used.

To define disease-associated populations of microglia more precisely, we took a single-cell RNAseq (scRNAseq) approach in the FNX model, which is not driven by any

* Correspondence: tuan.leng.tay@uniklinik-freiburg.de; gruen@ie-freiburg.mpg.de; marco.prinz@uniklinik-freiburg.de

†Tuan Leng Tay and Sagar contributed equally to this work.

[1]Institute of Neuropathology, Faculty of Medicine, University of Freiburg, Freiburg, Germany

[4]Max-Planck-Institute of Immunobiology and Epigenetics, Freiburg, Germany

Full list of author information is available at the end of the article

susceptibility gene. Indeed, a subset of disease-linked microglia from the ipsilateral FN was distinct from a homogenous cloud. Comparative analysis of single-cell transcriptomes across these three models of neurodegeneration furthermore established a strong conservation of the microglial gene regulatory profile ascribed to disease. Of high significance, we found temporal regulation of lesion-associated changes in our FNX model that distinguished microglia at peak and resolution of disease. In particular, we verified the emergence of a transient microglial cluster characterized by the upregulation of *Apoe* and *Ccl5* at the onset of recovery in situ. Collectively, our findings highlight a potential new interpretation of disease-associated gene regulation that may be critical to the restoration of CNS homeostasis mediated by microglial cells.

Materials and methods

Mice and treatments

$CX_3CR1^{GFP/+}$ [20] mice were bred in specific-pathogen-free facility and given chow and water ad libitum. Unilateral facial nerve axotomy (FNX) at the stylomastoid foramen was performed in 8 weeks old female $CX_3CR1^{GFP/+}$ mice described previously [43]. Only female mice were used to allow comparisons of the scRNAseq data in this study with the bulk RNAseq analyses performed before [43]. Mice were bred concurrently, received same-day operation and randomly assigned to each experimental group for sacrifice at the required time point. Animal experiments were approved by the Regional Council of Freiburg, Germany. Experimenters were blinded to all groups during data acquisition and analysis.

FACS

Mice were transcardially perfused with 20 ml ice-cold PBS. Pontine blocks were immediately cut in a coronal rodent brain matrix for acute isolation of single facial nuclei under the stereomicroscope. Brain tissue was gently mashed and resuspended in 20 ml ice-cold extraction buffer containing 1× HBSS, 1% fetal calf serum (FCS) and 1 mM EDTA, followed by the extraction of microglial cells in 5 ml 37% isotonic Percoll. Cells were labeled with antibodies CD45-BV421 (103,133, BioLegend), CD11b-BV605 (101,237, BioLegend) and MHC Class II-PE-Cy7 (107,630, BioLegend) in FACS buffer (1× PBS, 1% FCS). Single GFP+ CD45lo CD11b+ microglial cells were sorted into 384-well plates containing 240 nL of primer mix and 1.2 μl of Vapor-Lock (QIAGEN) PCR encapsulation barrier at the Influx™ cell sorter (Becton Dickinson) for subsequent RNA sequencing procedures.

Single-cell RNA amplification and library preparation

We used an automated and miniaturized version of the CEL-Seq2 protocol [18]. Sixteen libraries (1536 single cells) were sequenced on two lanes (pair-end multiplexing run, 100 bp read length) of an *Illumina HiSeq* 2500 sequencing system generating 243,638,747 sequence fragments.

Quantification of transcript abundance

For the FNX experiment, paired end reads were aligned to the transcriptome using bwa (version 0.6.2-r126) with default parameters [28]. The transcriptome contained all RefSeq gene models based on the mouse genome release mm10 downloaded from the UCSC genome browser comprising 31,201 isoforms derived from 23,538 gene loci [31]. All isoforms of the same gene were merged to a single gene locus. The 50 bp right mate of each read pair was mapped to the ensemble of all gene loci and to the set of 92 ERCC spike-ins in sense direction [4]. Reads that mapped to multiple loci were discarded. The 50 bp left read contains the barcode information: the first six bases corresponded to the unique molecular identifier (UMI) followed by six bases representing the cell specific barcode. The remainder of the left read contains a polyT stretch. Only the right read was used for quantification. For each cell barcode, the number of UMIs per transcript was counted and aggregated across all transcripts derived from the same gene locus. Based on binomial statistics, the number of observed UMIs was converted into transcript counts [15].

Single-cell RNA sequencing data analysis

Identification and visualization of different subpopulations as well as differential gene expression analysis was performed with the RaceID2 algorithm [16]. Out of 1536 cells sequenced in the FNX experiment, 944 cells passed the quality thresholds. The median, minimum and maximum number of genes identified per cell are 1560, 858 and 2658, respectively. Down-sampling to 1500 transcripts was used for data normalization. Clustering was performed using k-medoids clustering without outlier identification. Ten clusters were identified based on the saturation of the average within-cluster dispersion. To compare our disease-associated clusters with a recently described microglia type associated with neurodegenerative disease (DAM), we obtained the raw data from scRNAseq of all immune cells in wild type (WT) and Alzheimer's disease (AD) transgenic mouse brains [21]. The AD mouse model expressed five human familial AD gene mutations (FAD). Results were obtained from a mix of male and female mice which showed no difference due to sex. Raw count files (henceforth referred to as the "FAD data set") were downloaded from Gene Expression Omnibus (GEO): GSE98969 [21] and analyzed using the RaceID2 algorithm [16]. To exclude non-microglial cells from the FAD data set, only cells with UMI counts for *Cst3* (UMI > 10) and *Hexb* (UMI > 5) (as defined in [21]) prior to normalization were retained for further analysis. Perivascular macrophages and monocytes (*Cd74*, UMIs $\geq$5), granulocytes (*S100a9*, UMIs $\geq$50) and mature B-cells (*Cd79b*, UMIs $\geq$3) were removed from the dataset. Downsampling to 700 UMIs was performed for data normalization.

The t-distributed stochastic neighbor embedding (t-SNE) algorithm was used for dimensional reduction and cell cluster visualization [44]. Using the *phyper* function provided by the R software to perform a hypergeometric test, an enrichment score $[-\log_{10}(p\text{-value}+ 10^{-3})]$ was calculated for the FNX data to identify the enrichment of cells belonging to a group in a given cluster. Differentially expressed genes between the tail clusters (clusters 4, 8 and 9 in the FNX data) and cloud clusters were identified similar to a published method [2]. First, negative binomial distributions reflecting the gene expression variability within each subgroup were inferred based on the background model for the expected transcript count variability computed by RaceID2 [16]. Using these distributions, a P value for the observed difference in transcript counts between the two subgroups was calculated and multiple testing corrected by the Benjamini-Hochberg method.

The accession code for the FNX data set is GEO:GSE90975, https://www.ncbi.nlm.nih.gov/geo/query/acc.cgi?acc=GSE90975.

Gene set enrichment analysis
Gene IDs of the differentially expressed genes between the tail (clusters 4, 8 and 9) and cloud clusters in the FNX data were converted to Entrez IDs using the clusterProfiler package [46]. Gene set enrichment analysis was performed using the ReactomePA package [45]. The fold-change for each gene between the cloud and tail clusters was calculated using the diffexpnb function of the RaceID2 algorithm and given as an argument to the gsePathway function to calculate enriched gene sets in the tail clusters.

Comparative single-cell transcriptomic analysis
In addition to the comparison of our FNX data set with the DAM signature from the FAD scRNAseq study [21], we included the neurodegeneration response genes identified in another recent scRNAseq report based on the transgenic mouse model for severe neurodegeneration known as CK-p25 [30]. Male CK-p25 mice were analyzed. Withdrawal of doxycycline from the diet induces the CamKII promoter driven expression of p25, the calpain cleavage product of Cdk5 activator p35, and leads to apoptotic neuronal cell death. While the CK-p25 inducible mouse model is not based on genetic mutations associated with familial AD, the authors claimed that it recapitulates several aspects of AD pathology and the

transcriptional profile of FAD mice [30]. Data on neurodegeneration-associated differentially regulated genes identified in the respective FAD and CK-p25 studies were obtained from the Supplementary Table S3 (fold changes and P values; [21]) and Supplementary Table S4 (fold changes and Z scores, from which P values were calculated for the corresponding early and late response genes in Clusters 3 and 6; [30]). A total of 5820 genes were obtained after we overlapped the relevant genes in both studies with our FNX gene set for comparative assessment. Based on the Benjamini-Hochberg procedure, only genes with false discovery rate < 0.05 were considered for subsequent analysis.

Histology
Mice were transcardially perfused with 20 ml PBS. Brains were fixed overnight in 4% paraformaldehyde in PBS at 4°C and processed for frozen sectioning as before [43]. A coronal rodent brain matrix (RBM-2000C, ASI Instruments) was used to obtain consistent blocks of pontine regions that included both facial nuclei. Cryosections (14-μm) were collected from the entire facial nuclei on coated glass slides and stored at −20°C until use. Tissues were permeabilized in blocking solution (0.1% Triton-X 100, 5% bovine albumin, normal goat or normal donkey serum, and PBS) for 1 h at room temperature and incubated overnight at 4°C with primary antibodies: 1:200 rat anti-CD11b (ab8878, Abcam), 1:500 rabbit anti-IBA-1 (019–19,741, Wako), 1:200 goat anti-APOE (AB947, Merck), and 1:500 rabbit anti-CCL5 (RANTES) (710,001, ThermoFisher Scientific). Antigen retrieval was performed at 96 °C prior to APOE staining for 40 min in 10 mM citrate buffer at pH 9. Sections were incubated with corresponding secondary antibodies conjugated to 1:1000 Alexa Fluor 488 or Alexa Fluor 647 (Life Technologies) and 1:5000 nuclear counterstain 4′,6-diamidino-2-phenylindole (DAPI, Sigma) for 2 h at room temperature, and mounted in ProLong® Diamond Antifade Mountant (Life Technologies).

Microscopy and image analysis
GFP$^+$ microglia were imaged using a 20X / 0.75 NA objective lens on the Keyence BZ − 9000 inverted fluorescence microscope and quantified using the BZ-II Analyzer. Three brain sections per mouse were analyzed. Confocal images of immunohistological preparations were acquired with the SP8 STED-WS (Leica Microsystems) using a HCX PL HCL PL APO C 20X/0.75 NA glycerine objective lens and the LAS X software. DAPI and Alexa Fluors 488 and 647 were excited by the UV Diode Laser 405 nm, Argon Laser 488 nm and WL 647 nm, respectively, and detected in sequential and simultaneous acquisition settings with the HyD detectors

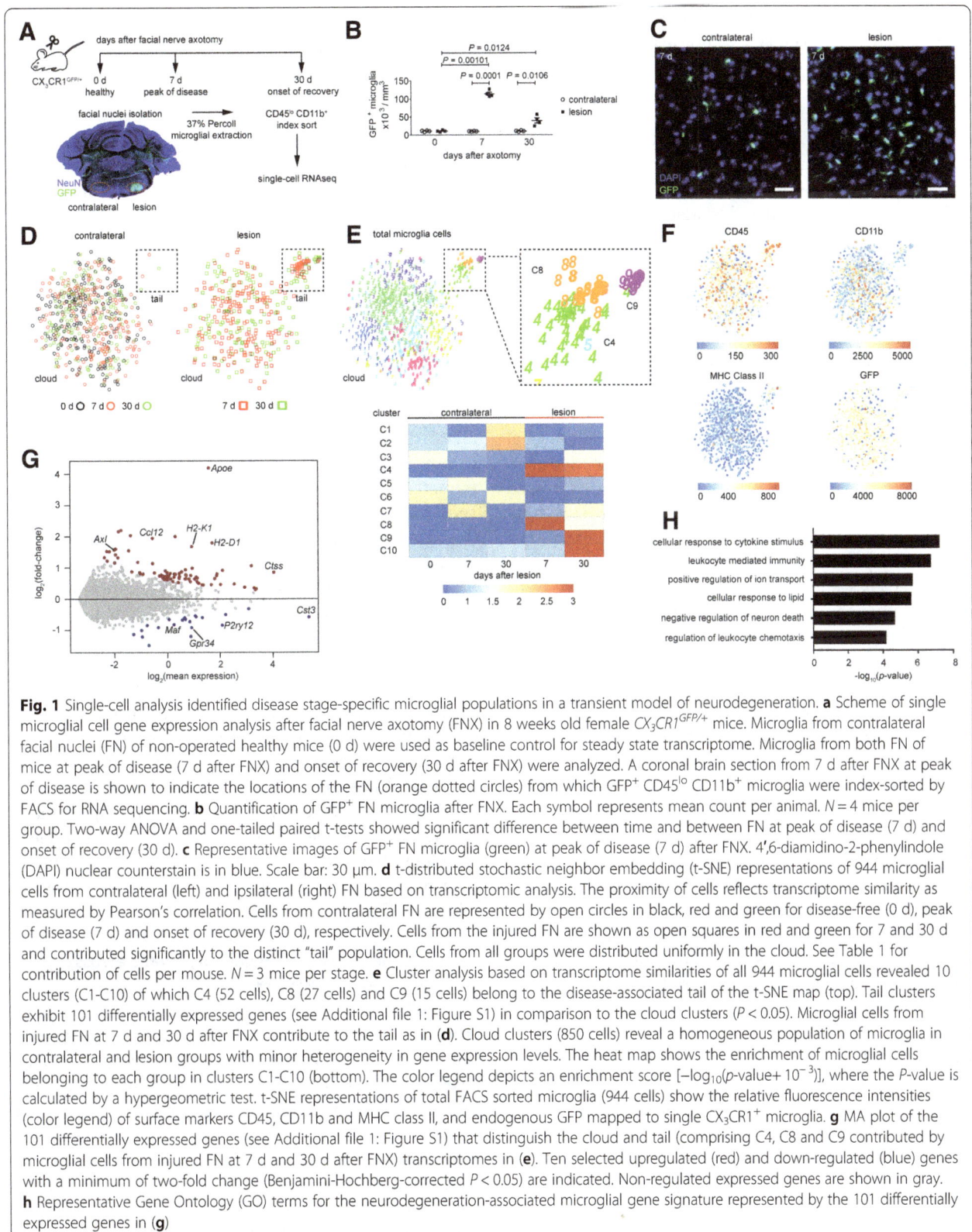

Fig. 1 Single-cell analysis identified disease stage-specific microglial populations in a transient model of neurodegeneration. **a** Scheme of single microglial cell gene expression analysis after facial nerve axotomy (FNX) in 8 weeks old female $CX_3CR1^{GFP/+}$ mice. Microglia from contralateral facial nuclei (FN) of non-operated healthy mice (0 d) were used as baseline control for steady state transcriptome. Microglia from both FN of mice at peak of disease (7 d after FNX) and onset of recovery (30 d after FNX) were analyzed. A coronal brain section from 7 d after FNX at peak of disease is shown to indicate the locations of the FN (orange dotted circles) from which GFP$^+$ CD45^{lo} CD11b$^+$ microglia were index-sorted by FACS for RNA sequencing. **b** Quantification of GFP$^+$ FN microglia after FNX. Each symbol represents mean count per animal. $N = 4$ mice per group. Two-way ANOVA and one-tailed paired t-tests showed significant difference between time and between FN at peak of disease (7 d) and onset of recovery (30 d). **c** Representative images of GFP$^+$ FN microglia (green) at peak of disease (7 d) after FNX. 4',6-diamidino-2-phenylindole (DAPI) nuclear counterstain is in blue. Scale bar: 30 μm. **d** t-distributed stochastic neighbor embedding (t-SNE) representations of 944 microglial cells from contralateral (left) and ipsilateral (right) FN based on transcriptomic analysis. The proximity of cells reflects transcriptome similarity as measured by Pearson's correlation. Cells from contralateral FN are represented by open circles in black, red and green for disease-free (0 d), peak of disease (7 d) and onset of recovery (30 d), respectively. Cells from the injured FN are shown as open squares in red and green for 7 and 30 d and contributed significantly to the distinct "tail" population. Cells from all groups were distributed uniformly in the cloud. See Table 1 for contribution of cells per mouse. $N = 3$ mice per stage. **e** Cluster analysis based on transcriptome similarities of all 944 microglial cells revealed 10 clusters (C1-C10) of which C4 (52 cells), C8 (27 cells) and C9 (15 cells) belong to the disease-associated tail of the t-SNE map (top). Tail clusters exhibit 101 differentially expressed genes (see Additional file 1: Figure S1) in comparison to the cloud clusters ($P < 0.05$). Microglial cells from injured FN at 7 d and 30 d after FNX contribute to the tail as in (**d**). Cloud clusters (850 cells) reveal a homogeneous population of microglia in contralateral and lesion groups with minor heterogeneity in gene expression levels. The heat map shows the enrichment of microglial cells belonging to each group in clusters C1-C10 (bottom). The color legend depicts an enrichment score [$-\log_{10}$(p-value+ 10^{-3})], where the P-value is calculated by a hypergeometric test. t-SNE representations of total FACS sorted microglia (944 cells) show the relative fluorescence intensities (color legend) of surface markers CD45, CD11b and MHC class II, and endogenous GFP mapped to single CX$_3$CR1$^+$ microglia. **g** MA plot of the 101 differentially expressed genes (see Additional file 1: Figure S1) that distinguish the cloud and tail (comprising C4, C8 and C9 contributed by microglial cells from injured FN at 7 d and 30 d after FNX) transcriptomes in (**e**). Ten selected upregulated (red) and down-regulated (blue) genes with a minimum of two-fold change (Benjamini-Hochberg-corrected $P < 0.05$) are indicated. Non-regulated expressed genes are shown in gray. **h** Representative Gene Ontology (GO) terms for the neurodegeneration-associated microglial gene signature represented by the 101 differentially expressed genes in (**g**)

in the gating mode. The pinhole was set to one airy unit. Image stacks were sampled with a pixel size of 142 nm and in 1 µm z-steps.

Statistical analysis

Data are presented as mean ± SEM. GraphPad Prism5 was used for multiple comparisons using 2-way ANOVA with Bonferroni correction and paired t-tests. Differences were considered statistically significant at $P < 0.05$.

Results and discussion

Single-cell analysis revealed stage-dependent microglial clusters during neurodegeneration

In our previous study, we reported that the rapid increase in microglial cells in response to FNX induced neurodegeneration was due to microglial clonal expansion [43]. In addition to accompanying morphological changes in microglia of the ipsilateral FN, we identified the differential regulation of 257 microglia-expressed genes in comparison to the contralateral FN by bulk microglia RNAseq [43]. While both clonal expansion and recovery of steady state microglial cell numbers by 60 d after FNX appeared to occur randomly, it was unclear whether the molecular programming of all microglia within the lesioned FN was homogeneous. To understand the relatedness of the cells based on their transcriptomes, we performed scRNAseq of microglia isolated from the contralateral and injured FN at stages representing disease-free (0 d), peak of disease (7 d after FNX) and onset of recovery following microgliosis (30 d after FNX) (Fig. 1a-c). At least 96 microglial cells were sorted for each experimental group per animal. After quality control, data from a total of 944 cells, from which 15,245 genes were quantified, were further analyzed using our RaceID2 algorithm [16] and depicted in t-distributed stochastic neighbor embedding (t-SNE) representations (Fig. 1d-f; Table 1). Microglia from all groups distributed uniformly in the "cloud", whereas cells that clustered separately in the

"tail" were derived solely from 7 and 30 d lesion groups, indicating that the tail comprises disease stage-specific microglia (Fig. 1d). This separation of disease-associated CNS immune cell populations agrees with a recent single-cell cytometry-based study [34]. Our transcriptome-based cluster analysis of all 944 microglial cells using the RaceID2 algorithm identified ten clusters (C1-C10), of which cells from C4, C8 and C9 mapped mainly to the tail (Fig. 1e). Other clusters (C1-C3, C5-C7, and C10) were identified within the cloud representing less distinct subpopulations of microglia with variations in the expression levels of similarly expressed genes (Fig. 1e). Analysis of surface markers revealed corresponding enrichment of the activation markers CD45 and MHC class II in cells within the tail (Fig. 1f). Notably, these differences at the levels of gene and protein expression did not correlate directly to cell morphology as most microglia within the injured FN appeared to have similarly retracted their ramifications and assumed amoeboid and rod-like shapes typical of activated microglia (Fig. 1c). Differential gene expression analysis of cloud versus tail clusters (Benjamini-Hochberg-corrected $P < 0.05$) identified 101 differentially expressed genes (Fig. 1g, Additional file 1: Figure S1). Gene Set Enrichment Analysis of all genes that distinguish the cloud and tail clusters revealed that gene sets corresponding to translation, degradation of the extracellular matrix and peptide ligand-binding receptors were upregulated, whereas gene sets related to membrane trafficking, intra-Golgi and retrograde Golgi-to-ER traffic, and fatty acid metabolism were down-regulated (Additional file 2: Figure S2). The genes upregulated during neurodegeneration were enriched for the Gene Ontology (GO) terms related to immune response, lipid mediation, neuronal cell death, and migration of microglia (Fig. 1h).

Common microglial gene regulatory profile across neurodegenerative diseases

The FNX paradigm represents a model for acute neurodegeneration where approximately 10–15% [7] of facial motoneurons in the FN die upon nerve transection, but clinical recovery is observed by two months [43]. We asked if our neurodegeneration-associated microglial gene signature would be identical across acute non-susceptibility gene-driven and transgene-induced chronic and destructive forms of neurodegeneration. A recent study based on scRNAseq of all immune cells in WT and AD transgenic mouse brains resulted in the identification of a unique microglia type associated with neurodegenerative diseases (DAM) [21]. The t-SNE representation of the Keren-Shaul et al. data (indicated as FAD for familial AD) resembles our FNX data set where the majority of the single-cell

Table 1 Contribution of facial nuclei microglia to single cell transcriptomic analysis

Group	CD45^{lo} CD11b^{+} GFP^{+} microglial cells						
	Mouse 1		Mouse 2		Mouse 3		Total
	Cloud	Tail	Cloud	Tail	Cloud	Tail	
0 d contralateral	61	2	31	0	105	4	203
7 d contralateral	76	1	77	2	60	1	217
7 d lesion	64	10	52	22	47	14	209
30 d contralateral	57	0	30	1	74	0	162
30 d lesion	37	6	30	3	50	27	153

Cloud clusters: C1-C3, C5-C7 and C10; tail clusters: C4, C8 and C9

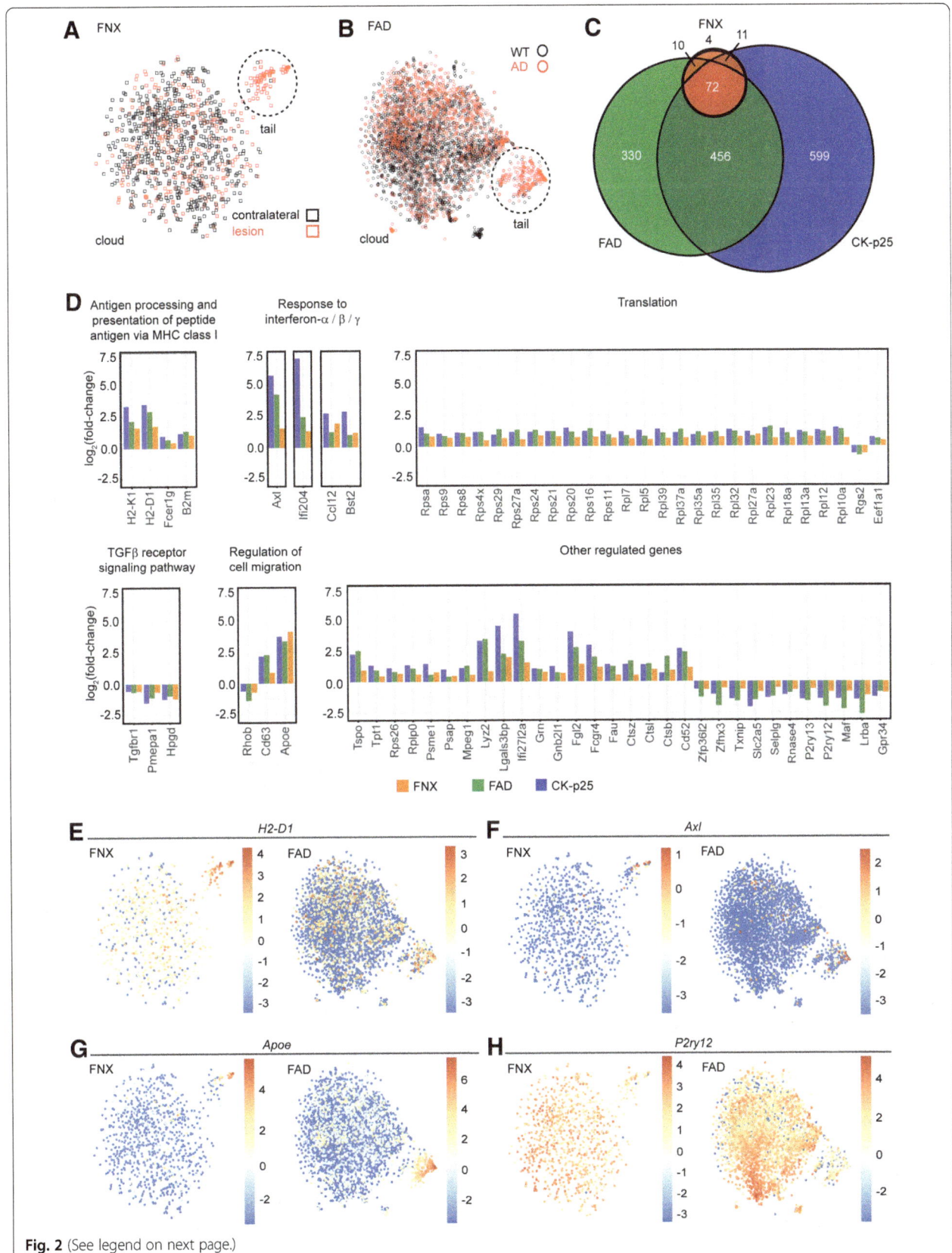

Fig. 2 (See legend on next page.)

(See figure on previous page.)

Fig. 2 Comparative analysis of single-cell microglial transcriptomes from acute and chronic neurodegeneration models unveiled a common gene regulatory signature. **a-b** t-SNE maps of **a** 944 microglial cells from FNX acute neurodegeneration in susceptibility gene-free $CX_3CR1^{GFP/+}$ mice (as in Fig. 1d-e) and **b** 3896 microglial cells from chronic neurodegeneration FAD model [21] based on RaceID2 transcriptomic analysis. Cells from contralateral (black square) and lesion (red square) FN and cells from wild type (WT) controls (black circle) and AD transgenic (red circle) mice are distributed uniformly in the clouds. Neurodegeneration-associated groups formed distinct tail populations (dotted circles). **c** Comparative differential gene expression analysis of disease-associated clusters in susceptibility gene-free FNX (orange), chronic FAD (green, [21]) and severe CK-p25 (blue; [30]) neurodegeneration models identified 72 common differentially regulated genes (red). See Table 2 and Additional file 5: Table S1 for details. **d** Log$_2$(fold-change) (y-axis) of 70 common neurodegeneration-associated genes (x-axis) identified in (**c**) that were similarly up- or down-regulated (represented as respective positive or negative values). Genes are categorized according to GO terms in panel titles. FNX (orange), FAD (green) and CK-p25 (blue). See also Table 2. **e-h** tSNE maps of common genes **e** H2-D1, **f** Axl, **g** Apoe, and **h** P2ry12 shown in (**d**) depict their single cell expression in the FNX and FAD data sets. Color legends represent log$_2$(transcript counts) across cells

transcriptomes from all groups were found in the cloud while subsets of microglia from lesion or AD groups were spatially distinct in the tail (Fig. 2a-b). Here, cloud and tail transcriptomes of the AD study were distinguished by differential expression of 109 genes (Benjamini-Hochberg-corrected $P < 0.05$) of which 29 genes were common to the differentially regulated genes identified in our FNX study (Additional file 3: Figure S3). The median number of unique molecular identifiers (UMIs) detected in the FNX and FAD studies were 3660.5 and 982, respectively (Additional file 4: Figure S4). In a transgenic mouse model for severe neurodegeneration known as CK-p25, upregulation of many disease-associated genes in microglia in the late response cluster of single-cell transcriptomic analysis [30] was reminiscent of the changes we observed in our tail transcriptomes. Comparison of differentially regulated DAM genes in all three models (detailed in the Methods) revealed an overlap of 72 common genes, with only 4 genes found to be FNX-specific (Fig. 2c; Table 2 and Additional file 5: Table S1). Analysis of the fold-change of the common genes showed that 70 of the genes were correspondingly up- or downregulated (Fig. 2d-h; Table 2). Similar to the outcome of a meta-analysis of transcriptomes from aging, primed and neurodegenerative conditions [19], our finding emphasizes that despite pathology-specific contextual differences, a strong consensus neurodegeneration-associated gene signature exists (Fig. 2c; Additional file 6: Table S2). We also validated our findings against a searchable database (http://research-pub.gene.com/BrainMyeloidLandscape) that is a curated compendium of mouse and human CNS myeloid cell expression profiles from various conditions of neurodegeneration or infection [9]. Taken together, this core signature we identified may hold promising therapeutic targets for relieving severe neuronal damage in related CNS disease phenotypes.

Recovery-associated microglial subset arises during injury resolution

Using the FNX model, we were able to track disease progression from peak of microgliosis (7 d after

FNX) to clinical recovery (60 d after FNX) that is accompanied by the resolution of microgliosis starting at 30 d [43]. Such kinetics of microgliosis are in sharp contrast to mouse models of chronic or severe neurodegeneration in which the resolution of microgliosis is not observed [21, 23, 30]. Notably, bulk RNAseq analysis revealed no change in gene regulation between the lesion and contralateral FN in at 60 d after FNX [43]. Closer examination of neurodegeneration-associated tail microglial cells revealed that cluster C9 comprises transcriptomes from the 30 d lesion group (Fig. 1d-e; Table 1). Strong upregulation of *apolipoprotein E (Apoe)* and *chemokine ligand 5 (Ccl5)* and down-regulation of *cystatin 3 (Cst3)* and *secreted protein acidic and rich in cysteine or osteonectin (Sparc)* in single microglial cells distinguished C9 from C4 and C8 in the tail (Figs. 1e, 3). High expression of *Apoe* and *Ccl5* is also in agreement with our previous findings from bulk RNAseq of sorted microglia from lesioned FN at 30 d after FNX [43]. The fraction of C9 microglia to all cells from 30 d lesion (Fig. 1d; Table 1) is reflected at the level of protein expression (Fig. 3f-g). Of note CCL5$^+$ CD11b$^+$ and APOE$^+$ IBA-1$^+$ microglial cells appear amoeboid, smaller, anucleated and possibly fragmented (Fig. 3f-g), suggesting a non-homeostatic (or transient and non-propagative) phenotype.

We believe that the interpretation of microglial upregulation of APOE during brain pathology is still up for dispute. High expression of APOE has been shown to be characteristic for a subtype of reactive microglia that appears in specific conditions of neurodegeneration in mice [6, 8, 19, 21, 23]. Multiple rodent studies demonstrated that genetic deletion or repression of APOE alleviated disease severity, as observed in the amelioration of experimental autoimmune encephalomyelitis (EAE) [25, 42], extension of lifespan in the SOD1 mouse model of amyotrophic lateral sclerosis [5], and protection from tau pathogenesis typical in AD [41]. These results thus

Table 2 Microglia regulated disease-associated genes in models of neurodegeneration

No.	Gene	log2(fold-change)			Adjusted P value		
		FNX	FAD	CK-p25	FNX	FAD	CK-p25
1	Apoe	4.19E+00	3.43E+00	3.80E+00	1.96E-23	1.77E-60	2.32E-11
2	Axl	1.57E+00	4.29E+00	5.83E+00	4.75E-05	2.72E-46	2.32E-11
3	B2m	1.07E+00	1.37E+00	1.20E+00	2.12E-16	1.02E-57	2.32E-11
4	Bst2	1.18E+00	1.01E+00	2.90E+00	3.49E-05	3.09E-07	2.32E-11
5	C1qa*	3.74E-01	-2.16E-01	5.68E-01	1.04E-04	3.53E-03	2.32E-11
6	Ccl12	1.94E+00	1.23E+00	2.75E+00	2.75E-21	1.26E-03	2.32E-11
7	Cd52	1.14E+00	2.40E+00	2.69E+00	4.66E-07	5.97E-33	2.32E-11
8	Cd63	9.04E-01	2.33E+00	2.21E+00	8.75E-06	2.57E-39	2.32E-11
9	Ctsb	9.16E-01	2.04E+00	6.88E-01	2.13E-20	8.08E-66	2.32E-11
10	Ctsl	9.88E-01	1.46E+00	1.38E+00	6.45E-13	1.89E-30	2.32E-11
11	Ctsz	5.05E-01	1.68E+00	1.41E+00	1.52E-03	5.34E-44	2.32E-11
12	Eef1a1	4.58E-01	6.10E-01	7.18E-01	9.07E-04	3.20E-04	2.32E-11
13	Fau	5.12E-01	1.24E+00	1.41E+00	1.76E-02	2.59E-11	2.32E-11
14	Fcer1g	4.58E-01	6.92E-01	9.87E-01	4.37E-03	1.51E-06	2.32E-11
15	Fcgr4	1.16E+00	2.00E+00	2.96E+00	8.84E-03	9.37E-04	2.32E-11
16	Fgl2	1.42E+00	2.77E+00	4.04E+00	4.92E-04	7.96E-08	2.32E-11
17	Gnb2l1	6.81E-01	7.51E-01	1.26E+00	4.40E-03	6.98E-08	2.32E-11
18	Gpr34	-9.12E-01	-8.58E-01	-1.26E+00	2.96E-08	2.66E-11	2.32E-11
19	Grn	8.04E-01	1.03E+00	1.08E+00	7.50E-14	3.61E-25	2.32E-11
20	H2-D1	1.80E+00	2.99E+00	3.56E+00	2.60E-10	7.01E-50	2.32E-11
21	H2-K1	1.68E+00	2.20E+00	3.41E+00	5.77E-37	2.25E-32	2.32E-11
22	Hpgd	-1.21E+00	-9.77E-01	-1.23E+00	7.06E-05	3.04E-05	2.32E-11
23	Ifi204	1.32E+00	2.47E+00	7.21E+00	4.99E-04	2.28E-04	2.32E-11
24	Ifi27l2a	1.55E+00	3.30E+00	5.47E+00	4.66E-07	2.99E-08	2.32E-11
25	Lgals3bp	2.00E+00	2.28E+00	4.52E+00	7.39E-37	1.74E-35	2.32E-11
26	Lrba	-1.13E+00	-2.65E+00	-1.47E+00	2.44E-03	7.66E-08	4.10E-09
27	Lyz2	8.53E-01	3.46E+00	3.32E+00	6.65E-03	1.21E-67	2.32E-11
28	Maf	-8.19E-01	-2.25E+00	-1.41E+00	1.64E-04	3.76E-23	2.63E-11
29	Mpeg1	5.59E-01	1.31E+00	1.14E+00	2.82E-04	8.63E-29	2.32E-11
30	P2ry12	-8.41E-01	-2.05E+00	-1.41E+00	2.14E-13	5.64E-59	2.32E-11
31	P2ry13	-6.05E-01	-1.59E+00	-1.44E+00	3.63E-03	4.10E-22	2.32E-11
32	Pmepa1	-6.52E-01	-1.11E+00	-1.53E+00	8.20E-04	2.17E-11	2.32E-11
33	Psap	4.64E-01	4.21E-01	1.02E+00	1.45E-04	2.44E-02	2.32E-11
34	Psme1	8.04E-01	5.71E-01	1.47E+00	7.52E-03	3.14E-02	2.32E-11
35	Rgs2	-6.02E-01	-7.74E-01	-5.98E-01	1.58E-04	1.55E-08	3.06E-05
36	Rhob	-7.27E-01	-1.40E+00	-6.28E-01	5.15E-05	9.17E-20	3.21E-04
37	Rnase4	-6.75E-01	-9.20E-01	-1.08E+00	8.20E-04	2.01E-14	2.32E-11
38	Rpl10a	6.46E-01	1.36E+00	1.50E+00	2.44E-03	3.72E-12	2.32E-11
39	Rpl12	7.46E-01	1.17E+00	1.29E+00	3.24E-04	1.56E-09	2.32E-11
40	Rpl13a	7.55E-01	1.09E+00	1.23E+00	2.49E-06	1.61E-15	2.32E-11
41	Rpl18a	6.44E-01	1.04E+00	1.41E+00	2.22E-05	7.63E-16	2.32E-11
42	Rpl23	6.51E-01	1.58E+00	1.47E+00	1.58E-04	1.06E-18	2.32E-11
43	Rpl27a	9.37E-01	8.14E-01	1.17E+00	6.52E-10	1.24E-05	2.32E-11
44	Rpl32	7.56E-01	1.20E+00	1.35E+00	8.07E-04	1.87E-16	2.32E-11
45	Rpl35	7.38E-01	1.17E+00	1.11E+00	1.12E-03	4.86E-11	2.32E-11
46	Rpl35a	8.16E-01	1.15E+00	9.27E-01	2.49E-06	2.42E-14	2.39E-11
47	Rpl37a	6.71E-01	1.37E+00	1.11E+00	4.87E-03	5.78E-20	2.32E-11
48	Rpl39	6.26E-01	1.07E+00	1.38E+00	1.25E-02	8.31E-13	2.32E-11
49	Rpl5	5.42E-01	8.10E-01	1.29E+00	3.72E-02	3.20E-04	2.32E-11
50	Rpl7	6.02E-01	8.72E-01	1.17E+00	2.19E-02	1.98E-08	2.32E-11
51	Rplp0	5.77E-01	1.10E+00	1.38E+00	1.85E-02	5.02E-13	2.32E-11
52	Rps11	6.63E-01	9.37E-01	1.20E+00	3.32E-04	2.20E-09	2.32E-11
53	Rps16	7.51E-01	1.44E+00	1.23E+00	3.32E-04	4.62E-16	2.32E-11
54	Rps20	7.23E-01	1.17E+00	1.50E+00	8.71E-04	3.02E-16	2.32E-11
55	Rps21	8.03E-01	1.23E+00	1.23E+00	1.52E-05	2.78E-22	2.32E-11
56	Rps24	8.74E-01	1.32E+00	1.17E+00	9.71E-08	5.90E-21	2.32E-11
57	Rps26	6.57E-01	8.33E-01	1.14E+00	1.96E-02	3.97E-06	2.47E-11
58	Rps27a	5.63E-01	1.34E+00	1.17E+00	1.36E-02	1.87E-09	2.32E-11
59	Rps29	6.77E-01	1.39E+00	9.57E-01	2.46E-06	9.47E-11	2.32E-11
60	Rps4x	5.01E-01	1.18E+00	1.17E+00	4.63E-02	2.42E-12	2.32E-11
61	Rps8	7.78E-01	1.11E+00	1.14E+00	1.35E-06	7.64E-11	2.32E-11
62	Rps9	7.07E-01	8.65E-01	1.05E+00	1.06E-06	5.45E-11	2.32E-11
63	Rpsa	8.22E-01	1.06E+00	1.58E+00	2.26E-05	2.46E-12	2.32E-11
64	Selplg	-5.06E-01	-1.23E+00	-1.32E+00	3.81E-05	9.76E-38	2.32E-11
65	Slc2a5	-8.45E-01	-1.51E+00	-2.06E+00	1.15E-02	1.13E-04	2.32E-11
66	Sparc*	3.25E-01	-8.36E-01	-3.89E-01	1.94E-04	3.78E-27	2.31E-04
67	Tgfbr1	-5.76E-01	-6.74E-01	-5.68E-01	9.62E-04	1.72E-07	1.10E-05
68	Tpt1	4.50E-01	9.61E-01	1.35E+00	5.97E-03	1.30E-06	2.32E-11
69	Tspo	9.50E-01	1.23E+00	2.24E+00	3.84E-02	1.32E-07	2.32E-11
70	Txnip	-6.23E-01	-1.59E+00	-1.41E+00	2.59E-02	1.49E-14	2.32E-11
71	Zfhx3	-5.44E-01	-1.98E+00	-1.05E+00	3.69E-03	1.64E-16	2.32E-11
72	Zfp36l2	-6.49E-01	-1.29E+00	-6.28E-01	4.77E-02	6.63E-03	1.54E-02
73	Actb	-3.20E-01	-3.54E-01	0.00E+00	2.95E-03	1.27E-07	1.00E+00
74	C1qb*	2.96E-01	-4.94E-01	0.00E+00	1.46E-03	1.48E-08	1.00E+00
75	Cst3	-5.89E-01	-2.29E-01	0.00E+00	1.20E-34	1.74E-05	1.00E+00
76	Ctsd	3.54E-01	1.45E+00	0.00E+00	4.62E-05	1.43E-63	1.00E+00
77	Ctss	8.52E-01	3.88E-01	0.00E+00	3.92E-18	1.30E-09	1.00E+00
78	Cx3cr1	-3.16E-01	-1.36E+00	0.00E+00	1.97E-02	4.56E-53	8.28E-01
79	Gm13826	6.19E-01	1.55E+00	5.08E-01	9.50E-03	9.92E-13	2.03E-01
80	Itgam*	7.58E-01	-1.12E+00	-1.20E-01	5.08E-07	2.42E-10	6.15E-01
81	Itm2b	4.82E-01	3.86E-01	0.00E+00	1.36E-06	1.07E-07	1.00E+00
82	Kctd12	-5.14E-01	-1.41E+00	-2.99E-01	1.86E-02	9.75E-04	1.64E-01
83	Ccl5	1.53E+00	-1.85E+00	5.53E+00	4.13E-04	9.43E-01	2.32E-11
84	Ctsh	6.51E-01	3.98E-01	8.67E-01	2.11E-04	1.01E-01	2.32E-11
85	Eif2ak2	7.74E-01	3.29E-02	4.49E-01	3.71E-02	8.63E-01	5.74E-03
86	Fcgr2b	7.56E-01	1.44E-01	8.37E-01	4.53E-02	8.87E-02	1.68E-06
87	Ifi30	7.45E-01	-4.93E-01	1.14E+00	2.16E-03	1.79E-01	1.91E-10
88	Irf7	1.61E+00	7.39E-01	5.05E+00	1.27E-05	5.39E-01	2.32E-11
89	Jun	-1.19E+00	-1.24E+00	-9.27E-01	1.00E-13	7.26E-02	5.20E-09
90	Ly6e	7.47E-01	-2.26E-02	1.44E+00	9.27E-12	7.85E-01	2.32E-11
91	Ly86	6.55E-01	2.40E-01	8.97E-01	2.15E-08	2.49E-01	2.32E-11
92	Socs3	1.02E+00	-1.07E+00	9.27E-01	1.85E-02	7.87E-01	4.47E-04
93	Xaf1	8.78E-01	1.59E+00	2.57E+00	1.12E-02	6.22E-01	2.32E-11
94	Fos	-1.48E+00	4.88E-01	-2.09E-01	2.07E-08	9.12E-01	6.66E-01
95	Jund	-9.09E-01	-5.15E-01	-8.07E-01	3.99E-04	5.62E-01	2.67E-01
96	Klf6	-6.95E-01	-4.14E-01	2.99E-01	3.37E-02	6.21E-01	3.68E-01
97	Sgk1	-6.59E-01	-3.13E-01	-3.29E-01	7.52E-03	4.39E-01	1.49E-01

Color code corresponds to Fig. 2c: common to FNX, FAD and CK-p25 (red); common to FNX and FAD (green); common to FNX and CK-p25 (blue); only regulated in FNX (orange). Negative values represent down-regulation. Asterisk (*) indicates different directionality of commonly regulated genes

suggest a detrimental role of APOE in neurodegeneration. Studies of human brain autopsies [36] and humanized mouse models of tauopathy [41] relating to AD have however shown that different isoforms of APOE may alternate between being a risk factor or neuroprotective. Since *Apoe* is highly expressed in mouse astrocytes and microglia [47] and mainly expressed by astrocytes in human [48], it is unclear if the ablation of APOE in some or all cell types contribute similarly to CNS pathology. In agreement with the observation that the upregulation of *Apoe* during the initial DAM activation in the FAD model is independent of triggering receptor expressed on myeloid cells 2 (Trem2) [21], the FNX-dependent upregulation of *Apoe* in cluster C9 from the onset of recovery corresponds with no change in *Trem2* expression (Additional file 5: Table S1). Our immunohistochemical results depicting C9 microglia that upregulate APOE (Fig. 3g) during recovery support the claim that switching on the TREM2-APOE pathway drives a non-homeostatic microglial phenotype [23]. However, could the higher frequency of *Apoe* upregulation during early disease stage in the FAD model [21] represent a recovery-promoting microglial subtype? In the EAE study, overall levels of APOE transcript and protein in rat spinal cord reduced at onset, elevated during peak, and plateaued at the end of disease [25]. Notably, a brain region-specific proteomic investigation of APOE protein levels and amyloid accumulation in three AD mouse models led the authors to predict that increased APOE detection drove amyloid clearance [40]. There are few clues to date regarding the functional or mechanistic role of the chemoattractant and activating cytokine CCL5 or RANTES [17] particularly in microglia. The down-regulation of *Cst3* seems to imply a loss of homeostatic microglial phenotype since it is typically considered a microglia signature gene [21]. Astrocyte-secreted SPARC protein was described to be antagonistic to synaptogenic function [24], however it is presently unclear if the down-regulation of *Sparc* in microglia during recovery plays a supportive role for synaptogenesis. Overall, it remains to be investigated whether microglia carrying the recovery-associated gene signature are targeted for removal by local apoptosis and/or emigration [43] during reinstatement of steady state microglial network that accompany CNS regeneration.

Conclusion

In conclusion, our combinatorial analysis of microglia gene expression profiles across neurodegeneration models strongly implicates APOE in disease modulation.

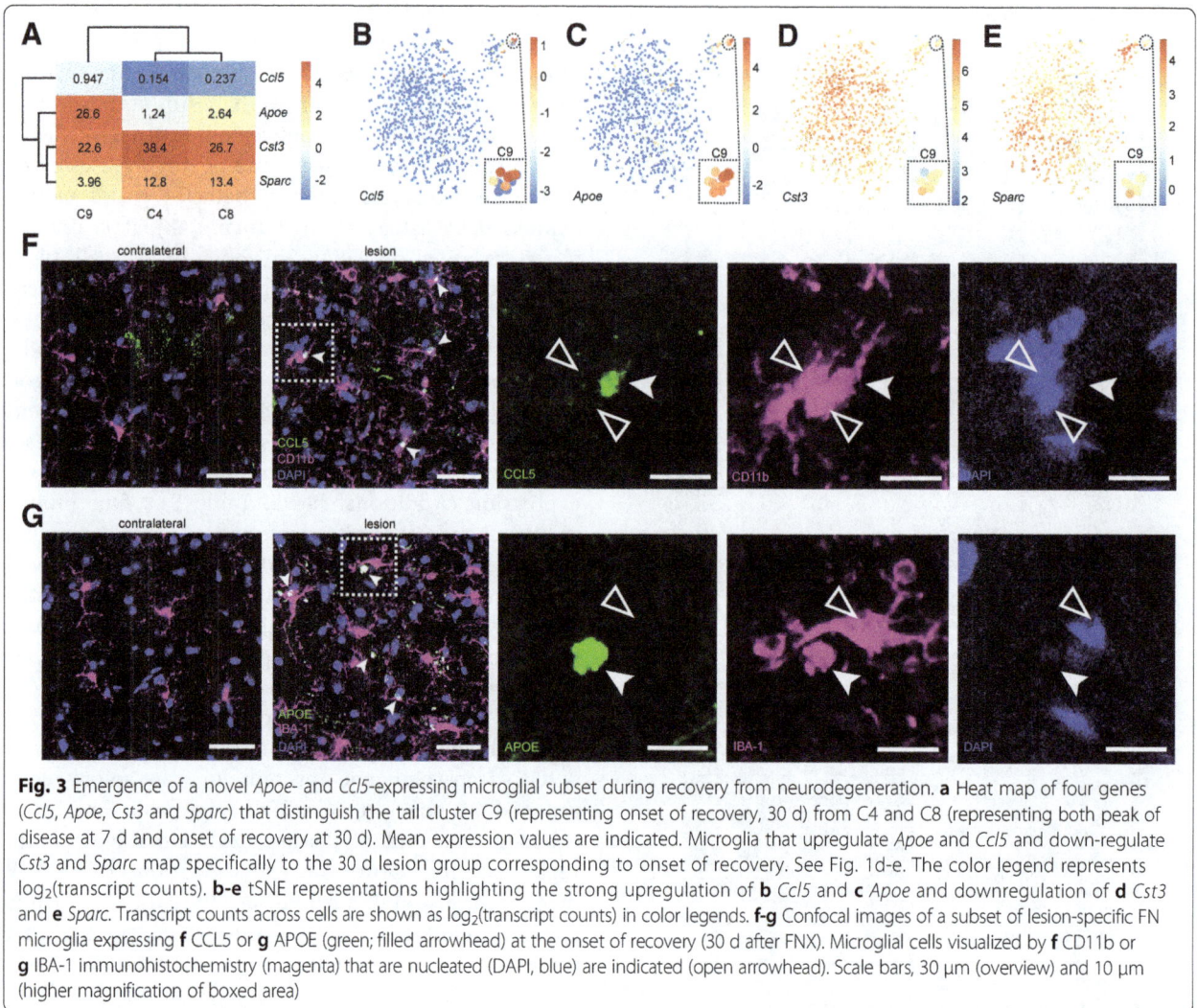

Fig. 3 Emergence of a novel *Apoe*- and *Ccl5*-expressing microglial subset during recovery from neurodegeneration. **a** Heat map of four genes (*Ccl5*, *Apoe*, *Cst3* and *Sparc*) that distinguish the tail cluster C9 (representing onset of recovery, 30 d) from C4 and C8 (representing both peak of disease at 7 d and onset of recovery at 30 d). Mean expression values are indicated. Microglia that upregulate *Apoe* and *Ccl5* and down-regulate *Cst3* and *Sparc* map specifically to the 30 d lesion group corresponding to onset of recovery. See Fig. 1d-e. The color legend represents $\log_2$(transcript counts). **b-e** tSNE representations highlighting the strong upregulation of **b** *Ccl5* and **c** *Apoe* and downregulation of **d** *Cst3* and **e** *Sparc*. Transcript counts across cells are shown as $\log_2$(transcript counts) in color legends. **f-g** Confocal images of a subset of lesion-specific FN microglia expressing **f** CCL5 or **g** APOE (green; filled arrowhead) at the onset of recovery (30 d after FNX). Microglial cells visualized by **f** CD11b or **g** IBA-1 immunohistochemistry (magenta) that are nucleated (DAPI, blue) are indicated (open arrowhead). Scale bars, 30 μm (overview) and 10 μm (higher magnification of boxed area)

However, our FNX model opens a new window for further investigation into the significance of this and other pathways during microglia-directed disease amelioration and recovery of CNS health.

Additional files

Additional file 1: Figure S1. Heat map of 101 differentially expressed genes that distinguish the cloud and tail (comprising C4, C8 and C9) transcriptomes from the FNX neurodegeneration model depicted across clusters 1 to 10 based on Benjamini-Hochberg-corrected $P < 0.05$. The color legend represents $\log_2$(transcript counts). (TIF 25531 kb)

Additional file 2: Figure S2. Gene Set Enrichment Analysis of all differentially expressed genes that distinguish the cloud and tail (comprising C4, C8 and C9) transcriptomes from the FNX neurodegeneration model depicted across clusters 1 to 10 based on Benjamini-Hochberg-corrected $P < 0.1$. The color legend represents the P-values. (TIF 25527 kb)

Additional file 3: Figure S3. MA plot of the 101 differentially expressed genes that distinguish the cloud and tail (in Fig. 1d-e) in the FNX neurodegeneration model. Genes that also distinguish the cloud and tail clusters in the FAD data set (in Fig. 2b) are indicated here as common

genes (blue). Upregulated (green) and down-regulated (red) genes with a minimum of two-fold change (Benjamini-Hochberg-corrected $P < 0.05$) and non-regulated expressed genes (gray) are shown. (TIF 25538 kb)

Additional file 4: Figure S4. Box plot of unique molecular identifiers (UMIs) detected from each single microglial cell in the FNX and FAD neurodegeneration models. (TIF 25520 kb)

Additional file 5: Table S1. Fold changes and adjusted P values of all 5820 genes included in the comparative transcriptomic analysis. (XLSX 479 kb)

Additional file 6: Table S2. Overlap of the 72 common differentially regulated genes (Fig. 2 and Table 2) with the consensus microglia gene expression signature induced by aging, primed and neurodegenerative conditions reported in Table S5 [19]. (XLSX 13 kb)

Acknowledgements

The authors thank Gen Lin for critical feedback and CEMT, University of Freiburg for excellent animal care. TLT was supported by the German Research Foundation (DFG, TA1029/1-1) and Ministry of Science, Research and the Arts of Baden-Württemberg (7532.21/2.1.6). MP is supported by the BMBF-funded competence network of multiple sclerosis (KKNMS), the Sobek Foundation, the Ernst-Jung Foundation, the DFG (SFB 992, SFB1160, SFB/TRR167, Reinhart-Koselleck-Grant) and the Ministry of Science, Research and Arts, Baden-Wuerttemberg (Sonderlinie "Neuroinflammation").

The article processing charge was funded by the German Research Foundation (DFG) and the University of Freiburg in the Open-Access Publishing funding programme.

Authors' contributions
TLT and MP conceived the study. TLT, S and JD performed the experiments and analyses. TLT, DG, and MP provided supervision. TLT and MP wrote the manuscript. All authors read and approved the final manuscript.

Competing interests
The authors declare that they have no competing interests.

Author details
[1]Institute of Neuropathology, Faculty of Medicine, University of Freiburg, Freiburg, Germany. [2]Cluster of Excellence BrainLinks-BrainTools, University of Freiburg, Freiburg, Germany. [3]Institute of Biology I, Faculty of Biology, University of Freiburg, Freiburg, Germany. [4]Max-Planck-Institute of Immunobiology and Epigenetics, Freiburg, Germany. [5]BIOSS Centre for Biological Signaling Studies, University of Freiburg, Freiburg, Germany.

References
1. Ajami B, Bennett JL, Krieger C, Tetzlaff W, Rossi FMV (2007) Local self-renewal can sustain CNS microglia maintenance and function throughout adult life. Nat Neurosci 10:1538–1543
2. Anders S, Huber W (2010) Differential expression analysis for sequence count data. Genome Biol 11:R106
3. Askew K, Li K, Olmos-Alonso A, Garcia-Moreno F, Liang Y, Richardson P et al (2017) Coupled proliferation and apoptosis maintain the rapid turnover of microglia in the adult brain. Cell Rep 18:391–405
4. Baker SC, Bauer SR, Beyer RP, Brenton JD, Bromley B, Burrill J et al (2005) The external RNA controls consortium: a progress report. Nat Meth 2:731–734
5. Butovsky O, Jedrychowski MP, Cialic R, Krasemann S, Murugaiyan G, Fanek Z et al (2015) Targeting miR-155 restores abnormal microglia and attenuates disease in SOD1 mice. Ann Neurol 77:75–99
6. Butovsky O, Jedrychowski MP, Moore CS, Cialic R, Lanser AJ, Gabriely G et al (2014) Identification of a unique TGF-β-dependent molecular and functional signature in microglia. Nat Neurosci 17:131–143
7. Canh M-Y, Serpe CJ, Sanders V, Jones KJ (2006) CD4(+) T cell-mediated facial motoneuron survival after injury: distribution pattern of cell death and rescue throughout the extent of the facial motor nucleus. J Neuroimmunol 181:93–99
8. Chiu IM, Morimoto ETA, Goodarzi H, Liao JT, O'Keeffe S, Phatnani HP et al (2013) A neurodegeneration-specific gene-expression signature of acutely isolated microglia from an amyotrophic lateral sclerosis mouse model. Cell Rep 4:385–401
9. Friedman BA, Srinivasan K, Ayalon G, Meilandt WJ, Lin H, Huntley MA et al (2018) Diverse brain myeloid expression profiles reveal distinct microglial activation states and aspects of Alzheimer's disease not evident in mouse models. Cell Rep 22:832–847
10. Füger P, Hefendehl JK, Veeraraghavalu K, Wendeln A-C, Schlosser C, Obermüller U et al (2017) Microglia turnover with aging and in an Alzheimer's model via long-term in vivo single-cell imaging. Nat Neurosci 20:1371–1376
11. Ginhoux F, Greter M, Leboeuf M, Nandi S, See P, Gokhan S et al (2010) Fate mapping analysis reveals that adult microglia derive from primitive macrophages. Science 330:841–845
12. Gomez Perdiguero E, Klapproth K, Schulz C, Busch K, Azzoni E, Crozet L et al (2015) Tissue-resident macrophages originate from yolk-sac-derived erythro-myeloid progenitors. Nature 518:547–551
13. Gómez-Nicola D, Fransen NL, Suzzi S, Perry VH (2013) Regulation of microglial proliferation during chronic neurodegeneration. J Neurosci 33:2481–2493
14. Grabert K, Michoel T, Karavolos MH, Clohisey S, Baillie JK, Stevens MP et al (2016) Microglial brain region-dependent diversity and selective regional sensitivities to aging. Nat Neurosci 19:504–516
15. Grün D, Kester L, van Oudenaarden A (2014) Validation of noise models for single-cell transcriptomics. Nat Meth. 11:637–640
16. Grün D, Muraro MJ, Boisset J-C, Wiebrands K, Lyubimova A, Dharmadhikari G et al (2016) De novo prediction of stem cell identity using single-cell transcriptome data. Cell Stem Cell 19:266–277
17. Gyoneva S, Ransohoff RM (2015) Inflammatory reaction after traumatic brain injury: therapeutic potential of targeting cell-cell communication by chemokines. Trends Pharmacol Sci 36:471–480
18. Hashimshony T, Senderovich N, Avital G, Klochendler A, de Leeuw Y, Anavy L et al (2016) CEL-Seq2: sensitive highly-multiplexed single-cell RNA-Seq. Genome Biol 17:77
19. Holtman IR, Raj DD, Miller JA, Schaafsma W, Yin Z, Brouwer N et al (2015) Induction of a common microglia gene expression signature by aging and neurodegenerative conditions: a co-expression meta-analysis. Acta Neuropathol Commun 3:31
20. Jung S, Aliberti J, Graemmel P, Sunshine MJ, Kreutzberg GW, Sher A et al (2000) Analysis of Fractalkine receptor CX3CR1 function by targeted deletion and green fluorescent protein reporter gene insertion. Mol Cell Biol 20:4106–4114
21. Keren-Shaul H, Spinrad A, Weiner A, Matcovitch-Natan O, Dvir-Szternfeld R, Ulland TK et al (2017) A Unique Microglia Type Associated with Restricting Development of Alzheimer's Disease. Cell 169:1276–1290.e17
22. Kierdorf K, Erny D, Goldmann T, Sander V, Schulz C, Gomez Perdiguero E et al (2013) Microglia emerge from erythromyeloid precursors via Pu.1- and Irf8-dependent pathways. Nat Neurosci 16:273–280
23. Krasemann S, Madore C, Cialic R, Baufeld C, Calcagno N, Fatimy El R et al (2017) The TREM2-APOE pathway drives the transcriptional phenotype of dysfunctional microglia in neurodegenerative diseases. Immunity 47:566–581
24. Kucukdereli H, Allen NJ, Lee AT, Feng A, Ozlu MI, Conatser LM et al (2011) Control of excitatory CNS synaptogenesis by astrocyte-secreted proteins Hevin and SPARC. Proc Natl Acad Sci U S A 108:E440–E449
25. Lavrnja I, Smiljanic K, Savic D, Mladenovic-Djordjevic A, Tesovic K, Kanazir S et al (2017) Expression profiles of cholesterol metabolism-related genes are altered during development of experimental autoimmune encephalomyelitis in the rat spinal cord. Sci Rep 7:2702
26. Lawson LJ, Perry VH, Dri P, Gordon S (1990) Heterogeneity in the distribution and morphology of microglia in the normal adult mouse brain. Neuroscience 39:151–170
27. Lawson LJ, Perry VH, Gordon S (1992) Turnover of resident microglia in the normal adult mouse brain. Neuroscience 48:405–415
28. Li H, Durbin R (2010) Fast and accurate long-read alignment with Burrows-Wheeler transform. Bioinformatics 26:589–595
29. Matcovitch-Natan O, Winter DR, Giladi A, Vargas Aguilar S, Spinrad A, Sarrazin S et al (2016) Microglia development follows a stepwise program to regulate brain homeostasis. Science 353:aad8670
30. Mathys H, Adaikkan C, Gao F, Young JZ, Manet E, Hemberg M et al (2017) Temporal tracking of microglia activation in neurodegeneration at single-cell resolution. Cell Rep 21:366–380
31. Meyer LR, Zweig AS, Hinrichs AS, Karolchik D, Kuhn RM, Wong M et al (2013) The UCSC genome browser database: extensions and updates 2013. Nucleic Acids Res 41:D64–D69
32. Mildner A, Schlevogt B, Kierdorf K, Böttcher C, Erny D, Kummer MP et al (2011) Distinct and non-redundant roles of microglia and myeloid subsets in mouse models of Alzheimer's disease. J Neurosci 31:11159–11171
33. Mildner A, Schmidt H, Nitsche M, Merkler D, Hanisch U-K, Mack M et al (2007) Microglia in the adult brain arise from Ly-6ChiCCR2+ monocytes only under defined host conditions. Nat Neurosci 10:1544–1553
34. Mrdjen D, Pavlovic A, Hartmann FJ, Schreiner B, Utz SG, Leung BP et al (2018) High-dimensional single-cell mapping of central nervous system immune cells reveals distinct myeloid subsets in health, aging, and disease. Immunity 48:380–386
35. Nimmerjahn A, Kirchhoff F, Helmchen F (2005) Resting microglial cells are highly dynamic surveillants of brain parenchyma in vivo. Science 308:1314–1318
36. Olah M, Patrick E, Villani A-C, Xu J, White CC, Ryan KJ et al (2018) A transcriptomic atlas of aged human microglia. Nat Commun 9:539
37. Olmos-Alonso A, Schetters STT, Sri S, Askew K, Mancuso R, Vargas-Caballero M et al (2016) Pharmacological targeting of CSF1R inhibits microglial proliferation and prevents the progression of Alzheimer's-like pathology. Brain 139:891–907
38. Prinz M, Priller J (2014) Microglia and brain macrophages in the molecular age: from origin to neuropsychiatric disease. Nat Rev Neurosci 15:300–312
39. Prinz M, Priller J, Sisodia SS, Ransohoff RM (2011) Heterogeneity of CNS

myeloid cells and their roles in neurodegeneration. Nat Neurosci 14: 1227–1235

40. Savas JN, Wang Y-Z, DeNardo LA, Martinez-Bartolome S, McClatchy DB, Hark TJ et al (2017) Amyloid accumulation drives proteome-wide alterations in mouse models of Alzheimer's disease-like pathology. Cell Rep 21:2614–2627

41. Shi Y, Yamada K, Liddelow SA, Smith ST, Zhao L, Luo W et al (2017) ApoE4 markedly exacerbates tau-mediated neurodegeneration in a mouse model of tauopathy. Nature 549:523–527

42. Shin S, Walz KA, Archambault AS, Sim J, Bollman BP, Koenigsknecht-Talboo J et al (2014) Apolipoprotein E mediation of neuro-inflammation in a murine model of multiple sclerosis. J Neuroimmunol 271:8–17

43. Tay TL, Mai D, Dautzenberg J, Fernández-Klett F, Lin G, Sagar et al (2017) A new fate mapping system reveals context-dependent random or clonal expansion of microglia. Nat Neurosci 20:793–803

44. van der Maaten L, Hinton G (2008) Visualizing data using t-SNE. J Mach Learn Res 9:2579–2605

45. Yu G, He Q-Y (2016) ReactomePA: an R/Bioconductor package for reactome pathway analysis and visualization. Mol BioSyst 12:477–479

46. Yu G, Wang L-G, Han Y, He Q-Y (2012) clusterProfiler: an R package for comparing biological themes among gene clusters. OMICS 16:284–287

47. Zhang Y, Chen K, Sloan SA, Bennett ML, Scholze AR, O'Keeffe S et al (2014) An RNA-sequencing transcriptome and splicing database of glia, neurons, and vascular cells of the cerebral cortex. J Neurosci 34:11929–11947

48. Zhang Y, Sloan SA, Clarke LE, Caneda C, Plaza CA, Blumenthal PD et al (2016) Purification and characterization of progenitor and mature human astrocytes reveals transcriptional and functional differences with mouse. Neuron 89:37–53

12

Decoding the synaptic dysfunction of bioactive human AD brain soluble Aβ to inspire novel therapeutic avenues for Alzheimer's disease

Shaomin Li[*] ⓘ, Ming Jin, Lei Liu, Yifan Dang, Beth L. Ostaszewski and Dennis J. Selkoe

Abstract

Pathologic, biochemical and genetic evidence indicates that accumulation and aggregation of amyloid β-proteins (Aβ) is a critical factor in the pathogenesis of Alzheimer's disease (AD). Several therapeutic interventions attempting to lower Aβ have failed to ameliorate cognitive decline in patients with clinical AD significantly, but most such approaches target only one or two facets of Aβ production/clearance/toxicity and do not consider the heterogeneity of human Aβ species. As synaptic dysfunction may be among the earliest deficits in AD, we used hippocampal long-term potentiation (LTP) as a sensitive indicator of the early neurotoxic effects of Aβ species. Here we confirmed prior findings that soluble Aβ oligomers, much more than fibrillar amyloid plaque cores or Aβ monomers, disrupt synaptic function. Interestingly, not all (84%) human AD brain extracts are able to inhibit LTP and the degree of LTP impairment by AD brain extracts does not correlate with Aβ levels detected by standard ELISAs. Bioactive AD brain extracts also induce neurotoxicity in iPSC-derived human neurons. Shorter forms of Aβ (including $A\beta_{1-37}$, $A\beta_{1-38}$, $A\beta_{1-39}$), pre-Aβ APP fragments (-30 to -1) and N-terminally extended Aβs (-30 to $+40$) each showed much less synaptotoxicity than longer Aβs ($A\beta_{1-42}$ - $A\beta_{1-46}$). We found that antibodies which target the N-terminus, not the C-terminus, efficiently rescued Aβ oligomer-impaired LTP and oligomer-facilitated LTD. Our data suggest that preventing soluble Aβ oligomer formation and targeting their N-terminal residues with antibodies could be an attractive combined therapeutic approach.

Keywords: Alzheimer's disease, Amyloid-beta protein, Synaptic plasticity, Long-term potentiation, Oligomers

Introduction

Alzheimer's disease (AD) is a neurodegenerative disorder characterized by progressive and irreversible cognitive decline. The pathological hallmarks of AD are the aberrant deposition of extracellular senile plaques comprised of amyloid-beta (Aβ) peptides and intracellular neurofibrillary tangles composed of altered forms of the tau protein. A growing body of evidence from genetic, in vivo imaging and biochemical studies has demonstrated that accumulation of oligomeric, diffusible assemblies of Aβ peptides, rather than mature amyloid fibrils, is the earliest pathogenic event in the ontogeny of AD [7, 43, 62, 70, 71].

Aβ peptides are generated throughout life from the amyloid precursor protein (APP) via a sequential, two-step proteolytic cleavage: first by β-site APP-cleaving enzyme 1 (BACE1), also called β-secretase, and then by the presenilin/γ-secretase complex [36, 49, 80]. Transgenic APP mutant mouse models showed that increasing β- or γ-secretase activity promotes the production of pathogenic Aβ and induces AD-like pathology, while decreasing their activities by inhibitors can reduce brain Aβ levels and ameliorate AD neuropathology and resultant behavioral deficits [9, 13]. Experimentally, the deposition of Aβ can be accelerated in the brains of APP-transgenic mice after intracerebral or intraperitoneal injection with Aβ aggregate-containing brain homogenate. This effect can be

* Correspondence: sli11@bwh.harvard.edu
Ann Romney Center for Neurologic Diseases, Department of Neurology, Brigham and Women's Hospital and Harvard Medical School, 60 Fenwood Road, Boston, MA 02115, USA

prevented by immunodepletion of Aβ from the injected materials, thereby supporting the direct role of Aβ as the seeding agent in this process [12, 40].

Symptomatically, the accumulation of Aβ is thought to play a fundamental role in triggering synaptic dysfunction in neurons and leading to their eventual loss. Synaptic failure is an early event in pathogenesis that can be detected in patients with mild cognitive impairment [2, 60]. Experimentally, soluble Aβ oligomers have been found to selectively block hippocampal long-term potentiation (LTP), widely believed to underlie learning and memory [26, 28, 29, 64, 71]. The impairment of synaptic plasticity can be detected before Aβ deposits in plaques in mouse models of AD [15, 31]. Importantly, active and passive Aβ immunotherapy has been shown to protect against the neuropathology and cognitive deficits observed in APP transgenic models of AD [20, 42] and prevent the soluble Aβ oligomers induced LTP impairment [27, 28].

Over the past two decades, several clinical trials that have attempted to reduce Aβ production by decreasing β- or γ-secretase activity or directly targeting Aβ by immunotherapy did not meet pre-specified clinical endpoints in mild to moderate AD patients, perhaps due to the presence of well-established amyloid and tau neuropathology and the complexity of accessing the most pathogenic Aβ species. The specific Aβ species that are most directly related to AD-type neurodegeneration in humans and precede dementia of the Alzheimer type have not been clearly identified. In this regard, numerous studies, including ours, have focused on soluble Aβ oligomers made from synthetic $Aβ_{40/42}$ peptides, secreted by FAD-mutant APP-expressing cells, or isolated directly from human (AD) cortex as to their effects on the hippocampal LTP and long-term synaptic depression (LTD), but the results have been variable and difficult to distil into a central conclusion. Here, we systematically compare the different sources, aggregation states of Aβ as well as various APP fragments that contain Aβ sequences and probe the experimental conditions which can affect the response of hippocampus to the complex array of AD-relevant assemblies.

Materials and methods
Mice
The Harvard Medical School and Brigham Women's hospital Standard Committee on Animals approved all experiments involving mice used for electrophysiology and biochemical assays. All mice (male and female) contained a mixed background of C57Bl/6 and 129. Animals were housed in a temperature-controlled room on a 12-h light/12-h dark cycle and had ad libitum access to food and water.

Hippocampal slice preparation
Mice (C57BL/6 × 129) were euthanized with Isoflurane at 2 to 3 months of age. Brains was quickly removed and submerged in ice-cold oxygenated sucrose-replaced artificial cerebrospinal fluid (ACSF) cutting solution (in mM) (206 sucrose, 2 KCl, 2 $MgSO_4$, 1.25 NaH_2PO_4, 1 $CaCl_2$, 1 $MgCl_2$, 26 $NaHCO_3$, 10 D-glucose, pH 7.4, 315 mOsm). Transverse slices (350 μm thickness) from the middle portion of each hippocampus were cut with a vibroslicer. After dissection, slices were incubated in ACSF that contained the following (in mM): 124 NaCl, 2 KCl, 2 $MgSO_4$, 1.25 NaH_2PO_4, 2.5 $CaCl_2$, 26 $NaHCO_3$, 10 D-glucose, pH 7.4, 310 mOsm, in which they were allowed to recover for at least 90 min before recording. A single slice was then transferred to the recording chamber and submerged beneath continuously perfusing ACSF that had been saturated with 95% O_2 and 5% CO_2. Slices were incubated in the recording chamber for 20 min before stimulation under room temperature (~ 26 °C).

Electrophysiological recordings
We used standard procedures to record field excitatory postsynaptic potentials (fEPSP) in the CA1 region of the hippocampus. A bipolar stimulating electrode (FHC Inc., Bowdoin, ME) was placed in the Schaffer collaterals to deliver test and conditioning stimuli. A borosilicate glass recording electrode filled with ACSF was positioned in stratum radiatum of CA1, 200~ 300 μm from the stimulating electrode. fEPSP in the CA1 region were induced by test stimuli at 0.05 Hz with an intensity that elicited a fEPSP amplitude 40–50% of maximum. Test responses were recorded for 30–60 min prior to beginning the experiment to assure stability of the response. Once a stable test response was attained, experimental treatments (Aβ species and/or antibodies) were added to the 10 mL ACSF perfusate, and a baseline was recorded for an additional 30 min. For the Anti-Aβ antibodies experiments, the antibodies: 3D6 (3 μg/ml), 266 (3 μg/ml), 82E1 (3 μg/ml), 6E10 (2 μg/ml), 4G8 (1 μg/ml), 2G3 (3 μg/ml), 21F12 (3 μg/ml) or R1282 (3 μg/ml) were added to the AD brain extract aliquots incubated with mixing for 30 min, then adding to the mixture to brain slice perfusion buffer. To induce LTP, two consecutive trains (1 s) of stimuli at 100 Hz separated by 20 s were applied to the slices, a protocol that induced LTP lasting approximately 1.5 h in wild-type mice of this genetic background. To induce LTD, 300 pulses were delivered at 1 Hz. The field potentials were amplified 100x using an Axon Instruments 200B amplifier and digitized with Digidata 1322A. Data were sampled at 10 kHz and filtered at 2 kHz. Traces were obtained by pClamp 9.2 and analyzed using the Clampfit 9.2 program. LTP and LTD values reported throughout were measured at 60 min after the conditioning stimulus unless stated otherwise.

Two-tailed Student's t-test and one-way analysis of variance (ANOVA) were used to determine statistical significance.

Human brain homogenate preparation

Homogenates of human brains were prepared as described elsewhere [64, 81]. Frozen brain tissue collected at Massachusetts Alzheimer's Disease Research Center (MADRC Neuropathology Core, Harvard, MA, USA) and Brigham and Women's Hospital under institutional review board-approved protocols. Frozen samples of temporal or frontal cortex (1 g) were allowed to thaw on ice, chopped into small pieces with a razor blade, and then homogenized with 25 strokes of a Dounce homogenizer (Fisher, Ottawa, ON, Canada) in 4 ml ice-cold 20 mM Tris–HCl, pH 7.4, containing 150 mM NaCl (Tris-buffered saline (TBS)) and protease inhibitors. Water-soluble Aβ was separated from membrane-bound and plaque Aβ by centrifugation at 175,000×g and 4 °C in a TLA 100 rotor (Beckman Coulter, Fullerton, CA, USA) for 30 min, and the supernatant (referred to as TBS extract) aliquoted and stored at − 80 °C. The ethical body approving this study was the Partners Institutional Review Board of the Partners Human Research Committee.

Production of induced neurons (iNs) from human induced pluripotent cells (iPSCs)

The YZ1 iPSC line was obtained from UCONN stem cell core [84] and used to prepare neurogenin 2 (Ngn2)-induced human neurons [86]. iPSCs were maintained in media containing DMEM/F12, Knockout Serum Replacement, pencillin/streptomycin/glutamine, MEM-NEAA, and 2-mercaptoethanol (all from Invitrogen, Carlsbad, CA) with addition of 10 μg/mL bFGF (Millipore, Billerica, MA) directly prior to media application. Neuronal differentiation was performed via doxycycline induced Neurogenin 2 system [86]. iPSCs were plated at a density of 95,000 cells/cm^2 for viral infection. Lentiviruses were obtained from Alstem with "ultrapure titres" and used at the following concentrations: pTet-O-NGN2-puro: 0.1 μl/50,000 cells; Tet-O-FUW-eGFP: 0.05 μl/ 50,000 cells; Fudelta GW-rtTA: 0.11 μl/50,000 cells. To induce Neurogenin 2 expression doxycycline is added on "iN day 1" at a concentration of 2 μg/ml. On iN day 2 puromycin is added at 10 mg/ml and is maintained in the media always thereafter. On iN day 4, cells were plated at 50,000 cells/well on matrigel (BD Biosciences, San Jose, CA)-coated Greiner 96 well microclear plates and maintained in media consisting of Neurobasal medium (Gibco), Glutamax, 20% Dextrose, MEM NEAA with B27, with BDNF, CNTF, GDNF (PeprpTech, Rocky Hill, NJ) each at a concentration of 10 ng/ml. At iN day 14 neurite number and expression of neural markers had reached near maximal levels. Thus, for experiments investigating the effects of AD brain extracts on neuronal viability iNs were used at iN day 21, a time point when iNs were fully mature.

Addition of AD brain extract to induced neurons (iNs) and live-cell imaging

Production and characterization of human brain extracts and induced neurons (iNs) from human induced pluripotent cells (iPSCs) as described previously [21]. Aliquots (two, 0.5 ml) of mock-immunodepleted (AD) or AW7-immunodepleted brain (ID-AD) extracts were thawed on ice for 30–60 min, vortexed, centrifuged at 16,000 g for 2 min, and buffer exchanged into neurobasal medium supplemented with B27/Glutamax using HiTrap 5 ml desalting column (GE Healthcare, Milwaukee, WI). AD and ID-AD extracts (1 ml) were applied to a desalting column using a 1 ml syringe at a flow rate of ~ 1 ml/min and eluted with culture medium using a peristaltic pump. Then, 0.5 ml fractions were collected. Prior experimentation revealed that the bulk of Aβ eluted in fractions 4 and 5. These two fractions were pooled – this pool is referred to as "exchanged extract". A small portion (50 μl) of the exchanged extract was taken for Aβ analysis and the reminder used in iN experiments.

Approximately 7 h prior to exchanging AD and ID-AD extracts into culture medium, iN day 21 neurons were placed in an IncuCyte Zoom live-cell imaging instrument (Essen Bioscience, Ann Arbor, MI). Four fields per well of a 96 well plate were imaged every 2 h for a total of 6 h. This analysis was used to define neurite length and branch points prior to addition of brain extracts. Buffer exchanged brain extracts were diluted 1:2 with culture medium. Half of the medium on iNs was removed (~ 100 μl) and replaced with 100 μl of 1:2 diluted buffer-exchanged extract – yielding a 1:4 diluted extract on iNs. Similarly, treatments using 1:8 and 1:16 diluted extracts were done in a similar manner. For long-term, continuous imaging, images of four fields per well were acquired every 2 h for 3 days (starting at iN day 21). Whole image sets were analyzed using Incucyte Zoom 2016A Software (Essen Bioscience, Ann Arbor, MI). The analysis job Neural Track was used to automatically define neurite processes and cell bodies based on phase contrast images. Typical settings were: Segmentation Mode - Brightness; Segmentation Adjustment - 1.2; Cell body cluster filter - minimum 500 μm^2; Neurite Filtering - Best; Neurite sensitivity - 0.4; Neurite Width - 2 μm. Total neurite length (in millimeters) and number of branch points were quantified and normalized to the average value measured during the 6 h' period prior to sample addition. Total neurite length is the summed length of neurites that extend from cell bodies, and number of branch points is the number of intersections of the neurites in image field.

Size exclusion chromatography (SEC)

Whole TBS extracts (250 µl) or their void volume SEC fractions (500 µl) were injected into either a Superdex 75 (10/30HR) column or a Superdex 200 (10/300GL) column (GE Healthcare) and eluted at a flow rate of 0.8 ml/min with 50 mm ammonium acetate, pH 8.5. The 1 ml fractions were collected; 0.5 ml of this material was used for ELISA, and the other 0.5 ml was lyophilized and used for Western blotting [65]. Samples were electrophoresed on 26-well, 4–12% polyacrylamide Bis-Tris gels using MES running buffer (Invitrogen), and proteins were transferred to 0.2 µm nitrocellulose filters, the filters microwaved, and Aβ detected using a mixture of mAbs 2G3,21F12 (each at 1 µg/ml) and 0.5 µg/ml of mAb 6E10. Membranes were rinsed and incubated for 1 h with fluorescein-conjugated goat anti-rabbit or anti-mouse IgG (1:5,000; Invitrogen), and bands visualized using a LiCor Odyssey Infrared System.

Cerebrospinal fluid sample collection and processing

Samples were collected from the L3/L4 interspace and transferred into nonabsorbing (polypropylene) tubes. CSF samples were mixed by gently inverting three or four times and then centrifuged at 400×g for 10 min. The crystal-clear supernatant was removed to a polypropylene tube and centrifuged at 2,000×g at 4 °C for 10 min, and aliquots of the supernatant were transferred to polypropylene storage tubes and stored at − 80 °C.

Cellular Aβ (7PA2 CM) preparations

Secreted human Aβ peptides were collected and prepared from the conditioned media (CM) of a CHO cell line (7PA2) that stably expresses human APP751 containing the V717F AD mutation [52] Cells were grown in Dulbecco's modified Eagle's medium (DMEM) containing 10% fetal bovine serum, 1% penicillin/streptomycin, 2 mM L-glutamine, and 200 mg/ml G418 for selection. Upon reaching ∼ 95% confluency, the cells were washed and cultured overnight (∼ 15 h) in serum-free medium. CM was collected, spun at 1500×g to remove dead cells and debris, and stored at 4 °C. The CM was concentrated 10-fold with a YM-3 Centricon filter [73]. The concentrated CM was pooled and aliquoted to produce a large number of identical medium samples for experiments. These concentrated 7PA2 CM aliquots were stored at − 80 °C until use. To prepare the N-terminal extension of Aβs, 7PA2 CM was first incubated with DE23 anion-exchange cellulose to bind and remove the highly charged APPs while leaving the various 4–17 kDa Aβ-immunoreactive products in solution. This APP pre-clearing step generated CM that could then be quantitatively immunodepleted of the NTE species with the pre-β antiserum. C8, an antiserum directed to the APP C-terminus, served as a negative control since it did not immunodeplete any of the Aβ-containing species found in 7PA2 CM.

Preparation of synthetic Aβ, including S26C dimers and dityrosine dimers

Synthetic Aβ(1–36), Aβ (1–37), Aβ(1–38), Aβ(1–39), Aβ(1–40), Aβ(1–42), Aβ (1–43), Aβ(1–45) and Aβ(1–46) all were purchased from AnaSpec (Fremont, CA). Synthetic Aβ(1–16) and Aβ (17–42) were purchased from rPeptide (Watkinsville, GA). Monomeric Aβ was prepared as described previously [72]. Aβ S26C-dimers were synthesized and purified using reverse-phase high performance liquid chromatography. Briefly, Aβ(1–40) was dissolved at 2 mg/ml in 50 mM Tris–HCl, pH 8.5, containing 7 M guanidinium HCl and 5 mM ethylenediamine tetraacetic acid, and incubated at room temperature overnight. The sample was then centrifuged at 16,000×g for 30 min and the upper 90% of supernatant applied to a Superdex 75 10/300 size exclusion column (GE Healthcare Biosciences, Pittsburgh, PA, USA), eluted at 0.5 ml/minute with 50 mM ammonium bicarbonate, pH 8.5, and absorbance monitored at 280 nm. Fractions of 0.5 ml were collected. The UV absorbance at 275 nm was determined for the peak fraction and the concentration of Aβ determined using ε_{275} = 1,361/M/cm [51]. Dityrosine cross-linked Aβ dimer $((A\beta(1–40))_{DiY})$ was prepared as reported previously and SEC-isolated as described above. The UV absorbance at 283 nm of the dimer peak fraction was measured and the concentration of DiY dimer determined using ε_{283} = 6,244/M/cm. $(A\beta(1–40)S26C)_2$ was prepared as described previously and the dimer was SEC-isolated as outlined above. The UV absorbance at 275 nm of the $(A\beta(1–40)S26C)_2$ peak was measured and the concentration of this dimer determined using ε_{275} = 2,722/M/cm .

Following collection and concentration determination, monomer and dimer peak fractions of the respective oligomer preparations were diluted to 48.5 µM and aliquots (20 µl) were immediately frozen on dry ice and then stored at − 80 °C. Once thawed, aliquots were used immediately either for characterization (using analytical SEC and electron microscopy) or as standards in the MSD or Erenna immunoassays.

Preparation of synthetic pre-Aβ and N-terminally extended Aβ peptides

Synthetic preAβ and N-Terminally Extended Aβ preparation were similar to previously described [68]. Five variants of preAβ and NTE-Aβ were produced with extensions of 10, 20, or 30 residues from the APP sequence added to the N-terminus of $A\beta_{1–40}$. The genes for N-terminally extended variants (by 10, 20, or 30 residues from APP) were produced through a stepwise extension of the synthetic $A\beta_{1–40}$ by PCR using oligonucleotides with the desired extensions with *E. coli* preferred codons. Aβ$_{1-40}$ and the N-terminally extended variants were expressed in *E. coli* (BL2 DE3 PLysS Star). The peptides were purified using ion exchange and size exclusion steps. The purity of the peptides was confirmed by SDS PAGE, RP-HPLC and MALDI-TOF mass spectrometry. Purified peptides were stored as lyophilized aliquots.

Aβ1-x, Aβx-40 and Aβx-42 enzyme-linked immunosorbent assays (ELISA)

Assays utilized the Meso Scale Discovery (MSD) platform and reagents from Meso Scale (Rockville, MD). MULTI-ARRAY® 96 well small-spot black microplates were coated with 3 µg/ml of monoclonal antibody 266 in tris buffered saline (TBS) and incubated at RT for 18 h. Monoclonal antibody 266 recognizes the mid-region of Aβ, thus enabling detection of both N- and C-terminally heterogeneous Aβ species. Binding sites that were unoccupied were blocked in 150 µl of 5% Blocker A (MSD) in TBS containing 0.05% tween 20 (TBST) and agitated at 400 rpm for 1 h and 22 ° C. Plates were washed 3 times with TBST and samples, and standards were applied in duplicate, and agitated at 400 rpm for 2 h and RT. After the capture phase, plates were washed 3 times with TBST and incubated with biotinylated antibody. To allow the detection of Aβ1-x or Aβx-42, we used biotinylated 3D6 (1 µg/ml) or 21F12 (1 µg/ml), respectively. Simultaneously, 1 µg/ml of the reporter reagent (SULFO-TAG Labelled Streptavidin) was added in ELISA diluent and incubated at RT with gentle agitation for 2 h. Finally, plates were washed 3 times with TBST and 2× MSD read buffer (150 µl per well) was applied to allow for electrochemiluminesence detection. A SECTOR imager was used to measure the intensity of emitted light, thus allowing quantitative measurement of analytes present in the samples.

Statistical analysis

The LTP and LTD values reported throughout were measured at 60 min after the conditioning stimulus unless stated otherwise. Results were expressed as means ± SEM from at least 4 independent biological samples. Two-tailed Student's t-test and one-way analysis of variance (ANOVA) were used to determine statistical significance throughout. For live-cell imaging experiments, samples and treatments were coded and tested in a blinded manner. Differences between groups were tested with One-way analysis of variance (ANOVA) with Bonferroni *post-hoc* tests or student's *t*-tests (* $p < 0.05$, ** $p < 0.01$, and *** $p < 0.001$).

Results

Soluble AD brain extracts rich in aqueously-soluble Aβ inhibit hippocampal LTP

We previously reported that soluble, human brain-derived Aβ oligomers inhibit hippocampal LTP [35, 64]. We first confirmed that some soluble Aβ-rich extracts of neuropathologically validated human (AD) cerebral cortex robustly and consistently inhibit hippocampal LTP while not altering basal synaptic transmission before the high-frequency stimulus (HFS) (control brain that were from age-matched neurologically normal human cortical extracts: $158 \pm 6\%$, $n = 8$ vs. AD brain: $130 \pm 4\%$, n = 8; p < 0.001) (Fig. 1a). However, cortical extracts from some other AD brains prepared using the identical procedure failed to inhibit LTP (control: $169 \pm 12\%$, $n = 6$, vs. AD: $165 \pm 9\%$, $n = 7$; $p > 0.05$) (Fig. 1b). Several other AD brain extracts also did not inhibit hippocampal LTP (4 out of 25, i.e. 16% of total tested AD brain. Figure 1c, red), while all non-AD brain extract did not impair LTP (Fig. 1c, blue). All clinical and neuropathological data of the AD patients and controls were listed on Additional file 1: Table S1. To verify whether the AD brain extracts that inhibited LTPs were soluble Aβ-dependent, we chose 7 AD brain extract samples that inhibited hippocampal LTP and immunodepleted their soluble Aβ by a high-titer polyclonal antiserum (AW7) to human Aβ (Additional file 1: Figure S1). Consistent with our previous finding [64], the immunodepleted AD brain extracts failed to inhibit LTP (Fig. 1d).

To further explore whether the AD brain extract-mediated impairment of LTP is dependent on the level of soluble Aβ [64], we plotted the mean LTP levels vs. the mean Aβ$_{x-42}$ and Aβ$_{x-40}$ concentrations determined by specific ELISAs (Fig. 1e, f). The impairment of LTP was weakly correlated with either [Aβ$_{x-42}$] ($R^2 = 0.04$, $p > 0.05$) or [Aβ$_{x-40}$] ($R^2 = 0.16$, p > 0.05). These results suggest that although AD brain Aβ levels are significantly higher than control brain levels, LTP impairment does not correlate directly with the total brain tissue Aβ level as detected by ELISA (Fig. 1e, f). Collectively, these results confirm previous findings that Aβ per se, not other components of the AD brain extracts, are responsible for the LTP impairment, but raise the possibility that Aβ conformation or assembly state, not simply the total Aβ monomer levels, may be another factor for its bioactivity.

Aβ oligomer-rich bioactive AD brain extracts induce neurotoxicity in iPSC-derived human neurons

To further verify whether bioactive AD brain extracts that inhibit hippocampal LTP can induce other forms of neurotoxicity, we employed a live-cell imaging paradigm using time-lapse video microscopy on an Essen IncuCyte apparatus to monitor the effects of the same AD brain extracts on iPSC-derived, neurogenin-induced human

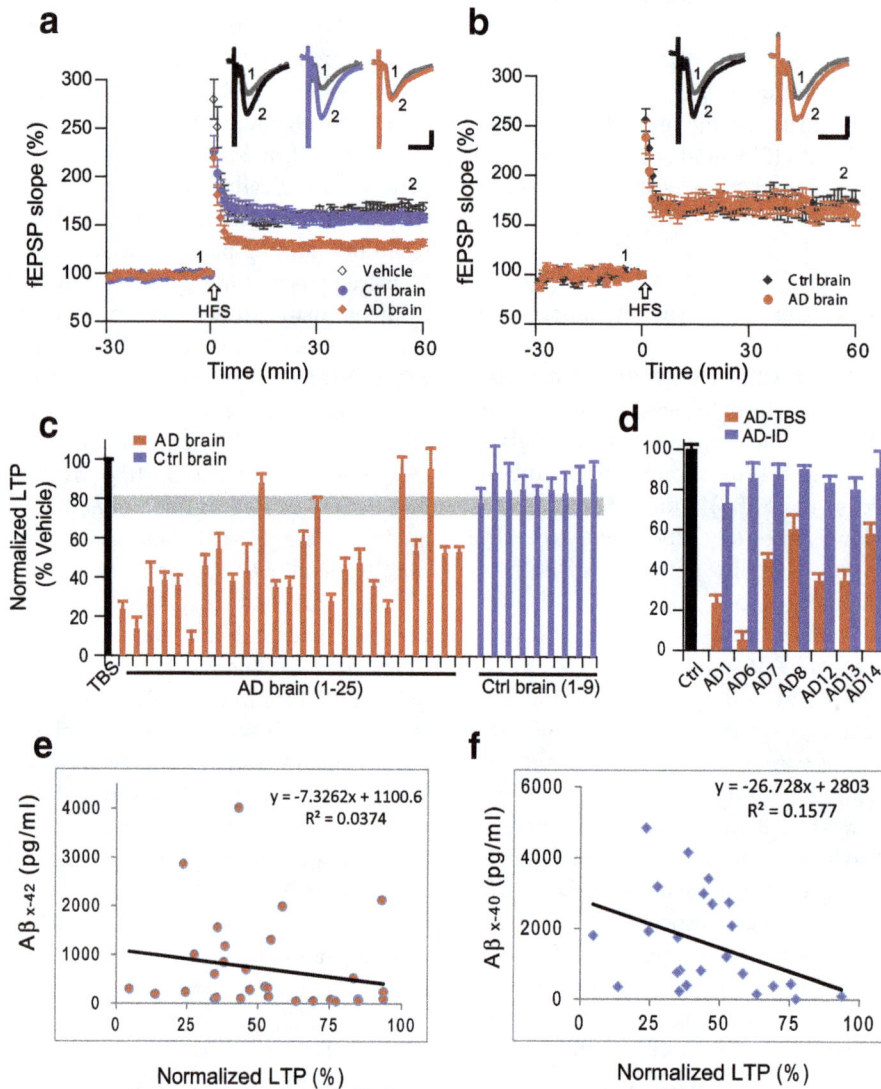

Fig. 1 Soluble Aβ extracted by homogenization in TBS from Alzheimer's disease brain alters hippocampal long-term potentiation. (**a**) LTP induction after treatment with vehicle (black open circles), control brain TBS extract (blue circles) and AD brain TBS extract (red diamonds) from one AD patient. (**b**) LTP after treatment with TBS extracts made from another control brain (black diamonds) or another AD brain (red circles). (**c**) Summary data of LTP results with one representative run with plain TBS buffer (black bar), 25 AD brain TBS extracts (red) and 9 control (non-AD) brain TBS extracts (blue). All LTP results represent values at 60 min post-HFS normalized to vehicle alone at that time point. Gray horizontal bar indicates the lowest LTP level from control brain. (**d**) LTP summary data of the AD TBS extracts (red) and their respective immunodepleted extracts (blue). (**e,f**) Correlations between LTP levels at 60 min and the respective [Aβ$_{x-42}$] (**e**) and [Aβ$_{x-40}$] (**f**) levels in the AD TBS extracts

neurons [86]. Consistent with the Aβ-impaired synaptic function, a bioactive AD brain extract (Fig. 1a) also induced marked deficits of neurites as regards their length (Fig. 2b: red) and branch point number (Fig. 2c: red), both of which were reduced 50–60% compared to identical treatment with a control brain extract (Fig. 2b, c: black). Applying the Aβ-immunodepleted aliquot from this bioactive AD brain extract, the neurite length and branch point number were normal (Fig 2a; Fig. 2b, c - tan). Interestingly, when we applied a non-bioactive AD brain extract (Fig. 1b) to the iPSC neurons, neurite length and branch points remained unchanged (Fig 2a; Fig. 2b, c -

blue), indicating that by both mouse hippocampal slice LTP and this human neuron assay, the inactive extract contains very low or no neurotoxic species. The Aβ-immunodepleted aliquot of this inactive AD sample was likewise inactive, as expected (Fig. 2b, c - light blue). These results suggest that Aβ-rich AD brain extracts interrupt both synaptic function and neurite intactness.

Soluble oligomers but not other Aβ forms inhibit hippocampal LTP

Aβ is pleomorphic and can populate a range of assemblies, with forms ranging from the monomer all the way

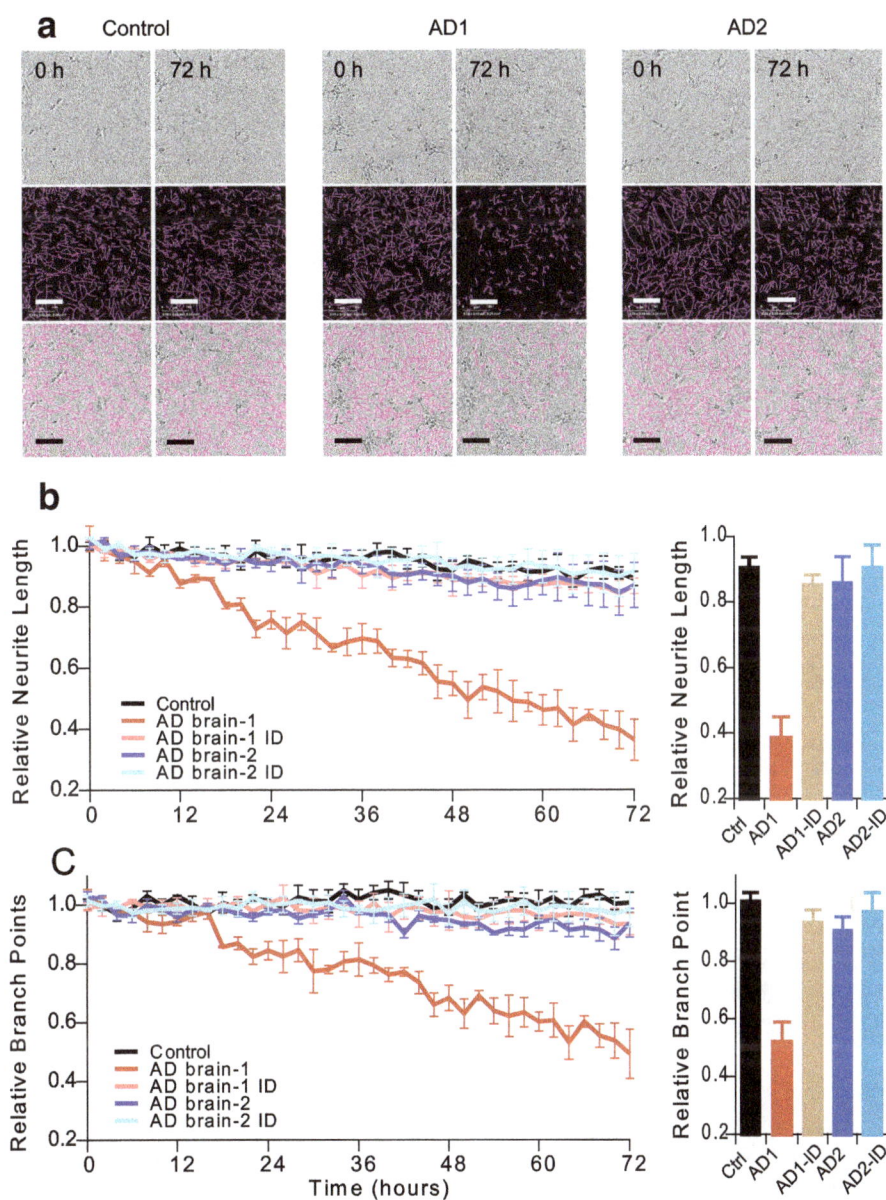

Fig. 2 Soluble Aβ extracts that either do or do not block LTP affect human neurites accordingly. IncuCyte live-cell video microscopy monitored the effect of AD brain extracts on iPSC-derived neurogenin-induced human neurons (iNs). On post-induction day 21, iNs were treated with Control TBS (Control: black) or AD extracts (colors) and the neurons imaged for 72 h. (**a**) Phase contrast images (top panel) at 0 and 72 h were analyzed using the incuCyte NeuronTrack algorithm to identify neurites (pseudocolored pink in middle panels). Identified neurites were superimposed on the phase contrast image (bottom panel). Scale bar, 100 μm. Each well of iNs was imaged for 6 h prior to addition of the extract and NeuroTrack measured neurite length and branch points at this baseline used to normalize neurite length measured at each interval after addition of extract. (**b,c**) Time course of change in neurite length (**b**) and branch points (**c**) after addition of AD brain extracts (red and blue) or immunodepleted sample (light brown and light blue, respectively) when compare to control brain extract (black). Summary results at 72 h treatments are shown on right

to the aggregates of insoluble ~ 8 nm fibrils found in amyloid plaques. In the past two decades, most studies have focused on aqueously soluble Aβ assemblies with sizes intermediate between monomer and fibrils [30]. To confirm our previous reports [64, 81], we chose four neuropathologically typical AD brains and two

age-matched control brains and prepared a series of Aβ-rich extracts: insoluble amyloid plaque cores and buffer-soluble fractions separated by Superdex 75 size-exclusion chromatography (SEC) that include the void volume (> 70 kDa), high molecular weight (HMW, 17~60 kDa), oligomers (6~16 kDa) and ~4 kDa monomers. Consistent with earlier findings [64], the plaque core-rich extracts did not alter LTP ($140 \pm 8\%$, $n = 6$ vs. vehicle alone $147 \pm 9\%$, $n = 7$, $p > 0.05$ (Fig. 3a), while Aβ oligomers released from the insoluble plaques by formic acid inhibited LTP ($116 \pm 5\%$, $n = 7$). Large soluble assemblies (void volume) from a Superdex 75 SEC column did not significantly alter LTP ($145 \pm 8\%$, $n = 8$ vs. vehicle alone: $158 \pm$ 8%, $n = 7$, $p > 0.05$) (Fig. 3b), but when the void volume fraction was incubated at 37 °C for 2 days, the large Aβ assemblies were dissociated into smaller Aβ oligomers that could inhibit hippocampal LTP ($122 \pm 4\%$, $n = 8$). Figure 3c summarizes the effects on LTP of SEC fractions isolated from AD and control brain extracts, confirming that smaller soluble Aβ oligomers confer LTP impairment.

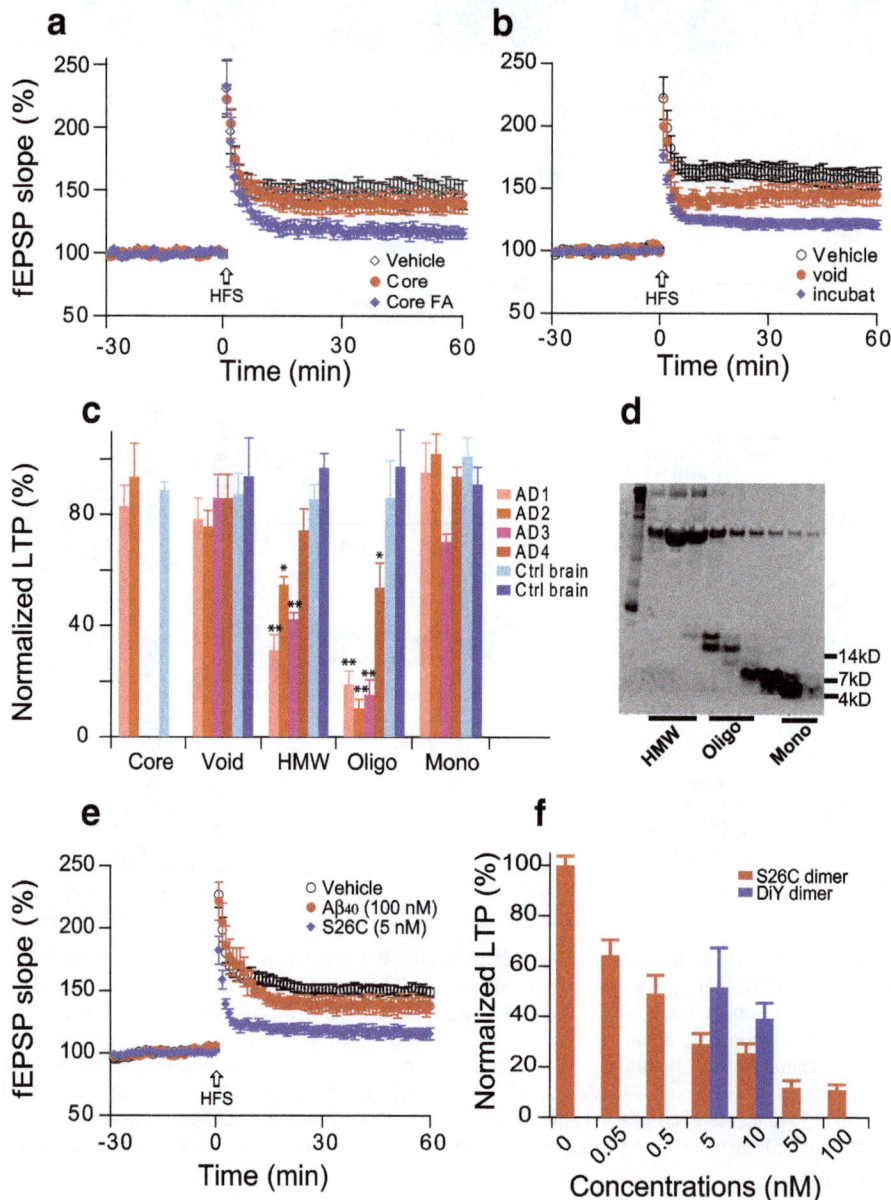

Fig. 3 Soluble Aβ oligomers inhibit hippocampal LTP. (**a**) Insoluble amyloid plaque cores from AD cortex fail to inhibit the LTP (red), while LTP was inhibited if an equivalent aliquot of the cores was solubilized in 88% formic acid and neutralized with NaOH (blue). (**b**) The void volume fraction of a Superdex 75 SEC chromatography of an AD cortex TBS extract (red) showed no significant LTP inhibition, but incubating the void volume fraction at 37 °C for 2 days released lower MW soluble Aβ oligomers that significantly impaired LTP (blue). (**c**) Summary LTP data of the indicated AD brain fractions ($n = 6\sim 8$). (**d**) Representative western blot shows different MW SEC fractions of soluble Aβ-rich AD cortical extracts; (**e**) Oxidized synthetic [Aβ$_{40}$-S26C]$_2$ dimers (blue diamonds) cause significant LTP inhibition but monomeric Aβ$_{1-40}$ does not (red); (**f**) Dose dependent LTP inhibition by oxidized synthetic [Aβ$_{40}$-S26C]$_2$ dimers (red), and dityrosine cross-linked Aβ1–40 dimers (DiY) (blue). *: $p < 0.05$; **: $p < 0.01$

To further verify these results, we used two synthetic crosslinked Aβ dimers [51]: S26C dimers (Aβ$_{1-40}$ with a cysteine residue in place of Ser^{26}, allowing formation of disulfide crosslinked dimers) and DiY dimers (wt Aβ$_{1-40}$, having a tyrosine at position 10, can be crosslinked to a dityrosine-linked dimer by oxidation). To assess the LTP effects of monomers and dimers, we used 100 nM Aβ$_{1-40}$ and 5 nM [S26C]$_2$ dimers. The 100 nM monomers had no effect on LTP (139 ± 7%, $n = 7$ vs. vehicle: 150 ± 4%, n = 7, p > 0.05) (Fig. 3e), while 20-fold less concentrated dimers significantly impaired LTP (116 ± 4%, $n = 7$). Figure 3f shows a dose-dependent LTP inhibition by [S26C]$_2$ dimer; a similar effect can be observed with the DiY dimers.

Soluble Aβ oligomers from other sources also inhibit hippocampal LTP

CSF is in direct contact with the extracellular space of the brain, and the principal species of Aβ that can be detected in CSF are aqueously soluble. To test whether the soluble Aβ from human brain plays a role in altering hippocampal LTP, we collected the CSF from the mild AD patients and concentrated them into 50 µl aliquots, then added one to the perfusion buffer (10 ml) of a mouse brain slice. LTP was significantly reduced by the AD CSF samples, while the CSF from age-matched non-AD controls produced no change vs. vehicle (Ctrl: 141 ± 4%, $n = 6$ vs. AD: 109 ± 6%, $n = 7$, $p < 0.001$) (Fig. 4a). When Aβ removed from the AD CSF by AW7 immunodepletion, hippocampal LTP was restored to the control level (135 ± 6%, $n = 6$).

To investigate whether Aβ isolated from APP tg mouse brain has an effect on LTP, we chose hAPP V717F mice generated by Mucke et al. [44], which have elevated levels of Aβ42 and Aβ42/40 ratio and develop Aβ deposits and plaque formation at 8 months of age. The brains of five 7-months-old J20 mice and 5 wild-type littermates were harvested, and Aβ extracts were prepared similarly to the AD brain extracts. The J20 but not the wild-type extracts impaired hippocampal LTP (150 ± 7%, $n = 5$ vs. 107 ± 3%, $n = 7$, $p < 0.001$), and the LTP inhibition was Aβ-dependent because immunodepleted J20 brain extract had no effect on LTP (146 ± 12%, n = 6) (Fig. 4b).

Another Aβ source is naturally secreted, soluble amyloid-β oligomers generated in a cell culture model termed 7PA2 cells, which express hAPP with the familial AD "Indiana" mutation (APPV717F). These cells secrete

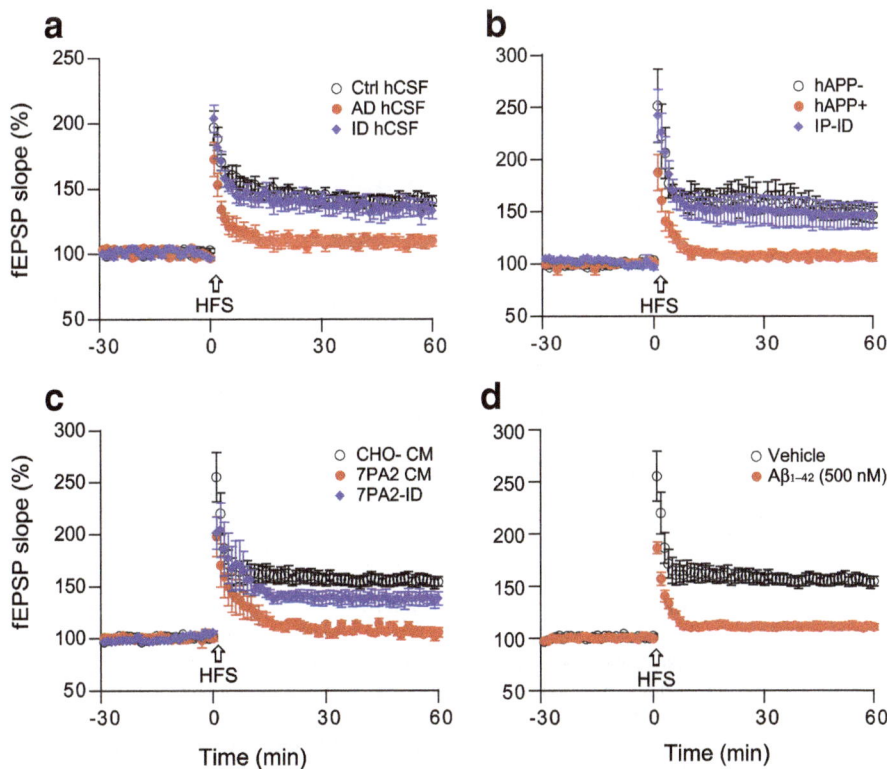

Fig. 4 Soluble Aβ oligomers from other sources also inhibit hippocampal LTP. Several sources of soluble Aβ included (**a**) AD patient CSF; (**b**) APP tg mouse of AD (J20 mice); (**c**) cell secreted human soluble Aβ; and (**d**) synthetic Aβ$_{1-42}$ peptide, effect on hippocampal LTP. All these impaired hippocampal LTP (red), while the inhibition of LTP by the 3 biological sources was prevented by removing soluble Aβ via immunodepletion (blue)

Aβ dimers and trimers [52] but have also been shown to secrete some N-terminally extended monomers that extend from aa − 31 to aa 40 and 42 (based on Aβ numbering) [77]. In line with other sources of Aβ, the 7PA2 CM (total Aβ 1514 ± 824 pg/ml) inhibited LTP (156 ± 5%, n = 6 vs. 106 ± 4%, n = 7, p < 0.001) (Fig. 4c). Immunodepleting Aβ prevented the inhibition of LTP to control levels (138 ± 7%, n = 7). Lastly, the widely used synthetic Aβ$_{1-42}$ peptide (500 nM) significantly impaired hippocampal LTP (156 ± 5%, n = 6 vs. 111 ± 3%, n = 7, p < 0.001) (Fig. 4d). These results suggest that multiple sources of soluble Aβ, wherever from human or rodent and cell derived or synthetic, can specifically and significantly inhibit hippocampal LTP.

Certain soluble Aβ fragments inhibit hippocampal LTP

Amyloidogenic processing of the amyloid precursor protein (APP) by β- and γ-secretases generates several biologically active products, including different Aβ fragments and the APP intracellular domain. It has been found that Aβ37, Aβ38, Aβ39, Aβ40, Aβ42, Aβ43 can all be detected in human cerebrospinal fluid [23, 66], while even longer, more hydrophobic Aβ peptides (Aβ45, Aβ46) can be found in cell lysate [53]. To examine the potential effects of these various species, 200 nM concentrations of Aβ$_{1-37}$ to Aβ$_{1-46}$, were added to the hippocampal slice perfusate for 30 min prior to a HFS that would induce LTP. Aβ$_{1-37}$, Aβ$_{1-38}$ and Aβ$_{1-39}$ and Aβ$_{1-40}$ peptides had little or no significant effect on LTP. Aβ$_{1-42}$, Aβ$_{1-43}$, Aβ$_{1-45}$, and Aβ$_{1-46}$ each significantly inhibited LTP (Fig. 5a, c). We speculated that Aβ$_{1-46}$ might be more potent than Aβ$_{1-42}$ in inhibiting LTP, so we tried different concentrations of Aβ$_{1-46}$: (200 nM, 100 nM, and 50 nM), but the degree of LTP impairment did not differ significantly (data not shown).

In addition to variable C-terminally truncated Aβ species, N-terminally truncated Aβs were also found in AD brain [6]. To assess whether the N-terminally truncated Aβs have any effect on the hippocampal LTP, we chose Aβ$_{1-16}$ and Aβ$_{17-42}$ to test their bioactivity on the brain slices. Consistent with short form of Aβ$_{1-37}$, the Aβ$_{1-16}$ (200 nM) has no significant effect on the LTP (146 ± 5%, $n = 7$ vs. 156 ± 6%, n = 7, $p > 0.05$, Fig. 5b, c). Interestingly, the Aβ$_{17-42}$ (200 nM) has a partial effect on the LTP (127 ± 5%, n = 7 vs. 156 ± 6%, n = 7, $p < 0.01$, Fig. 5b, c), this result further suggests that the hydrophobic C-terminal of Aβ$_{1-42}$ may initiate the Aβ aggregation to form the toxic Aβ species.

We previously reported the existence of APP proteolytic fragments released by certain cultured cells that

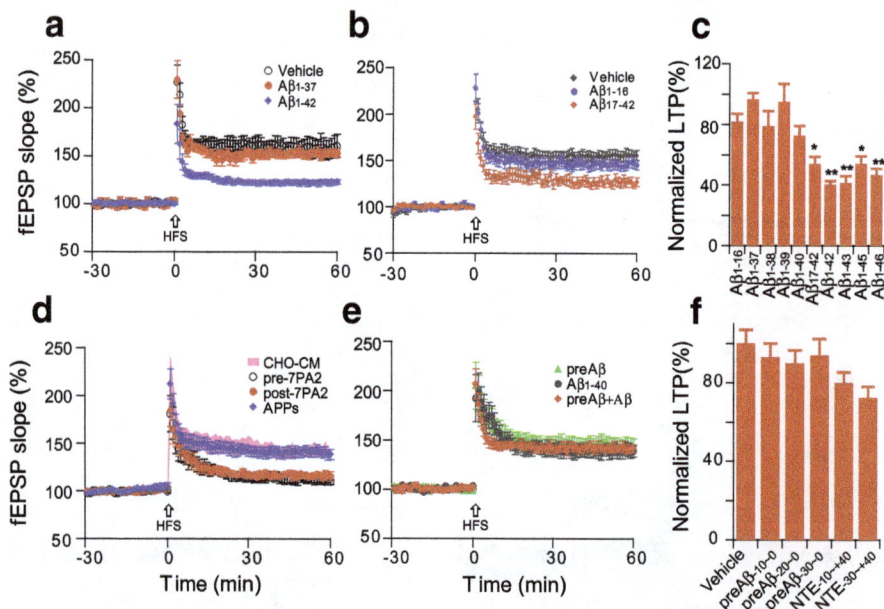

Fig. 5 Soluble Aβ peptides with longer C-termini confer greater synaptic toxicity. (**a**) The short Aβ$_{1-37}$ synthetic peptide did not impair hippocampal LTP at concentrations of 200 nM (red, $n = 7$, $p > 0.05$), while the same dose of the longer Aβ$_{1-42}$ peptide showed significant inhibition (blue, n = 6, $p < 0.001$); (**b**) N-terminally truncated synthetic Aβ$_{1-16}$ and Aβ$_{17-42}$ effect on the hippocampal LTP. (**c**) Summary data of LTP effects of Aβ peptides of increasing lengths at 200 nM concentrations; (**d**) The whole 7PA2 CM as well as immunoprecipitated NTE-Aβs (black open circles, n = 7, $p < 0.001$) and the CM remaining CM after depletion of APPs by DE23 resin (red circles, n = 7, $p < 0.001$) all inhibit LTP, while the isolated APPs alone (blue diamonds, n = 7, $p > 0.05$) does not; (**e**) Treatment of slices with synthetic pre-Aβ (− 30 to − 1) does not facilitate synthetic Aβ$_{1-40}$ to induce synaptotoxicity, that is to say, a synthetic APP-34 to − 1 fragment added to an Aβ$_{1-40}$ peptide does not inhibit LTP (n = 6, p > 0.05); (**f**) Summary data of synthetic peptides containing or not various lengths (− 10. -20, − 30) of APP prior to the Aβ1–40 Asp1 start site (called "preAβ") and N-terminal extension on Aβ1–40 do not inhibit LTP. (n = 6~ 8). *: $p < 0.05$; **: $p < 0.01$

contain the entire Aβ region plus a variable-length N-terminal extension (NTE), including a species beginning at least 34 residues N-terminal to the Asp1 start site of Aβ. We found that such NTE-Aβ monomers are secreted along with Aβ monomers and dimers by CHO cells stably expressing the FAD APP V717F mutation (called 7PA2 cells), and they contribute to the impairment of LTP by the 7PA2 CM [77]. Here, we showed that whole 7PA2 CM (0.5x, fresh made 7PA2 CM or called pre-7PA2; the total Aβs concentration by ELISA is 757 pg/ml) and the CM after depleting it of secreted APPs-α with DE23 resin (called post-7PA2) blocked LTP, while the APPs fraction itself did not alter LTP (Fig. 5d). In order to characterize certain pre-Aβ (the APP fragments before the Aβ starting point of APP_{672}) fragments of APP (-30 to -1, -20 to -10, -10 to -10) and also Aβ species having such N-terminal extensions (-30 to $+40$, and -10 to $+40$), we applied these peptides at 1 μM concentrations; the preAβs and short form NTEs did not inhibit LTP (Fig. 5e, f). Then, we combined the $preAβ_{-20\ to\ -1}$ peptide with the $Aβ_{1-40}$ peptide; the mixed peptides did not cause $Aβ_{1-40}$ to induce synaptic dysfunction (Fig. 5e). These results suggest that pre-Aβ, $Aβ_{1-16}$, $Aβ_{1-37}$, $Aβ_{1-39}$ and NTE (-30 to $+40$), all of which are relatively more hydrophilic than the synaptotoxic $Aβ_{1-42}$, are not synaptotoxic, whereas the longer forms ($Aβ_{1-42}$ to $Aβ_{1-46}$) that are more hydrophobic and more prone to aggregate were toxic species.

Antibodies to the N-terminus of Aβ prevent the LTP inhibition

Active immunization with synthetic Aβ peptides or passive infusions of humanized anti-Aβ monoclonal antibodies has been widely investigated as an immunotherapeutic approach to treat and prevent clinical AD. To examine this approach in tightly-controlled, reductionist experiments, we conducted a series of studies of hippocampal LTP and LTD in the absence or presence of antibodies raised to various human APP sequences within and flanking the Aβ region. The antibodies and their epitopes were 3D6 (requires a free Asp1 at the Aβ N-terminus), 82E1 (recognizes a free Asp1 at the Aβ N-terminus), 6E10 (to aa 3–8), 266 (to aa 13–28), 4G8 (to aa 17–24), 2G3 (requires a free Gly40 at the end of aa 33~ 40), 21F12 (requires a free Ile42 at the end of aa 33~ 42) and polyclonal antibody R1282 (principally recognizes epitopes in the N-terminal third of Aβ). To test the effects of these antibodies in rescuing Aβ-impaired LTP, we first tested each antibody (at 1–3 μg/ml) itself whether has any effect on the hippocampal LTP (Additional file 1: Figure S2), then added each antibody to an AD brain extract previously shown to inhibit LTP and incubated with mixing for 30 min before adding the mixture to the slice perfusion buffer. The N-terminal antibody 3D6 but not the C-terminal antibodies 2G3 and 21F12 fully prevented LTP

impairment by the soluble Aβ oligomer-rich AD extract (Fig. 6a, b). These results further supported that the N-terminally, not those C-terminally targeted antibodies of Aβ could neutralize Aβ-mediated synaptotoxicity and reduce the pathology of AD model mice [64, 83].

Another feature of synaptic plasticity is represented by long-term depression (LTD), an electrophysiological response known to correlate with dendritic spine shrinkage and synapse collapse [4, 78]. It has become widely used to assess Aβ-induced synaptic dysfunction after we first demonstrated that soluble Aβ oligomers of several sources could facilitate a persistent LTD upon a weak low-frequency (1 cps × 300 s) stimulation that usually fails to induce LTD [10, 16, 34, 38, 50, 56]. Again, two Asp1 N-terminus-specific antibodies, 3D6 and 82E1, but not the C-terminal antibodies 2G3 and 21F12, prevented the Aβ-facilitated LTD (Fig. 6c, d). A broad N-terminal region antibody, 6E10, and a mid-region antibody, 4G8, only partially prevented the Aβ-facilitated LTD. These results further support that the N-terminus of $Aβ_{1-42}$ plays a crucial role in triggering synaptic dysfunction.

Discussion

Here, we have performed a systematic comparative analysis of numerous features of the well-known inhibition of hippocampal synaptic plasticity by soluble oligomers of human Aβ. Our results complement and extend previous studies from our and other laboratories that found that soluble Aβ oligomers inhibit hippocampal LTP and induce synapse and neurite loss, including by oligomers isolated directly from AD cortex. We show here that Aβ inhibition of LTP is not conferred by monomers but rather by soluble oligomer-rich preparations. We also found that APP proteolytic fragments just prior to the Aβ N-terminus, the short Aβ peptides $Aβ_{1-16}$ through $Aβ_{1-40}$ and the N-terminally extended peptide -30 to Aβ40 ($APP641-711$ of APP_{770}) all failed to significantly inhibit LTP, while the longer, more hydrophobic peptides $Aβ_{1-42}$ through $Aβ_{1-46}$ were synaptotoxic. Two different N-terminal antibodies recognizing the free Asp1, 3D6 and 82E1, but not two C-terminal antibodies, could prevent Aβ oligomer impairment of LTP.

Cerebral Aβ accumulation and aggregation are early pathological events in AD, starting some 2 to 3 decades or more before the onset of readily detectable clinical symptoms [5, 18, 19, 67]. Although insoluble, fibrillar aggregates of Aβ constitute the neuropathological hallmark of AD, the number of plaques and the levels of insoluble Aβ correlate weakly with the local extent of synaptic and neuronal loss and thus with cognitive impairment in humans [45, 47]. On the other hand, the levels of soluble assemblies (oligomers) of Aβ appear to correlate better with disease progression in both rodent models and AD subjects [8, 32, 39, 64]. In AD model

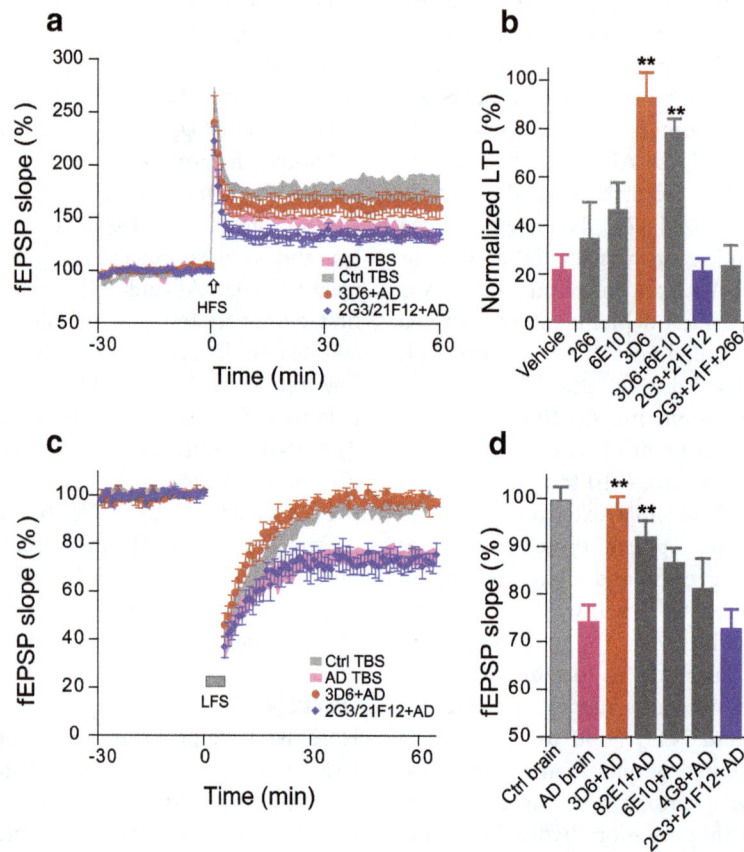

Fig. 6 N-terminal antibodies prevent interruption of hippocampal synaptic plasticity by soluble Aβ-rich brain extract. (**a**) Asp1 N-terminus specific Aβ antibody, 3D6 (red circles), not the C-terminal-specific antibodies 2G3 + 21F12 (blue diamonds) prevent the AD brain TBS extract (purple traces) from inhibiting LTP. (**b**) Summary data of antibodies to different Aβ epitopes as to their effect on AD brain TBS extract impairment of LTP ($N \geq 6$ recordings for each antibody). (**c**) N-terminal antibody 3D6 (red circles), not the C-terminal target antibodies, 2G3 + 21F12 (blue diamond) prevent the AD brain extract (purple traces) from facilitating LTD. (**d**). Summary data of antibodies to different Aβ epitopes as to their effect on the AD brain extract's facilitation of LTD ($N > 5$ recordings for each antibody). *: $p < 0.05$; **: $p < 0.01$

mice, spatial learning and memory have been shown to be impaired in nearly all models of Aβ overproduction by transgenic APP expression, and the onset of the cognitive decline occurred close to that of brain amyloid deposition [76]. Despite the genetic evidence suggesting a pivotal role for Aβ, considerable controversy still exists about its precise pathogenic role in AD [46]. This may be due to a lack of reliable approaches for the early AD diagnosis. For example, a sensitive method to detect the Aβ oligomers and its conformations can clarify this controversy, as some Aβ oligomer-detecting techniques (such as sodium dodecyl sulfate (SDS) polyacrylamide gel electrophoresis (PAGE)) may be relatively insensitive or even lead to artifacts [75]. The fact that brain Aβ levels measured by largely monomer-specific ELISAs did not correlate closely with degree of synaptotoxicity is not surprising; in contrast, special immunoassays that selectively detect soluble Aβ oligomers can readily distinguish extracts of AD vs. age-matched normal brain [14, 59, 74, 82].

The amyloid plaques consist of different variants of the Aβ peptide, with the most abundant being $Aβ_{1-40}$ and $Aβ_{1-42}$. AD brain specimen analyses have revealed numerous N-terminal or C-terminal truncated or modified Aβ species in addition to the full-length $Aβ_{1-40}$ and $Aβ_{1-42}$ [17, 37, 54, 55]. The sequential hydrolysis of APP by γ-secretase in AD generates a step-wise series of Aβ peptides terminating in residues 49, 48, 46, 45, 43, 42, 40, 39, 38 and 37 [53, 69]. Here we found that synthetic Aβ fragments longer than 1–40, including $Aβ_{1-42}$, $Aβ_{1-43}$, $Aβ_{1-45}$ and $Aβ_{1-46}$, confer significant impairment of LTP, while the shorter forms of $Aβ_{1-16}$, $Aβ_{1-37}$, $Aβ_{1-38}$, $Aβ_{1-39}$ and $Aβ_{1-40}$ have little effect on synaptic function. It is generally accepted that $Aβ_{1-42}$ plays a more pivotal role in AD pathogenesis than $Aβ_{1-40}$ because of its much higher aggregation propensity and thus neurotoxicity [58]. It has been considered that the C- terminal hydrophobic residues in $Aβ_{42}$ are a driving force for protein misfolding and self-assembly, leading to stabilization of neurotoxic low-order oligomers (dimers and larger)

[1, 48, 83]. One report showed that $Aβ_{1-42}$ and $Aβ_{1-43}$ were selectively deposited principally in senile plaques while shorter Aβ peptides such as Aβ1–37, 1–38, 1–39, and Aβ1–40 were deposited more in leptomeningeal blood vessels [22]. The longer forms of Aβs likely have a greater propensity to aggregate into oligomers and bind to the cell membrane because of their longer hydrophobic C-termini residues. And the shorter forms have been shown in some studies to have anti-amyloidogenic properties [33].

In addition to the above C-terminally heterogeneous Aβ species, N-terminally extended Aβ (NTE-Aβ) monomers with up to 9 residue extensions also have been detected in human plasma [24]. We previously reported that the CM of 7PA2 cells (CHO cells expressing the hAPP V717F FAD mutation) that is rich in NTE-Aβ variants as well as Aβ monomers and dimers could block hippocampal LTP. Immunodepletion of the NTE monomers with a pre-Aβ region polyclonal antibody prevented the 7PA2 CM-mediated LTP impairment, and removing all Aβ species with a pan-Aβ antiserum R1282 prevented the LTP impairment, suggesting that the monomeric N-terminally extended APP fragments containing the entire Aβ region can impair LTP [77].

To further compare the effects of N-termini vs. C-termini of Aβ on synaptic plasticity, we used several epitope-specific antibodies. We found that antibodies to the N-terminus starting with a free Asp1 (3D6 and 82E1) could fully rescue the impaired LTP and enhanced LTD caused by AD-TBS extracts, while two C-terminal antibodies (2G3 and 21F12) had no effect. The mid-region targeted antibodies (6E10, 266 and 4G8) had minor effects that did not reach significance. These results confirm previous reports including ours that antibodies which target the N-terminus, but not those targeting the C-terminus, can neutralize Aβ-mediated synaptotoxicity and reduce Aβ plaque load [3, 64, 83], thus leading to most anti-Aβ antibodies in clinical trials targeting the N-terminus or mid-region. However, several earlier studies using C-terminal antibodies, deglycosylated antibodies (D-2H6) and naturally occurring auto-antibodies against Aβ (NAbs–Aβ), were reported to significantly reduce Aβ burden and reverse cognitive deficits in AD mouse model [11, 25, 79]. The differential effects of N-terminal vs C-terminal anti-Aβ antibodies may be due to experimental paradigm differences in AD mouse models, such as dosing, administration mode or ages of treatment. The hydrophobic C-terminus of $Aβ_{42}$ which forms part of the core structure of the aggregates is then inaccessible to antibodies, while the N-terminus is exposed and is considered an avenue neurotoxic neutralization [48, 83, 85]. Therefore, C-terminal antibodies may be more active in the preclinical stages of AD, by binding to low aggregated (more soluble) Aβ

oligomers, whereas N-terminal antibodies may better access highly aggregated Aβ oligomers and fibrils (associated with a later disease state).

Although others find the seeding activity of AD brain-derived Aβ to be at least 100 times more potent than that of Aβ from CSF or synthetic Aβ in young APP transgenic mice, we find that all sources inhibit hippocampal LTP in brain slices [12, 40]. Together with the fact that C-terminal Aβ antibodies did not rescue the Aβ-impaired synaptic function in vitro, while C-terminal antibodies could improve cognitive function in APP Tg mice [11, 25, 79]. Such discrepancies may be due to the experimental paradigm. Our experimental conditions in slice LTP studies are reductionist compared to the complexities of Aβ production, aggregation and clearance that are dynamic in vivo, as well as effects of the blood-brain barrier and Aβ-degrading enzymes which are not considered in hippocampal slices. These factors will need to be addressed in further in vivo LTP studies to verify our conclusions. Another possibility is the different readout: the synaptic plasticity in present study vs. the behavior or cerebral β-amyloidosis in others. Additional specific functional biomarker (i.e. integrative EEG, event-related potentials and oscillations) that correlated with cognition or β-amyloidosis will clarify the present conclusion.

Unfortunately, several antibodies targeting Aβ have failed in clinical trials, including bapineuzumab [57], a humanized monoclonal antibody directed against the N-terminus of Aβ that recognizes the amyloid beta 1–5 region [41], similar to murine monoclonal antibody 3D6. The reasons are likely attributable to its very low dosing in the trials due to the first appearance in AD immunotherapy of amyloid-related imaging abnormality-edema (ARIA-E). The relatively late symptomatic stage (mild-moderate AD) of subjects in this and other antibody trials could also contribute to a failure to significantly slow cognitive decline. More recent trials that began treating at early or very early symptomatic stages of AD and used substantial doses of N-terminally-directed antibodies appear to clear amyloid plaques and lead to some apparent slowing of cognitive decline [61, 63]. Our results indicated that preventing soluble Aβ oligomer formation and targeting their N-terminal residues with antibodies could be an attractive combined therapeutic approach.

Conclusions

In this study, we have performed a systematic comparative analysis of numerous features of the well-knowninhibition of hippocampal synaptic plasticity by soluble oligomers of human Aβ. Our results provide evidence that preventing soluble Aβ oligomer formation and targeting their N-terminal residues with antibodies could be an attractive combined therapeutic approach.

Acknowledgments

We thank Drs. Dominic Walsh and Zemin Wang for their expert advice. We thank Nina Shepardson and Molly Rajsombath for preparing 7PA2 CM and CHO- CM, Wei Hong and Ting Yang for preparing AD and control brain TBS extracts, Marty Fernandez for preparing $A\beta_{1-45}$ and $A\beta_{1-46}$ and Tiernan O'Malley for preparing S26C dimers and DiY dimers. Supported by Alzheimer's Association NIRG-12-242825 (S.L) and NIH grant AG006173 (D.J.S).

Authors' contributions

SL carried out electrophysiological experiments and analyzed the data. MJ carried out living-cell imaging study. LL and BLO prepared the Aβs fragments. YD performed the ELISA experiments. SL designed the experiments and wrote the paper. DJS advised the experimental design and edited the manuscript. All authors read and approved the final manuscript.

Competing interests

DJS is a director of and consultant to Prothena Biosciences. The other authors declare that they have no conflicts of interest.

References

1. Ahmed M, Davis J, Aucoin D, Sato T, Ahuja S, Aimoto S et al (2010) Structural conversion of neurotoxic amyloid-beta(1-42) oligomers to fibrils. Nat Struct Mol Biol 17:561–567
2. Arendt T (2009) Synaptic degeneration in Alzheimer's disease. Acta Neuropathol 118:167–179
3. Bard F, Barbour R, Cannon C, Carretto R, Fox M, Games D et al (2003) Epitope and isotype specificities of antibodies to beta -amyloid peptide for protection against Alzheimer's disease-like neuropathology. Proc Natl Acad Sci U S A 100:2023–2028
4. Bastrikova N, Gardner GA, Reece JM, Jeromin A, Dudek SM (2008) Synapse elimination accompanies functional plasticity in hippocampal neurons. Proc Natl Acad Sci U S A 105:3123–3127
5. Bateman RJ, Xiong C, Benzinger TL, Fagan AM, Goate A, Fox NC et al (2012) Clinical and biomarker changes in dominantly inherited Alzheimer's disease. N Engl J Med 367:795–804
6. Bayer TA, Wirths O (2014) Focusing the amyloid cascade hypothesis on N-truncated Aβ peptides as drug targets against Alzheimer's disease. Acta Neuropathol 127:787–801
7. Bilousova T, Miller CA, Poon WW, Vinters HV, Corrada M, Kawas C et al (2016) Synaptic Amyloid-β Oligomers Precede p-Tau and Differentiate High Pathology Control Cases. Am J Pathol 186:185–198
8. Brody DL, Jiang H, Wildburger N, Esparza TJ (2017) Non-canonical soluble amyloid-beta aggregates and plaque buffering: controversies and future directions for target discovery in Alzheimer's disease. Alzheimers Res Ther 9(1):62. https://doi.org/10.1186/s13195-017-0293-3
9. Chang WP, Huang X, Downs D, Cirrito JR, Koelsch G, Holtzman DM et al (2011) Beta-secretase inhibitor GRL-8234 rescues age-related cognitive decline in APP transgenic mice. FASEB J 25:775–784
10. Chen X, Lin R, Chang L, Xu S, Wei X, Zhang J et al (2013) Enhancement of long-term depression by soluble amyloid β protein in rat hippocampus is mediated by metabotropic glutamate receptor and involves activation of p38MAPK, STEP and caspase-3. Neuroscience 253:435–443
11. Dodel R, Balakrishnan K, Keyvani K, Deuster O, Neff F, Andrei-Selmer LC et al (2011) Naturally occurring autoantibodies against beta-amyloid: investigating their role in transgenic animal and in vitro models of Alzheimer's disease. J Neurosci 31:5847–5854
12. Eisele YS, Obermüller U, Heilbronner G, Baumann F, Kaeser SA, Wolburg H et al (2010) Peripherally applied Abeta-containing inoculates induce cerebral beta-amyloidosis. Science 330:980–982
13. Fowler SW, Chiang AC, Savjani RR, Larson ME, Sherman MA, Schuler DR et al (2014) Genetic modulation of soluble Aβ rescues cognitive and synaptic impairment in a mouse model of Alzheimer's disease. J Neurosci 34:7871–7885
14. Herskovits AZ, Locascio JJ, Peskind ER, Li G, Hyman BT. (2013) A Luminex assay detects amyloid β oligomers in Alzheimer's disease cerebrospinal fluid. PLoS one. 2013 Jul 2;8(7):e67898
15. Hsia AY, Masliah E, McConlogue L, Yu GQ, Tatsuno G, Hu K et al (1999) Plaque-independent disruption of neural circuits in Alzheimer's disease mouse models. Proc Natl Acad Sci U S A 96:3228–3233
16. Hu NW, Nicoll AJ, Zhang D, Mably AJ, O'Malley T, Purro SA et al (2014) mGlu5 receptors and cellular prion protein mediate amyloid-β-facilitated synaptic long-term depression in vivo. Nat Commun 5:3374
17. Iwatsubo T, Odaka A, Suzuki N, Mizusawa H, Nukina N, Ihara Y (1994) Visualization of A beta 42(43) and A beta 40 in senile plaques with end-specific A beta monoclonals: evidence that an initially deposited species is A beta 42(43). Neuron 13:45–53
18. Jack CR Jr, Knopman DS, Jagust WJ, Shaw LM, Aisen PS, Weiner MW et al (2010) Hypothetical model of dynamic biomarkers of the Alzheimer's pathological cascade. Lancet Neurol 9(1):119–128
19. Jansen WJ, Ossenkoppele R, Knol DL, Tijms BM, Scheltens P et al (2015) Prevalence of cerebral amyloid pathology in persons without dementia: a meta-analysis. JAMA 313:1924–1938
20. Janus C, Pearson J, McLaurin J, Mathews PM, Jiang Y, Schmidt SD et al (2000) A beta peptide immunization reduces behavioural impairment and plaques in a model of Alzheimer's disease. Nature 408:979–982
21. Jin M, O'Nuallain B, Hong W, Boyd J, Lagomarsino VN, O'Malley TT, et al. (2018) An in vitro paradigm to assess potential anti-Aβ antibodies for Alzheimer's disease. Nat Commun. 2018 Jul 11;9(1):2676
22. Kakuda N, Miyasaka T, Iwasaki N, Nirasawa T, Wada-Kakuda S, Takahashi-Fujigasaki J et al (2017) Distinct deposition of amyloid-β species in brains with Alzheimer's disease pathology visualized with MALDI imaging mass spectrometry. Acta Neuropathol Commun 5(1):73. https://doi.org/10.1186/s40478-017-0477-x
23. Kakuda N, Shoji M, Arai H, Furukawa K, Ikeuchi T, Akazawa K et al (2012) Altered γ-secretase activity in mild cognitive impairment and Alzheimer's disease. EMBO Mol Med. 4:344–352
24. Kaneko N, Yamamoto R, Sato TA, Tanaka K (2014) Identification and quantification of amyloid beta-related peptides in human plasma using matrix-assisted laser desorption/ionization time-of-flight mass spectrometry. Proc Jpn Acad Ser B Phys Biol Sci 90:104–117
25. Karlnoski RA, Rosenthal A, Alamed J, Ronan V, Gordon MN, Gottschall PE et al (2008) Deglycosylated anti-Abeta antibody dose-response effects on pathology and memory in APP transgenic mice. J Neuroimmune Pharmacol 3:187–197
26. Kasza Á, Penke B, Frank Z, Bozsó Z, Szegedi V, Hunya Á, et al. (2017) Studies for Improving a Rat Model of Alzheimer's Disease: Icv Administration of Well-Characterized β-Amyloid 1-42 Oligomers Induce Dysfunction in Spatial Memory. Molecules. 22(11). Pii: E2007
27. Klyubin I, Betts V, Welzel AT, Blennow K, Zetterberg H, Wallin A et al (2008) Amyloid beta protein dimer-containing human CSF disrupts synaptic plasticity: prevention by systemic passive immunization. J Neurosci 28:4231–4237
28. Klyubin I, Walsh DM, Lemere CA, Cullen WK, Shankar GM, Betts V et al (2005) Amyloid beta protein immunotherapy neutralizes Abeta oligomers that disrupt synaptic plasticity in vivo. Nat Med 11:556–561
29. Lambert MP, Barlow AK, Chromy BA, Edwards C, Freed R, Liosatos M et al (1998) Diffusible, nonfibrillar ligands derived from Abeta1-42 are potent central nervous system neurotoxins. Proc Natl Acad Sci U S A 95:6448–6453
30. Lannfelt L, Möller C, Basun H, Osswald G, Sehlin D, Satlin A et al (2014) Perspectives on future Alzheimer therapies: amyloid-β protofibrils - a new target for immunotherapy with BAN2401 in Alzheimer's disease. Alzheimers Res Ther 6(2):16. https://doi.org/10.1186/alzrt246
31. Larson J, Lynch G, Games D, Seubert P (1999) Alterations in synaptic transmission and long-term potentiation in hippocampal slices from young and aged PDAPP mice. Brain Res 840:23–35
32. Lesné S, Koh MT, Kotilinek L, Kayed R, Glabe CG, Yang A et al (2006) A specific amyloid-beta protein assembly in the brain impairs memory. Nature 440:352–357
33. Levites Y, Das P, Price RW, Rochette MJ, Kostura LA, McGowan EM, Murphy MP, Golde TE (2006) Anti-Abeta42- and anti-Abeta40-specific mAbs attenuate amyloid deposition in an Alzheimer disease mouse model. J Clin Invest 116(1):193–201
34. Li S, Hong S, Shepardson NE, Walsh DM, Shankar GM, Selkoe D (2009) Soluble oligomers of amyloid Beta protein facilitate hippocampal long-term depression by disrupting neuronal glutamate uptake. Neuron 62:788–801
35. Li S, Jin M, Koeylsperger T, Shepardson NE, Shankar GM, Selkoe DJ (2011) Soluble Aβ oligomers inhibit long-term potentiation through a mechanism

involving excessive activation of extrasynaptic NR2B-containing NMDA receptors. J Neurosci 31:6627–6638

36. Lichtenthaler SF, Haass C, Steiner H (2011) Regulated intramembrane proteolysis--lessons from amyloid precursor protein processing. J Neurochem 117:779–796

37. Lyons B, Friedrich M, Raftery M, Truscott R (2016) Amyloid Plaque in the Human Brain Can Decompose from Aβ(1-40/1-42) by Spontaneous Nonenzymatic Processes. Anal Chem 88(5):2675–2684

38. Ma T, Du X, Pick JE, Sui G, Brownlee M, Klann E (2012) Glucagon-like peptide-1 cleavage product GLP-1(9-36) amide rescues synaptic plasticity and memory deficits in Alzheimer's disease model mice. J Neurosci 32: 13701–13708

39. Mc Donald JM, Savva GM, Brayne C, Welzel AT, Forster G, Shankar GM et al (2010) The presence of sodium dodecyl sulphate-stable Abeta dimers is strongly associated with Alzheimer-type dementia. Brain 133(Pt 5):1328–1341

40. Meyer-Luehmann M, Coomaraswamy J, Bolmont T, Kaeser S, Schaefer C, Kilger E et al (2006) Exogenous induction of cerebral beta-amyloidogenesis is governed by agent and host. Science 313:1781–1784

41. Miles LA, Crespi GA, Doughty L, Parker MW (2013) Bapineuzumab captures the N-terminus of the Alzheimer's disease amyloid-beta peptide in a helical conformation. Sci Rep 3:1302. https://doi.org/10.1038/srep01302

42. Morgan D, Diamond DM, Gottschall PE, Ugen KE, Dickey C, Hardy J et al (2000) A beta peptide vaccination prevents memory loss in an animal model of Alzheimer's disease. Nature 408:982–985

43. Mroczko B, Groblewska M, Litman-Zawadzka A, Kornhuber J, Lewczuk P (2018) Amyloid β oligomers (AβOs) in Alzheimer's disease. J Neural Transm (Vienna) 125:177–191

44. Mucke L, Masliah E, Yu GQ, Mallory M, Rockenstein EM, Tatsuno G et al (2000) High-level neuronal expression of abeta 1-42 in wild-type human amyloid protein precursor transgenic mice: synaptotoxicity without plaque formation. J Neurosci 20:4050–4058

45. Mufson EJ, Malek-Ahmadi M, Snyder N, Ausdemore J, Chen K, Perez SE (2016) Braak stage and trajectory of cognitive decline in noncognitively impaired elders. Neurobiol Aging 43:101–110

46. Mullane K, Williams M (2013) Alzheimer's therapeutics: continued clinical failures question the validity of the amyloid hypothesis-but what lies beyond? Biochem Pharmacol 85:289–305

47. Nelson PT, Braak H, Markesbery WR (2009) Neuropathology and cognitive impairment in Alzheimer disease: a complex but coherent relationship. J Neuropathol Exp Neurol 68:1–14

48. Nisbet RM, Nigro J, Breheney K, Caine J, Hattarki MK, Nuttall SD (2013) Central amyloid-β-specific single chain variable fragment ameliorates Aβ aggregation and neurotoxicity. Protein Eng Des Sel 26:571–580

49. O'Brien RJ, Wong PC (2011) Amyloid precursor protein processing and Alzheimer's disease. Annu Rev Neurosci 34:185–204

50. Olsen KM, Sheng M (2012) NMDA receptors and BAX are essential for Aβ impairment of LTP. Sci rep 2:225. https://doi.org/10.1038/srep00225

51. O'Malley TT, Oktaviani NA, Zhang D, Lomakin A, O'Nuallain B, Linse S et al (2014) Aβ dimers differ from monomers in structural propensity, aggregation paths and population of synaptotoxic assemblies. Biochem J 461:413–426

52. Podlisny MB, Ostaszewski BL, Squazzo SL, Koo EH, Rydell RE, Teplow DB et al (1995) Aggregation of secreted amyloid beta-protein into sodium dodecyl sulfate-stable oligomers in cell culture. J Biol Chem 270:9564–9570

53. Qi-Takahara Y, Morishima-Kawashima M, Tanimura Y, Dolios G, Hirotani N, Horikoshi Y et al (2005) Longer forms of amyloid beta protein: implications for the mechanism of intramembrane cleavage by gamma-secretase. J Neurosci 25:436–445

54. Roher AE, Kokjohn TA, Clarke SG, Sierks MR, Maarouf CL, Serrano GE et al (2017) APP/Aβ structural diversity and Alzheimer's disease pathogenesis. Neurochem Int 110:1–13

55. Rostagno A, Neubert TA, Ghiso J (2018) Unveiling Brain Aβ Heterogeneity Through Targeted Proteomic Analysis. Methods Mol Biol 1779:23–43

56. Salgado-Puga K, Rodríguez-Colorado J, Prado-Alcalá RA, Peña-Ortega F (2017) Subclinical Doses of ATP-Sensitive Potassium Channel Modulators Prevent Alterations in Memory and Synaptic Plasticity Induced by Amyloid-β. J Alzheimers Dis 57:205–226

57. Salloway S, Sperling R, Fox NC, Blennow K, Klunk W, Raskind M et al (2014) Two phase 3 trials of bapineuzumab in mild-to-moderate Alzheimer's disease. N Engl J Med 370:322–333

58. Sato M, Murakami K, Uno M, Nakagawa Y, Katayama S, Akagi K et al (2013) Site-specific inhibitory mechanism for amyloid β42 aggregation by catechol-type flavonoids targeting the Lys residues. J Biol Chem 288:23212–23224

59. Savage MJ, Kalinina J, Wolfe A, Tugusheva K, Korn R, Cash-Mason T et al (2014) A sensitive aβ oligomer assay discriminates Alzheimer's and aged control cerebrospinal fluid. J Neurosci 34:2884–2897

60. Selkoe DJ (2002) Alzheimer's disease is a synaptic failure. Science 298:789–791

61. Selkoe DJ. (2018) Light at the end of the amyloid tunnel. Biochemistry, 2018 Oct 1. doi: https://doi.org/10.1021/acs.biochem.8b00985

62. Selkoe DJ, Hardy J (2016) The amyloid hypothesis of Alzheimer's disease at 25 years. EMBO Mol Med 8:595–608

63. Sevigny J, Chiao P, Bussière T, Weinreb PH, Williams L, Maier M et al (2016) The antibody aducanumab reduces Aβ plaques in Alzheimer's disease. Nature 537:50–56

64. Shankar GM, Li S, Mehta TH, Garcia-Munoz A, Shepardson NE, Smith I et al (2008) Amyloid-beta protein dimers isolated directly from Alzheimer's brains impair synaptic plasticity and memory. Nat Med 14:837–842

65. Shankar GM, Welzel AT, McDonald JM, Selkoe DJ, Walsh DM (2011) Isolation of low-n amyloid β-protein oligomers from cultured cells, CSF, and brain. Methods Mol Biol 670:33–44

66. Soares HD, Gasior M, Toyn JH, Wang JS, Hong Q, Berisha F et al (2016) The γ-Secretase Modulator, BMS-932481, Modulates Aβ Peptides in the Plasma and Cerebrospinal Fluid of Healthy Volunteers. J Pharmacol Exp Ther 358: 138–150

67. Sperling RA, Aisen PS, Beckett LA, Bennett DA, Craft S, Fagan AM et al (2011) Toward defining the preclinical stages of Alzheimer's disease: recommendations from the National Institute on Aging-Alzheimer's Association workgroups on diagnostic guidelines for Alzheimer's disease. Alzheimers Dement 7:280–292

68. Szczepankiewicz O, Linse B, Meisl G, Thulin E, Frohm B, Sala Frigerio C et al (2015) N-Terminal Extensions Retard Aβ42 Fibril Formation but Allow Cross-Seeding and Coaggregation with Aβ42. J Am Chem Soc 137:14673–14685

69. Takami M, Nagashima Y, Sano Y, Ishihara S, Morishima-Kawashima M, Funamoto S et al (2009) gamma-Secretase: successive tripeptide and tetrapeptide release from the transmembrane domain of beta-carboxyl terminal fragment. J Neurosci 29:13042–13052

70. Viola KL, Klein WL (2015) Amyloid β oligomers in Alzheimer's disease pathogenesis, treatment, and diagnosis. Acta Neuropathol 129:183–206

71. Walsh DM, Klyubin I, Fadeeva JV, Cullen WK, Anwyl R, Wolfe MS et al (2002) Naturally secreted oligomers of amyloid beta protein potently inhibit hippocampal long-term potentiation in vivo. Nature 416:535–539

72. Walsh DM, Thulin E, Minogue AM, Gustavsson N, Pang E, Teplow DB et al (2009) A facile method for expression and purification of the Alzheimer's disease-associated amyloid beta-peptide. FEBS J 276:1266–1281

73. Walsh DM, Townsend M, Podlisny MB, Shankar GM, Fadeeva JV, El Agnaf O et al (2005) Certain inhibitors of synthetic amyloid beta-peptide (Abeta) fibrillogenesis block oligomerization of natural Abeta and thereby rescue long-term potentiation. J Neurosci 25:2455–2462

74. Wang-Dietrich L, Funke SA, Kühbach K, Wang K, Besmehn A, Willbold S et al (2013) The amyloid-β oligomer count in cerebrospinal fluid is a biomarker for Alzheimer's disease. J Alzheimers Dis 34:985–994

75. Watt AD, Perez KA, Rembach A, Sherrat NA, Hung LW, Johanssen T et al (2013) Oligomers, fact or artefact? SDS-PAGE induces dimerization of β-amyloid in human brain samples. Acta Neuropathol 125:549–564

76. Webster SJ, Bachstetter AD, Nelson PT, Schmitt FA, Van Eldik LJ (2014) Using mice to model Alzheimer's dementia: an overview of the clinical disease and the preclinical behavioral changes in 10 mouse models. Front Genet 5: 88. https://doi.org/10.3389/fgene.2014.00088

77. Welzel AT, Maggio JE, Shankar GM, Walker DE, Ostaszewski BL, Li S et al (2014) Secreted amyloid β-proteins in a cell culture model include N-terminally extended peptides that impair synaptic plasticity. Biochemistry 53:3908–3921

78. Wiegert JS, Oertner TG (2013) Long-term depression triggers the selective elimination of weakly integrated synapses. Proc Natl Acad Sci U S A 110(47): E4510–E4519

79. Wilcock DM, Alamed J, Gottschall PE, Grimm J, Rosenthal A, Pons J et al (2006) Deglycosylated anti-amyloid-beta antibodies eliminate cognitive

deficits and reduce parenchymal amyloid with minimal vascular consequences in aged amyloid precursor protein transgenic mice. J Neurosci 26:5340–5346

80. Wolfe MS, Xia W, Ostaszewski BL, Diehl TS, Kimberly WT, Selkoe DJ (1999) Two transmembrane aspartates in presenilin-1 required for presenilin endoproteolysis and gamma-secretase activity. Nature 398:513–517

81. Yang T, Li S, Xu H, Walsh DM, Selkoe DJ (2017) Large Soluble Oligomers of Amyloid β-Protein from Alzheimer Brain Are Far Less Neuroactive Than the Smaller Oligomers to Which They Dissociate. J Neurosci 37:152–163

82. Yang T, O'Malley TT, Kanmert D, Jerecic J, Zieske LR, Zetterberg H et al (2015) A highly sensitive novel immunoassay specifically detects low levels of soluble Aβ oligomers in human cerebrospinal fluid. Alzheimers Res Ther 7(1):14

83. Zago W, Buttini M, Comery TA, Nishioka C, Gardai SJ, Seubert P et al (2012) Neutralization of soluble, synaptotoxic amyloid β species by antibodies is epitope specific. J Neurosci 32:2696–2702

84. Zeng H, Guo M, Martins-Taylor K, Wang X, Zhang Z, Park JW et al (2010) Specification of region-specific neurons including forebrain glutamatergic neurons from human induced pluripotent stem cells. PLoS One 5(7):e11853 Epub 2010/08/06

85. Zhang Y, Chen X, Liu J, Zhang Y (2015) The protective effects and underlying mechanism of an anti-oligomeric Aβ42 single-chain variable fragment antibody. Neuropharmacology 99:387–395

86. Zhang Y, Pak C, Han Y, Ahlenius H, Zhang Z, Chanda S et al (2013) Rapid single-step induction of functional neurons from human pluripotent stem cells. Neuron 78:785–798

13

Tectal glioma as a distinct diagnostic entity: a comprehensive clinical, imaging, histologic and molecular analysis

Anthony P. Y. Liu[1], Julie H. Harreld[2], Lisa M. Jacola[3], Madelyn Gero[3], Sahaja Acharya[4], Yahya Ghazwani[1], Shengjie Wu[5], Xiaoyu Li[6], Paul Klimo Jr[7,8,9,10], Amar Gajjar[1], Jason Chiang[6*] and Ibrahim Qaddoumi[1*]

Abstract

Tectal glioma (TG) is a rare low-grade tumor occurring predominantly in the pediatric population. There has been no detailed analysis of molecular alterations in TG. Risk factors associated with inferior outcome and long-term sequelae of TG have not been well-documented. We retrospectively studied TGs treated or referred for review at St. Jude Children's Research Hospital (SJCRH) between 1986 and 2013. Longitudinal clinical data were summarized, imaging and pathology specimen centrally reviewed, and tumor material analyzed with targeted molecular testing and genome-wide DNA methylation profiling. Forty-five patients with TG were included. Twenty-six (57.8%) were male. Median age at diagnosis was 9.9 years (range, 0.01–20.5). Median follow-up was 7.6 years (range, 0.5–17.0). The most common presenting symptoms were related to increased intracranial pressure. Of the 22 patients treated at SJCRH, 19 (86%) required cerebrospinal fluid diversion and seven (32%) underwent tumor-directed surgery. Five patients (23%) received radiation therapy and four (18%) systemic therapy. Ten-year overall and progression-free survival were $83.9 \pm 10.4\%$ and $48.7 \pm 14.2\%$, respectively. Long-term morbidities included chronic headaches, visual symptoms and neurocognitive impairment. Lesion $\geq 3cm^2$, contrast enhancement and cystic changes at presentation were risk factors for progression. Among those with tumor tissue available, 83% showed growth patterns similar to pilocytic astrocytoma and 17% aligned best with diffuse astrocytoma. *BRAF* duplication (a marker of *KIAA1549-BRAF* fusion) and *BRAF* V600E mutation were detected in 25% and 7.7%, respectively. No case had histone H3 K27M mutation. DNA methylation profile of TG was distinct from other brain tumors. In summary, TG is an indolent, chronic disease with unique clinical and molecular profiles and associated with long term morbidities. Large size, contrast enhancement and cystic changes are risk factors for progression.

Keywords: Tectal glioma, Imaging findings, Prognostic factors, Histopathology, DNA methylation profiling, Long-term follow-up

Introduction

Tectal glioma (TG) is a rare tumor with a predilection for the pediatric population [18]. It involves critical locations in the brainstem including superior and inferior colliculi and the narrow passage of aqueduct of Sylvius. TG may be diagnosed by its typical appearance on imaging and, if biopsied, as a low-grade glioma (LGG)

histologically. Given the usual indolent course and risk associated with resection in such an eloquent area, the general recommendation is close observation after CSF diversion for hydrocephalus. Many studies on patient outcome are based on neurosurgical series with possible bias [5, 8, 9, 16, 17, 20, 22, 25, 26, 28, 32, 38, 42, 43, 45, 48]. Data on progression predictors, long-term morbidities, and molecular features of this peculiar group of LGG are lacking. We report comprehensively the clinical, neurocognitive, imaging, histologic and molecular features of TG cases treated or reviewed at St. Jude Children's Research Hospital (SJCRH) over three decades. We found that while clinically indolent, TG is associated

* Correspondence: jason.chiang@stjude.org; ibrahim.qaddoumi@stjude.org
[6]Department of Pathology, St. Jude Children's Research Hospital, 262 Danny Thomas Place, MS 250, Memphis 38105-3678, TN, USA
[1]Department of Oncology, St. Jude Children's Research Hospital, 262 Danny Thomas Place, MS 260, Memphis 38105-3678, TN, USA
Full list of author information is available at the end of the article

with significant long-term morbidities. Although morphologically similar to pilocytic astrocytoma (PA) of other sites of the central nervous system, TG shows a distinct DNA methylation profile. We have identified large size, contrast enhancement and cystic changes as risk factors for progression.

Material and methods
Study population
Forty-five patients with TG treated ($n = 22$) or referred for case review ($n = 23$) at SJCRH between January 1986 and December 2017 were reviewed. Diagnosis was based on typical imaging findings (tumor intrinsic to or centered in the tectal plate) and supported by histopathology when available. Comprehensive clinical, imaging and histopathologic data were reviewed as available. Long-term morbidities, including those affecting neurocognitive function were summarized.

MRI and image analysis
MR images acquired at diagnosis and first progression, if applicable, were centrally reviewed by a board-certified neuroradiologist (JHH). Each tumor was measured in three orthogonal planes, assessed for T1 and T2 signal intensity and circumscription, and graded for the proportions of cystic and/or enhancing tumor components and enhancement avidity at each time-point. The relative apparent diffusion coefficient (rADC) was calculated relative to normal-appearing cerebellum [23]. Progressive disease (PD) was defined as an increase of ≥25% in the product of the two greatest perpendicular diameters compared to baseline [49].

Histopathologic and molecular studies
The histopathology of cases with available tissue ($n = 30$) was centrally reviewed by a board-certified neuropathologist (JC). For immunohistochemistry, we used antibodies against GFAP (Ventana, 760–4345, prediluted), Olig2 (Cell Marque, 387 M-15, diluted 1:50), neurofilament (Ventana, 760–2661, prediluted), and Ki67 (Dako, M7240, diluted 1:100). Histone H3 K27M mutant proteins were detected with a rabbit polyclonal antibody (EMD Millipore, ABE419, diluted 1:600). *BRAF* V600E mutant protein was detected with a mouse monoclonal antibody (Ventana, 790–4855, prediluted). Chromosome 7q34 duplication, a surrogate marker for *KIAA1549-BRAF* fusion, was detected by interphase fluorescence in situ hybridization (iFISH) with a probe developed in-house (information available upon request).

Genome-wide DNA methylation profiling and analysis
Genomic DNA (≥250 ng from each sample) was extracted from formalin-fixed paraffin-embedded (FFPE) tissue from nine TG samples with adequate tissue and

analyzed using Illumina Infinium MethylationEPIC BeadChip arrays in accordance with the manufacturer's instructions. Nineteen non-NF1 hypothalamic PAs (HTPAs, $n = 9$) and cerebellar PAs (CBPAs, $n = 10$) were also retrieved from the institutional tumor bank for comparison. Reference methylation profiles of 8 brain tumor entities (rosette-forming glioneuronal tumor, dysembryoplastic neuroepithelial tumor, ganglioglioma, subependymal giant cell astrocytoma, *MYB*-altered low-grade glioma, histone H3 K27M-mutant diffuse midline glioma, and IDH-mutant diffuse astrocytoma / oligodendroglioma) and normal tissue from the hypothalamus, pons, cerebellum and white matter were obtained from publicly available database for comparison [6]. Array data analysis was performed using R v.3.5.0 with several packages from Bioconductor [36]. Raw signal intensities were obtained from IDAT files by using minfi package v.1.26.0 and normalized by performing background correction and a dye-bias correction for both color channels with the functional normalization method [2, 13]. Poor quality ($P > 0.01$) and failed probes ($n = 29{,}567$) were removed from the downstream analysis. The following filtering criteria were applied: removal of probes targeting the X and Y chromosomes ($n = 8971$), removal of probes containing single-nucleotide polymorphism ($n = 13{,}776$), and removal of probes not mapping uniquely to the human reference genome (hg19) allowing for one mismatch ($n = 3965$). In total, 400,253 probes targeting CpG sites were kept. Beta-values of the 1000 most variable CpG sites were derived for further analysis. t-SNE analysis was performed using Rtsne package v.0.13 with theta $= 0.0$ [24, 44]. Agglomerative nesting hierarchical clustering analysis was performed using cluster package v.2.0.7-1 with Euclidean distances and a generalized average method [27].

Neuropsychologic evaluation
Cognitive assessments performed at SJCRH were reviewed ($n = 10$) for evidence of long-term neurocognitive impairment. For patients with multiple assessments, data from the most recent assessment were used. The cognitive domains most consistently included for analysis were global intelligence, working memory, processing speed, and academics (i.e., word reading and math calculation). Global intelligence (estimated or full-scale IQ score) was assessed with age-appropriate Wechsler scale or the Differential Abilities Scale, Second Edition [11, 47]. Working memory and processing speed were assessed with age appropriate Wechsler scale. Academics were assessed with Woodcock-Johnson Tests of Achievement, Wide Range Achievement Test, or Wechsler Individual Achievement Test [19, 46, 50]. All age-standardized scores were converted to z-scores

(mean = 0 and standard deviation = 1). Impairment was defined as a z-score ≥ -1.33 (ninth percentile).

Statistical analysis

Statistical analysis was performed with R v.3.5.0. The date of diagnosis was defined as the date of the MRI on which the tumor was first detected. Progressive disease (PD) was defined by radiologic progression, together with clinical deterioration and/or a need for intervention. Tumor size and rADC were compared between baseline and progression by paired t-test. Survival analysis was performed with the Kaplan-Meier method. Overall survival (OS) was determined as the duration between diagnosis and death from any cause or last follow-up, whichever was earlier. Progression-free survival (PFS) was determined as the duration between diagnosis and the first detection of PD, death from any cause, or last follow-up, whichever was earlier. Variables were analyzed for their impact on survival by the log-rank test or the Cox proportional hazards model.

Results

Demographic and presenting features

Forty-five patients with TG were included in this study (Fig. 1, Additional file 1: Figure S1). Twenty-six (58%) were males, and the median age of diagnosis was 9.9 years (range, 0.01–20.5). Among the 22 patients treated at SJCRH, two had neurofibromatosis type-1 (NF1) and four were diagnosed incidentally: one through antenatal ultrasound and three with failed vision screening (Additional file 2: Table S1). The other patients most commonly presented with headaches (*n* = 11) (Fig. 1). The median duration of symptoms before diagnosis was 0.46 year (range, 1 week-7.3 years). In the three patients for whom presentation preceded diagnosis by ≥6 years, a ventriculoperitoneal (VP) shunt was inserted for hydrocephalus because of a presumed aqueductal stenosis seen on CT; TG was diagnosed only after subsequent MRI (performed because of seizures in two patients and diplopia in one). One out of the 13 patients who underwent complete imaging with MRI brain and spine at diagnosis had evidence of metastasis.

CSF diversion and surgical and nonsurgical interventions

CSF diversion was required in 19/22 (86%) patients, being performed at presentation in all cases (Fig. 1, Table 1). The initial procedure was an endoscopic third ventriculostomy (ETV) in 10 patients and VP shunting in nine; an Ommaya reservoir was also inserted in eight patients who underwent ETV. Of those who underwent VP shunting, six (67%) required shunt revisions (range, 1–12 times) and one eventually required an ETV. Two patients had a subdural hematoma due to over-shunting, requiring evacuation. Of the patients who had ETV upfront, two (20%)

experienced failure necessitating VP shunt placement. Tumor-directed surgery was performed in seven (32%) patients treated at SJCRH. Three had biopsies (two upfront, one at progression), three underwent gross-total resection (GTR) (one upfront, two at progression), and one underwent resection of a spinal metastasis at progression. Two of the patients who underwent GTR developed profound neurologic morbidities due to stroke. Five patients (23%) received focal radiotherapy at 54–55.8Gy: as upfront adjuvant therapy in two cases and at progression in three. One patient suffered from symptomatic radionecrosis requiring steroid and bevacizumab. Systemic therapy was used in four patients (18%) at progression, including one who received RT; a carboplatin-containing regimen was adopted in three out of these patients.

Disease progression, patient outcome, and long-term morbidities

During the follow-up period (median, 7.64 years; range, 0.51–16.98), seven patients (32%) treated at SJCRH experienced progression, including two (9%) with metastasis (Table 1). Four patients had a single progression, whereas the remainder experienced two to four progressions. Of the two patients with metastasis, one had known metastatic deposit at the infundibular recess at diagnosis. The second patient did not undergo spinal MRI at diagnosis and was found to have infundibular and spinal metastasis 4 months after diagnosis. The median duration from diagnosis to first progression was 0.68 years (range, 0.28–8.98). Three patients (14%), including two with PD, died (of suicide, obstructive hydrocephalus and suspected shunt failure). This translates into a 5/10-year OS and PFS of 100%/83.9 ± 10.4%, and 76.8 ± 9.1%/48.7 ± 14.2% (Fig. 2). Patients with TG reported significant long-term morbidities, including persistent headaches and visual symptoms (Fig. 1). Cognitive assessments were completed and at a median age of 14.96 years (range, 4.5–24.92) and at a median 5.63 years (range, 0.44–9.55) after diagnosis. Impaired scores were most frequently identified in processing speed (7 out of 7 scores; 100%), working memory (2 out of 7; 28.6%) and academics (math, 3 out of 7, 42.9%). (Fig. 1, Additional file 3: Table S2).

Imaging features and predictors of progression

Imaging was available for review in 22 patients (19 patients treated at SJCRH and 3 seen for review). Images obtained at diagnosis revealed that nine patients (40.9%) had lesions confined to the tectal plate, whereas 13 (59.1%) had lesions extending to adjacent structures such as the tegmentum and thalami (Fig. 1, Additional file 4: Table S3). Mean tumor measurements at diagnosis were 4.3(±4.05) cm^2. All lesions were isointense or hypointense on T1-weighted images and most were

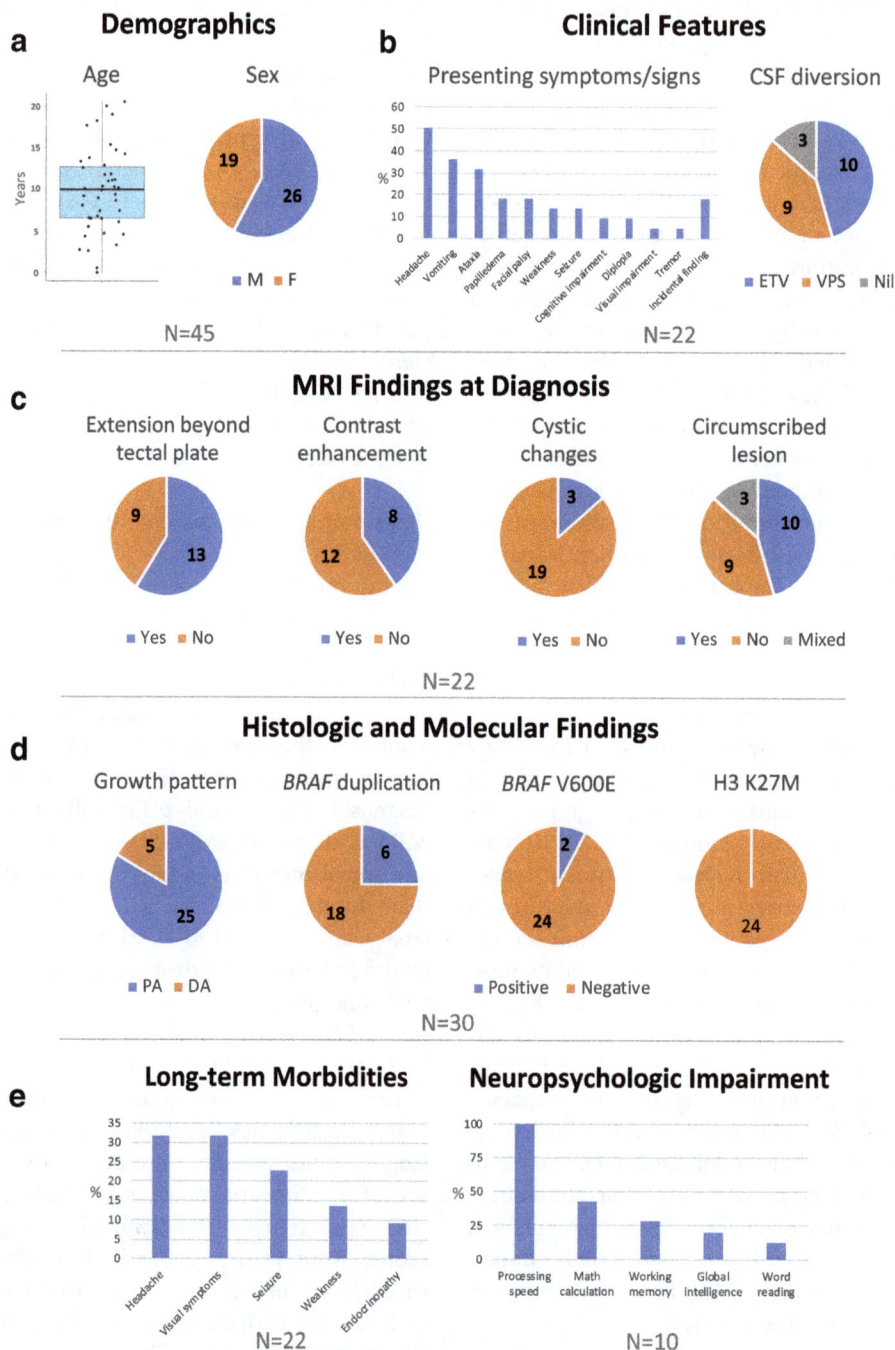

Fig. 1 a Demographics, **b** clinical features, **c** imaging characteristics, **d** histologic and molecular findings, and **e** long-term morbidities in patients with tectal glioma

hyperintense on T2-weighted sequences (Fig. 3). Contrast enhancement was detected in 8/20 (40%) and cystic changes in 3/22 (14%), the presence of both were significantly correlated with lesions ≥3cm^2 ($P = 0.027$ and 0.043 respectively). In those who had diffusion-weighted imaging (DWI, $n = 18$), the mean (±SD) relative apparent diffusion coefficient (rADC) was 1.69 (±0.47). Lesions with measured area greater than 3cm^2 ($P = 0.023$),

contrast enhancement ($P = 0.039$), and cystic changes ($P = 0.037$) at diagnosis predicted inferior PFS (Fig. 2). Other radiologic parameters, including tumor extent, tumor circumscription, and rADC values, as well as clinical parameters, namely sex, presenting symptoms, symptom duration before diagnosis and need for CSF diversion, were not significantly associated with PFS. In comparison of sequential MR images at diagnosis

Table 1 Interventions and outcomes for patients treated at SJCRH

No.	CSF diversion (no. of revision[s])	Ommaya	Surgery	Chemotherapy	RT	Indication for adjuvant	Long-term sequelae	Outcome	Duration of follow-up (y)
1	VPS (1)	No	Bx upfront	Nil	54 Gy	Upfront	Seizure; memory issues	Alive with SD	12.67
2	VPS (6)	No	Bx at progression, then repeated drainage of cyst; and GTR×2	POG9060 (ifosfamide)	55.8 Gy	Multiple PD	Learning difficulties	Died of shunt failure	6.78
3	VPS (subdural)	No	Nil	Nil	Nil	N/A	HA + diplopia	Died of obstructive hydrocephalus	7.72
4	VPS (12) → ETV (1)	No	Nil	Carboplatin + tamoxifen	Nil	PD	HA, N, V, nystagmus, OA, VF defect, R CN VII deficit, hypopituitarism	Died of suicide	10.72
5	VPS (subdural)	No	Nil	Nil	Nil	N/A	Nil	Alive with SD	16.98
6	VPS	No	Nil	Nil	Nil	N/A	Spastic quadriplegic CP, epilepsy, severe mental retardation,	Alive with SD	13.97
7	VPS (2)	No	Bx upfront, then resection of spinal metastasis at progression	1. Carboplatin + vincristine + temozolomide 2. Lomustine + procarbazine + vincristine	Nil	PD (metastasis)	GHD, epilepsy off medications	Alive with SD	11.24
8	Nil	No	Nil	Nil	Nil	N/A	Migraine	Alive with SD	11.28
9	ETV → VPS at progression	No	Bx upfront, resection at progression (complicated by hemorrhagic stroke)	Nil	54 Gy	Upfront	L hemiparesis, bilateral CN IV and VI palsy	Alive with NED	10.31
10	ETV → VPS (1)	Yes	Bx at progression	1. Carboplatin + vincristine + temozolomide 2. Vinblastine 3. Selumetinib	Nil	PD (metastasis)	HA	Alive with SD on treatment	9.37
11	VPS (2)	No	Bx upfront inconclusive; 2 more Bxs at progression	Nil	54 Gy RT necrosis requiring steroid/bevacizumab	PD	Pathological fracture due to steroid use	Alive with SD	9.57
12	Nil	No	Nil	Nil	54 Gy	PD	Headache, L ptosis, xerostomia, ADHD	Alive with SD	7.56
13	VPS (2)	No	Nil	Nil	Nil	N/A	Seizure, bilateral exotropia, delay, learning difficulty, NF-1 related	Alive with SD	9.81
14	ETV	Yes	Nil	Nil	Nil	N/A	Nil	Alive with SD	5.46
15	ETV	Yes	Nil	Nil	Nil	N/A	Intermittent exotropia bilaterally	Alive with SD	5.81
16	Nil	No	Nil	Nil	Nil	N/A	Migraine	Alive with SD	4.94

Table 1 Interventions and outcomes for patients treated at SJCRH *(Continued)*

No.	CSF diversion (no. of revision[s])	Ommaya	Surgery	Chemotherapy	RT	Indication for adjuvant	Long-term sequelae	Outcome	Duration of follow-up (y)
17	ETV	Yes	Nil	Nil	Nil	N/A	Memory problem, NF-1 related	Alive with SD	4.51
18	ETV	Yes	Nil	Nil	Nil	N/A	HA? Migraine	Alive with SD	3.64
19	ETV	Yes	Nil	Nil	Nil	N/A	Abnormal EEG	Alive with SD	1.49
20	ETV	Yes	Nil	Nil	Nil	N/A	Nil	Alive with SD	1.49
21	ETV	Yes	Nil	Nil	Nil	N/A	Nil	Alive with SD	1.24
22	ETV	No	Bx upfront	Nil	Nil	N/A	Nil	Alive with SD	0.51

ADHD attention-deficit hyperactivity disorder, *Bx* biopsy, *CP* cerebral palsy, *CSF* cerebrospinal fluid, *CN* cranial nerve, *ETV* endoscopic third ventriculostomy, *GHD* growth hormone deficiency, *GTR* gross total resection, *HA* headache, *L* left, *N* nausea, *NF-1* neurofibromatosis type 1, *OA* optic atrophy, *PD* progressive disease, *R* right, *RT* radiotherapy, *SD* stable disease, *V* vomiting, *VF* visual field, *VPS* ventriculo-peritoneal shunt, *y* year(s)

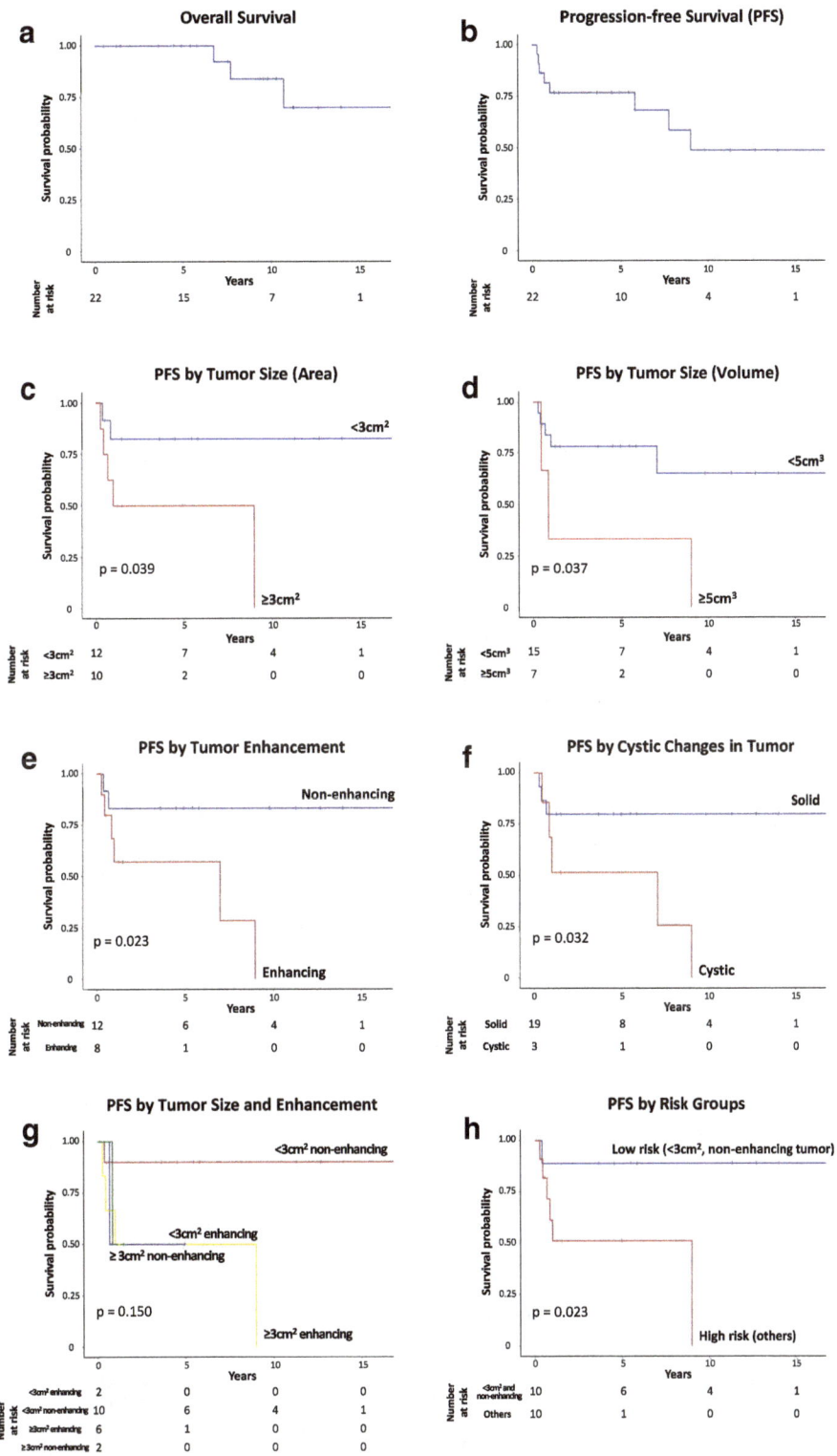

Fig. 2 a Overall survival and **b** progression-free survival of patients with longitudinal follow-up in our cohort. **c-h** Imaging predictors of progression-free survival

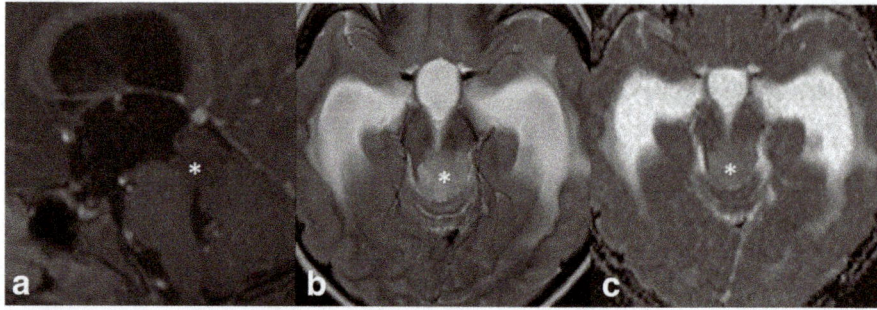

Fig. 3 Typical MRI features of tectal glioma. **a** Sagittal post-contrast T1-weighted image shows a typical non-enhancing, T1 hypointense lesion obstructing the cerebral aqueduct (*). **b** Axial T2-weighted image shows typical T2 hyperintensity of the lesion (*), and periventricular CSF accumulation indicative of hydrocephalus. **c** on ADC map, tectal gliomas (*) are typically high in signal ("facilitated" diffusion)

and progression ($n = 8$) (Additional file 5: Table S4), mean tumor measurements were 5.48 (±5.54) cm^2 and 9.61 (±8.35) cm^2, respectively, with mean increase of 88.19 (±51.49) %. All lesions enhanced at progression, with further increases in the extent and avidity of enhancement in those with pre-existing enhancement. One additional lesion (for a total of four out of eight) developed cystic change at progression, and intra-tumoral hemorrhage was evident in one patient. No significant alteration in rADC was observed at progression ($P = 0.760$).

Histopathologic and molecular features

Thirty patients had tumor tissue available for pathology review. They included seven patients treated at SJCRH and 23 referred for case review (Figs 1 and 4, Additional file 6: Table S5). Sixteen patients had tumor samples from initial diagnosis available and 14 had samples obtained at progression. All specimens were classified as LGG and showed bland cytology. Twenty-five samples (83%) displayed histopathological features similar to PA (WHO grade I). These tumors had a non-infiltrative growth pattern with biphasic, alternating loose and more compact architecture, similar to PAs of other sites. The tumor cells had piloid morphology. Microcystic regions, Rosenthal fibers and eosinophilic granular bodies were frequent findings. Five (17%) had histopathological features aligned best with diffuse astrocytoma (DA) (WHO grade II). These tumors had a diffusely infiltrative growth pattern similar to DAs of other sites. Only 1/14 samples obtained at progression (7.1%) exhibited a DA growth pattern, suggesting that such finding does not equate an increased risk of progression. *BRAF* duplication consistent with the presence of *KIAA1549-BRAF* fusion was present in 6/24 samples (25%), whereas *BRAF* V600E mutation was detected in 2/26 samples (7.7%). All eight samples with *BRAF* alterations exhibited a PA-like growth pattern. In contrast, none of the 24 samples evaluated harbored the histone H3 K27M mutation.

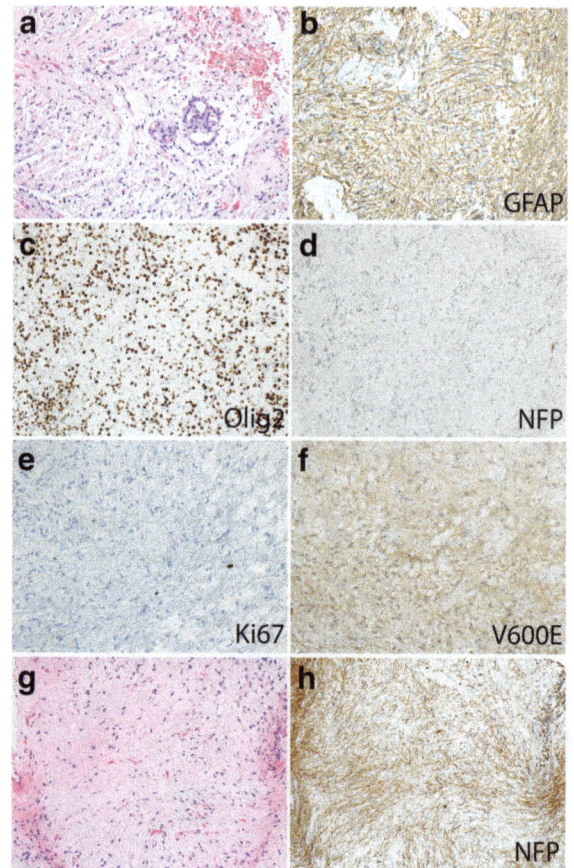

Fig. 4 Histologic features of tectal glioma. **a** Most tectal gliomas demonstrate typical morphologic features of pilocytic astrocytoma, including alternating loose and more compact architecture, bland cytology, Rosenthal fibers, and sclerotic vessels, as well as glomeruloid microvascular proliferation. **b**, **c** The tumor cells are diffusely and strongly positive for GFAP and Olig2. **d** Occasional entrapped axons are highlighted by neurofilament (NFP) staining. **e** Ki67 labeling is minimal. **f** *BRAF* V600E mutant protein is detected by immunohistochemical staining in a few cases. **g** Occasionally, tectal glioma may have a more diffuse growth pattern, similar to that of a diffuse astrocytoma, with numerous entrapped axons (highlighted by NFP staining, **h**)

The prognostic value of *BRAF* alterations could not be meaningfully interpreted with the limited sample size.

Genome-wide DNA methylation profiling

Analysis of genomic DNA methylation profiles by t-SNE plot and unsupervised cluster analysis demonstrated that TG harbors methylation patterns distinct from PAs of nearby sites (cerebellum, CBPA, and hypothalamus, HTPA) and also other brain tumors including rosette-forming glioneuronal tumor (RGNT), dysembryoplastic neuro-epithelial tumor (DNET), ganglioglioma (GG), sube-pendymal giant cell astrocytoma (SEGA), *MYB*-altered LGG, histone H3 K27M-mutant diffuse midline glioma (DMG), and IDH-mutant diffuse astrocytoma (AIDH) / oligodendroglioma (OIDH), and normal tissue from the hypothalamus (Hyp), pons, cerebellum (CB) and white matter (WM) (Fig. 5).

Discussion

We have reported imaging findings, histopathology, molecular analysis and outcomes of children with TG compiled over a period of three decades. The presentation of TG is often typified by symptoms of raised intracranial pressure and delayed diagnosis, with most reports describing a lead time of 3–6 months [1, 4, 5, 8, 15, 16, 37, 39, 41, 43, 45]. Misdiagnosis of TG as aqueductal stenosis based on CT, as in three of our patients, was common and was associated with even longer symptom

durations before TG diagnosis [5]. The more widespread application of MRI for neuroimaging has resulted in incidental diagnoses of TG [1, 14, 17, 22, 26, 32–34, 41, 42, 48]. TG was an incidental finding in up to 27% of patients in various series and in an even higher percentage when MRI was part of a structured surveillance, as in children with NF1 [14, 33]. Whether TG diagnosis in this context is truly beneficial for patient outcomes remains uncertain [40].

Initial treatment of pediatric TG presented with obstructive hydrocephalus involves CSF diversion. VPS use has been associated with frequent failures, the need for revision, issues with MR compatibility, and over-shunting [4, 8, 15, 16, 28, 41]. Consequently, ETV has replaced shunt insertion as the preferred method of CSF diversion [9, 20, 26, 48]. Ommaya reservoirs can be safely inserted during ETV, allowing emergent CSF withdrawal in the event of ETV failure [10]. Concomitant tumor resection is best avoided because of its inherent risks [25]. Lapras and colleagues reported their experience in resecting 12 tectal plate lesions upfront, with GTR being achieved in nine patients and partial resection in three [25]. However, this accomplishment was at the expense of a vegetative state and death in one patient and surgical complications requiring early re-operation in four others, as well as other complications including visual-field defects, Parinaud syndrome, and mutism in further patients. Other studies reserved tumor biopsy/resection for disease progression [22, 43].

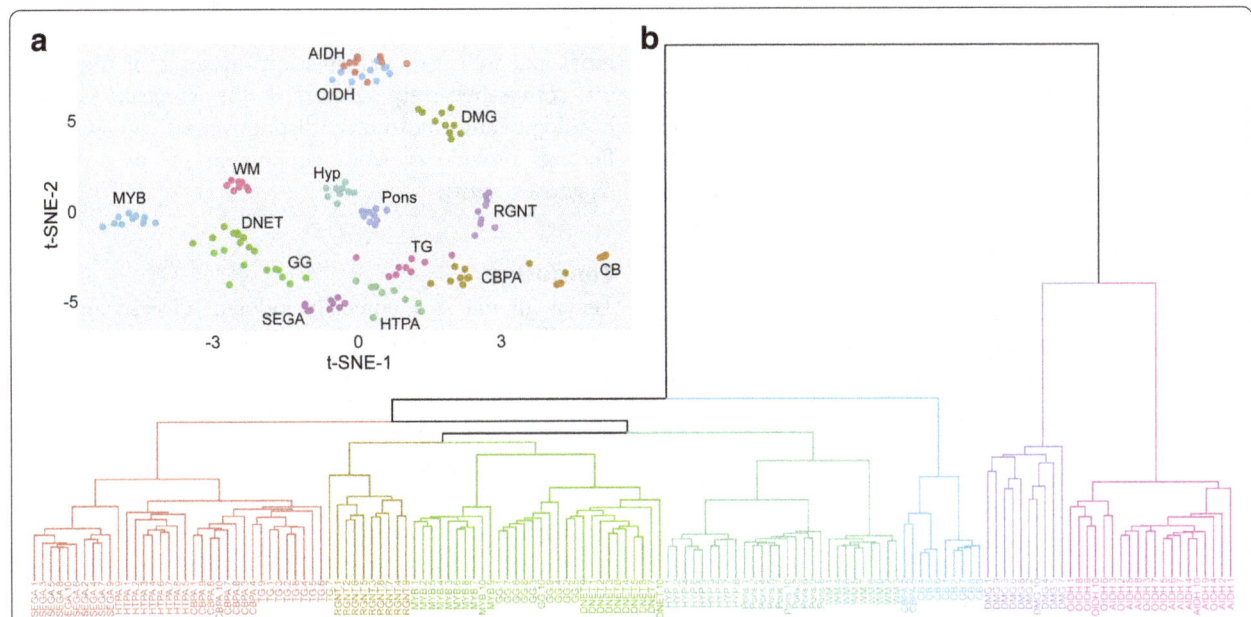

Fig. 5 Genome-wide DNA methylation profiling support tectal glioma as a molecularly distinct entity. **a** t-SNE plot and **b** dendrogram of unsupervised cluster analysis comparing DNA methylation profile of tectal glioma with those of 10 other brain tumor entities including PAs of nearby sites (cerebellum, CBPA, and hypothalamus, HTPA), rosette-forming glioneuronal tumor (RGNT), dysembryoplastic neuroepithelial tumor (DNET), ganglioglioma (GG), subependymal giant cell astrocytoma (SEGA), *MYB*-altered LGG, histone H3 K27M-mutant diffuse midline glioma (DMG) and IDH-mutant diffuse astrocytoma (AIDH) / oligodendroglioma (OIDH), and normal tissue from hypothalamus (Hyp), pons, cerebellum (CB) and white matter (WM) demonstrate that tectal glioma forms a distinct cluster

Similar to our cohort, around one-third of patients in the literature eventually required tumor-directed surgery, and visual deficits, gaze palsies, and intracranial hemorrhages remained significant complications. In view of the significant surgical morbidities, biopsy or resection of TG should only be reserved for tumors with an atypical radiographic appearance, and for debulking as well as to guide targeted treatment (such as *BRAF* and *MEK* inhibitors) at progression [5, 39, 42].

Adjuvant therapy with chemotherapy and/or focal radiation is often employed in patients with PD [4, 5, 14, 17, 21, 25, 30, 32, 34, 38, 41–43, 45]. In our study, significant predictors of progression included tumor size greater than $3cm^2$, contrast enhancement and cystic changes at diagnosis, confirming the suggestions of previous reports [22, 34, 43]. To evaluate the role of adjuvant therapy and treatment outcome, we extensive reviewed clinical reports on pediatric TG (< 21 years at diagnosis, 5 or more patients) and combined with data from our cohort (Additional file 7: Table S6) [1, 4, 5, 7–9, 14–17, 20–22, 25, 26, 28, 30, 32–34, 37–39, 41–43, 45, 48]. Among 26 studies reporting details of adjuvant therapy, 56/463 patients (12.1%) received focal radiation with doses of 50.2–56.8Gy, whereas 26/463 (5.6%) received systemic therapy [1, 4, 5, 8, 9, 14–17, 21, 25, 26, 28, 30, 32–34, 37–39, 41–43, 45, 48]. Patient outcomes were reported in 28 studies, with 495/508 patients (97.4%) surviving for average durations ranging from 2 to 10 years at follow-up [1, 4, 5, 8, 9, 14–17, 20–22, 25, 26, 28, 30, 32–34, 37–39, 41–43, 45, 48]. In the studies describing PD (*n* = 24), 121 of 453 patients (26.7%) displayed clinical and/or radiographic PD, with the average duration from diagnosis to progression ranging from 3 months to 7.8 years [1, 4, 5, 8, 9, 14–17, 20–22, 28, 30, 32–34, 38, 39, 41–43, 48]. Of the 13 patients who died, eight died of PD (one had high-grade glioma [HGG]), one died of metastatic neuroblastoma, one died of VPS infection, and three deaths were from our series discussed earlier. These data suggest that the vast majority of children with TG, despite the risk of progression in a quarter, are long-term survivors with salvage adjuvant treatment. Such findings are striking in the context of most TG not being surgically removed and the extent of resection being one of the most important prognostic factors in other LGGs [35].

The unique clinical behavior of TG might be explained by its anatomical location and the differences in tumor biology among LGGs from various body sites. In our study, we for the first time interrogated the molecular distinctiveness of TG by performing targeted studies (of *BRAF* alterations and histone mutations) and genome-wide DNA methylation profiling. The frequency of *KIAA1549-BRAF* fusion (by the presence of *BRAF* locus duplication on iFISH) in TG (25%) appeared to be lower than that in PAs from the cerebellum (92%) and supratentorium (59%), whereas the frequency of *BRAF* V600E mutation (7.7%) appeared to be intermediate between the two (0% and 10% respectively) [3, 52]. Despite the extra-tectal extension of a proportion of tumors, the lack of histone H3 K27M mutations in all 24 samples supported the biological distinctiveness of TG from other midline diffuse gliomas of the brainstem, which are often characterized by such histone mutations and a more aggressive clinical course. DNA methylation profiling has established a role in defining clinically relevant subgroups in CNS tumors such as medulloblastoma, ependymoma and HGG [12, 31, 51]. Our comparison of the methylation profiles of TG and cerebellar/hypothalamic PAs revealed molecular heterogeneity among these morphologically similar lesions, further supporting the biological uniqueness of TG.

Pediatric TG should be considered a chronic disease, in which care for long-term morbidities is of paramount importance. Caregivers should be informed of the common long term morbidities in patients with TG including chronic headache, persistent visual symptoms and neurocognitive impairments [1, 4, 14, 16, 20, 22, 25, 28, 29, 39, 43, 48]. Neuropsychologic assessments in our cohort suggested areas of deficit in working memory, processing speed and academics, specifically math, thus adding to prior reports of problems in visual attention deficits, behavior problems, and academic achievement, calling for neuropsychologic evaluation as standard of care in patients with TG [1, 14]. Despite the retrospective nature of our analysis and limitation on available material and follow-up information on some of the cases, we comprehensively addressed the clinical, imaging, histologic and molecular distinctiveness of TG. Our findings provide evidence supporting TG as a distinct diagnostic entity.

Conclusion

Tectal glioma is a clinically indolent disease and biologically distinct from other LGGs. Symptoms are frequently due to obstructive hydrocephalus and diagnosis can be made based on typical MRI features. CSF diversion by ETV is sufficient for most patients. Disease progression may be predicted by size, contrast enhancement and cystic change on initial MRI. Long-term follow-up for morbidities including neuropsychologic impairments is necessary for patients with this chronic illness.

Additional files

Additional file 1: Figure S1. Number of patients who underwent clinical, radiologic and pathologic review in our cohort. (TIF 881 kb)

Additional file 2: Table S1. Demographics and presenting symptoms in patients treated at SJCRH. (DOCX 23 kb)

Additional file 3: Table S2. Characteristics of patients who underwent neuropsychologic testing in our cohort. (DOCX 22 kb)

Additional file 4: Table S3. Centrally reviewed diagnostic imaging features in our study cohort. (DOCX 27 kb)

Additional file 5: Table S4. Evolution of imaging features at disease progression. (DOCX 24 kb)

Additional file 6: Table S5. Histopathologic features and molecular findings. (DOCX 24 kb)

Additional file 7: Table S6. Summary of literature on pediatric tectal glioma. (DOCX 47 kb)

Acknowledgements
The authors would like to thank Emily Walker in the Hartwell Center of St. Jude Children's Research Hospital for her technical support on genomic DNA methylation profiling, Raven Holcomb and Alice Slusher in the Department of Pathology for their assistant in performing immunohistochemistry and tissue processing, Susana Raimondi and James Dalton in the Department of Pathology for their assistance in performing fluorescence in situ hybridization, Matthew Lear at St. Jude Biorepository for his assistance in providing study material, Dianne Scott and Stacey Davis in the Department of Pathology for administrative support, and Keith A. Laycock, PhD, ELS for scientific editing of the manuscript.

Funding
JC receives research support from the American Lebanese Syrian Associated Charities (ALSAC) through the Department of Pathology of St. Jude Children's Research Hospital.

Authors' contributions
APYL, JHH, LMJ, MG, SA, SW, PK, AG, JC and IQ analyzed and interpreted the results. JHH performed central review of the imaging findings. JC performed central pathology review. LMJ and MG reviewed and analyzed the neuropsychological assessment data. APYL, YG, JC and IQ collected the patient cohort. SW performed statistical analysis. XL and JC performed molecular analysis. APYL, JHH, LMJ, MG, XL, JC and IQ wrote the manuscript. All authors read and approved the final manuscript.

Competing interests
The authors declare that they have no competing interests.

Author details
[1]Department of Oncology, St. Jude Children's Research Hospital, 262 Danny Thomas Place, MS 260, Memphis 38105-3678, TN, USA. [2]Department of Diagnostic Imaging, St. Jude Children's Research Hospital, Memphis, TN, USA. [3]Department of Psychology, St. Jude Children's Research Hospital, Memphis, TN, USA. [4]Department of Radiation Oncology, St. Jude Children's Research Hospital, Memphis, TN, USA. [5]Department of Biostatistics, St. Jude Children's Research Hospital, Memphis, TN, USA. [6]Department of Pathology, St. Jude Children's Research Hospital, 262 Danny Thomas Place, MS 250, Memphis 38105-3678, TN, USA. [7]Department of Surgery, St. Jude Children's Research Hospital, Memphis, TN, USA. [8]Department of Neurosurgery, University of Tennessee Health Science Center, Memphis, TN, USA. [9]Le Bonheur Neuroscience Institute, Le Bonheur Children's Hospital, Memphis, TN, USA. [10]Semmes Murphey Clinic, Memphis, TN, USA.

References
1. Aarsen FK, Arts WF, Van Veelen-Vincent ML, Lequin MH, Catsman-Berrevoets CE (2014) Long-term outcome in children with low grade tectal tumours and obstructive hydrocephalus. Eur J Paediatr Neurol 18:469–474
2. Aryee MJ, Jaffe AE, Corrada-Bravo H, Ladd-Acosta C, Feinberg AP, Hansen KD, Irizarry RA (2014) Minfi: a flexible and comprehensive bioconductor package for the analysis of Infinium DNA methylation microarrays. Bioinformatics 30:1363–1369. https://doi.org/10.1093/bioinformatics/btu049
3. Bergthold G, Bandopadhayay P, Hoshida Y, Ramkissoon S, Ramkissoon L, Rich B, Maire CL, Paolella BR, Schumacher SE, Tabak B (2015) Expression profiles of 151 pediatric low-grade gliomas reveal molecular differences associated with location and histological subtype. Neuro-Oncology 17:1486–1496
4. Bowers DC, Georgiades C, Aronson LJ, Carson BS, Weingart JD, Wharam MD, Melhem ER, Burger PC, Cohen KJ (2000) Tectal gliomas: natural history of an indolent lesion in pediatric patients. Pediatr Neurosurg 32:24–29
5. Boydston WR, Sanford RA, Muhlbauer MS, Kun LE, Kirk E, Dohan JFC, Schweitzer JB (1991) Gliomas of the Tectum and periaqueductal region of the mesencephalon. Pediatr Neurosurg 17:234–238
6. Capper D, Jones DTW, Sill M, Hovestadt V, Schrimpf D, Sturm D, Koelsche C, Sahm F, Chavez L, al RDE (2018) DNA methylation-based classification of central nervous system tumours. Nature 555:469–474. https://doi.org/10.1038/nature26000
7. Dabscheck G, Prabhu SP, Manley PE, Goumnerova L, Ullrich NJ (2015) Risk of seizures in children with tectal gliomas. Epilepsia 56:e139–e142. https://doi.org/10.1111/epi.13080
8. Dağlıoğlu E, Çataltepe O, Akalan N (2003) Tectal gliomas in children: the implications for natural history and management strategy. Pediatr Neurosurg 38:223–231
9. Diaz RJ, Girgis FM, Hamiltonn MG (2014) Endoscopic third ventriculostomy for hydrocephalus due to tectal glioma. Can J Neurol Sci 41:476–481
10. Drake J, Chumas P, Kestle J, Pierre-Kahn A, Vinchon M, Brown J, Pollack IF, Arai H (2006) Late rapid deterioration after endoscopic third ventriculostomy: additional cases and review of the literature. J Neurosurg Pediatr 105:118–126
11. Elliott CD (2007) Differential ability scales, 2nd edn. Harcourt Assessment, City, San Antonio, TX
12. Ellison DW, Kocak M, Dalton J, Megahed H, Lusher ME, Ryan SL, Zhao W, Nicholson SL, Taylor RE, Bailey S et al (2011) Definition of disease-risk stratification groups in childhood medulloblastoma using combined clinical, pathologic, and molecular variables. Journal of clinical oncology : official journal of the American Society of Clinical Oncology 29:1400–1407. https://doi.org/10.1200/jco.2010.30.2810
13. Fortin JP, Labbe A, Lemire M, Zanke BW, Hudson TJ, Fertig EJ, Greenwood CM, Hansen KD (2014) Functional normalization of 450k methylation array data improves replication in large cancer studies. Genome Biol 15:503. https://doi.org/10.1186/s13059-014-0503-2
14. Gass D, Dewire M, Chow L, Rose SR, Lawson S, Stevenson C, Pai AL, Jones B, Sutton M, Lane A (2015) Pediatric tectal plate gliomas: a review of clinical outcomes, endocrinopathies, and neuropsychological sequelae. J Neuro-Oncol 122:169–177
15. Gomez-Gosalvez F, Menor F, Morant A, Clemente F, Escriva P, Carbonell J, Mulas F (2000) Tectal tumours in paediatrics. A review of eight patients Revista de neurologia 33:605–611
16. Grant GA, Avellino AM, Loeser JD, Ellenbogen RG, Berger MS, Roberts TS (1999) Management of intrinsic gliomas of the tectal plate in children. Pediatr Neurosurg 31:170–176
17. Griessenauer CJ, Rizk E, Miller JH, Hendrix P, Tubbs RS, Dias MS, Riemenschneider K, Chern JJ (2014) Pediatric tectal plate gliomas: clinical and radiological progression, MR imaging characteristics, and management of hydrocephalus. J Neurosurg Pediatr 13:13–20
18. Guillamo J-S, Doz F, Delattre J-Y (2001) Brain stem gliomas. Curr Opin Neurol 14:711–715
19. Jastak S, Wilkinson G (1984) Wide Range Achievement Test - Revised. Jastak Associates, City, Wilmington, DE
20. Javadpour M, Mallucci C (2004) The role of neuroendoscopy in the management of tectal gliomas. Childs Nerv Syst 20:852–857
21. Kaufmann A, Gerber NU, Kandels D, Azizi AA, Schmidt R, Warmuth-Metz M, Pietsch T, Kortmann R-D, Gnekow AK, Grotzer MA (2018) Management of

Primary Tectal Plate low-Grade Glioma in pediatric patients: results of the multicenter treatment study SIOP-LGG 2004. Neuropediatrics

22. Kershenovich A, Silman Z, de Rungs D, Koral K, Gargan L, Weprin B (2016) Tectal lesions in children: a long-term follow-up volumetric tumor growth analysis in surgical and nonsurgical cases. Pediatr Neurosurg 51:69–78

23. Koral K, Alford R, Choudhury N, Mossa-Basha M, Gargan L, Gimi B, Gao A, Zhang S, Bowers DC, Koral KM (2014) Applicability of apparent diffusion coefficient ratios in preoperative diagnosis of common pediatric cerebellar tumors across two institutions. Neuroradiology 56:781–788

24. Krijthe J (2015) Rtsne: T-Distributed Stochastic Neighbor Embedding using a Barnes-Hut Implementation, https://github.com/jkrijthe/Rtsne

25. Lapras C, Bognar L, Turjman F, Villanyi E, Mottolese C, Fischer C, Jouvet A, Guyotat J (1994) Tectal plate gliomas. Part I: microsurgery of the tectal plate gliomas. Acta Neurochir 126:76–83

26. Li KW, Roonprapunt C, Lawson HC, Abbott IR, Wisoff J, Epstein F, Jallo GI (2005) Endoscopic third ventriculostomy for hydrocephalus associated with tectal gliomas. Neurosurg Focus 18:1–4

27. Maechler M, Rousseeuw P, Struyf A, Hubert M, Hornik K (2018) Cluster: cluster analysis basics and extensions. R package version 2.0.7-1.:

28. May PL, Blaser SI, Hoffman HJ, Humphreys RP, Harwood-Nash DC (1991) Benign intrinsic tectal "tumors" in children. J Neurosurg 74:867–871

29. Mohme M, Fritzsche FS, Mende KC, Matschke J, Löbel U, Kammler G, Westphal M, Emami P, Martens T (2018) Tectal gliomas: assessment of malignant progression, clinical management, and quality of life in a supposedly benign neoplasm. Neurosurg Focus 44:E15

30. Mottolese C, Szathmari A, Beuriat PA, Frappaz D, Jouvet A, Hermier M (2015) Tectal plate tumours. Our experience with a paediatric surgical series Neurochirurgie 61:193–200. https://doi.org/10.1016/j.neuchi.2013.12.007

31. Pajtler KW, Witt H, Sill M, Jones DT, Hovestadt V, Kratochwil F, Wani K, Tatevossian R, Punchihewa C, Johann P (2015) Molecular classification of ependymal tumors across all CNS compartments, histopathological grades, and age groups. Cancer Cell 27:728–743

32. Pollack IF, Pang D, Albright AL (1994) The long-term outcome in children with late-onset aqueductal stenosis resulting from benign intrinsic tectal tumors. J Neurosurg 80:681–688

33. Pollack IF, Shultz B, Mulvihill JJ (1996) The management of brainstem gliomas in patients with neurofibromatosis 1. Neurology 46:1652–1660

34. Poussaint TY, Kowal JR, Barnes PD, Zurakowski D, Anthony DC, Goumnerova L, Tarbell NJ (1998) Tectal tumors of childhood: clinical and imaging follow-up. Am J Neuroradiol 19:977–983

35. Qaddoumi I, Sultan I, Gajjar A (2009) Outcome and prognostic features in pediatric gliomas : a review of 6212 cases from the surveillance, epidemiology and end results (SEER) database. Cancer 115:5761–5770. https://doi.org/10.1002/cncr.24663

36. R Core Team (2018) R: A language and environment for statistical computing https://www.R-project.org/

37. Ramelli GP, Cortesi C, Boscherini D, Faggin R, Bianchetti MG (2011) Age-dependent presentation of tectal plate tumors: preliminary observations. J Child Neurol 26:377–380

38. Ramina R, Coelho Neto M, Fernandes YB, Borges G, Honorato DC, Arruda WO (2005) Intrinsic tectal low grade astrocytomas: is surgical removal an alternative treatment? Long-term outcome of eight cases. Arq Neuropsiquiatr 63:40–45

39. Robertson PL, Muraszko KM, Brunberg JA, Axtell RA, Dauser RC, Turrisi AT (1995) Pediatric midbrain tumors: a benign subgroup of brainstem gliomas. Pediatr Neurosurg 22:65–73

40. Roth J, Keating RF, Myseros JS, Yaun AL, Magge SN, Constantini S (2012) Pediatric incidental brain tumors: a growing treatment dilemma. J Neurosurg Pediatr 10:168–174

41. Squires LA, Allen JC, Abbott R, Epstein FJ (1994) Focal tectal tumors management and prognosis. Neurology 44:953–953

42. Stark AM, Fritsch MJ, Claviez A, Dörner L, Mehdorn HM (2005) Management of tectal glioma in childhood. Pediatr Neurol 33:33–38

43. Ternier J, Wray A, Puget S, Bodaert N, Zerah M, Sainte-Rose C (2006) Tectal plate lesions in children. J Neurosurg Pediatr 104:369–376

44. van der Maaten LJP, Hinton GE (2008) Visualizing High-Dimensional Data Using t-SNE. Journal of Machine Learning ResearchNov (9): 2579–2605

45. Vandertop WP, Hoffman HJ, Drake JM, Humphreys RP, Rutka JT, Amstrong DC, Becker LE (1992) Focal midbrain tumors in children. Neurosurgery 31: 186-194

46. Wechsler D (2009) Wechsler individual achievement test, 3rd edn. Psychological Corporation, City, San Antonio, TX

47. Wechsler D (2014) Wechsler intelligence scale for children, 5th edn. Pearson, City, Bloomington, MN

48. Wellons Iii JC, Tubbs RS, Banks JT, Grabb B, Blount JP, Oakes WJ, Grabb PA (2002) Long-term control of hydrocephalus via endoscopic third ventriculostomy in children with tectal plate gliomas. Neurosurgery 51:63–68

49. Wen PY, Chang SM, Van den Bent MJ, Vogelbaum MA, Macdonald DR, Lee EQ (2017) Response assessment in Neuro-oncology clinical trials. J Clin Oncol 35:2439–2449. https://doi.org/10.1200/JCO.2017.72.7511

50. Woodcock RW, KS MG, Mather N (2001) Woodcock-Johnson III tests of achievement. Riverside Publishing, City, Itasca, IL

51. Wu G, Diaz AK, Paugh BS, Rankin SL, Ju B, Li Y, Zhu X, Qu C, Chen X, Zhang J et al (2014) The genomic landscape of diffuse intrinsic pontine glioma and pediatric non-brainstem high-grade glioma. Nat Genet 46:444–450. https://doi.org/10.1038/ng.2938

52. Zhang J, Wu G, Miller CP, Tatevossian RG, Dalton JD, Tang B, Orisme W, Punchihewa C, Parker M, al QI (2013) Whole-genome sequencing identifies genetic alterations in pediatric low-grade gliomas. Nat Genet 45:602–612

14

Analysis of cerebrospinal fluid metabolites in patients with primary or metastatic central nervous system tumors

Leomar Y. Ballester[1,2,6*] (iD), Guangrong Lu[2], Soheil Zorofchian[1], Venkatrao Vantaku[4], Vasanta Putluri[5], Yuanqing Yan[2], Octavio Arevalo[3], Ping Zhu[2], Roy F. Riascos[3,6], Arun Sreekumar[4], Yoshua Esquenazi[2,6], Nagireddy Putluri[4*] and Jay-Jiguang Zhu[2,6]

Abstract

Cancer cells have altered cellular metabolism. Mutations in genes associated with key metabolic pathways (e.g., isocitrate dehydrogenase 1 and 2, *IDH1/IDH2*) are important drivers of cancer, including central nervous system (CNS) tumors. Therefore, we hypothesized that the abnormal metabolic state of CNS cancer cells leads to abnormal levels of metabolites in the CSF, and different CNS cancer types are associated with specific changes in the levels of CSF metabolites. To test this hypothesis, we used mass spectrometry to analyze 129 distinct metabolites in CSF samples from patients without a history of cancer ($n = 8$) and with a variety of CNS tumor types ($n = 23$) (i.e., glioma IDH-mutant, glioma-IDH wildtype, metastatic lung cancer and metastatic breast cancer). Unsupervised hierarchical clustering analysis shows tumor-specific metabolic signatures that facilitate differentiation of tumor type from CSF analysis. We identified differences in the abundance of 43 metabolites between CSF from control patients and the CSF of patients with primary or metastatic CNS tumors. Pathway analysis revealed alterations in various metabolic pathways (e.g., glycine, choline and methionine degradation, dipthamide biosynthesis and glycolysis pathways, among others) between IDH-mutant and IDH-wildtype gliomas. Moreover, patients with IDH-mutant gliomas demonstrated higher levels of D-2-hydroxyglutarate in the CSF, in comparison to patients with other tumor types, or controls. This study demonstrates that analysis of CSF metabolites can be a clinically useful tool for diagnosing and monitoring patients with primary or metastatic CNS tumors.

Keywords: CSF, Metabolites, Brain tumor, Glioma, Hydroxyglutarate, Liquid biopsy

Introduction

Alterations in cellular metabolism are a critical part of cancer cell biology [8]. Studies of cellular metabolism have shown a variety of metabolic alterations in cancer [5, 9, 15, 22]. In the presence of oxygen, energy production in normal cells occurs primarily through oxidative phosphorylation. In contrast, anaerobic glycolysis followed by lactic acid fermentation, is utilized to produce energy in the absence of oxygen. However, many cancer cells produce energy through glycolysis and lactic acid fermentation, even in the presence of oxygen,

a phenomenon called the Warburg effect [11]. Metabolic alterations in cancer cells can be useful in the diagnosis and monitoring of cancer patients. For example, the Warburg effect leads to an increased rate of glycolysis that is accompanied by an increase in glucose uptake, this becomes the basis for the use of fluorodeoxyglucose as a tracer for positron emission tomography (PET) studies [14].

Mutations in genes involved in important metabolic pathways, such as isocitrate dehydrogenase 1 and 2 (*IDH1/IDH2*), are important cancer drivers (e.g., gliomas and leukemias) [19]. *IDH1/IDH2* mutations are associated with the production of an oncogenic metabolite, D-2-hydroxyglutarate (D-2-HG), which appears to be a critical aspect of tumor development [5, 21]. Increased levels of D-2-HG have been demonstrated in *IDH1/IDH2* mutant cells and culture media [5]. The survival of patients with IDH-mutant gliomas is

* Correspondence: leomar.y.ballester@uth.tmc.edu; putluri@bcm.edu
[1]Department of Pathology and Laboratory Medicine, University of Texas Health Science Center at Houston, 6431 Fannin St., MSB 2.136, Houston, TX 77030, USA
[4]Department of Molecular and Cellular Biology, Baylor College of Medicine, 120D, Jewish Building, One Baylor Plaza, Houston, TX 77030, USA
Full list of author information is available at the end of the article

Table 1 Patient characteristics

Patient ID	Age at time of CSF collection	LP vs OM	Sex	Race	Diagnosis	CSF cytology	MRI
1	42	LP	F	Unk	Chiari I malformation	N/A	Neg
2	47	LP	F	W	Aneurysm	N/A	Neg
3	56	LP	F	Unk	Left trigeminal neuralgia.	N/A	Neg
4	37	LP	F	Unk	Benign cyst	N/A	Neg
5	56	LP	M	W	Motor neuron disease	Neg	Neg
6	52	LP	F	Unk	Hydrocephalus	Neg	Neg
7	36	LP	M	AA	Hydrocephalus	Neg	Neg
8	20	LP	F	Unk	Pseudotumor cerebri	Neg	Neg
9	37	LP	F	W	Glioblastoma,IDH-WT	Neg	Pos
10	56	LP	M	W	Glioblastoma,IDH-WT	Neg	N/A
11	77	LP	M	His	Glioblastoma,IDH-WT	N/A	N/A
12	61	LP	F	W	Glioblastoma,IDH-WT	Neg	Pos
13	50	LP	M	W	Glioblastoma,IDH-WT	Neg	Pos
14	47	LP	M	A	Glioblastoma,IDH-WT	N/A	N/A
15	54	LP	M	A	Glioblastoma,IDH-WT	N/A	N/A
16	76	LP	F	Unk	Metastatic Lung Cancer	Neg	N/A
17	77	LP	M	A	Metastatic Lung Cancer	rare atypical cells	Pos
18	60	LP	F	W	Metastatic Lung Cancer	Neg	Pos
19	63	LP	F	W	Metastatic Lung Cancer	Neg	Pos
20	70	LP	M	W	Metastatic Lung Cancer	Neg	Pos
21	60	LP	F	Unk	Metastatic Lung Cancer	Neg	Pos
22	61	LP	F	W	Metastatic Lung Cancer	Neg	N/A
23	59	OM	F	A	Metastatic breast cancer	suspcious for lobular breast CA	Neg
24	59	LP	F	His	Metastatic breast cancer	consistent with metastatic carcinoma	Neg
25	62	LP	F	Unk	Metastatic breast cancer	negative	Pos
26	38	LP	F	His	Metastatic breast cancer	negative	Pos
27	73	OM	F	W	Metastatic breast cancer	negative	Pos
28	28	LP	M	W	Glioblastoma,IDH-mutant	N/A	N/A
29–30		OM				N/A	N/A
31	56	LP	M	Unk	Glioblastoma,IDH-mutant	Neg	Pos
32–33		OM				Neg	Pos
34	32	LP	M	W	Glioblastoma,IDH-mutant	atypical cells present	Pos
35–37		OM				Neg	Pos
38	23	LP	M	W	Glioblastoma,IDH-mutant	Neg	Pos
39–40		OM				Neg	Pos

significantly better than that of patients with IDH-wildtype gliomas. As a result, the WHO classification for central nervous system tumors was recently modified to include mutations in *IDH1/IDH2* as a critical part of the diagnosis of infiltrating gliomas [13]. Also, genes frequently mutated in CNS tumors (e.g., *PTEN*, *PI3K*) have known effects in metabolic pathways. For example, activation of the PI3K/AKT/mTOR pathway leads to increased translation of the hypoxia inducible factor 1α (HIF1α), increased glucose uptake, and increased uptake of essential amino acids [7]. Similarly, the transcription factor Myc can increase the expression of many metabolic enzymes [7].

The tools currently utilized for the diagnosis and monitoring of patients with CNS tumors include CNS imaging, evaluation of tumor cells in the cerebrospinal fluid (CSF-cytology) and brain biopsies. However, CNS imaging studies lack specificity, CSF-cytology has extremely poor sensitivity, and brain biopsies are an

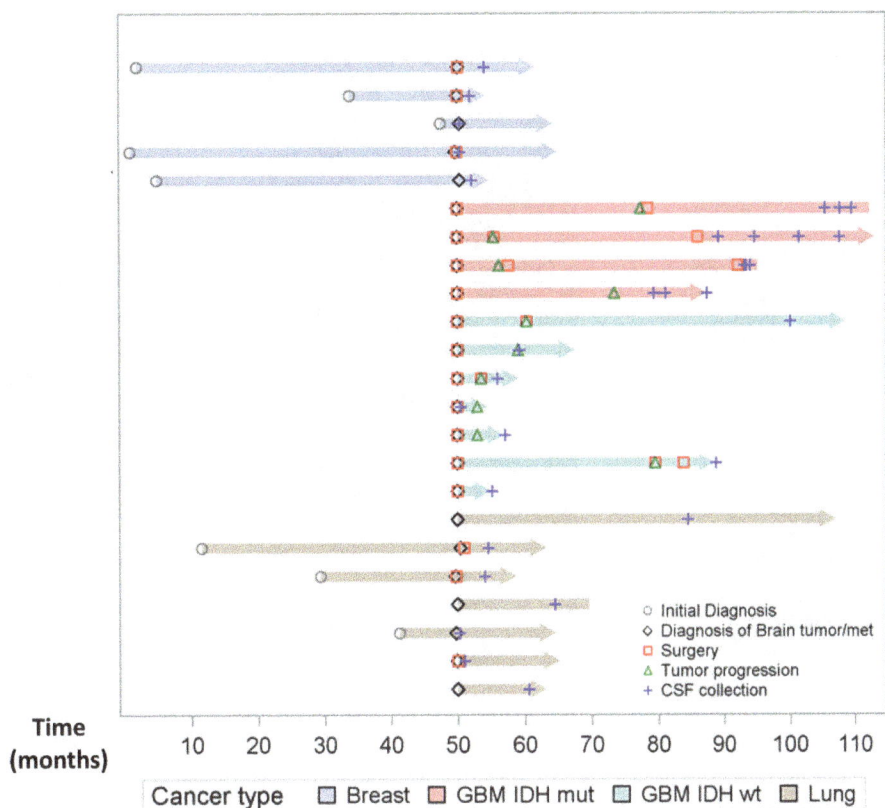

Fig. 1 Swimmer plot depicting CSF sample collections for each patient. Each bar represents one subject included in the study. The blue crosses represent CSF collections. Surgery is indicated by the red square. Grey circles represent the initial diagnosis. The X-axis represents months. For some patients with metastatic disease (i.e., breast and lung cancer) the initial diagnosis of the systemic malignancy occured many months before the development of CNS disease

invasive procedure. Therefore, there is a critical need for more specific and less invasive methods for diagnosing and monitoring patients with CNS tumors. In particular, minimally invasive methods that inform aspects of CNS tumor biology that influence treatment decisions. Although it is recognized that metabolic alterations are common in cancer cells, it remains unclear to what extent the analysis of cellular metabolites in biofluids can be utilized in the clinical management of cancer patients. Several studies have demonstrated differences in circulating metabolites in the blood of patients with a variety of cancer types [3, 20]. However, blood is not an ideal fluid for detecting biomarkers in patients with CNS tumors [2, 6]. In contrast, studies have shown that the cerebrospinal fluid (CSF) is a better source of CNS-tumor-derived biomarkers [6, 10, 17]. In fact, elevated levels of D-2-HG have been demonstrated in the CSF of patients with IDH-mutant gliomas [10]. Differences in the levels of citric acid and lactic acid in the CSF of gliomas of different histologic grade have also been shown [16].

Considering the preliminary evidence showing alterations in metabolites in CNS tumors [10, 12] we decided to perform a comprehensive analysis of 129 metabolites in the CSF of patients with a variety of CNS tumor types. We analyzed the levels of metabolites in the context of CNS imaging and CSF-cytology results, routine clinical assays performed in the evaluation of patients with CNS malignancies. Our results provide insight into metabolic pathways that are altered in IDH-mutant gliomas in comparison to IDH-wildtype gliomas. Also, our data demonstrates elevated levels of D-2-HG in the CSF of patients with IDH-mutant gliomas. In summary, our data supports the idea that analysis of metabolites in the CSF can help in the diagnosis and monitoring of patients with CNS tumors.

Methods

Patients

The study was approved by the institutional review board (IRB). All patients provided informed consent for participation of their samples in research. CSF was collected via lumbar puncture (LP) or intraventricular catheter (Ommaya reservoir, OM). Samples from patients with glioblastoma IDH-WT ($n = 7$), IDH-mutant ($n = 4$; 13 samples), metastatic lung cancer ($n = 7$) or metastatic breast cancer

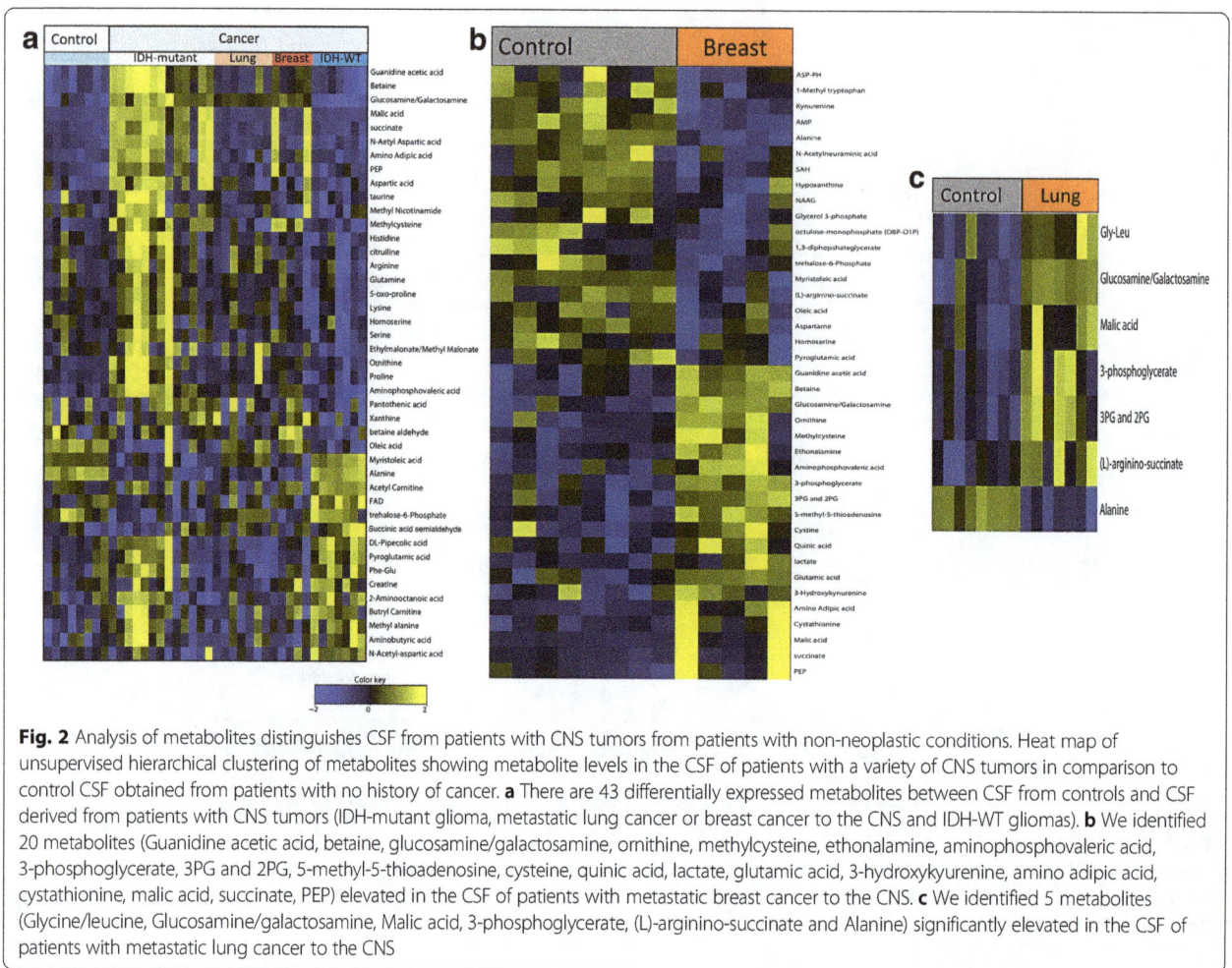

Fig. 2 Analysis of metabolites distinguishes CSF from patients with CNS tumors from patients with non-neoplastic conditions. Heat map of unsupervised hierarchical clustering of metabolites showing metabolite levels in the CSF of patients with a variety of CNS tumors in comparison to control CSF obtained from patients with no history of cancer. **a** There are 43 differentially expressed metabolites between CSF from controls and CSF derived from patients with CNS tumors (IDH-mutant glioma, metastatic lung cancer or breast cancer to the CNS and IDH-WT gliomas). **b** We identified 20 metabolites (Guanidine acetic acid, betaine, glucosamine/galactosamine, ornithine, methylcysteine, ethonalamine, aminophosphovaleric acid, 3-phosphoglycerate, 3PG and 2PG, 5-methyl-5-thioadenosine, cysteine, quinic acid, lactate, glutamic acid, 3-hydroxykyurenine, amino adipic acid, cystathionine, malic acid, succinate, PEP) elevated in the CSF of patients with metastatic breast cancer to the CNS. **c** We identified 5 metabolites (Glycine/leucine, Glucosamine/galactosamine, Malic acid, 3-phosphoglycerate, (L)-arginino-succinate and Alanine) significantly elevated in the CSF of patients with metastatic lung cancer to the CNS

($n = 5$) to the CNS were included (Table 1). All CSF samples from patients with CNS tumors were acquired during the course of the patient's treatment (Fig. 1). Samples from patients with no history of cancer were included as controls ($n = 8$). All gliomas were sequenced for mutations in *IDH1* or *IDH2*. Contrast-enhanced brain MR with optimum 2D/3D images matching the CSF collection date were available for 23 of the 31 patients. MRI scans were interpreted as positive or negative for tumor by a neuroradiologist. Patient characteristics are included in Table 1.

CSF-cytology

CSF was collected via LP or OM. Samples were processed within 2 h from collection time, and centrifuged at 1000 g for 10 min at 4 °C. The cell pellet was discarded and the CSF supernatant was aliquoted and immediately stored at − 80 °C. For CSF-cytology examination the CSF was centrifuged at 1500 rpm for 5 min. The supernatant was discarded and the cell pellet was resuspended in RPMI. Two – six drops of fluid were pipetted into cytospin chambers and the chambers centrifuged at 700 rpm for 7 min into one albumin-covered slide. The slides

were stained with Wright-Giemsa and examined by a board certified cytopathologist.

Imaging

Contrast-enhanced brain MR with optimum 2D/3D images were available for 23 patients. The images were analyzed for the presence of tumor by a board certified neuroradiologist.

Metabolomic analysis

Targeted Metabolic profiling by LC-MS Single Reaction Monitoring (SRM) was used to characterize metabolites. We measured the metabolites using three different chromatographic methods (Additional file 1: Supplementary methods A-C), in each method metabolites were normalized with the spiked internal standards and data were log2-transformed. For each metabolite in the normalized dataset, a two-tailed t-test was used to compare their expression levels between two groups and ANOVA was used to compare more than two groups for their expression levels. Differentially expressed metabolites were identified after adjusting p-values for multiple hypothesis testing

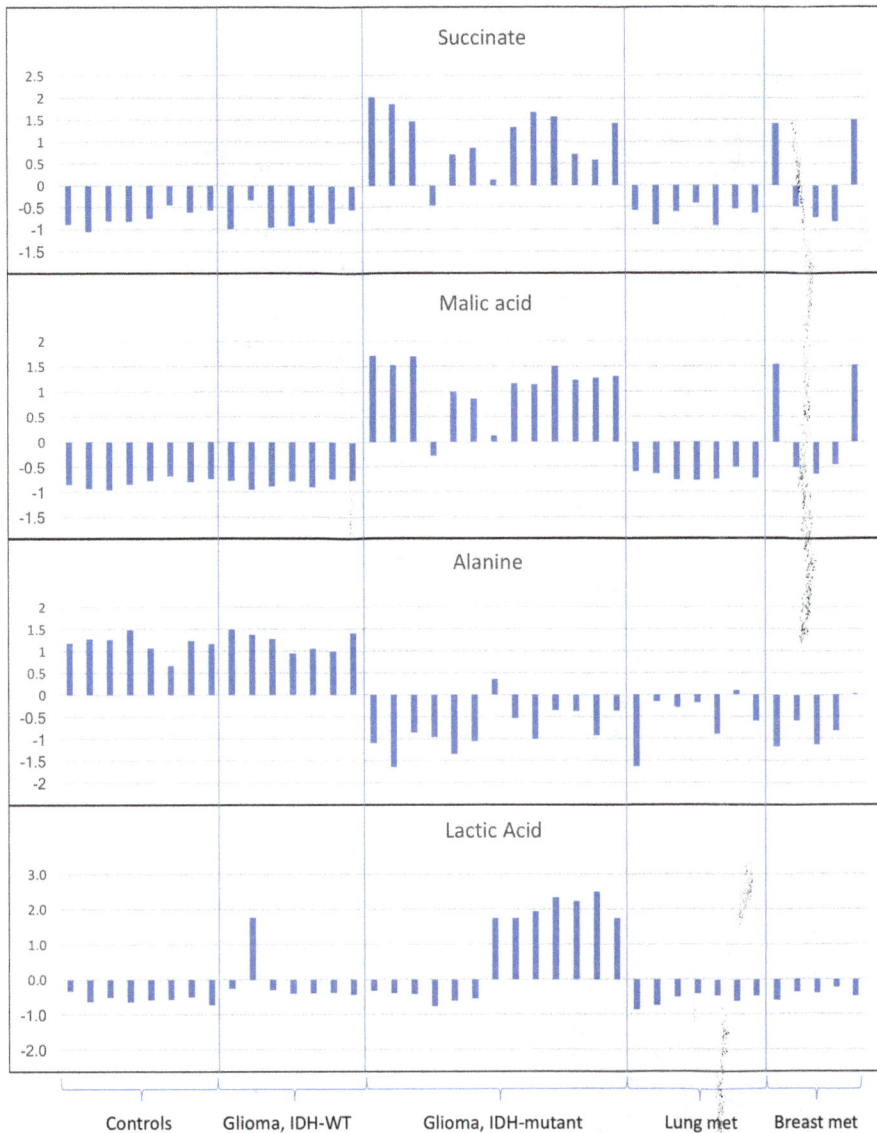

Fig. 3 Differences in the levels of specific CSF metabolites. Differences in the levels of succinate, malic acid, alanine and lactic acid between 40 CSF samples from patients with no history of cancer (controls) or patients with gliomas IDH-WT, gliomas IDH-mutant, or metastatic lung or breast cancer to the CNS. Succinate and malic acid are elevated in all but one of the samples from patients with IDH-mutant glioma, in comparison to patients with IDH-WT gliomas, or controls. In contrast, alanine levels are reduced in CSF samples from patients with IDH-mutant gliomas or metastatic lung or breast carcinomas, in comparison to control CSF samples. Lactic acid levels were elevated in a subset of CSF samples from patients with IDH-mutant gliomas, in comparison to controls or patients with other cancer types. The Y-axis represents normalized log2 transformed values

using the Benjamini-Hochberg method [1] and a False Discovery Rate (FDR) of < 0.25. A hierarchical cluster of the differentially expressed metabolites was generated using the R statistical system (https://www.r-project.org/). We have identified 129 metabolites. AUC (area under the receiver operating characteristic curve) as well as its 95% confidence interval was evaluated by the "DeLong" method with "pROC" package in R (Version 3.4.2) computing environment. The data was log2-transformed and normalized with internal standards on a per-sample, per-method basis.

Results

Patients and clinical characteristics

CSF ($n = 40$) from 31 patients; 13 males and 18 females with age ranging from 20 to 77 years old were included. CSF-cytology results were available for 22/31 patients. One out of three (1/3) available CSF-cytology results from patients with an IDH-mutant glioma was reported as "atypical cells present", 2/5 CSF-cytology results from patients with metastatic breast cancer were reported as "suspicious" or "consistent" with metastatic carcinoma and 1/7 CSF-cytology results from patients with metastatic lung cancer were reported as

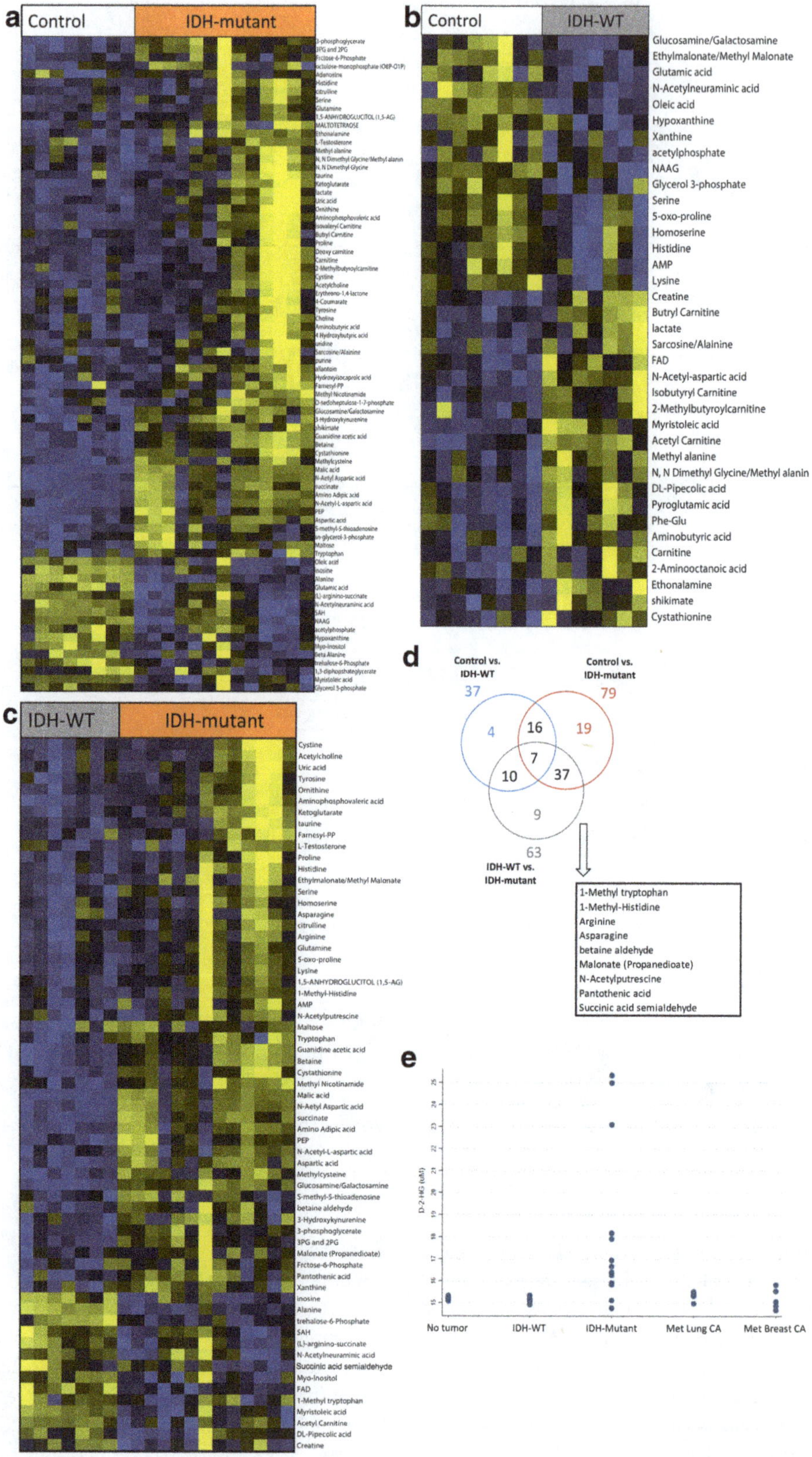

Fig. 4 (See legend on next page.)

"atypical cells present". CSF-cytology results were available for 3/7 patients with IDH-WT gliomas, the 3 samples were reported as negative for tumor cells. CSF-cytology results for 4/8 control patients were available and the result was negative for tumor cells. In total, there were 14 instances in which CSF samples were reported as negative for tumor cells, but the MRI results demonstrated the presence of tumor involving the CNS (Table 1).

Altered metabolites in the CSF of patients with CNS tumors

Using targeted metabolomics, we detected 129 named metabolites (in positive ionization and negative ionization mode) in the CSF of individuals with no cancer history. Differences in the abundance of 43 metabolites were found between CSF from control patients and CSF from patients with a history of a primary or metastatic CNS tumor. (Fig. 2a; FDR adjusted $p < 0.25$). By mapping the 43 altered metabolites into known metabolic pathways, we identified several pathways significantly affected, including glycine, arginine, choline, nitrogen metabolism and glycolysis (Additional file 2: Figure S1).

A heat map depicting the unsupervised hierarchical clustering of samples is shown in Additional file 3: Figure S2. Tricarboxylic acid (TCA) cycle metabolites were found to be elevated in the CSF of patients with CNS tumors including malic acid and succinate. Succinate, malic acid and lactic acid were particularly elevated in IDH-mutant gliomas (Fig. 3). In addition, phosphoenolpyruvate (PEP) levels were elevated in the CSF of patients with IDH-mutant gliomas in comparison to patients with IDH-wildtype tumors (Fig. 4). We also found elevations in amino adipic acid in the CSF of patients with IDH-mutant gliomas. Acetylcarnitine and shikimate were elevated in the CSF of patients with IDH-WT gliomas in comparison to CSF from controls. In the case of patients with metastatic breast cancer, we identified the levels of 20 metabolites to be elevated in the CSF (Fig. 2b). Also, we identified 5 metabolites (Glycine/leucine, Glucosamine/galactosamine, Malic acid, 3-phosphoglycerate, (L)-arginino-succinate and Alanine) significantly elevated in the CSF of patients with metastatic lung cancer in comparison to CSF from controls (Fig. 2c).

CSF metabolites in IDH-mutant versus IDH-WT gliomas

We identified 37 differential CSF metabolites between IDH-WT gliomas and controls, 79 differential metabolites between IDH-mutant gliomas and controls, and 63 differential metabolites between IDH-WT and IDH-mutant gliomas (Fig. 4). Further analysis identified several metabolites (1-methyl tryptophan, 1-methyl-histidine, arginine, asparagine, N-acetylputrescine, succinic acid semialdehyde, malonate, betaine aldehyde and pantothenic acid) that are associated with the presence of an *IDH1* mutation (Fig. 4d). In addition, we detected higher D-2HG levels in the CSF of patients with IDH-mutant gliomas (Fig. 4e). These metabolites were further analyzed individually for the area under the curve (AUC), in the receiver operator characteristics (ROC) curve, to evaluate the ability of each metabolite to discriminate IDH-mutant from IDH-WT gliomas. Individual metabolites were found to have a significant AUC between 0.724–0.888 (Fig. 5). Taken together, the 10 metabolites had a combined AUC of 0.918. While D-2-HG, malic acid and succinate levels were higher in IDH-mutant gliomas, the levels of alanine where significantly elevated in patients with IDH-WT gliomas compared to IDH-mutant tumors (Fig. 3).

Lumbar puncture versus intraventricular catheter

We compared the levels of metabolites in CSF collected by lumbar puncture (LP) and CSF collected from an intraventricular catheter (Ommaya reservoir, OM). The was done by fitting a linear mixed effect model and conducting the likelihood ratio test. To account for the multiplicity, the p value was adjusted by Benjamini and Hochberg method [1]. An adjusted p value of less than 0.05 was considered statistically significant. We did not observe statistically significant differences in the levels of metabolites in samples obtained via LP versus OM (Table 1).

Discussion

Our data shows that it is possible to discriminate CSF from patients with CNS tumors from CSF obtained from patients with non-neoplastic conditions. There are 14 CSF samples that were reported as negative for tumor by CSF-cytology, even when tumor was detected on the MRI, highlighting the limited sensitivity of CSF-cytology for detecting CNS malignancies, and the need for more sensitive and specific methodology to evaluate patients with CNS tumors. Only 1/12 (~ 8%) patients with a metastatic CNS tumor had a positive CSF-cytology result. Our results demonstrate that analysis of CSF metabolites could help identify patients with primary or metastatic CNS tumors, even in the absence of detectable tumor cells in the CSF.

Metabolites in nitrogen metabolism and aminoacyl-tRNA biosynthesis were elevated in the CSF of patients with CNS

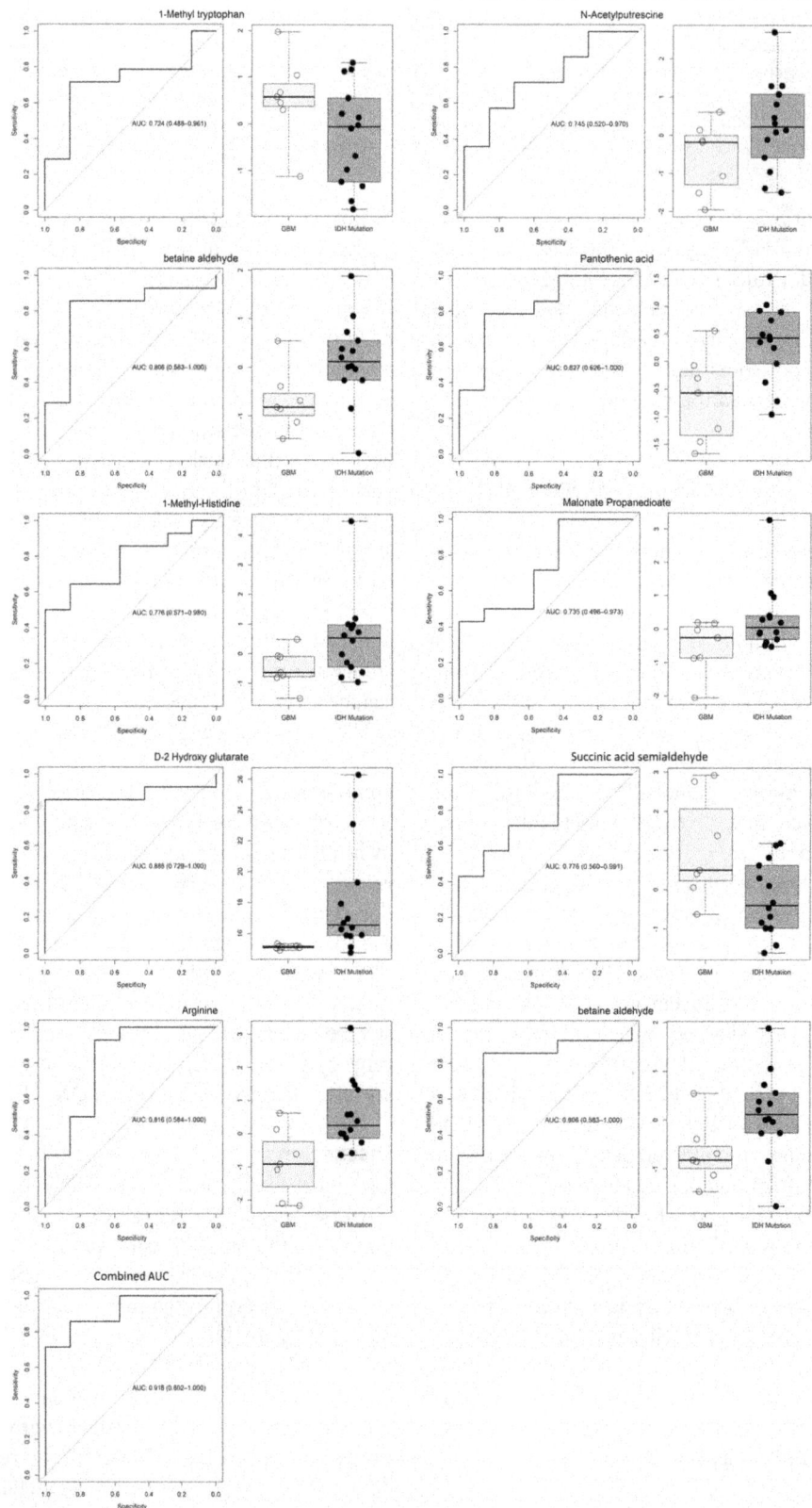

Fig. 5 (See legend on next page.)

(See figure on previous page.)
Fig. 5 Area under the ROC curve. The levels of 10 metabolites are significantly different between IDH-mutant and IDH-WT gliomas. The area under the ROC curve for these metabolites individually and combined is shown. The area under the ROC curve for these 10 metabolites ranged from 0.724 to 0.888. In combination, the area under the ROC curve for the 10 metabolites was 0.918. The levels of these metabolites in CSF can help discriminate patients with IDH-mutant gliomas from IDH-WT gliomas

tumors. Also, glycine, serine threonine, alanine, aspartate and glutamate were present at significantly different levels in the CSF of patients with tumor when compared to controls. These data show that the metabolism of non-essential aminoacids is altered in the CSF of patients with brain tumors and elevations of these amino acids in the CSF could indicate a neoplastic process. Acetylcarnitine and shikimate were elevated in the CSF of patients with IDH-WT-gliomas in comparison to control CSF, an observation that is consistent with a previous report that analyzed CSF from 10 patients with gliomas [12].

It is not surprising that several of the altered metabolites are involved in the TCA cycle. Malic acid and succinate were particularly elevated in IDH-mutant gliomas, consistent with dysregulation of the TCA cycle in these tumors. These data indicate that TCA metabolite alterations in the CSF of patients with IDH-mutant gliomas could be helpful in distinguishing IDH-mutant from IDH-WT tumors. Also, our data shows higher D-2-HG levels in the CSF of patients with IDH-mutant gliomas, consistent with prior reports [5, 10, 18]. In addition, phosphoenolpyruvate (PEP) levels were elevated in the CSF of patients with IDH-mutant gliomas in comparison to patients with IDH-wildtype tumors. Elevated PEP levels have been previously described in glioblastoma tissue samples [4].

To our knowledge, this study is one of the most comprehensive analysis of CSF metabolites in patients with different types of primary or metastatic CNS tumors [12, 16, 23]. Our results show that it is possible to discriminate CSF from patients with IDH-mutant or IDH-WT gliomas and metastatic carcinomas, from patients with non-neoplastic conditions. One limitation of our study is that CSF samples were obtained during or after the patient's treatment. Although the treatment for IDH-mutant and IDH-wildtype gliomas is similar, it is possible that some of the changes in metabolites in CSF could be influenced by the patient's treatment. Therefore, additional studies with CSF obtained prior to therapeutic intervention will be greatly informative. It is important to highlight that metabolomic analysis can be performed with ~100uL of CSF in less than 24 h, and our results provide evidence for tumor-specific metabolic signatures that can help in discriminating neoplastic from non-neoplastic disease. Although studies have postulated differences in CSF biomarkers associated with collection method [10], we did not observe statistically significant differences in the levels of metabolites in samples obtained via LP versus intraventricular catheter. These suggests that although the collection method might influence the levels of

some metabolites, it does not have significant effect on the levels of all metabolites. In conclusion, our data suggest that metabolomic analysis of CSF can provide clinically useful information with a fast turn-around-time, which could be helpful in the evaluation of patients with CNS tumors. This method can serve to complement the measurements of other tumor biomarkers (e.g., circulating tumor DNA) and increase the sensitivity and specificity of CSF analysis as a liquid biopsy approach for patients with CNS malignancies.

Acknowledgments
Baylor College of Medicine Metabolomics core with funding from the NIH (P30 CA125123), CPRIT Proteomics and Metabolomics Core Facility (D.P.E.), (RP170005), and Dan L. Duncan Cancer Center. This research also supported by American Cancer Society (ACS) Award 127430-RSG-15-105-01-CNE (N.P.), NIH U01 CA167234 (A.S.K) and NIH R01CA220297 (N.P.). U01CA179674 (A.S.K), RP120092 (ASK), Agilent Foundation and Brockman Foundation.

Disclosure
The authors have no conflict of interest to disclose.

Author details
[1]Department of Pathology and Laboratory Medicine, University of Texas Health Science Center at Houston, 6431 Fannin St., MSB 2.136, Houston, TX 77030, USA. [2]Department of Neurosurgery, University of Texas Health Science Center at Houston, 6431 Fannin St., MSB 2.136, Houston, TX 77030, USA. [3]Department of Radiology, University of Texas Health Science Center at Houston, Houston, TX 77030, USA. [4]Department of Molecular and Cellular Biology, Baylor College of Medicine, 120D, Jewish Building, One Baylor Plaza, Houston, TX 77030, USA. [5]Advanced Technology Core, Baylor College of Medicine, Houston, TX 77030, USA. [6]Memorial Hermann Hospital, Houston, TX 77030, USA.

References
1. Benjamini Y, Hochberg Y (1995) Controlling the false discovery rate: a practical and powerful approach to multiple testing 57:289–300. https://doi.org/10.2307/2346101
2. Bettegowda C, Sausen M, Leary RJ, Kinde I, Wang Y, Agrawal N, Bartlett BR, Wang H, Luber B, Alani RM, Antonarakis ES, Azad NS, Bardelli A, Brem H, Cameron JL, Lee CC, Fecher LA, Gallia GL, Gibbs P, Le D, Giuntoli RL, Goggins M, Hogarty MD, Holdhoff M, Hong S-M, Jiao Y, Juhl HH, Kim JJ, Siravegna G, Laheru DA, Lauricella C, Lim M, Lipson EJ, Marie SKN, Netto GJ, Oliner KS, Olivi A, Olsson L, Riggins GJ, Sartore-Bianchi A, Schmidt K, Shih L-M, Oba-Shinjo SM, Siena S, Theodorescu D, Tie J, Harkins TT, Veronese S, Wang T-L, Weingart JD, Wolfgang CL, Wood LD, Xing D, Hruban RH, Wu J, Allen PJ, Schmidt CM, Choti MA, Velculescu VE, Kinzler KW, Vogelstein B, Papadopoulos N, Diaz LA (2014) Detection of circulating tumor DNA in early- and late-stage human malignancies. Sci Transl Med 6:224ra24–224ra24. https://doi.org/10.1126/scitranslmed.3007094
3. Chen Y, Ma Z, Min L, Li H, Wang B, Zhong J, Dai L (2015) Biomarker identification and pathway analysis by serum metabolomics of lung cancer. Biomed Res Int 2015:183624–183629. https://doi.org/10.1155/2015/183624

4. Chinnaiyan P, Kensicki E, Bloom G, Prabhu A, Sarcar B, Kahali S, Eschrich S, Qu X, Forsyth P, Gillies R (2012) The Metabolomic signature of malignant Glioma reflects accelerated anabolic metabolism. Cancer Res 72:5878–5888. https://doi.org/10.1158/0008-5472.CAN-12-1572-T

5. Dang L, White DW, Gross S, Bennett BD, Bittinger MA, Driggers EM, Fantin VR, Jang HG, Jin S, Keenan MC, Marks KM, Prins RM, Ward PS, Yen KE, Liau LM, Rabinowitz JD, Cantley LC, Thompson CB, Vander Heiden MG, Su SM (2009) Cancer-associated IDH1 mutations produce 2-hydroxyglutarate. Nature 462:739–744. https://doi.org/10.1038/nature08617

6. De Mattos-Arruda L, Mayor R, Ng CKY, Weigelt B, nez-Ricarte FMI, Torrejon D, Oliveira M, Arias A, Raventos C, Tang J, Guerini-Rocco E, ez EMIN-SA, Lois S, N OMI, La Cruz de X, Piscuoglio S, Towers R, Vivancos A, Peg V, Cajal SRY, Carles J, Rodon J, Lez-Cao MIAGA, Tabernero J, Felip E, Sahuquillo J, Berger MF, Cortes J, Reis-Filho JS, Seoane J (2015) Cerebrospinal fluid-derived circulating tumour DNA better represents the genomic alterations of brain tumours than plasma Nat Commun 6:1–6. https://doi.org/10.1038/ncomms9839

7. DeBerardinis RJ, Lum JJ, Hatzivassiliou G, Thompson CB (2008) The biology of cancer: metabolic reprogramming fuels cell growth and proliferation. Cell Metab 7:11–20. https://doi.org/10.1016/j.cmet.2007.10.002

8. Ferreira LMR (2010) Cancer metabolism: the Warburg effect today. Exp Mol Pathol 89:372–380. https://doi.org/10.1016/j.yexmp.2010.08.006

9. Haq R, Shoag J, Andreu-Perez P, Yokoyama S, Edelman H, Rowe GC, Frederick DT, Hurley AD, Nellore A, Kung AL, Wargo JA, Song JS, Fisher DE, Arany Z, Widlund HR (2013) Oncogenic BRAF regulates oxidative metabolism via PGC1α and MITF. Cancer Cell 23:302–315. https://doi.org/10.1016/j.ccr.2013.02.003

10. Kalinina J, Ahn J, Devi NS, Wang L, Li Y, Olson JJ, Glantz M, Smith T, Kim EL, Giese A, Jensen RL, Chen CC, Carter BS, Mao H, He M, Van Meir EG (2016) Selective detection of the D-enantiomer of 2-Hydroxyglutarate in the CSF of Glioma patients with mutated Isocitrate dehydrogenase. Clin Cancer Res 22:6256–6265. https://doi.org/10.1158/1078-0432.CCR-15-2965

11. Kim J-W, Dang CV (2006) Cancer's molecular sweet tooth and the Warburg effect: figure 1. Cancer Res 66:8927–8930. https://doi.org/10.1158/0008-5472.CAN-06-1501

12. Locasale JW, Melman T, Song S, Yang X, Swanson KD, Cantley LC, Wong ET, Asara JM (2012) Metabolomics of human cerebrospinal fluid identifies signatures of malignant Glioma. Mol Cell Proteomics 11:M111.014688–M111.014612. https://doi.org/10.1074/mcp.M111.014688

13. Louis DN, Ohgaki H, Wiestler OD, Cavenee WK, Ellison DW, Figarella-Branger D, Perry A, Reifenberger G, Deimling von A (2016) WHO classification of Tumours of the central nervous system, 4 ed. WHO

14. Miles KA (2008) Warburg revisited: imaging tumour blood flow and metabolism. Cancer Imaging 8:81–86. https://doi.org/10.1102/1470-7330.2008.0011

15. Mishra P, Tang W, Putluri V, Dorsey TH, Jin F, Wang F, Zhu D, Amable L, Deng T, Zhang S, Killian JK, Wang Y, Minas TZ, Yfantis HG, Lee DH, Sreekumar A, Bustin M, Liu W, Putluri N, Ambs S (2018) ADHFE1 is a breast cancer oncogene and induces metabolic reprogramming. J Clin Invest 128:323–340. https://doi.org/10.1172/JCI93815

16. Nakamizo S, Sasayama T, Shinohara M, Irino Y, Nishiumi S, Nishihara M, Tanaka H, Tanaka K, Mizukawa K, Itoh T, Taniguchi M, Hosoda K, Yoshida M, Kohmura E (2013) GC/MS-based metabolomic analysis of cerebrospinal fluid (CSF) from glioma patients. J Neuro-Oncol 113:65–74. https://doi.org/10.1007/s11060-013-1090-x

17. Pentsova EI, Shah RH, Tang J, Boire A, You D, Briggs S, Omuro A, Lin X, Fleisher M, Grommes C, Panageas KS, Meng F, Selcuklu SD, Ogilvie S, Distefano N, Shagabayeva L, Rosenblum M, DeAngelis LM, Viale A, Mellinghoff IK, Berger MF (2016) Evaluating Cancer of the central nervous system through next-generation sequencing of cerebrospinal fluid. J Clin Oncol 34:2404–2415. https://doi.org/10.1200/JCO.2016.66.6487

18. Reitman ZJ, Jin G, Karoly ED, Spasojevic I, Yang J, Kinzler KW, He Y, Bigner DD, Vogelstein B, Yan H (2011) Profiling the effects of isocitrate dehydrogenase 1 and 2 mutations on the cellular metabolome. PNAS 108:3270–3275. https://doi.org/10.1073/pnas.1019393108

19. Reitman ZJ, Yan H (2010) Isocitrate dehydrogenase 1 and 2 mutations in Cancer: alterations at a crossroads of cellular metabolism. JNCI Journal of the National Cancer Institute 102:932–941. https://doi.org/10.1093/jnci/djq187

20. Shen J, Ye Y, Chang DW, Huang M, Heymach JV, Roth JA, Wu X, Zhao H (2017) Circulating metabolite profiles to predict overall survival in advanced non-small cell lung cancer patients receiving first-line chemotherapy. Lung Cancer 114:70–78. https://doi.org/10.1016/j.lungcan.2017.10.018

21. Sonoda Y, Tominaga T (2014) 2-hydroxyglutarate accumulation caused by IDHmutation is involved in the formation of malignant gliomas. Expert Rev Neurother 10:487–489. https://doi.org/10.1586/ern.10.19

22. Terunuma A, Putluri N, Mishra P, Mathé EA, Dorsey TH, Yi M, Wallace TA, Issaq HJ, Zhou M, Killian JK, Stevenson HS, Karoly ED, Chan K, Samanta S, Prieto D, Hsu TYT, Kurley SJ, Putluri V, Sonavane R, Edelman DC, Wulff J, Starks AM, Yang Y, Kittles RA, Yfantis HG, Lee DH, Ioffe OB, Schiff R, Stephens RM, Meltzer PS, Veenstra TD, Westbrook TF, Sreekumar A, Ambs S (2014) MYC-driven accumulation of 2-hydroxyglutarate is associated with breast cancer prognosis. J Clin Invest 124:398–412. https://doi.org/10.1172/JCI71180

23. Yoo BC, Lee JH, Kim K-H, Lin W, Kim JH, Park JB, Park HJ, Shin SH, Yoo H, Kwon JW, Gwak H-S (2017) Cerebrospinal fluid metabolomic profiles can discriminate patients with leptomeningeal carcinomatosis from patients at high risk for leptomeningeal metastasis. Oncotarget 8:101203–101214. https://doi.org/10.18632/oncotarget.20983

15

NMDA receptors mediate synaptic depression, but not spine loss in the dentate gyrus of adult amyloid Beta (Aβ) overexpressing mice

Michaela Kerstin Müller[1], Eric Jacobi[1], Kenji Sakimura[3], Roberto Malinow[4] and Jakob von Engelhardt[1,2]* (iD)

Abstract

Amyloid beta (Aβ)-mediated synapse dysfunction and spine loss are considered to be early events in Alzheimer's disease (AD) pathogenesis. N-methyl-D-aspartate receptors (NMDARs) have previously been suggested to play a role for Amyloid beta (Aβ) toxicity. Pharmacological block of NMDAR subunits in cultured neurons and mice suggested that NMDARs containing the GluN2B subunit are necessary for Aβ-mediated changes in synapse number and function in hippocampal neurons. Interestingly, NMDARs undergo a developmental switch from GluN2B- to GluN2A-containing receptors. This indicates different functional roles of NMDARs in young mice compared to older animals. In addition, the lack of pharmacological tools to efficiently dissect the role of NMDARs containing the different subunits complicates the interpretation of their specific role. In order to address this problem and to investigate the specific role for Aβ toxicity of the distinct NMDAR subunits in dentate gyrus granule cells of adult mice, we used conditional knockout mouse lines for the subunits GluN1, GluN2A and GluN2B. Aβ-mediated changes in synaptic function and neuronal anatomy were investigated in several-months old mice with virus-mediated overproduction of Aβ and in 1-year old 5xFAD mice. We found that all three NMDAR subunits contribute to the Aβ-mediated decrease in the number of functional synapses. However, NMDARs are not required for the spine number reduction in dentate gyrus granule cells after chronic Aβ-overproduction in 5xFAD mice. Furthermore, the amplitude of synaptic and extrasynaptic NMDAR-mediated currents was reduced in dentate gyrus granule of 5xFAD mice without changes in current kinetics, suggesting that a redistribution or change in subunit composition of NMDARs does not play a role in mediating Amyloid beta (Aβ) toxicity. Our study indicates that NMDARs are involved in AD pathogenesis by compromising synapse function but not by affecting neuron morphology.

Keywords: NMDA receptor, Amyloid Beta, Alzheimer's disease, GluN2B, GluN2A

Introduction

Amyloid beta (Aβ) deposition in the brain of Alzheimer Disease (AD) patients initiates a cascade of events that trigger synaptic dysfunction, spine loss and ultimately neuronal death (reviewed in [26]). Indeed, the amount of soluble Aβ correlates highly with the state of cognitive impairment in AD patients [49, 52, 58, 97]. However,

despite intense research, it is not well understood how Aβ induces early disease pathologies.

Several studies suggested that Aβ-toxicity is mediated via an influence on NMDAR function or expression [29, 36, 37, 79]. NMDARs are known to play an important role for synaptic plasticity in the healthy brain (reviewed in [88]). Therefore, it has been speculated that altered NMDAR signalling is involved in the pathogenesis of several neurological diseases including AD (reviewed in [42]). Consistently, one of the two types of FDA (U.S. Food and Drug Administration) approved AD therapies targets NMDARs. Thus, the partial NMDAR antagonist Memantine alleviates cognitive impairments in

* Correspondence: engelhardt@uni-mainz.de
[1]Institute of Pathophysiology, University Medical Center of the Johannes Gutenberg University Mainz, 55128 Mainz, Germany
[2]Synaptic Signalling and Neurodegeneration, German Center for Neurodegenerative Diseases (DZNE), 53127 Bonn, Germany
Full list of author information is available at the end of the article

moderate-severe AD patients [68, 73, 83, 100]. However, antagonists that are selective for specific NMDAR sub-units would be more effective as AD treatment than the unselective blocker Memantine.

NMDARs are tetramers composed of two obligatory GluN1 subunits and combinations of subunits GluN2A-D and/or GluN3A-B subunits [12, 39, 56]. NMDARs containing different GluN2 subunits differ in their expression profile and function [57, 91, 97]. GluN1, GluN2A and GluN2B are the predominant subunits that are expressed in excitatory neurons of the adult rodent forebrain [57, 98], forming diheteromeric GluN1/GluN2A- and GluN1/GluN2B- as well as triheteromeric GluN1/GluN2A/GluN2B containing NMDARs [50, 77, 86]. The GluN2A subunit is postnatally upregulated [57] and thought to be the major synaptic sub-unit of homomeric NMDARs of excitatory forebrain neurons in adult mice. In contrast, the GluN2B subunit is also expressed in forebrain neurons of newborn mice, but thought to be present in the majority of extrasynaptic NMDARs [18, 24, 27, 63, 87]. The activation of synaptic NMDARs has been shown to exert protective function [25]. In contrast, activation of extrasynaptic NMDARs activates apoptotic signalling cascades [25, 78].

It has been shown that the GluN2B subunit is involved in the Aβ-mediated synaptic dysfunction and spine loss of cultured neurons [7, 30, 40, 74, 79]. However, studies on Aβ-toxicity in cultured neurons that are prepared from newborn mice may well overestimate the contribution of the GluN2B subunit since they predominantly express this subunit [55, 91, 92]. However, blockade of NMDARs with ifenprodil or radiprodil, antagonists specific for diheteromeric GluN1/GluN2B-containing NMDARs, or deletion of the GluN2B subunit rescued Aβ-induced long-term-potentiation (LTP) deficits [31, 64–66, 70]. This suggests that the GluN2B subunit plays a role for Aβ-toxicity also in the adult brain. It remains to be shown if the GluN2B subunit is also involved in other alterations that are known to be mediated by Aβ-overproduction like changes in basal synaptic function and in the morphology of neurons such as in spine loss, since contrasting data have been published [30, 41, 66, 79, 82].

Little is known about the mechanisms how NMDARs are involved in Aβ-toxicity. Several mechanisms have been proposed including that Aβ may directly bind to NMDARs and influence their gating [14, 43]. Additionally, Aβ-mediated Calcium-influx via NMDARs leads to the formation of reactive oxygen species (ROS) and initializes oxidative stress [13]. An alternative hypothesis suggests that an Aβ-mediated redistribution of NMDARs may increase the vulnerability of neurons to higher extracellular glutamate levels, similar to what has been shown for Huntington's disease [53]. Thus, a relative upregulation of the number of extrasynaptic GluN2B-containig NMDARs, which activate apoptotic pathways [47, 71, 87], and

downregulation of, eventually more neuroprotective, synaptic GluN2A-containing NMDARs [8, 47, 89], could explain an increased susceptibility to excitotoxicity. Aβ indeed decreases NMDAR expression on the cell surface of neurons from post-mortem AD patients [33, 35, 54, 72]. However, it is not clear which NMDAR subunit is affected, whether synaptic or extrasynaptic NMDARs are downregulated, and finally if Aβ induces changes in NMDAR distribution in the adult brain.

To investigate the role of NMDARs for Aβ-toxicity in adult mice, we used conditional NMDAR knockout mice. Changes in synaptic function and neuronal morphology in response to subacute Aβ-overproduction was investigated by a virus-mediated expression of Aβ for several weeks in dentate gyrus (DG) granule cells of adult mice. The DG was chosen as region of interest, since LTP, which is inhibited by Aβ, occurs in CA1 and DG. Since Aβ plaques form in the DG before they appear in CA1 area, we focused on this brain area. The influence of chronic Aβ overproduction was investigated in 1-year old 5xFAD mice. We found that NMDARs indeed play a major role for the influence of Aβ on the number of functional synapses, but not on the Aβ-mediated change in spine number after chronic Aβ overproduction. Moreover, Aβ reduces the expression of NMDARs at both synaptic and extrasynaptic sites without a major influence on subunit composition.

Material & Methods
Animals
Mouse experiments were performed according to the German Animal Welfare Act and the Regierungspräsidium Karlsruhe as well as the Landesuntersuchungsamt Rhineland-Palatinate. All procedures followed the "Principles of laboratory animal care" (NIH publication No. 86–23, revised 1985). Mice had access to food and water ad libitum. The conditional NMDAR knockout mouse lines GluN1$^{fl/fl}$ [59], GluN2A $^{fl/fl}$ [19] and GluN2B$^{fl/fl}$ [60, 93], in which the grin1, grin2a and grin2b genes are flanked by loxP sites, were used for conditional deletion of the different NMDAR subunits. Mice of both sexes were used. The 5xFAD mouse line [60] was used as a mouse model for AD and crossbred with the conditional NMDAR knockout mice lines. Only female mice were used from these mouse lines. Deletion of NMDAR subunits in the conditional knockout mice was achieved by injection of recombinant adeno-associated viruses (rAAVs) expressing Cre-recombinase into the DG (rAAV-Syn-Cre-T2A-EGFP).

rAAV production and stereotactic injection
pAAV-CaMKII-T2A-tdTom plasmid was used to subclone Aβ overexpressing DNA (C-terminal 100 (CT100)) from a sindbis virus backbone [36] in an rAAV vector.

A mutated CT100 DNA construct containing an isoleucine to phenylalanine switch at amino acid position 716, named CT100(I716F), was constructed via site-directed-mutagenesis (Quik Change II kit from Agilent Technologies, USA) from the pAAV-CaMKII-CT100-T2A-tdTom plasmid to produce pAAV-CaMKII-CT100(I716F)-T2A-tdTom for increased $A\beta_{42/40}$ overexpression [21]. The following constructs were expressed in rAAVs and used in the study: rAAV-CaMKII-tdTom (control cells), rAAV-CaMKII-CT100/CT100(I716F)-T2A-td-Tom (CT100 or CT100(I716F) overexpression), rAAV-Syn-Cre-T2A-GFP (NMDAR subunit deletion) and rAAV-Syn-Cre-T2A-GFP + rAAV-CaMKII-CT100/CT100(I716F)-T2A-tdTom (NMDAR subunit deletion and CT100 or CT100(I716F) overexpression) (Fig. 1b and Additional file 1: S1b). Co-injection of control- and Cre-expressing-rAAVs could thus be differentiated by red and green fluorescence (Fig. 1a).

Plasmids used for rAAV1/2 production were amplified with the Qiagen Maxi Kit Plus (Qiagen, Germany). HEK293T cells were transfected with the DNA plasmids with a standard $CaCl_2$ transfection protocol and the rAAV was purified via heparin columns (GE Healthcare, England) using standard procedures.

rAAVs were stereotactically injected into the DG through a thin glass capillary using the following coordinates according to bregma: anteroposterior, − 3 mm; mediolateral, ±3 mm; dorsoventral, − 3.5 mm from the skull surface.

Preparation of acute slices

Mice were deeply anesthetized with 3% isoflurane and cardially perfused with ice-cold slicing solution (212 mM sucrose, 26 mM $NaHCO_3$, 1.25 mM NaH_2PO_4, 3 mM KCl, 0.2 mM $CaCl_2$, 7 mM $MgCl_2$ and 10 mM glucose). Brains were quickly removed and 250 μm thick acute transverse slices were cut in ice-cold slicing Solution with the help of a tissue slicer (slicer: Sigmann Elektronik, Germany; razor blade: Personna, USA). Acute brain slices were immediately transferred to a slice holding chamber with 37 °C ACSF (125 mM NaCl, 25 mM $NaHCO_3$, 1.25 mM NaH_2PO_4, 2.5 mM KCl, 2 mM $CaCl_2$,1 mM $MgCl_2$ and 25 mM glucose) and incubated for 15 min. The holding chamber was slowly cooled down to RT and slices were incubated for 45 min before being used in experiments.

Electrophysiology

Acute transverse slices were completely submerged and continuously perfused with carbogen-saturated artificial cerebral spine fluid (ACSF, see supplemental methods) at RT with a flow-rate of 1 ml/min. Slices were imaged with an Olympus BX51WI upright microscope (Olympus, Japan) fitted with a 4× air (Plan N, NA 0.1; Olympus, Japan) and 40× water-immersion (LUMPlan FI/IR, NA 0.8w; Olympus, Japan) objective. Electrical signals were acquired at 10 kHz for miniature excitatory post-synaptic current (mEPSC) recordings and 50 kHz for all other recordings using an EPC10 amplifier (HEKA, Germany), connected to a probe and PC. Electrical signals were recorded with the help of Patchmaster software (HEKA, Germany). No correction for liquid junction potential was done. For A/N ratios, paired pulse ratio recordings and firing patterns, 10 μM SR95531 hydrobromide (Biotrend, Germany) were added to the ACSF. 1 μM TTX (Biotrend, Germany) and 50 μM APV (Biotrend, Germany) were additionally added in mEPSC recordings. For NMDAR decay experiments 10 μM SR95531 hydrobromide was added with 50 μM CNQX.

For extracellular stimulation of the medial perforant path, the stimulus was generated by a stimulus isolator (WPI, USA) connected with the EPC10 amplifier and triggered by the Patchmaster software. A chlorinated silver wire located inside a borosilicate glass capillary filled with ACSF was used as stimulation electrode. For nucleated patches, cells were slowly pulled out of the slice while simultaneously applying negative pressure after reaching the whole cell configuration. Thus, the nucleus covered with cell membrane was pulled out of the slice and navigated in front of a theta glass tubing mounted onto a piezo translator (PI, Germany). A 1 ms pulse of 1 mM glutamate application solution (in mM): 135 NaCl, 10 HEPES, 5.4 KCl, 1.8 CaCl2, 5 glucose, 0.01 CNQX, 0.01 glycine (pH 7.2) was applied via one pipe of the theta glass. The other pipe contained the application solution without glutamate.

Morphological analysis

Cells used for morphological analysis were filled with an intracellular solution containing 0.1–0.5% biocytin (Sigma Aldrich, USA) through the patch-pipette while recording. Acute slices were fixed in 4% Histofix (Carl Roth, Germany) after recording. 2–10 days later, slices were washed in 1× PBS (phosphate buffered saline), permeabilized in 0.2% PBST (0.2% Triton in 1× PBS) and stained overnight with a Streptavidin-coupled Alexa594-conjugated antibody (life technologies, USA). Slices from 5xFAD mice were additionally stained with an Alexa488-coupled 6E10 Antibody (Covance, USA) for Aβ plaque staining. After washing in 1× PBS, slices were mounted in ProLong Gold Antifade (life technologies, USA).

Neurons were imaged with a fixed-stage Leica TCS SP5 II microscope (Leica, Germany) and the Leica LAS AF Lite Software (Leica, Germany). Z-stacks from whole neurons were imaged with a 40× oil-immersion objective (Leica, Germany) with the following parameters: voxel size x/y = 0.758 μm, z = 0.209 μm. Z-stacks from dendrites were taken with a 63× oil-immersion objective (Leica, Germany) with the following parameters: voxel size x/y = 0.08 μm, z = 0.168 μm.

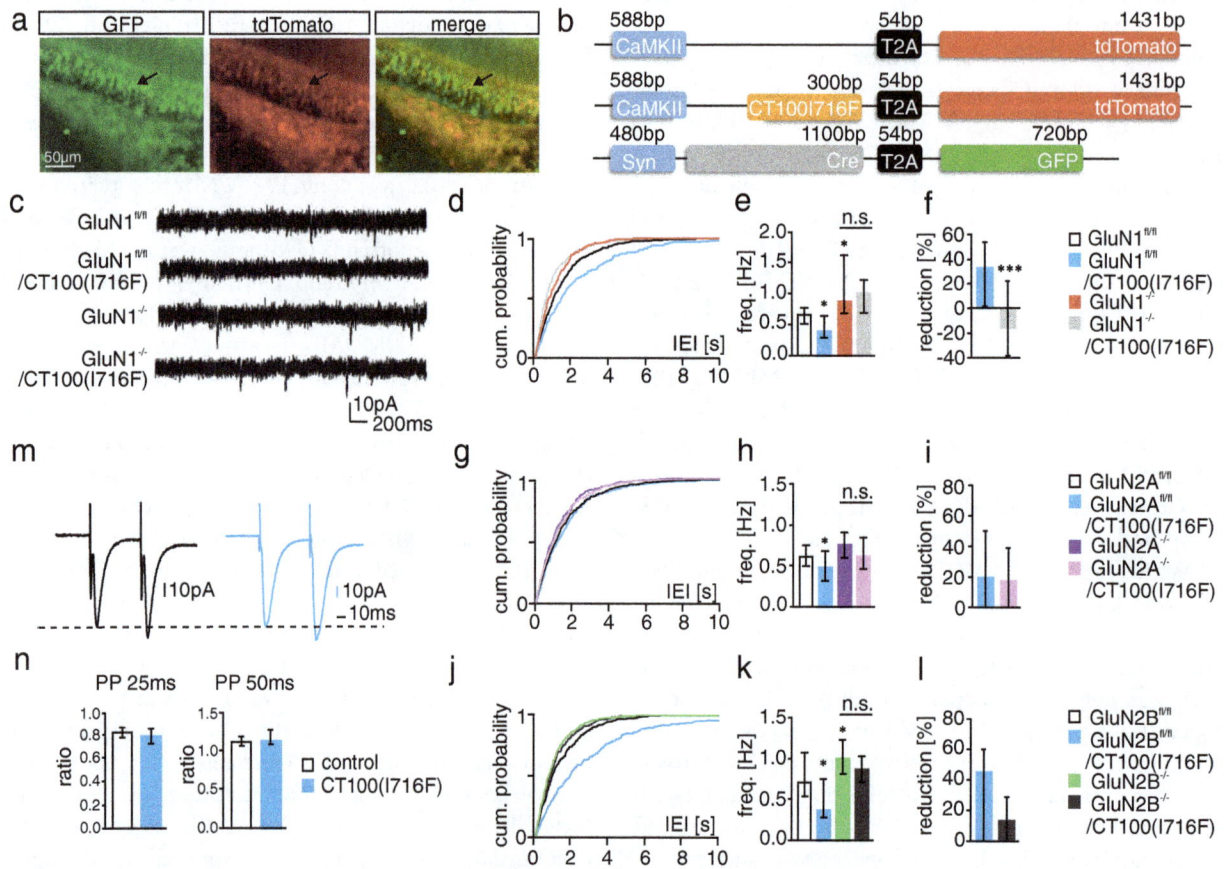

Fig. 1 CT100(I716F)-mediated synaptic depression in granule cells of adult mice is NMDAR dependent. **a** Double infection with rAAV-Syn-Cre-T2A-GFP and rAAV-CaMKII-CT100(I716F)-T2A-tdTomato in DG neurons. The arrowhead points to a double-infected DG granule cell. **b** pAAV constructs were used to express CT100(I716F) or Cre-recombinase or tdTomato as control. **c** Example traces of mEPSC recordings from GluN1$^{fl/fl}$ mice injected with the different AAV constructs as indicated. **d + e** CT100(I716F) increases inter-event-interval (IEI) and reduces mEPSC frequency in DG granule cells in cells of GluN1$^{fl/fl}$ mice. Deletion of GluN1 (GluN1$^{-/-}$) increases mEPSC frequency. Overexpression of CT100(I716F) does not significantly reduce mEPSC frequency in GluN1$^{-/-}$ granule cells. **f** To test if the effect of CT100(I716F) in GluN1$^{fl/fl}$ neurons is different from that in GluN1$^{-/-}$ granule cells, we calculated the respective percent of CT100(I716F)-mediated reduction in mEPSC frequency. The mEPSC frequency is smaller in GluN1$^{fl/fl}$/CT100(I716F) than in GluN1$^{fl/fl}$ cells (blue bar) and slightly bigger in GluN1$^{-/-}$/CT100(I716F) than in GluN1$^{-/-}$ cells (gray bar). The reduction in GluN1$^{fl/fl}$ cells is significantly bigger than the effect of CT100(I716F) in GluN1$^{-/-}$ granule cells. **g + h** CT100(I716F) reduces mEPSC frequency in DG granule cells in cells of GluN2A$^{fl/fl}$ mice, but does not significantly reduce mEPSC frequency in GluN2A$^{-/-}$ granule cells. **i** The CT100(I716F)-mediated decrease in mEPSC frequency in GluN2A$^{fl/fl}$ cells is not significantly different from the decrease in GluN2A$^{-/-}$ cells. **j + k** CT100(I716F) increases IEI and reduces mEPSC frequency in DG granule cells of GluN2B$^{fl/fl}$ mice. Deletion of GluN2B (GluN2B$^{-/-}$) increases mEPSC frequency. Overexpression of CT100(I716F) does not significantly reduce mEPSC frequency in GluN2B$^{-/-}$ granule cells. **l** The CT100(I716F)-mediated decrease in mEPSC frequency in GluN2B$^{fl/fl}$ cells is not significantly different from the decrease in GluN2B$^{-/-}$ cells. **m** Example traces of paired-pulse recordings (PPR) with pairs of inter-stimulus intervals (ISI) of 25 ms **n** The PPR of the amplitudes of two currents evoked with 25 ms or 50 ms ISIs is not different in control cells and CT100(I716F)-overexpressing cells. ISIs are shown on the top of the quantification. Bar graphs show median ± IQR. * = $p < 0.05$, ** = $p < 0.01$, *** = $p < 0.001$; cum. = cumulative

Z-stacks of DG granule cells were semi-automatically traced with Neuronstudio (CNIC, Mount Sinai School of Medicine, USA) and Sholl analysis was performed. Dendritic spines were also counted semi-automatically with Neuronstudio.

Analysis and statistics

Analysis of electrophysiological experiments was carried out using Clampfit (Molecular Devices, USA), IGOR Pro (WaveMetrix, USA), Microsoft Office Excel (Microsoft,

USA) and GraphPad Prism (GraphPad software, USA). For mEPSC analysis, the minianalysis plugin of the Clampfit software was used. For Firing pattern and NMDAR decay analysis, IGOR Pro was used with the Patcher's Power Tools and Neuromatic analysis package (MPI for biophysical chemistry, Germany and Jason Rothman, http://www.neuromatic.thinkrandom.com/). Morphological datasets were analyzed using the NeuronStudio software. Amira (FEI, USA) was used for blind deconvolution to improve image quality for spine analysis.

Statistics were performed with Graphpad Prism 6 (Graphpad, USA). Sholl analysis was statistically evaluated with a two-way ANOVA (analysis of variance with Tukey test for multiple comparisons). Datasets were tested for statistical significance with Mann-Whitney (MW) or Kruskal-Wallis (followed by Dunn's posttest) tests. Data is depicted as median ± interquartile ranges (IQR). Sholl analysis is shown as Mean ± standard error of the mean (SEM). P values < 0.05 were considered statistically significant (* = $p < 0.05$, ** = $p < 0.01$, *** = $p < 0.001$). All figures were prepared with Corel Draw X7 (Corel, Canada).

Results

NMDARs are involved in CT100-induced changes of synaptic function in young mice

Synaptic dysfunction, one of the earliest events in AD pathology [51], is thought to be caused by overproduction of toxic Aβ species [30, 95]. To induce Aβ-toxicity, we overexpressed Aβ in the DG of adult mice using a virus-mediated approach. To this end, we injected rAAVs that expressed the penultimate Aβ precursor CT100 (Additional file 1: S1a), which is known to reduce functional synapse number of neurons in organotypic slice cultures [67]. However, CT100 overexpression for three (data not shown, Table 1) and 9–10 weeks (Table 1 and Additional file 1: S1d) did not affect the number of functional synapses in adult mice, as mEPSC frequency in infected granule cells was unaffected compared to that in control cells. This was surprising because CT100 overexpression with a sindbis virus in organotypic slice

cultures has been shown to induce synaptic dysfunction 24 h post infection [36, 67]. Since organotypic brain slices are prepared from newborn mice, we wondered if neurons in the brains of younger mice are more susceptible to Aβ-toxicity. We thus injected rAAVs overexpressing CT100 into the DG of young mice (P7) and indeed observed a decrease in mEPSC frequency in CT100-overexpressing cells 9–10 weeks post injection (Table 1 and Additional file 1: S1f), possibly suggesting that Aβ-toxicity reduces with brain development. However, infection efficacy and Aβ-overproduction may also change with development, which could explain the observed age-dependency.

To investigate the role of NMDARs in Aβ-mediated changes in synapse number and function, we deleted NMDARs subunits by injection of a Cre-recombinase expressing rAAV (rAAV-Syn-Cre-T2A-GFP) into the DG of mice, in which the gene encoding the GluN1 subunit (*grin1*) is flanked by *loxP* sites (GluN1$^{fl/fl}$ mice). The ratio of NMDAR-mediated to AMPAR-mediated current amplitudes (NMDA/AMPA ratio) was significantly decreased (86.83%) three weeks post injection, indicating a nearly complete loss of NMDARs (Additional file 2: S4a, b and Table 2).

In the next step, NMDARs were deleted in parallel with overexpression of Aβ to investigate whether NMDARs play a role in Aβ-mediated changes in synaptic function in young mice. To this end, one week old GluN1$^{fl/fl}$ mice were injected with the following viruses: rAAV-CaMKII-tdTom (control cells = GluN1$^{fl/fl}$), rAAV-CaMKII-CT100-T2A-tdTom (CT100 overexpression), rAAV-Syn-Cre-T2A-GFP (GluN1 deletion: GluN1$^{-/-}$) and rAAV-Syn-Cre-T2A-GFP +

Table 1 mEPSC recordings of CT100-overexpressing DG granule cells

Adult mice					
3w pi	Control ($n = 22$)		CT100 ($n = 11$)		
Frequency [Hz]	0.59 [0.37–0.77]		0.48 [0.44–0.71]		MW test: $p = 0.9074$
10w pi	Control ($n = 40$)		CT100 ($n = 19$)		
Frequency [Hz]	0.71 [0.4–0.92]		0.54 [0.42–0.77]		MW test $p = 0.21$
Young mice					
9w pi	Control (n = 56)		CT100 (n = 26)		
Frequency [Hz]	0.81 [0.51–1.02]		0.61 [0.41–0.81]		MW test: $p = 0.047$
GluN1$^{fl/fl}$ 9w pi	Control (n = 34)	CT100 (n = 10)	GluN1$^{-/-}$ (n = 21)	GluN1$^{-/-}$ + CT100 (n= 9)	
Frequency [Hz]	0.69 [0.55–0.83]	0.37 [0.32–0.55]	0.99 [0.76–1.22]	1.18 [1.08–1.47]	Kruskal-Wallis: $p < 0.0001$; Dunn's posttest: control vs CT100 $p = 0.04$; control vs GluN1$^{-/-}$ $p = 0.0045$; GluN1$^{-/-}$ vs GluN1$^{-/-}$ + CT100 $p = 0.7895$
Amplitude [pA]	10.47 [9.27–11.53]	10.47 [9.94–11.53]	14.85 [12.96–16.09]	12.4 [10.99–13.81]	Kruskal-Wallis: $p < 0.0001$; Dunn's posttest: control vs CT100 $p > 0.9999$; control vs GluN1$^{-/-}$ $p < 0.0001$; GluN1$^{-/-}$ vs GluN1$^{-/-}$ + CT100 $p = 0.336$

Table 2 NMDAR-mediated currents in 5xFAD DG granule cells and virus-infected cells

	Control (n = 16)	GluN1$^{-/-}$ (n = 15)	
NMDAR/AMPAR ratio	1 ± 0.65	0.13 ± 0.04	MW test: p < 0.0001
	WT (n = 22)	5xFAD (n = 29)	
NMDAR/AMPAR ratio	1.18 [0.79–1.77]	0.72 [0.43–1.2]	MW test: $p = 0.0029$
	WT (n = 18)	5xFAD (n = 25)	
Decay tau [ms]	62.91 [57.75–67.48]	66.51 [59.2–72.86]	MW test: $p = 0.0969$
	WT (n = 23)	5xFAD (n = 22)	
Extrasynaptic amplitude [pA]	125.3 [85.8–178.6]	77.57 [43.12–101.2]	MW test: $p = 0.0003$
	WT (n = 23)	5xFAD (n = 22)	
Deactivation [ms]	74.76 [63.62–88.33]	79.43 [71.22–104.3]	MW test: $p = 0.1712$

rAAV-CaMKII-CT100-T2A-tdTom (GluN1$^{-/-}$ and CT100 overexpression) (Additional file 1: S1a). Nine weeks after rAAV injection, mEPSCs were recorded from infected DG granule cells. In accordance with the results shown above, mEPSC frequency was reduced in CT100 overexpressing DG granule cells (Additional file 3: S2c, blue bar). Furthermore, an increase in mEPSC frequency and amplitude was observed in GluN1$^{-/-}$ cells (red bar). Since deletion of GluN1 per se increased mEPSC frequency, we tested for an involvement of NMDARs in Aβ-toxicity by comparing GluN1$^{-/-}$ cells with CT100/GluN1$^{-/-}$ cells. Importantly, mEPSC frequency of CT100 expressing GluN1$^{-/-}$ cells was not significantly different from the mEPSC frequency in GluN1$^{-/-}$ cells (Additional file 3: S2c, grey bar and Table 1). This indicates that NMDARs mediate the Aβ-induced reduction in the number of functional synapses. However, we cannot exclude that NMDARs and Aβ affect functional synapse number via independent parallel pathways. While performing electrophysiological recordings, neurons were filled with biocytin to subsequently perform morphological analysis. Interestingly, spine density was increased in dendrites of Aβ-overexpressing DG granule cells with no change in the distribution of stubby, thin and mushroom spines (Additional file 3: S2d, g, Tables 3 and 4). Thus, unexpectedly, Aβ increased the number of spines while in parallel reducing the number of functional synapses.

CT100(I716F) overexpression reduces the number of functional synapses in adult mice

One intention of the study was to investigate the role of NMDARs for Aβ-toxicity in adult mice (12–16 weeks of age), i.e. at an age when the composition of NMDARs is

similar to the composition in aging. However, CT100 overexpression was ineffective in adult mice (see above). We therefore generated a mutated version of CT100, in which isoleucine (I) at position 716 was exchanged to phenylalanine (F) (CT100(I716F)). This mutation alters the γ-secretase cleavage site and is known to increase the production of the toxic Aβ$_{42}$ [28, 81]. Expression of CT100(I716F) in primary hippocampal cultures increased Aβ in the supernatant as verified by dot blot analysis (data not shown). Overexpression of CT100(I716F) induced a decrease in mEPSC frequency three weeks after rAAV injection into the DG of adult mice (Fig. 1e, h, k and Table 5). Thus, the increased production of Aβ$_{42}$ resulting from the I716F mutation indeed affected synaptic function stronger than the unmutated CT100. To investigate whether the reduction in mEPSC frequency results from a decreased release probability, we investigated the paired pulse ratio (PPR) of medial perforant path synapses. CT100(I716F) did not affect the PPR (Fig. 1n and Table 6). This indicates that Aβ decreases mEPSC frequency by reducing synapse number or by increasing the number of synapses devoid of AMPAR (i.e silent synapses) [94]. Previous studies suggested that Aβ alters neuronal excitability [6, 90]. We therefore investigated intrinsic active and passive electrophysiological properties of DG granule cells (Additional file 4: S3). CT100(I716F) overexpression did not change threshold potential, action potential (AP) amplitude, duration, afterhyperpolarisation (AHP) and input resistance. Firing frequency, as well as early- and late adaptation were also not different between CT100(I716F) expressing DG granule cells and control cells (Additional file 4: S3b, c and Table 7). Thus, three-week

Table 3 Morphological analysis of CT100-overexpressing DG granule cells

GluN1$^{fl/fl}$ 9w pi

Spine numbers	Control (n = 23)	CT100 (n = 6)	GluN1$^{-/-}$ (n= 23)	GluN1$^{-/-}$ + CT100 (n = 10)	
	1.54 [1.25–1.84]	2.22 [1.95–2.37]	1.73 [1.54–1.9]	1.51 [1.34–1.62]	Kruskal-Wallis: $p = 0.0015$; Dunn's posttest: control vs CT100 $p = 0.0026$; control vs GluN1$^{-/-}$ $p = 0.1332$; GluN1$^{-/-}$ vs GluN1$^{-/-}$ + CT100 $p = 0.1119$

Table 4 Values for spine morphology in CT100 and CT100(I716F) overexpression experiments

	Spine morphology distribution [%]		
	Stubby	Thin	Mushroom
9w pi CT100 in P7 floxed GluN1			
Control (23)	0.29 [0.26–0.31]	0.62 [0.6–0.67]	0.09 [0.47–0.11]
CT100 (6)	0.36 [0.27–0.4]	0.59 [0.54–0.64]	0.06 [0.04–0.09]
GluN1$^{-/-}$ (10)	0.29 [0.23–0.35]	0.6 [0.57–0.7]	0.07 [0.05–0.1]
GluN1$^{-/-}$ + CT100 (23)	0.27 [0.23–0.32]	0.64 [0.62–0.67]	0.07 [0.05–0.11]
Kruskal Wallis test (Dunn's posttest)	$P = 0.1972$ (Control vs CT100: $p = 0.4813$ Control vs GluN1-/-: $p > 0.9999$; GluN1−/− vs GluN1−/− + CT100: $p > 0.9999$)	$P = 0.1433$ (Control vs CT100: $p = 0.6288$; Control vs GluN1$^{-/-}$: $p > 0.9999$; GluN1$^{-/-}$ vs GluN1$^{-/-}$ + CT100: $p = 0.5863$)	$P = 0.8439$ (Control vs CT100: $p > 0.9999$; Control vs GluN1$^{-/-}$: $p > 0.9999$; GluN1$^{-/-}$ + CT100: $p > 0.9999$)
DG granule cells GluN1$^{-/-}$ line			
Control (49)	0.32 [0.27–0.36]	0.61 [0.54–0.64]	0.08 [0.05–0.10]
CT100(I716F) (19)	0.29 [0.27–0.33]	0.63 [0.59–0.66]	0.08 [0.06–0.08]
GluN1$^{-/-}$ (22)	0.32 [0.26–0.39]	0.56 [0.49–0.64]	0.1 [0.06–0.14]
GluN1$^{-/-}$ + CT100(I716F) (28)	0.32 [0.27–0.37]	0.61 [0.55–0.67]	0.07 [0.05–0.85]
Kruskal Wallis test (Dunn's posttest)	$p = 0.529$ (Control vs CT100(I716F): $p = 0.53$; Control vs GluN1$^{-/-}$: $p > 0.9999$; GluN1$^{-/-}$ vs GluN1$^{-/-}$ + CT100(I716F): $p > 0.9999$)	$p = 0.198$ (Control vs CT100(I716F): $p = 0.5339$; Control vs GluN1$^{-/-}$: $p = 0.8345$; GluN1$^{-/-}$ vs GluN1$^{-/-}$ + CT100(I716F): $p = 0.3877$)	$p = 0.1098$ (Control vs CT100(I716F): $p > 0.9999$; Control vs GluN1$^{-/-}$: $p = 0.2132$; GluN1$^{-/-}$ vs GluN1$^{-/-}$ + CT100(I716F): $p = 0.0511$)
DG granule cells GluN2A$^{fl/fl}$ line			
Control (11)	0.35 [0.32–0.37]	0.57 [0.53–0.62]	0.08 [0.03–0.11]
CT100(I716F) (17)	0.36 [0.29–0.38]	0.57 [0.52–0.62]	0.07 [0.06–0.11]
GluN2A$^{-/-}$ (26)	0.38 [0.34–0.42]	0.54 [0.49–0.58]	0.1 [0.06–0.18]
GluN2A$^{-/-}$ + CT100(I716F) (21)	0.34 [0.3–0.38]	0.55 [0.52–0.61]	0.1 [0.08–0.13]
Kruskal Wallis test (Dunn's posttest)	$p = 0.1208$ (Control vs CT100(I716F): $p > 0.999$; Control vs GluN1$^{-/-}$: $p = 0.9455$; GluN1$^{-/-}$ vs GluN1$^{-/-}$ + CT100(I716F): $p = 0.0586$)	$p = 0.2321$ (Control vs CT100(I716F): $p > 0.9999$; Control vs GluN1$^{-/-}$: $p = 0.2893$; GluN1$^{-/-}$ vs GluN1$^{-/-}$ + CT100(I716F): $p = 0.7813$)	$p > 0.1487$ (Control vs CT100(I716F): $p > 0.9999$; Control vs GluN1$^{-/-}$: $p > 0.9999$; GluN1$^{-/-}$ vs GluN1$^{-/-}$ + CT100(I716F): $p = 0.4372$)
DG granule cells GluN2B$^{fl/fl}$ line			
Control (31)	0.36 [0.33–0.42]	0.55 [0.49–0.58]	0.08 [0.06–0.111]
CT100(I716F) (45)	0.32 [0.28–0.4]	0.59 [0.53–0.6442]	0.07 [0.05–0.1]
GluN2B$^{-/-}$ (29)	0.33 [0.28–0.39]	0.56 [0.49–0.6]	0.11 [0.09–0.14]
GluN2B$^{-/-}$ + CT100(I716F) (16)	0.37 [0.33–0.44]	0.57 [0.5–0.6]	0.07 [0.04–0.09]
Kruskal Wallis test (Dunn's posttest)	$P = 0.0105$ (Control vs CT100(I716F): $p = 0.0277$; Control vs GluN2B$^{-/-}$: $p = 0.043$; GluN2B$^{-/-}$ vs GluN2B$^{-/-}$ + CT100(I716F): $p = 0.1063$)	$P = 0.0319$ (Control vs CT100(I716F): $p = 0.0112$; Control vs GluN2B$^{-/-}$: $p = 0.6837$; GluN2B$^{-/-}$ vs GluN2B$^{-/-}$ + CT100(I716F): $p > 0.9999$)	$P = 0.0002$ (Control vs CT100(I716F): $p > 0.9999$; Control vs GluN2B$^{-/-}$: $p = 0.0066$; GluN2B$^{-/-}$ vs GluN2B$^{-/-}$ + CT100(I716F): $p = 0.0048$)

Table 5 mEPSC recordings of CT100(I716F)-overexpressing DG granule cells

GluN1^fl/fl	Control (n = 26)	CT100(I716F) (n = 33)	GluN1^-/- (n = 24)	GluN1^-/- + CT100(I716F) (n = 21)	
Frequency [Hz]	0.66 [0.52–0.77]	0.42 [0.3–0.64]	0.89 [0.69–1.63]	1.02 [0.68–1.23]	Kruskal-Wallis: $p < 0.0001$; Dunn's posttest: control vs CT100(I716F) $p = 0.029$; control vs GluN1^-/- $p = 0.044$; GluN1^-/- vs CT100(I716F) $p > 0.99$
Percentual reduction		0.36 [0.02–0.55]		−0.15 [−0.38–0.23]	$p = 0.0137$
Amplitude [pA]	10.81 [10.03–11.47]	10.62 [10.02–11.13]	11.2 [10.34–12.44]	11.05 [9.78–12]	Kruskal-Wallis: $p = 0.3076$; Dunn's posttest: control vs CT100(I716F) $p > 0.99$; control vs GluN1^-/- $p = 0.75$; GluN1^-/- vs CT100(I716F) $p > 0.99$
GluN2A^fl/fl	Control (n = 36)	CT100(I716F) (n = 37)	GluN2A^-/- (n = 24)	GluN2A^-/- + CT100(I716F) (n = 19)	
Frequency [Hz]	0.61 [0.5–0.75]	0.5 [0.31–0.68]	0.76 [0.6–0.92]	0.62 [0.46–0.85]	Kruskal-Wallis: $p = 0.0004$; Dunn's posttest: control vs CT100(I716F) $p = 0.0468$; control vs GluN2A^-/- $p = 0.149$; GluN2A^-/- vs CT100(I716F) $p = 0.485$
Percentual reduction		0.19 [−0.1–0.51]		0.18 [−0.11–0.39]	$p = 0.27$
Amplitude [pA]	9.67 [8.46–10.32]	9.83 [9.3–10.82]	10.47 [9.29–12.96]	10.44 [9.84–11.95]	Kruskal-Wallis: $p = 0.013$; Dunn's posttest: control vs CT100(I716F) $p = 0.844$; control vs GluN2A^-/- $p = 0.75$; GluN2A^-/- vs CT100(I716F) $p > 0.99$
GluN2B^fl/fl	Control (n = 28)	CT100(I716F) (n = 25)	GluN2B^-/- (n = 27)	GluN2B^-/- + CT100(I716F) (n = 26)	
Frequency [Hz]	0.71 [0.53–1.08]	0.39 [0.28–0.75]	1.01 [0.81–1.23]	0.87 [0.72–1.03]	Kruskal-Wallis: $p < 0.0001$; Dunn's posttest: control vs CT100(I716F) $p = 0.013$; control vs GluN2B^-/- $p = 0.018$; GluN2B^-/- vs CT100(I716F) $p = 0.497$
Percentual reduction		0.45 [−0.06–0.6]		0.14 [−0.02–0.29]	$p = 0.1$
Amplitude [pA]	9.58 [8.61–10.26]	9.65 [8.43–10.51]	9.8 [9.2–10.61]	11.59 [10.16–12.69]	Kruskal-Wallis: $p < 0.0001$; Dunn's posttest: control vs CT100(I716F) $p > 0.9999$; control vs GluN2B^-/- $p > 0.9999$; GluN2B^-/- vs GluN2B^-/- + CT100(I716F) $p = 0.0033$

Table 6 Values of PPR of CT100(I716F)-overexpressing DG granule cells

	WT (n = 20)	CT100(I716F) (n = 20)	
25 ms ISI	0.84 [0.78–0.88]	0.81 [0.74–0.87]	MW-test: $p = 0.2423$
50 ms ISI	1.1 [1.05–1.17]	1.13 [1.07–1.26]	MW-test: $p = 0.201$

overproduction of Aβ did not influence the active and passive properties of DG granule cells, but decreased the number of functional synapses.

NMDARs are required for the Aβ-mediated reduction in functional synapse number in adult mice

We next asked whether NMDARs are involved in the Aβ-mediated changes in synapse function in adult mice. To this end, mEPSCs were recorded in three different mouse strains, each with conditional deletion of either GluN1, GluN2A, or GluN2B (GluN1$^{fl/fl}$, GluN2A$^{fl/fl}$ and GluN2B$^{fl/fl}$). Conditional deletion of the subunits has been induced by injection of either one or two viruses: rAAV-CaMKII-tdTom (control cells = GluN1$^{fl/fl}$, GluN2A$^{fl/fl}$ or GluN2B$^{fl/fl}$), rAAV-CaMKII-CT100(I716F)-T2A-tdTom (CT100(I716F) overexpression), rAAV-Syn-Cre-T2A-GFP (GluN1$^{-/-}$ or GluN2A$^{-/-}$ or GluN2B$^{-/-}$ granule cells) and rAAV-Syn-Cre-T2A-GFP + rAAV-CaMKII-CT100(I716F)--T2A-tdTom (NMDAR subunit deletion together with CT100(I716F) overexpression) (Fig. 1a). Synaptic currents were recorded three weeks after virus injection. CT100(I716F) overexpression significantly decreased mEPSC frequency by 20–45% without affecting mEPSC amplitude (Fig. 1e, h, k, Additional file 2: S4d, f, h and Table 5). Deletion of the GluN1 subunit as well as deletion of the GluN2B subunit increased mEPSC frequency (Fig. 1e, n and Table 5) similar to the observations in young mice. Importantly, overexpression of CT100(I716F) in GluN1$^{-/-}$, GluN2A$^{-/-}$ and

GluN2B$^{-/-}$ granule cells did not significantly reduce mEPSC frequency (Fig. 1e, h, k and Table 5). Deletion of GluN1 abolished the effect of Aβ overproduction almost completely: the CT100(I716F)-mediated mEPSC frequency reduction in GluN1$^{-/-}$ cells was significantly smaller than the reduction in wildtype cells (Fig. 1f). This indicates that the effect of Aβ on the number of functional synapses is mediated via NMDARs (since there are nearly no functional NMDARs in GluN1$^{-/-}$ cells; Additional file 2: S4b and Table 2). The deletion of only GluN2A or GluN2B had a smaller impact on the effect of CT100(I716F) on mEPSC frequency (Fig. 1i, l).

CT100(I716F) overexpression and NMDAR subunit knockout did not affect total length and arborisation of granule cell dendrites except for subtle changes in dendritic complexity in CT100(I716F) overexpressing cells compared to GluN2B$^{-/-}$ cells (Fig. 2a, b, Additional file 5: S5 and Table 8). Interestingly, Aβ overproduction via CT100(I716F) for 3 weeks did not influence the number of spines (Fig. 2c–f and Table 8) despite the Aβ-mediated reduction in functional synapse number (reduction in mEPSC frequency; Fig. 1e, h, k). This suggests that Aβ increases the number of silent synapses. The deletion of the GluN1 or GluN2B subunit reduced spine number (Fig. 2d, f and Table 8). Together with the increased mEPSC frequency (Fig. 1e, k), this indicates that deletion of GluN1 or GluN2B decreases silent synapse number. Spine morphology was not affected as shown by unaltered distributions of stubby, thin and mushroom spines in the GluN1$^{fl/fl}$ and GluN2A$^{fl/fl}$ line, but small changes were observed in the GluN2B$^{fl/fl}$ line (Fig. 2g, i, j and Table 4).

NMDARs are not required for the spine loss in 5xFAD mice

Our data so far showed that Aβ-overproduction for three weeks decreases the number of functional synapses and that NMDARs are required for this effect. There

Table 7 Intrinsic and firing properties of CT100(I716F) overexpressing DG granule cells

	3w pi CT100(I716F)		
	Control	CT100(I716F)	
	n = 31	n = 20	
Passive properties			
Input resistance [mΩ]	182 [140–211.5]	170 [129.5–184]	MW test: $p = 0.2418$
Active properties			
AP threshold [mV]	−37.27 [−39.18 - -33.78]	−35.84 [− 39.04 - -30.2]	MW test: $p = 0.5246$
AP width [ms]	1.26 [1.2–1.32]	1.24 [1.15–1.28]	MW test: $p = 0.3286$
AP amplitude [mV]	94.03 [90.88–97.7]	91.25 [87.12–95.74]	MW test: $p = 0.1308$
AHP [mV]	−13.83 [−16–58- -10]	−13.76 [−15.77- - 11.23]	MW test: $p = 0.7964$
Firing properties			
Firing frequency [Hz]	22 [16–26]	20.5 [17.25–23.75]	MW test: $p = 0.7484$
Early adaptation [%]	451.7 [356–563.4]	391.4 [347.1–543.1]	MW test: $p = 0.6064$
Late adaptation [%]	41.98 [24.16–61.51]	42.37 [20.43–102.4]	MW test: $p = 0.8231$

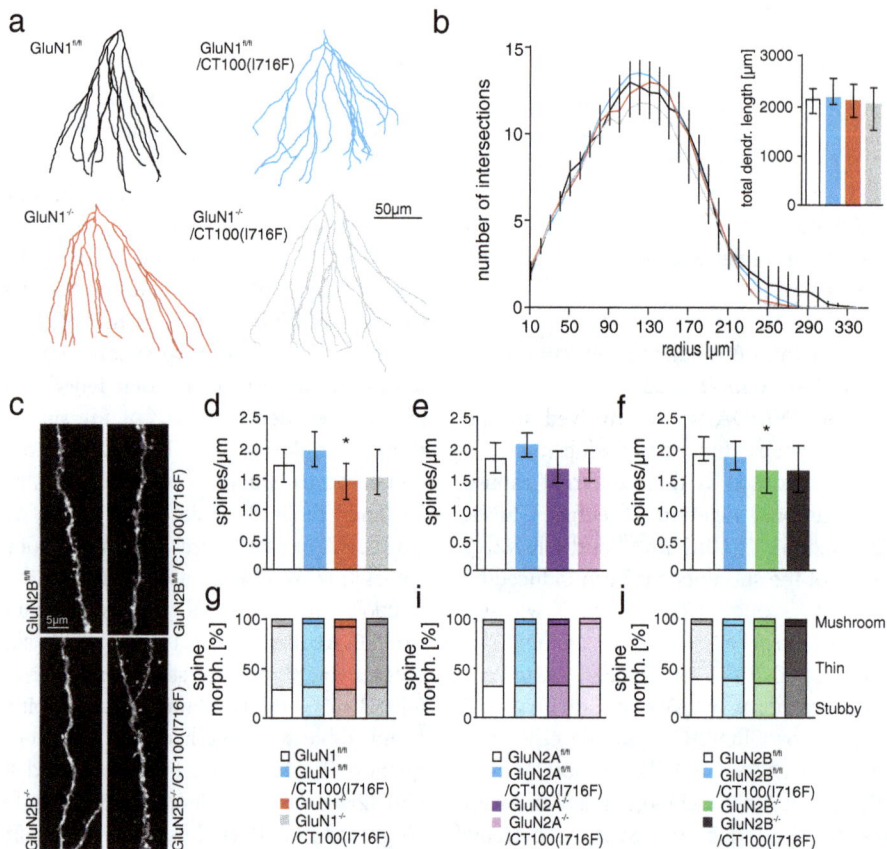

Fig. 2 CT100(I716F) overexpression does not affect morphology of granule cells in adult mice. **a** Examples of traced DG granule cells after biocytin filling. **b** Sholl analysis shows that neither CT100(I716F)-overexpression nor GluN1 knockout affects the number of intersections of granule cell dendrites. There is no difference in the total dendritic length of neurons in the different groups. **c** Examples of maximum intensity projections of z-stacks of GluN2B$^{fl/fl}$, GluN2B$^{fl/fl}$/CT100(I716F), GluN2B$^{-/-}$ and GluN2B$^{-/-}$/CT100(I716F) granule cell dendrites. **d + e + f** Spine number is not affected after three weeks of CT100(I716F)-overexpression. Spine number is reduced in GluN1$^{-/-}$ (**d**), and GluN2B$^{-/-}$ (**f**) granule cells. **g + i + j** The distribution of stubby, thin and mushroom spines is slightly affected by CT100(I716F)-overexpression and/or NMDAR subunit knockout with fewer thin spines in GluN2B$^{fl/fl}$ vs GluN2B$^{-/-}$; GluN2B$^{-/-}$ vs GluN2B$^{-/-}$/CT100(I716F) and an increase in stubby spines in GluN2A$^{-/-}$ vs GluN2A$^{-/-}$/CT100(I716F); GluN2B$^{fl/fl}$ vs GluN2B$^{fl/fl}$/CT100(I716F); GluN2B$^{fl/fl}$ vs GluN2B$^{-/-}$. Bar graphs show median ± IQR. * = $p < 0.05$, ** = $p < 0.01$, *** = $p < 0.001$; morph. = morphology

was no decrease in spine number, which, however, is an early event in AD pathogenesis that correlates well with cognitive impairment [84]. The absence of a spine loss in CT100(I716F)-expressing cells may be explained by the relatively short time-period of CT100(I716F) expression and perhaps by a moderate Aβ overproduction using the virus-mediated approach. To analyze the role of NMDARs for Aβ-mediated spine loss, we thus employed 5xFAD mice, in which mutations in the *APP* and *PSEN1* genes result in the accumulation of high levels of Aβ$_{42}$ [60]. In 12 months old 5xFAD mice, we detected Aβ plaques throughout the DG in close proximity to the investigated cells (Fig. 3a). Spine density and spine morphology was not changed in granule cells of six-month-old 5xFAD mice (Additional file 6: S6d, e and Table 9). Consistently, there was no change in mEPSC frequency, but we found an increase in mEPSC

amplitude (Additional file 6: S6g and Table 10). In contrast, spine density and mEPSC frequency were significantly reduced in granule cells of one-year-old 5xFAD mice (Fig. 3g, k, Tables 9 and 10). Spine density reduction in 5xFAD mice was not due to loss of a specific morphological spine subtype (Fig. 3m and Table 11). Sholl analysis revealed no difference in dendritic arborization and total dendritic length between 5xFAD and WT mice (Fig. 3h, i and Table 9).

To investigate the role of NMDARs in Aβ-mediated synapse dysfunction and spine density reduction, 5xFAD mice were bred with conditional NMDAR KO lines (GluN1$^{fl/fl}$, GluN2A$^{fl/fl}$, and GluN2B$^{fl/fl}$ mice). Cre-recombinase expressing rAAVs were injected into the DG of nine-month old 5xFAD/GluN1$^{fl/fl}$, 5xFAD/GluN2A$^{fl/fl}$ and 5xFAD/GluN2B$^{fl/fl}$ mice and littermate controls (GluN1$^{fl/fl}$, GluN2A$^{fl/fl}$ and GluN2B$^{fl/fl}$) to induce

Table 8 Morphology of CT100(I716F)-overexpressing DG granule cells

GluN1$^{fl/fl}$

	Control	CT100(I716F)	GluN1$^{-/-}$	GluN1$^{-/-}$ + CT100(I716F)	Statistics
Spine numbers	Control (n = 51) 1.7 [1.45–1.97]	CT100(I716F) (n = 20) 1.96 [1.69–2.27]	GluN1$^{-/-}$ (n = 22) 1.46 [1.16–1.72]	GluN1$^{-/-}$ + CT100(I716F) (n = 28) 1.51 [1.23–1.98]	Kruskal-Wallis: p = 0.0008; Dunn's posttest: control vs CT100 p = 0.1308 control vs GluN1$^{-/-}$ p = 0.0381; GluN1$^{-/-}$ vs GluN1$^{-/-}$ + CT100 p > 0.99
Total dendritic length [μm]	Control (n = 15) 2106 [1843–2325]	CT100(I716F) (n = 27) 2155 [2018–2533]	GluN1$^{-/-}$ (n = 17) 2090 [1782–2418]	GluN1$^{-/-}$ + CT100(I716F) (n = 22) 2019 [1495–2343]	Kruskal-Wallis: p = 0.0195; Dunn's posttest: control vs CT100 p > 0.99 control vs GluN1$^{-/-}$ p > 0.99; GluN1$^{-/-}$ vs GluN1$^{-/-}$ + CT100 p > 0.99

GluN2A$^{fl/fl}$

	Control	CT100(I716F)	GluN2A$^{-/-}$	GluN2A$^{-/-}$ + CT100(I716F)	Statistics
Spine numbers	Control (n = 11) 1.81 [1.56–1.09]	CT100(I716F) (n = 17) 2.97 [1.84–2.25]	GluN2A$^{-/-}$ (n = 26) 1.65 [1.42–1.95]	GluN2A$^{-/-}$ + CT100(I716F) (n = 21) 1.67 [1.46–1.96]	Kruskal-Wallis: p = 0.0015; Dunn's posttest: control vs CT100 p = 0.3366 control vs GluN2A$^{-/-}$ p = 0.5077; GluN2A$^{-/-}$ vs GluN2A$^{-/-}$ + CT100 p > 0.9999
Total dendritic length [μm]	Control (n = 16) 2162 [1657–2391]	CT100(I716F) (n = 17) 1889 [1577–2155]	GluN2A$^{-/-}$ (n = 17) 1862 [1528–2254]	GluN2A$^{-/-}$ + CT100(I716F) (n = 18) 2046 [1885–2189]	Kruskal-Wallis: p = 0.337; Dunn's posttest: control vs CT100 p = 0.5642 control vs GluN2A$^{-/-}$ p = 0.6218; GluN2A$^{-/-}$ vs GluN2A$^{-/-}$ + CT100 p = 0.6027

GluN2B$^{fl/fl}$

	Control	CT100(I716F)	GluN2B$^{-/-}$	GluN2B$^{-/-}$ + CT100(I716F)	Statistics
Spine numbers	Control (n = 31) 1.91 [1.8–2.2]	CT100(I716F) (n = 45) 1.88 [1.65–2.13]	GluN2B$^{-/-}$ (n = 29) 1.63 [1.29–2.06]	GluN2B$^{-/-}$ + CT100(I716F) (n = 16) 1.55 [1.18–1.87]	Kruskal-Wallis: p = 0.0021; Dunn's posttest: control vs CT100 p = 0.7884 control vs GluN2B$^{-/-}$ p = 0.0151; GluN2B$^{-/-}$ vs GluN2B$^{-/-}$ + CT100 p > 0.99
Total dendritic length [μm]	Control (n = 29) 2248 [2013–2577]	CT100(I716F) (n = 26) 2223 [1882–2364]	GluN2B$^{-/-}$ (n = 23) 2336 [2064–26811]	GluN2B$^{-/-}$ + CT100(I716F) (n = 16) 1882 [1668–2437]	Kruskal-Wallis: p = 0.1092; Dunn's posttest: control vs CT100 p = 0.6198 control vs GluN2B$^{-/-}$ p > 0.9999; GluN2B$^{-/-}$ vs GluN2B$^{-/-}$ + CT100 p = 0.1049

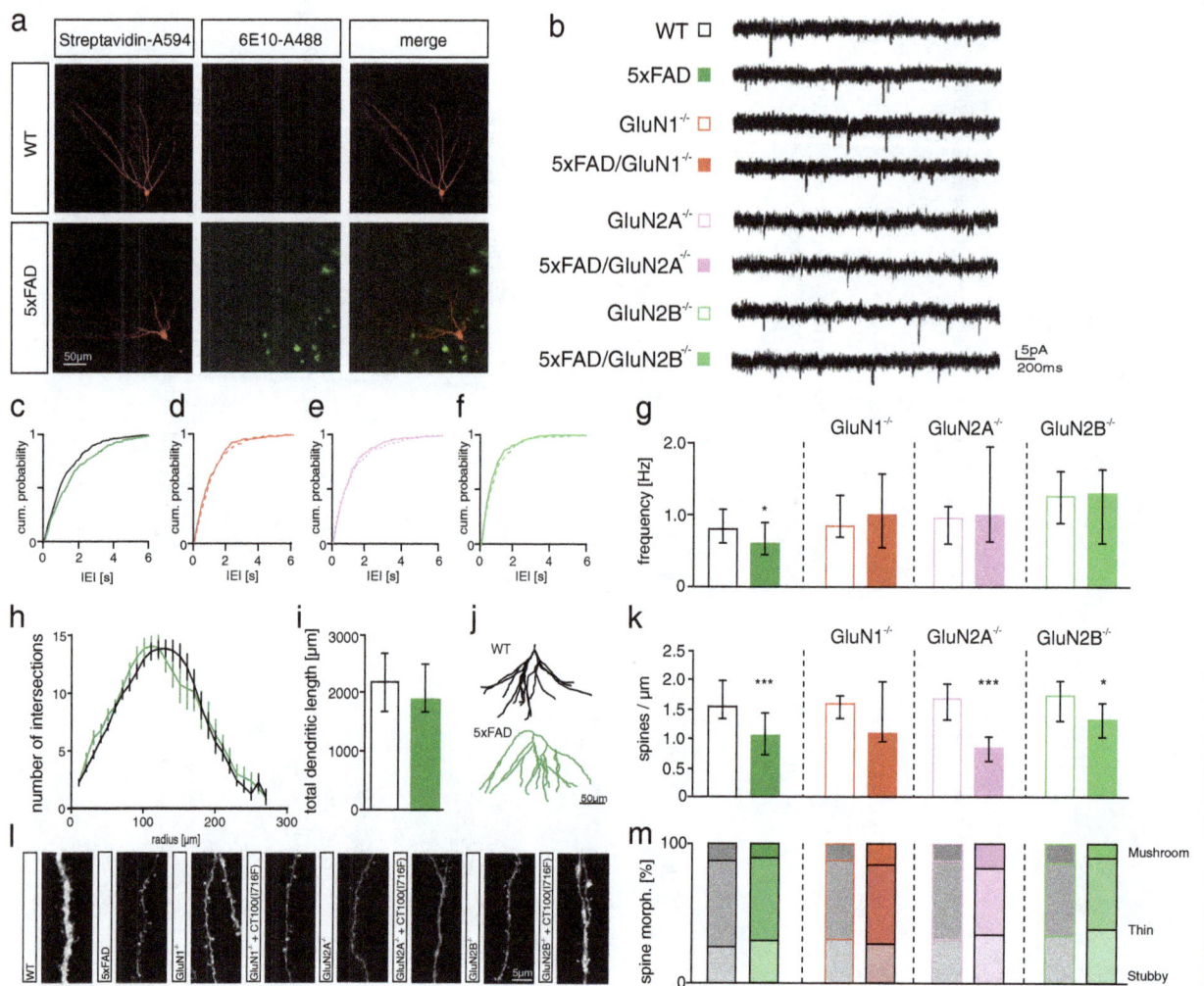

Fig. 3 The synaptic depression in DG granule cells of 5xFAD mice is NMDAR dependent. **a** Biocytin filled granule cells (red) in brain slices of WT and 5xFAD mice. Aβ plaques in 5xFAD mice were visualized using a 6E10-coupled A488 antibody. No plaques are seen in WT mice. **b** Example traces of mEPSC recordings from granule cells of WT and 5xFAD mice with NMDAR subunit deletions. **c + d + e + f** Cumulative probability of the IEIs is shifted towards larger IEIs in cells of 5xFAD mice, but not in cells of 5xFAD/GluN1$^{-/-}$, 5xFAD/GluN2A$^{-/-}$ and 5xFAD/GluN2B$^{-/-}$ mice. **g** mEPSC frequency is reduced in granule cells of 5xFAD mice. There is no difference in mEPSC frequency in granule cells of GluN1$^{-/-}$ and 5xFAD/GluN1$^{-/-}$, GluN2A$^{-/-}$ and 5xFAD/GluN2A$^{-/-}$ or GluN2B$^{-/-}$ and 5xFAD/GluN2B$^{-/-}$ mice. **h** The number of intersections is not changed in granule cells of 5xFAD mice. Number of intersections: Mean ± SEM. **i** Total dendritic length is not affected in granule cells of 5xFAD mice. **j** Examples of traced DG granule cells from one year old 5xFAD mice and WT littermates. **k** Spine number is decreased in granule cells of 5xFAD mice. There is a trend to a reduced spine numbers in 5xFAD/GluN1$^{-/-}$ cells and a significantly decreased spine number in 5xFAD/GluN2A$^{-/-}$ and 5xFAD/GluN2B$^{-/-}$ granule cells. **l** Example images of maximum intensity projections of z-stacks from the different conditions analyzed for the spine counting. **m** Quantification of spine morphology distribution indicates that the decrease in spine number in DG granule cells of 5xFAD mice is not due to a loss of a specific spine subtype except for the 5xFAD/GluN2A$^{-/-}$ cells, in which thin spines were reduced. Bar graphs show median ± IQR. * = $p < 0.05$, ** = $p < 0.01$, *** = $p < 0.001$; cum. = cumulative; morph. = morphology

NMDAR subunit deletion (GluN1$^{-/-}$, GluN2A$^{-/-}$ and GluN2B$^{-/-}$ cells). There was no difference in mEPSC frequency between GluN1$^{-/-}$ and 5xFAD/GluN1$^{-/-}$ granule cells (Fig. 3g, red bars and Table 10). Similarly, the mEPSC frequency was not different between GluN2A$^{-/-}$ and 5xFAD/GluN2A$^{-/-}$ granule cells as well as between GluN2B$^{-/-}$ and 5xFAD/GluN2B$^{-/-}$ granule cells (Fig. 3g, light green bars and Table 10). Thus, NMDARs are required for the reduction in the

number of functional synapses in paradigms with short-time (with CT100(I716F) expression for three weeks) and chronic Aβ-overproduction (in 5xFAD mice). In fact, the protection that was induced by NMDAR subunit deletion was more evident in 5xFAD mice than in cells with CT100(I716F) expression. In addition, the deletion of only one subunit (GluN2A or GluN2B) was sufficient to abolish the influence of Aβ on functional synapse number in 5xFAD mice.

Table 9 Morphological analysis of the 5xFAD mouse model

6 m DG			
Spine numbers	WT (n = 17)	5xFAD (n = 20)	
	1.25 [0.93–1.56]	1.36 [1–1.6]	MW-test: $p = 0.8923$
Total dendritic length	WT ($n = 13$)	5xFAD (n = 20)	
	2707 [2131–3003]	2425 [2134–2630]	MW-test: $p = 0.1275$
1a DG			
Spine numbers	WT (n = 27)	5xFAD (n = 28)	
	1.54 [1.35–1.99]	1.07 [0.73–1.46]	MW-test: p < 0.0001
	GluN1$^{-/-}$ ($n = 6$)	5xFAD/GluN1$^{-/-}$ ($n = 12$)	
	1.62 [1.36–1.76]	1.13 [0.96–2.02]	MW-test: $p = 0.325$
	GluN2A$^{-/-}$ (n = 12)	5xFAD/GluN2A$^{-/-}$ ($n = 10$)	
	1.7 [1.36–1.98]	0.87 [0.64–1.04]	MW-test: $p = 0.0001$
	GluN2B$^{-/-}$ (n = 28)	5xFAD/GluN2B$^{-/-}$ (n = 13)	
	1.73 [1.29–1.96]	1.33 [1.02–1.6]	MW-test: $p = 0.0165$
Total dendritic length [µm]	WT (n = 22)	5xFAD (n = 19)	
	2222 [1704–2660]	1882 [1708–2480]	MW-test: $p = 0.4763$

Knockout of GluN1, GluN2A or GluN2B per se did not affect spine density of granule cells. Importantly, deletion of GluN2A or GluN2B did not prevent the reduction in spine number in dendrites of granule cells in 5xFAD mice (Fig. 3k, light green bars and Table 9). The highly variable spine number in 5xFAD/GluN1$^{-/-}$ cells reduces the informative value of the non-significant difference to the spine number in GluN1$^{-/-}$ cells (Fig. 3k, red bars and Table 9). This hampers conclusions about the role of GluN1. However, the strong trend to reduced

spine numbers in 5xFAD/GluN1$^{-/-}$ cells indicates that NMDARs play a small role in the Aβ-mediated spine number reduction, in contrast to their requirement for the Aβ-mediated changes in functional synapse number.

Aβ decreases surface expression of NMDARs

Results from the experiments described above showed that NDMARs are involved in Aβ-mediated changes of synapse function in adult mice. However, changes in the expression of NMDARs altered the number of functional

Table 10 mEPSC recordings from the 5xFAD mouse model

6 m DG			
	WT (n = 24)	5xFAD (n = 23)	
Frequency [Hz]	0.73 [0.44–0.91]	0.66 [0.45–1.2]	MW-test: $p = 0.6612$
Amplitude [pA]	10.08 [9.15–10.52]	10.64 [10.15–11.7]	MW-test: $p = 0.0013$
1a DG			
	WT (n = 27)	5xFAD (n = 21)	
Frequency [Hz]	0.80 [0.61–1.07]	0.61 [0.44–0.89]	MW-test: $p = 0.026$
Amplitude [pA]	10.44 [8.54–11.95]	11.2 [8.94–11.86]	MW-test: $p = 0.47$
	GluN1$^{-/-}$ (n = 17)	5xFAD/ GluN1$^{-/-}$ (n = 17)	
Frequency [Hz]	0.85 [0.68–1.26]	1.02 [0.55–1.56]	MW-test: $p = 0.8119$
Amplitude [pA]	11.2 [10.24–12.84]	10.43 [9.66–12.31]	MW-test: $p = 0.394$
	GluN2A$^{-/-}$ (n = 23)	5xFAD/ GluN2A$^{-/-}$ (n = 17)	
Frequency [Hz]	0.97 [0.61–1.13]	1.01 [0.64–1.98]	MW-test: $p = 0.2802$
Amplitude [pA]	9.0 [8.38–9.93]	9.45 [8.97–10.72]	MW-test: $p = 0.1626$
	GluN2B$^{-/-}$ (n = 21)	5xFAD/ GluN2B$^{-/-}$ (n = 16)	
Frequency [Hz]	1.26 [0.89–1.61]	1.31 [0.6–1.63]	MW-test: p > 0.999
Amplitude [pA]	11.63 [10.72–12.14]	10.06 [9.88–12.92]	MW-test: $p = 0.3232$

Table 11 Overview of values for spine morphology in 5xFAD mice

	Spine Morphology distribution [%]		
	Stubby	Thin	Mushroom
6 m 5xFAD DG			
WT (17)	0.31 [0.25–0.34]	0.6 [0.56–0.64]	0.1 [0.06–0.1]
5xFAD (18)	0.32 [0.27–0.35]	0.58 [0.56–0.61]	0.1 [0.09–0.11]
Mann-Whitney test	$p = 0.4$	$p = 0.142$	$p = 0.85$
1a 5xFAD DG			
WT (29)	0.26 [0.22–0.35]	0.64 [0.6–0.7]	0.08 [0.04–0.11]
5xFAD (28)	0.32 [0.23–0.38]	0.59 [0.23–0.38]	0.09 [0.06–0.16]
Mann-Whitney test	$p = 0.32$	$p = 0.13$	$p = 0.14$
GluN1$^{-/-}$ (7)	0.32 [0.27–0.39]	0.56 [0.45–0.62]	0.12 [0.12–0.16]
5xFAD/GluN21$^{-/-}$ (12)	0.29 [0.25–0.31]	0.57 [0.47–0.63]	0.14 [0.12–0.21]
Mann-Whitney test	$p = 0.16$	$p = 0.526$	$p = 0.29$
GluN2A$^{-/-}$ (12)	0.31 [0.24–0.36]	0.58 [0.47–0.64]	0.13 [0.09–0.17]
5xFAD/GluN2A$^{-/-}$ (10)	0.39 [0.32–0.5]	0.39 [0.29–0.46]	0.19 [0.14–0.26]
Mann-Whitney test	$p = 0.02$	$p = 0.002$	$p = 0.025$
GluN2B$^{-/-}$ (15)	0.35 [0.27–0.4]	0.53 [0.45–0.62]	0.1 [0.08–0.14]
5xFAD/GluN2B$^{-/-}$ (11)	0.42 [0.34–0.52]	0.47 [0.37–0.54]	0.13 [0.1–0.16]
Mann-Whitney test	$p = 0.0362$	$p = 0.0687$	$p = 0.3565$

synapses also in control mice. Thus, an important question is if Aβ reduces the number of functional synapses by influencing the surface expression of NMDARs. To address this question, we investigated synaptic and extrasynaptic NMDAR-mediated currents in granule cells of one-year-old 5xFAD mice. The NMDAR/AMPAR ratio was reduced in 5xFAD mice when compared to that in WT littermates (Fig. 4a, b and Table 2). This suggests that the number of synaptic NMDARs is markedly reduced in one-year-old 5xFAD mice considering the reduction in frequency of AMPAR-mediated mEPSCs (Fig. 3g). The gating kinetics of NMDARs depend on their subunit composition. For example, the deactivation time-constant of GluN1/GluN2A-containing NMDARs is 14 times smaller than that of GluN1/GluN2B-containing NMDARs [86]. Consequently, the deactivation time-constant of triheteromeric GluN1/GluN2A/GluN2B-containining NMDARs is with 78.7 ms in between that of the diheteromeric NMDARs [86]. Decay time constant of synaptic NMDAR-mediated currents was unaltered in one-year-old 5xFAD mice (Fig. 4c, d and Table 2). As the decay time constant of synaptic NMDAR-mediated currents is mainly determined by the deactivation time constant, this result suggests that the subunit composition of synaptic NMDARs was not changed in 5xFAD mice. It has been shown that extrasynaptic NMDARs play an important role for mediating neuron dysfunction and cell death in various brain diseases that are connected to over-activation of NMDARs (for review see [62]). We studied extrasynaptic NMDAR-mediated currents by ultra-fast application of

glutamate onto nucleated patches of granule cells from one-year-old 5xFAD and WT mice. The amplitude of extrasynaptic NMDAR-mediated currents was decreased in 5xFAD mice (Fig. 4e, f and Table 2), showing that Aβ overexpression reduces also the number of extrasynaptic NMDARs. The deactivation time constant was not changed in granule cells of 5xFAD mice (Fig. 4g, h and Table 2), indicating that the subunit composition of extrasynaptic NMDARs is not affected by Aβ-overproduction.

Discussion

The open-channel NMDAR blocker Memantine has been shown to improve cognitive abilities in moderate-to-severe AD patients [68, 100]. A series of studies using rodent neurons additionally suggested that NMDARs are involved in the pathophysiology of AD [74, 79]. Importantly, there is evidence that NMDARs mediate Aβ-induced changes in synaptic function and neuronal morphology [45, 70, 74, 99]. However, conclusions about the role of NMDARs in Aβ-toxicity were mostly drawn from studies using cultured neurons, which are relatively immature, and mostly by using pharmacological tools. Thus, these studies do not allow drawing unequivocal conclusions about the contribution of NMDAR subunits to Aβ toxicity.

We show in this study that NMDARs are required for the Aβ-induced reduction of functional synapse number in adult mice. Thus, deletion of either subunit was sufficient to protect granule cells from loss of functional synapses in 5XFAD mice. Interestingly, deletion of GluN2A was effective in 1 year old 5XFAD mice, but

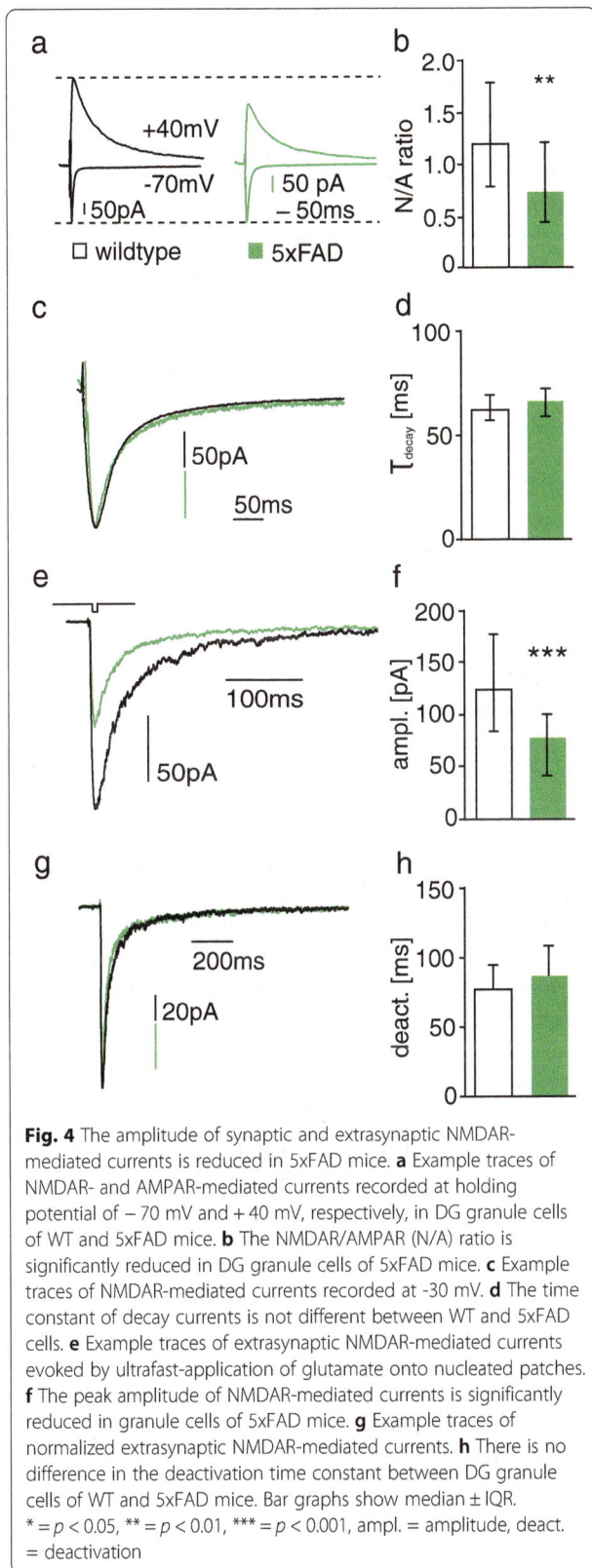

Fig. 4 The amplitude of synaptic and extrasynaptic NMDAR-mediated currents is reduced in 5xFAD mice. **a** Example traces of NMDAR- and AMPAR-mediated currents recorded at holding potential of − 70 mV and + 40 mV, respectively, in DG granule cells of WT and 5xFAD mice. **b** The NMDAR/AMPAR (N/A) ratio is significantly reduced in DG granule cells of 5xFAD mice. **c** Example traces of NMDAR-mediated currents recorded at -30 mV. **d** The time constant of decay currents is not different between WT and 5xFAD cells. **e** Example traces of extrasynaptic NMDAR-mediated currents evoked by ultrafast-application of glutamate onto nucleated patches. **f** The peak amplitude of NMDAR-mediated currents is significantly reduced in granule cells of 5xFAD mice. **g** Example traces of normalized extrasynaptic NMDAR-mediated currents. **h** There is no difference in the deactivation time constant between DG granule cells of WT and 5xFAD mice. Bar graphs show median ± IQR. * = p < 0.05, ** = p < 0.01, *** = p < 0.001, ampl. = amplitude, deact. = deactivation

did not prevent reduction of functional synapse number in CT100(I716F)-expressing cells of 4–5 months old mice. Perhaps the role of GluN2A for Aβ toxicity was different between 4 and 5 months and 1 year old mice because of an aging dependent upregulation of GluN2A. Age dependent changes in subunit expression may also explain why previous studies had shown that block of NMDARs with non-selective or GluN2B-specific antagonists, but not GluN2A-preferring antagonists prevent the Aβ-mediated depression of synaptic current amplitudes in organotypic slice cultures [37].

Virus-mediated deletion of NMDARs per se increases the number of functional synapses in DG granule cells as evidenced by the increase in mEPSC frequency. This was most pronounced in cells with deletion of the GluN2B subunit for three months. This is in line with previous studies on the influence of NMDARs on functional synapse number of cortical, CA1 and CA3 neurons [1, 19, 22, 96] and suggests that the GluN2B-mediated reduction of functional synapse number is a widespread homeostatic plasticity mechanism that controls the strength of neuronal communication in different neuron types. The underlying mechanism for the increase in the number of functional synapses is most likely an NMDAR-mediated Ca^{2+}-influx, which activates intracellular signaling molecules such as such as PKA and CaMKII leading to an upregulation of AMPAR number on the cell surface and in synapses [32, 76]. GluN2B-containing NMDARs are not only involved in the homeostatic control of functional synapse number, but also in the activity-dependent long-term plasticity of synaptic strength in mature neurons. Thus, genetic deletion of the GluN2B subunit reduces synaptic LTP [93]. Interestingly, GluN2B-containing NMDARs are required for the Aβ-induced reduction of synaptic long-term potentiation [70].

Our experiments with adult 5xFAD mice showed that GluN2A and GluN2B are dispensable for the Aβ-induced spine reduction. This is in line with some studies showing that block of GluN2B-containing NMDARs does not prevent Aβ-mediated spine loss [23, 82], but contrasts the finding of others that the GluN2B subunit mediates spines loss [82]. However, a general role of NMDARs in Aβ-induced spine reduction was found in other studies [4, 66, 74, 99]. Differences in in the maturity of neurons may well account for the contrasting findings of these studies and our study. NMDARs contributed to the Aβ-induced spine reduction in immature cultured neurons (studies mentioned above), but not in the brain of adult mice as shown in our study. The impact of NMDARs on neuron morphology in general may decrease with development. The morphology of immature cultured neurons is more flexible and spine stability lower than in mature neurons of the adult brain, suggesting that the mechanisms that control neuron morphology and spine density may well differ between immature and mature neurons. Indeed, block of NMDARs with APV for 14 days decreases spine density in cultured neurons [10]. Genetic deletion of the GluN2B subunit during developmental stages at which the rate of changes in neuron morphology is still high results in reduced spine number and alterations in dendrite arborization of CA1, CA3 and DG granule cells [2, 15, 17, 19]. Similarly, we observed a lower number of spines three weeks after deletion of the GluN2B subunit in 3–4 months old mice. However, after chronic GluN2B deletion for three months in one year old mice this effect vanished. This may indicate that the influence of GluN2B decreases with brain age or alternatively that the absence of GluN2B function for longer a time-period is compensated by other mechanisms that influence spine density such as BDNF-signaling [46, 69], or activation of voltage-gated-Ca-channels [80].

Differences in the spine stability may also explain that Aβ overproduction for three weeks with a virus-mediated approach did not reduce spine density in adult mice (this study), but decreased spine density in organotypic slice cultures already after 2–7 days [30, 99]. However, there are several other possible differences between young and adult brains that may account for the age-dependent decrease in Aβ-toxicity, such as differences in virus-infection efficacy or Aβ-expression levels in infected neurons. The bigger effect of Aβ overproduction on spine density or synaptic function in some studies using organotypic slices of young mice than in our study with adult mice may also be explained by the different types of viruses that were used. Thus, Aβ overproduction may be more pronounced when using Sindbis viruses [37, 99] than when using rAAVs (this study) for CT100 overexpression. In addition, the mode of application determines extent and velocity of Aβ-toxicity. Thus, repeated Aβ-application into the DG of 1-year-old mice over 6 days is neurotoxic [5]. It is likely that peak Aβ concentration is higher in this approach than in brains with 10-weeks virus-mediated CT100 overexpression or in 6 months-old 5xFAD mice. We did observe a spine number reduction in granule cells of 12-months old 5xFAD mice. Again, the mechanisms that reduce spine number may differ between the direct application of high doses of Aß and the more chronic Aβ overproduction in 5xFAD mice, which might better resemble the pathological situation in the brain of AD patients. Differences in the mechanisms of Aβ-toxicity between immature and mature neurons and/or high and lower Aβ-concentration could explain that GluN2B-containing NMDARs are required for the Aβ-mediated spine reduction in cultured neurons [30, 75, 99], but not in 5xFAD mice. In conclusion, other studies and our findings suggest that pathophysiological mechanisms of Aβ-toxicity change with brain maturation. Of note, a possible higher Aβ-toxicity in immature than in adult brains is not at odds with the fact that AD is a disease of elderly people. Thus, Aβ

concentration may increase with age. In addition, chronically elevated Aβ levels may be necessary to induce toxicity leading to AD.

Our results so far lead to the question: What is the possible link of Aβ and NMDARs? Aβ may alter NMDAR activity by different mechanisms: 1. direct interaction with NMDARs [11], 2. increased ambient glutamate levels (due to reduced glutamate reuptake) [45], or by changes in NMDAR expression [79]. Direct binding of Aß to or next to NMDARs influences their function of localization [13, 40]. For example, Aß has been shown to directly activate recombinant GluN2A- and GluN2B-containing NMDARs expressed in Xenopus oocytes [85]. An augmented and potentially toxic calcium influx may be the consequence from the direct Aβ with NMDAR interaction or increased ambient glutamate levels [3]. Interestingly, this effect is subunit-dependent in cultured cortical neurons: Activation of GluN2B-containing NMDARs elevates, whereas activation of GluN2A-containing NMDARs reduces intracellular calcium levels upon stimulation with Aß [16]. Interestingly, there is also evidence that activation of NMDARs by Aß may not require ion-flux via the channel pore suggesting a metabotropic function of NMDARs when activated by Aß [4, 37]. There are several proposed mechanisms by which Aβ may affect the expression of NMDARs on the cell surface. For example, Aβ reduces the expression of synaptic NMDARs in cultured neurons and Tg2576 mice possibly by activation of α-7 nicotinic receptors, which promotes receptor internalization in a PP2B and STEP-dependent fashion [38, 79]. Another mechanism may be the Aβ-mediated depletion of EphB2, which has been shown to reduce surface expression of NMDARs on DG granule cells [9]. Consistently, the current amplitude of synaptic NMDAR-mediated currents is reduced in DG granule cells of adult 5xFAD mice (this study) and CA1 neurons in organotypic slices that were infected with CT100-expressing viruses [37]. In contrast to the study of Kessels and colleagues, in which CT100 reduced preferentially the current amplitude of GluN2B-containing NMDARs, we did not find any indication for changes in the subunit composition [37, 67]. This difference may be well explained by a smaller contribution of GluN2B-containing NMDARs to synaptic currents in mature neurons than in immature neurons of organotypic slices. It has been hypothesized that the reduction in synaptic NMDAR number results not only from increased receptor internalization, but also from redistribution from synaptic to extrasynaptic sites [79]. A redistribution of NMDARs may contribute to Aβ-toxicity as the activation of synaptic NMDARs is thought to stimulate pro-survival signaling in neurons, whereas that of extrasynaptic NMDARs induces neuron apoptosis [25, 44], but see also: [101]. In fact, a redistribution of NMDARs is thought to play a role for the pathophysiology of another neurodegenerative disease, e.g. in Huntington's disease. Thus, exposure of neurons to huntingtin decreases the expression of synaptic NMDARs [53, 61] and increases the expression of extrasynaptic GluN2B-containing NMDARs [53]. We analyzed currents mediated by extrasynaptic NMDARs to investigate if a similar receptor redistribution is also involved in AD. Interestingly, we observed a reduction in the amplitude of extrasynaptic NMDAR-mediated currents again without indication for changes in the subunit composition. This rules out that the toxic influence of Aβ results from a redistribution of NMDARs from synaptic to extrasynaptic sites or from a change in the composition of extrasynaptic NMDARs with a relative increase in GluN2B-containing NMDARs. In fact, the decay time constant of synaptic NMDAR-mediated currents was in a similar range to the time constant of extrasynaptic NMDAR-mediated currents (62 ms and 76 ms, respectively), suggesting that the composition of synaptic and extrasynaptic NMDARs is very similar.

Our observation that synaptic and extrasynaptic NMDAR-mediated current amplitudes reduced to a similar extent without changes in subunit composition is in accordance with findings from a post-mortem study of the brain of human AD patients and healthy controls. In this study the authors revealed a comparable downregulation of the GluN2A and GluN2B subunit in hippocampus, temporal and cingulate cortex [34]. However, other studies were indicative for a downregulation in the expression of preferentially GluN2B-containing NMDARs in the hippocampus of AD patients [54]. The fact that we did not observe changes in spine number three months after genetic deletion of the GluN2B and GluN1 subunit makes it is unlikely that the downregulation of synaptic or extrasynaptic NMDARs is responsible for the Aβ-mediated reduction in functional synapses and spine number. It is rather the activation of the remaining NMDARs that contributes to the Aβ-mediated changes in functional synapse number and NMDAR-independent mechanisms that mediate the spine loss of granule cells in adult mice. The NMDAR downregulation may therefore even reduce the effect of Aβ on functional synapse number.

Conclusion

Using conditional NMDAR subunit KO mice, we showed that NMDARs are required for the influence of Aβ on the number of functional synapses of dentate gyrus granule cells. However, they were not responsible for the reduction in spine number that are observed after chronic Aβ-overproduction. Similar observations were made in somatosensory neurons (data not shown), indicating that the role of NMDARs in Aβ-toxicity is not specific for the dentate gyrus. Our data suggest that pharmacological block of NMDARs may reduce the influence of Aβ on synaptic function at early AD stages, but most likely does not prevent the changes in neuron morphology that are seen at later AD stages. This could also explain why the low affinity NMDAR antagonist Memantine alleviates cognitive

symptoms to some extent, but does not halt or reverse the progression of AD [20, 48].

Additional files

Additional file 1: S1. AAV-CT100 overexpression leads to synaptic depression in young mice. **a** pAAV constructs used for control conditions (tdTomato) and for stable co-expression of a fluorescent marker and CT100 (tdTomato) or Cre-recombinase (GFP). **b** Example traces of mEPSC recordings from adult and young control or CT100-overexpressing DG granule cells. **c + d** CT100 overexpression for 9 weeks does not reduce mEPSC frequency and does not change the cumulative propability of inter-event-intervals (IEIs) in DG granule cells from adult mice. **e + f** CT100 overexpression for 9 weeks reduces mEPSC frequency in DG granule cells from younger mice (injected at P7). Bar graphs show median ± IQR. * = p < 0.05, ** = p < 0.01, *** = p < 0.001 (PDF 1550 kb)

Additional file 2: S4. NMDAR subunit deletion does not influence mEPSC peak amplitude in DG granule cells. **a** Example traces of NMDAR/AMPAR (N/A) ratio recordings three weeks after injection of AAV-Cre-T2A-GFP. **b** N/A ratio is strongly reduced three weeks after NMDAR deletion (GluN1$^{-/-}$) in comparison to cells injected with a control virus (AAV-T2A-tdTom = GluN1$^{fl/fl}$). **c-h** CT100(I716F) overexpression does not influence peak amplitude (blue bars). Peak amplitude is increased in GluN2B$^{-/-}$ compared to GluN2B$^{-/-}$/CT100(I716F) DG granule cells. Bar graphs show median ± IQR. * = p < 0.05, ** = p < 0.01, *** = p < 0.001, norm. = normalized, cum. = cumulative, ampl. = amplitude (PDF 1391 kb)

Additional file 3: S2. Synaptic depression induced by CT100 overexpression is NMDAR dependent in young mice. **a** Example traces of mEPSC recordings from mice injected with AAV-Tom (GluN1$^{fl/fl}$), AAV-CT100-T2A-Tom (GluN1$^{fl/fl}$/CT100), AAV-Cre-T2A-GFP (GluN1$^{-/-}$) or co-injected with AAV-CT100-T2A-Tom and AAV-Cre-T2A-GFP (GluN1$^{-/-}$/CT100). **b** Cumulative probability of inter-event-interval (IEI) is shifted to longer IEIs in CT100(I716F) overexpressing cells. **c** mEPSC frequency is reduced in CT100-overexpressing and increased in GluN1$^{-/-}$ DG granule cells. There is no difference between GluN1$^{-/-}$ cells and GluN1$^{-/-}$/CT100 DG granule cells. **e + f** Peak amplitude is increased in GluN1$^{-/-}$ cells compared to GluN1$^{fl/fl}$ cells. Cumulative probability of the amplitude is shifted towards larger amplitues in GluN1$^{-/-}$ neuons. **d** CT100 increased the spine number of DG granule cells from slices of young mice. **g** The quantification of the spine morphology distribution shows no significant difference between the groups. Bar graphs show median ± IQR. * = p < 0.05, ** = p < 0.01, *** = p < 0.001; cum. = cumulative; morph. = morphology (PDF 1485 kb)

Additional file 4: S3. Active and passive properties of DG granule cells are not altered by CT100(I716F) overexpression. **a** Example traces of action potentials (APs) from control and CT100(I716F)-overexpressing DG granule cells. **b** CT100(I716F) overexpression does not alter the intrinsic properties threshold, amplitude, half-amplitude (HA) duration, afterhyperpolarization (AHP) and input resistance of DG granule cells compared to control cells. **c** Firing frequency, early- and late adaptation do not differ between control and CT100(I716F)-overexpressing DG granule cells. **d** Example traces of firing patterns of control and CT100(I716F) DG granule cells. Bar graphs show median ± IQR. (PDF 146 kb)

Additional file 5: S5. CT100(I716F) overexpression does not influence total dendritic length in adult mice. **a** Examples of traced DG granule cells of the GluN2A$^{fl/fl}$ mouse line. **b** The number of intersections analyzed by Sholl analysis is not changed by CT100(I716F) overexpression, GluN2A subunit deletion and GluN2A deletion in combination with CT100(I716F) overexpression. Mean ± SEM. Total dendritic length is not different between the groups. **c** Examples of traced DG granule cells of the GluN2B$^{fl/fl}$ mouse line. **d** Sholl analysis of the number of intersections shows subtle changes in dendritic complexity in GluN2B$^{-/-}$/CT100(I716F) cells compared to their respective control (GluN2B$^{-/-}$). Mean ± SEM. Total dendritic length is not different between the groups. Bar graphs show median ± IQR; dendr. = dendritic, morph. = morphology (PDF 133 kb)

Additional file 6: S6. Functional and structural properties are not affected in six-month old 5xFAD mice. **a** Examples of traced DG granule cells of six-month old WT and 5xFAD mice. **b** The number of intersections per radius is not changed as revealed by a Sholl analysis of cells from 5xFAD and WT mice. Mean ± SEM. **c** Total dendritic length is also not changed. **d + e** Spine number and spine morphology is not affected in DG granule cells of 5xFAD compared to WT mice. **f** mEPSC example traces of WT and 5xFAD granule cells. **g + h** mEPSC frequency is not changed in 5xFAD compared to WT granule cells, but peak amplitude is increased. Bar graphs show median ± IQR. * = $p < 0.05$, ** = $p < 0.01$, *** = $p < 0.001$; dendr. = dendritic, morph. = morphology (PDF 100 kb)

Additional file 7: Table S1. mEPSC recordings of CT100-overexpressing DG granule cells. **Table S2.** Morphological analysis of CT100-overexpressing DG granule cells. **Table S3.** mEPSC recordings of CT100(I716F)-overexpressing DG granule cells. **Table S4.** Morphology of CT100(I716F)-overexpressing DG granule cells. **Table S5.** Values of PPR of CT100(I716F)-overexpressing DG granule cells. **Table S6.** mEPSC recordings from the 5xFAD mouse model. **Table S7.** Morphological analysis of the 5xFAD mouse model. **Table S8.** Intrinsic and firing properties of CT100(I716F) overexpressing DG granule cells. **Table S9.** NMDAR-mediated currents in 5xFAD DG granule cells and virus-infected cells. **Table S10.** Values for spine morphology in CT100 and CT100(I716F) overexpression experiments. **Table S11.** Overview of values for spine morphology in 5xFAD mice. (DOCX 49 kb)

Abbreviations
ACSF: Artificial cerebral spine fluid; AD: Alzheimer Disease; AHP: Afterhyperpolarisation; AMPAR: α-amino-3-hydroxy-5-methyl-4-isoxazolepropionic acid receptor; AP: Action potential; Aβ: Amyloid Beta; CT100: C-terminal 100; DG: Dentate gyrus; LTP: Long-term-potentiation; mEPSC: miniature excitatory post-synaptic current; NMDA/AMPA ratio: NMDAR-mediated to AMPAR-mediated current amplitude ratio; NMDARs: N-methyl-D-aspartate receptors; PPR: Paired-pulse ratio; rAAVs: Recombinant adeno-associated viruses; SD: Standard deviation

Acknowledgements
We thank Benjamin Schieb, Barbara Biesalski and Dr. Viola Nordström for technical help. We further thank the Light Microscopy Facility of the DKFZ Heidelberg for support with confocal imaging.

Funding
The work was supported by a grant from the Fritz Thyssen foundation to JvE (Az. 10.15.1.017MN) and a NIH grant to RM (NIH grant AG032132).

Authors' contributions
MKM, EJ performed experiments. MKM, EJ and JvE analyzed and interpreted the results. MKM and EJ performed statistical analysis. MKM, EJ, RM, and JvE designed the study. MKM, EJ, KS, RM, and JvE wrote the manuscript and approved the final manuscript

Competing interests
The authors declare that they have no conflict of interest.

Author details
[1]Institute of Pathophysiology, University Medical Center of the Johannes Gutenberg University Mainz, 55128 Mainz, Germany. [2]Synaptic Signalling and Neurodegeneration, German Center for Neurodegenerative Diseases (DZNE), 53127 Bonn, Germany. [3]Department of Cellular Neurobiology, Brain Research Institute, Niigata University, Niigata 951-8585, Japan. [4]Center for Neural Circuits and Behavior, Department of Neuroscience and Section for Neurobiology, Division of Biology, University of California at San Diego, San Diego, CA, USA.

References
1. Adesnik H et al (2008) NMDA receptors inhibit synapse unsilencing during brain development. Proc Natl Acad Sci U S A 105(14):5597–5602
2. Akashi K et al (2009) NMDA receptor GluN2B (GluR epsilon 2/NR2B) subunit is crucial for channel function, postsynaptic macromolecular organization, and actin cytoskeleton at hippocampal CA3 synapses. J Neurosci 29(35): 10869–10882
3. Alberdi E et al (2010) Amyloid beta oligomers induce Ca2+ dysregulation and neuronal death through activation of ionotropic glutamate receptors. Cell Calcium 47(3):264–272
4. Birnbaum JH et al (2015) Calcium flux-independent NMDA receptor activity is required for Abeta oligomer-induced synaptic loss. Cell Death Dis 6:e1791
5. Brouillette J et al (2012) Neurotoxicity and memory deficits induced by soluble low-molecular-weight amyloid-beta1-42 oligomers are revealed in vivo by using a novel animal model. J Neurosci 32(23):7852–7861
6. Busche MA et al (2012) Critical role of soluble amyloid-beta for early hippocampal hyperactivity in a mouse model of Alzheimer's disease. Proc Natl Acad Sci U S A 109(22):8740–8745
7. Calabrese B et al (2007) Rapid, concurrent alterations in pre- and postsynaptic structure induced by naturally-secreted amyloid-beta protein. Mol Cell Neurosci 35(2):183–193
8. Chen Q et al (2007) Differential roles of NR2A- and NR2B-containing NMDA receptors in activity-dependent brain-derived neurotrophic factor gene regulation and limbic epileptogenesis. J Neurosci 27(3):542–552
9. Cisse M et al (2011) Reversing EphB2 depletion rescues cognitive functions in Alzheimer model. Nature 469(7328):47–52
10. Collin C, Miyaguchi K, Segal M (1997) Dendritic spine density and LTP induction in cultured hippocampal slices. J Neurophysiol 77(3):1614–1623
11. Cousins SL et al (2009) Amyloid precursor protein 695 associates with assembled NR2A- and NR2B-containing NMDA receptors to result in the enhancement of their cell surface delivery. J Neurochem 111(6):1501–1513
12. Cull-Candy S, Brickley S, Farrant M (2001) NMDA receptor subunits: diversity, development and disease. Curr Opin Neurobiol 11(3):327–335
13. De Felice FG et al (2007) Abeta oligomers induce neuronal oxidative stress through an N-methyl-D-aspartate receptor-dependent mechanism that is blocked by the Alzheimer drug memantine. J Biol Chem 282(15):11590–11601
14. Domingues A et al (2007) Toxicity of beta-amyloid in HEK293 cells expressing NR1/NR2A or NR1/NR2B N-methyl-D-aspartate receptor subunits. Neurochem Int 50(6):872–880
15. Espinosa JS et al (2009) Uncoupling dendrite growth and patterning: single-cell knockout analysis of NMDA receptor 2B. Neuron 62(2):205–217
16. Ferreira IL et al (2012) Amyloid beta peptide 1-42 disturbs intracellular calcium homeostasis through activation of GluN2B-containing N-methyl-d-aspartate receptors in cortical cultures. Cell Calcium 51(2):95–106
17. Gambrill AC, Barria A (2011) NMDA receptor subunit composition controls synaptogenesis and synapse stabilization. Proc Natl Acad Sci U S A 108(14): 5855–5860
18. Gladding CM, Raymond LA (2011) Mechanisms underlying NMDA receptor synaptic/extrasynaptic distribution and function. Mol Cell Neurosci 48(4): 308–320
19. Gray JA et al (2011) Distinct modes of AMPA receptor suppression at developing synapses by GluN2A and GluN2B: single-cell NMDA receptor subunit deletion in vivo. Neuron 71(6):1085–1101
20. Grossberg GT (2005) Rationalizing therapeutic approaches in Alzheimer's disease. CNS Spectr 10(11 Suppl 18):17–21
21. Guardia-Laguarta C et al (2010) Clinical, neuropathologic, and biochemical profile of the amyloid precursor protein I716F mutation. J Neuropathol Exp Neurol 69(1):53–59
22. Hall BJ, Ripley B, Ghosh A (2007) NR2B signaling regulates the development of synaptic AMPA receptor current. J Neurosci 27(49):13446–13456
23. Hanson JE et al (2014) Chronic GluN2B antagonism disrupts behavior in wild-type mice without protecting against synapse loss or memory impairment in Alzheimer's disease mouse models. J Neurosci 34(24):8277–8288
24. Hardingham GE, Bading H (2010) Synaptic versus extrasynaptic NMDA receptor signalling: implications for neurodegenerative disorders. Nat Rev Neurosci 11(10):682–696

25. Hardingham GE, Fukunaga Y, Bading H (2002) Extrasynaptic NMDARs oppose synaptic NMDARs by triggering CREB shut-off and cell death pathways. Nat Neurosci 5(5):405–414

26. Hardy J, Selkoe DJ (2002) The amyloid hypothesis of Alzheimer's disease: progress and problems on the road to therapeutics. Science 297(5580):353–356

27. Harris AZ, Pettit DL (2007) Extrasynaptic and synaptic NMDA receptors form stable and uniform pools in rat hippocampal slices. J Physiol 584(Pt 2):509–519

28. Herl L et al (2009) Mutations in amyloid precursor protein affect its interactions with presenilin/gamma-secretase. Mol Cell Neurosci 41(2):166–174

29. Hsia AY et al (1999) Plaque-independent disruption of neural circuits in Alzheimer's disease mouse models. Proc Natl Acad Sci U S A 96(6):3228–3233

30. Hsieh H et al (2006) AMPAR removal underlies Abeta-induced synaptic depression and dendritic spine loss. Neuron 52(5):831–843

31. Hu NW et al (2009) GluN2B subunit-containing NMDA receptor antagonists prevent Abeta-mediated synaptic plasticity disruption in vivo. Proc Natl Acad Sci U S A 106(48):20504–20509

32. Husi H, Grant SG (2001) Isolation of 2000-kDa complexes of N-methyl-D-aspartate receptor and postsynaptic density 95 from mouse brain. J Neurochem 77(1):281–291

33. Hynd MR, Scott HL, Dodd PR (2001) Glutamate(NMDA) receptor NR1 subunit mRNA expression in Alzheimer's disease. J Neurochem 78(1):175–182

34. Hynd MR, Scott HL, Dodd PR (2004) Differential expression of N-methyl-D-aspartate receptor NR2 isoforms in Alzheimer's disease. J Neurochem 90(4):913–919

35. Jacob CP et al (2007) Alterations in expression of glutamatergic transporters and receptors in sporadic Alzheimer's disease. J Alzheimers Dis 11(1):97–116

36. Kamenetz F et al (2003) APP processing and synaptic function. Neuron 37(6):925–937

37. Kessels HW, Nabavi S, Malinow R (2013) Metabotropic NMDA receptor function is required for beta-amyloid-induced synaptic depression. Proc Natl Acad Sci U S A 110(10):4033–4038

38. Kurup P et al (2010) Abeta-mediated NMDA receptor endocytosis in Alzheimer's disease involves ubiquitination of the tyrosine phosphatase STEP61. J Neurosci 30(17):5948–5957

39. Kutsuwada T et al (1992) Molecular diversity of the NMDA receptor channel. Nature 358(6381):36–41

40. Lacor PN et al (2007) Abeta oligomer-induced aberrations in synapse composition, shape, and density provide a molecular basis for loss of connectivity in Alzheimer's disease. J Neurosci 27(4):796–807

41. Lambert MP et al (1998) Diffusible, nonfibrillar ligands derived from Abeta1-42 are potent central nervous system neurotoxins. Proc Natl Acad Sci U S A 95(11):6448–6453

42. Lau CG, Zukin RS (2007) NMDA receptor trafficking in synaptic plasticity and neuropsychiatric disorders. Nat Rev Neurosci 8(6):413–426

43. Le WD et al (1995) Cell death induced by beta-amyloid 1-40 in MES 23.5 hybrid clone: the role of nitric oxide and NMDA-gated channel activation leading to apoptosis. Brain Res 686(1):49–60

44. Leveille F et al (2008) Neuronal viability is controlled by a functional relation between synaptic and extrasynaptic NMDA receptors. FASEB J 22(12):4258–4271

45. Li S et al (2009) Soluble oligomers of amyloid Beta protein facilitate hippocampal long-term depression by disrupting neuronal glutamate uptake. Neuron 62(6):788–801

46. Lin B et al (2005) Theta stimulation polymerizes actin in dendritic spines of hippocampus. J Neurosci 25(8):2062–2069

47. Liu Y et al (2007) NMDA receptor subunits have differential roles in mediating excitotoxic neuronal death both in vitro and in vivo. J Neurosci 27(11):2846–2857

48. Lopez OL et al (2009) Long-term effects of the concomitant use of memantine with cholinesterase inhibition in Alzheimer disease. J Neurol Neurosurg Psychiatry 80(6):600–607

49. Lue LF et al (1999) Soluble amyloid beta peptide concentration as a predictor of synaptic change in Alzheimer's disease. Am J Pathol 155(3):853–862

50. Luo J et al (1997) The majority of N-methyl-D-aspartate receptor complexes in adult rat cerebral cortex contain at least three different subunits (NR1/NR2A/NR2B). Mol Pharmacol 51(1):79–86

51. Masliah E et al (1994) Synaptic and neuritic alterations during the progression of Alzheimer's disease. Neurosci Lett 174(1):67–72

52. McLean CA et al (1999) Soluble pool of Abeta amyloid as a determinant of severity of neurodegeneration in Alzheimer's disease. Ann Neurol 46(6):860–866

53. Milnerwood AJ et al (2010) Early increase in extrasynaptic NMDA receptor signaling and expression contributes to phenotype onset in Huntington's disease mice. Neuron 65(2):178–190

54. Mishizen-Eberz AJ et al (2004) Biochemical and molecular studies of NMDA receptor subunits NR1/2A/2B in hippocampal subregions throughout progression of Alzheimer's disease pathology. Neurobiol Dis 15(1):80–92

55. Mizuta I et al (1998) Developmental expression of NMDA receptor subunits and the emergence of glutamate neurotoxicity in primary cultures of murine cerebral cortical neurons. Cell Mol Life Sci 54(7):721–725

56. Monyer H et al (1992) Heteromeric NMDA receptors: molecular and functional distinction of subtypes. Science 256(5060):1217–1221

57. Monyer H et al (1994) Developmental and regional expression in the rat brain and functional properties of four NMDA receptors. Neuron 12(3):529–540

58. Naslund J et al (2000) Correlation between elevated levels of amyloid beta-peptide in the brain and cognitive decline. JAMA 283(12):1571–1577

59. Niewoehner B et al (2007) Impaired spatial working memory but spared spatial reference memory following functional loss of NMDA receptors in the dentate gyrus. Eur J Neurosci 25(3):837–846

60. Oakley H et al (2006) Intraneuronal beta-amyloid aggregates, neurodegeneration, and neuron loss in transgenic mice with five familial Alzheimer's disease mutations: potential factors in amyloid plaque formation. J Neurosci 26(40):10129–10140

61. Okamoto S et al (2009) Balance between synaptic versus extrasynaptic NMDA receptor activity influences inclusions and neurotoxicity of mutant huntingtin. Nat Med 15(12):1407–1413

62. Parsons MP, Raymond LA (2014) Extrasynaptic NMDA receptor involvement in central nervous system disorders. Neuron 82(2):279–293

63. Petralia RS et al (2010) Organization of NMDA receptors at extrasynaptic locations. Neuroscience 167(1):68–87

64. Rammes G et al (2011) Therapeutic significance of NR2B-containing NMDA receptors and mGluR5 metabotropic glutamate receptors in mediating the synaptotoxic effects of beta-amyloid oligomers on long-term potentiation (LTP) in murine hippocampal slices. Neuropharmacology 60(6):982–990

65. Rammes G et al (2017) Involvement of GluN2B subunit containing N-methyl-d-aspartate (NMDA) receptors in mediating the acute and chronic synaptotoxic effects of oligomeric amyloid-beta (Abeta) in murine models of Alzheimer's disease (AD). Neuropharmacology 123:100–115

66. Rammes G et al (2018) The NMDA receptor antagonist Radiprodil reverses the synaptotoxic effects of different amyloid-beta (Abeta) species on long-term potentiation (LTP). Neuropharmacology 140:184–192

67. Reinders NR et al (2016) Amyloid-beta effects on synapses and memory require AMPA receptor subunit GluA3. Proc Natl Acad Sci U S A 113(42):E6526–E6534

68. Reisberg B et al (2003) Memantine in moderate-to-severe Alzheimer's disease. N Engl J Med 348(14):1333–1341

69. Rex CS et al (2007) Brain-derived neurotrophic factor promotes long-term potentiation-related cytoskeletal changes in adult hippocampus. J Neurosci 27(11):3017–3029

70. Ronicke R et al (2011) Early neuronal dysfunction by amyloid beta oligomers depends on activation of NR2B-containing NMDA receptors. Neurobiol Aging 32(12):2219–2228

71. Rumbaugh G, Vicini S (1999) Distinct synaptic and extrasynaptic NMDA receptors in developing cerebellar granule neurons. J Neurosci 19(24):10603–10610

72. Sandhu FA et al (1993) NMDA and AMPA receptors in transgenic mice expressing human beta-amyloid protein. J Neurochem 61(6):2286–2289

73. Schneider LS et al (2011) Lack of evidence for the efficacy of memantine in mild Alzheimer disease. Arch Neurol 68(8):991–998

74. Shankar GM et al (2007) Natural oligomers of the Alzheimer amyloid-beta protein induce reversible synapse loss by modulating an NMDA-type glutamate receptor-dependent signaling pathway. J Neurosci 27(11):2866–2875

75. Shankar GM et al (2008) Amyloid-beta protein dimers isolated directly from Alzheimer's brains impair synaptic plasticity and memory. Nat Med 14(8):837–842

76. Sheng M (2001) The postsynaptic NMDA-receptor--PSD-95 signaling complex in excitatory synapses of the brain. J Cell Sci 114(Pt 7):1251

77. Sheng M et al (1994) Changing subunit composition of heteromeric NMDA receptors during development of rat cortex. Nature 368(6467):144–147

78. Sinor JD et al (2000) NMDA and glutamate evoke excitotoxicity at distinct cellular locations in rat cortical neurons in vitro. J Neurosci 20(23):8831–8837

79. Snyder EM et al (2005) Regulation of NMDA receptor trafficking by amyloid-beta. Nat Neurosci 8(8):1051–1058

80. Stanika RI, Flucher BE, Obermair GJ (2015) Regulation of postsynaptic stability by the L-type Calcium Channel CaV1.3 and its interaction with PDZ proteins. Curr Mol Pharmacol 8(1):95–101

81. Suarez-Calvet M et al (2014) Autosomal-dominant Alzheimer's disease mutations at the same codon of amyloid precursor protein differentially alter Abeta production. J Neurochem 128(2):330–339

82. Tackenberg C et al (2013) NMDA receptor subunit composition determines beta-amyloid-induced neurodegeneration and synaptic loss. Cell Death Dis 4:e608

83. Tariot PN et al (2004) Memantine treatment in patients with moderate to severe Alzheimer disease already receiving donepezil: a randomized controlled trial. JAMA 291(3):317–324

84. Terry RD et al (1991) Physical basis of cognitive alterations in Alzheimer's disease: synapse loss is the major correlate of cognitive impairment. Ann Neurol 30(4):572–580

85. Texido L et al (2011) Amyloid beta peptide oligomers directly activate NMDA receptors. Cell Calcium 49(3):184–190

86. Tovar KR, McGinley MJ, Westbrook GL (2013) Triheteromeric NMDA receptors at hippocampal synapses. J Neurosci 33(21):9150–9160

87. Tovar KR, Westbrook GL (1999) The incorporation of NMDA receptors with a distinct subunit composition at nascent hippocampal synapses in vitro. J Neurosci 19(10):4180–4188

88. Traynelis SF et al (2010) Glutamate receptor ion channels: structure, regulation, and function. Pharmacol Rev 62(3):405–496

89. Tu W et al (2010) DAPK1 interaction with NMDA receptor NR2B subunits mediates brain damage in stroke. Cell 140(2):222–234

90. Varga E et al (2014) Abeta(1-42) enhances neuronal excitability in the CA1 via NR2B subunit-containing NMDA receptors. Neural Plast 2014:584314

91. Vicini S et al (1998) Functional and pharmacological differences between recombinant N-methyl-D-aspartate receptors. J Neurophysiol 79(2):555–566

92. von Engelhardt J et al (2007) Excitotoxicity in vitro by NR2A- and NR2B-containing NMDA receptors. Neuropharmacology 53(1):10–17

93. von Engelhardt J et al (2008) Contribution of hippocampal and extra-hippocampal NR2B-containing NMDA receptors to performance on spatial learning tasks. Neuron 60(5):846–860

94. Voronin LL, Cherubini E (2004) 'Deaf, mute and whispering' silent synapses: their role in synaptic plasticity. J Physiol 557(Pt 1):3–12

95. Walsh DM et al (2005) The role of cell-derived oligomers of Abeta in Alzheimer's disease and avenues for therapeutic intervention. Biochem Soc Trans 33(Pt 5):1087–1090

96. Wang CC et al (2011) A critical role for GluN2B-containing NMDA receptors in cortical development and function. Neuron 72(5):789–805

97. Wang J et al (1999) The levels of soluble versus insoluble brain Abeta distinguish Alzheimer's disease from normal and pathologic aging. Exp Neurol 158(2):328–337

98. Watanabe M et al (1992) Developmental changes in distribution of NMDA receptor channel subunit mRNAs. Neuroreport 3(12):1138–1140

99. Wei W et al (2010) Amyloid beta from axons and dendrites reduces local spine number and plasticity. Nat Neurosci 13(2):190–196

100. Winblad B, Poritis N (1999) Memantine in severe dementia: results of the 9M-best study (benefit and efficacy in severely demented patients during treatment with memantine). Int J Geriatr Psychiatry 14(2):135–146

101. Zhou X et al (2013) NMDA receptor-mediated excitotoxicity depends on the coactivation of synaptic and extrasynaptic receptors. Cell Death Dis 4:e560

16

Hypoxic pre-conditioning suppresses experimental autoimmune encephalomyelitis by modifying multiple properties of blood vessels

Sebok K. Halder, Ravi Kant and Richard Milner*

Abstract

While hypoxic pre-conditioning protects against neurological disease the underlying mechanisms have yet to be fully defined. As chronic mild hypoxia (CMH, 10% O_2) triggers profound vascular remodeling in the central nervous system (CNS), the goal of this study was to examine the protective potential of hypoxic pre-conditioning in the experimental autoimmune encephalomyelitis (EAE) model of multiple sclerosis (MS) and then determine how CMH influences vascular integrity and the underlying cellular and molecular mechanisms during EAE. We found that mice exposed to CMH at the same time as EAE induction were strongly protected against the development of EAE progression, as assessed both at the clinical level and at the histopathological level by reduced levels of inflammatory leukocyte infiltration, vascular breakdown and demyelination. Mechanistically, our studies indicate that CMH protects, at least in part, by enhancing several properties of blood vessels that contribute to vascular integrity, including reduced expression of the endothelial activation molecules VCAM-1 and ICAM-1, maintained expression of endothelial tight junction proteins ZO-1 and occludin, and upregulated expression of the leukocyte inhibitory protein laminin-111 in the vascular basement membrane. Taken together, these data suggest that optimization of BBB integrity is an important mechanism underlying the protective effect of hypoxic pre-conditioning.

Keywords: Endothelial, Laminin, Hypoxic pre-conditioning, Experimental autoimmune encephalomyelitis, Blood-brain barrier

Introduction

Multiple sclerosis (MS) is the most common neurological disease in the young-middle age population, affecting more than 400,000 people in the United States [9, 44]. At the pathological level, MS is an autoimmune disease in which inflammatory leukocytes directed against myelin antigens, infiltrate the CNS (brain and spinal cord) to establish a chronic inflammatory response that results in demyelination and axonal degeneration [16, 27]. Strong evidence demonstrates that alterations in vascular properties at an early stage of disease onset play a central role in the initiation and maintenance of MS pathogenesis by permitting leukocyte infiltration into the CNS [18, 25, 39, 40]. CNS blood vessels are unique in forming an extremely tight barrier between the blood and parenchymal tissue (termed blood-brain barrier (BBB) or blood-spinal cord barrier (BSCB) depending on location), which confers high electrical resistance and low permeability properties, thus protecting neural cells from potentially harmful blood components [1, 23, 38]. The integrity of the BBB/BSCB is regulated at a number of levels including: (i) inter-endothelial tight junction proteins, (ii) the vascular basal lamina comprising a mixture of extracellular matrix (ECM) proteins, and (iii) the influence of astrocyte end-feet and pericytes [5, 7, 37, 45].

Pre-conditioning describes the phenomenon whereby exposure to a mild stimulus for a period of time confers protection against a subsequent stronger insult. In the study of ischemic stroke it is well established that pre-conditioning with mild hypoxia protects against the

* Correspondence: rmilner@scripps.edu
Department of Molecular Medicine, MEM-151, The Scripps Research Institute, 10550 North Torrey Pines Road, La Jolla, CA 92037, USA

development of ischemic infarct [10, 34, 43]. Interestingly, several years ago, the Dore-Duffy lab demonstrated that hypoxic pre-conditioning may also protect against the progression of experimental autoimmune encephalomyelitis (EAE), an animal model of MS. [8] In that study, chronic exposure of mice to 10% O_2 (chronic mild hypoxia, CMH) suppressed clinical severity of EAE, which correlated with reductions in both leukocyte adherence to cerebral blood vessels and their infiltration into the CNS. Despite the profound protection that hypoxic pre-conditioning affords, the cellular and molecular mechanisms underlying this protection have yet to be fully defined. Recent work suggests that CMH protects in part, by inducing an anti-inflammatory milieu in the spinal cord of EAE affected mice, as defined by reduced levels of infiltrating CD4+ T lymphocytes and delayed Th17-specific cytokine response, correlating with increased levels of regulatory T cells (Tregs) and the anti-inflammatory cytokine IL-10 [15].

In addition to exerting an anti-inflammatory effect on cells of the immune system, because CMH promotes a robust vascular remodeling response in the CNS [26, 30, 36], it is possible that it might also protect against EAE by modifying the properties of blood vessels. In particular, several lines of evidence suggest that CMH enhances the integrity of CNS blood vessels. First, CMH reduces the adherence of circulating leukocytes to the endothelium of cerebral blood vessels in mouse models of MS and ischemic stroke [8, 43]. Second, CMH triggers strong upregulation of endothelial tight junction proteins at the BBB [3, 20, 30]. Third, we have recently found that CMH also stimulates enhanced expression of the ECM protein laminin in the basement membranes of cerebral blood vessels [21], a protein which prevents leukocyte transmigration across blood vessel walls by virtue of its anti-adhesive properties on this cell type [41]. In light of these observations, the goal of this study was to examine the protective potential of CMH in a relapsing-remitting EAE model of MS and then determine how CMH influences vascular integrity and the different cellular and molecular components underlying this integrity. Specifically, we wanted to define how CMH influences vascular expression of the following parameters during EAE progression: (i) endothelial activation molecules that mediate leukocyte adherence to the endothelium, vascular cell adhesion molecule-1 (VCAM-1) and intercellular adhesion molecule-1 (ICAM-1), (ii) the tight junction proteins ZO-1 and occludin, and (iii) vascular ECM proteins thought to be important for regulating leukocyte infiltration into the CNS.

Materials and methods
Animals
The studies described have been reviewed and approved by The Scripps Research Institute (TSRI) Institutional Animal Care and Use Committee. Wild-type female SJL/J mice were purchased from JAX labs and maintained under pathogen-free conditions in the closed breeding colony of TSRI.

Experimental autoimmune encephalomyelitis (EAE)
EAE was performed using a protocol and materials provided by Hooke Laboratories (Lawrence, MA). Briefly, 10 week old SJL/J female mice were immunized sub-cutaneously with 200 μl of 1 mg/ml $PLP_{139-151}$ peptide emulsified in complete Freund's adjuvant (CFA) containing 1 mg/ml Mycobacterium tuberculosis in both the base of the tail and upper back. This protocol leads to robust induction of clinical EAE 10–15 days following immunization in which mice reach peak disease before making significant recovery (remission), but then follow a cyclical relapsing-remitting course [32, 33]. Animals were monitored daily for clinical signs and scored as follows: 0-no symptoms; 1-flaccid tail; 2-paresis of hind limbs; 3-paralysis of hind limbs; 4-quadriplegia; 5-death. Clinical EAE data were assessed using one-way analysis of variance (ANOVA) followed by post-hoc Student's test, in which $p < 0.05$ was defined as statistically significant. For histological analysis, disease-free controls or EAE mice maintained under normoxic or hypoxic conditions were euthanized during the peak phase of disease, typically 14–15 days post-immunization.

Chronic hypoxia model
Following immunization with $PLP_{139-151}$ peptide, mice, housed 4 to a cage, were randomly divided into two groups: one was placed into a hypoxic chamber (Biospherix, Redfield, NY) maintained at 10% O_2 for the duration of the experiment, while the control group was kept in the same room under similar conditions except that they were kept at ambient sea-level oxygen levels (normoxia, approximately 21% O_2 at sea-level). Every day, the chamber was briefly opened to allow for clinical assessment of mice and cage cleaning and food and water replacement.

Immunohistochemistry and antibodies
Immunohistochemistry was performed on 10 μm frozen sections of cold phosphate buffer saline (PBS) perfused tissues as described previously [35]. Rat monoclonal antibodies from BD Pharmingen (La Jolla, CA) reactive for the following antigens were used in this study: CD31 (clone MEC13.3), MECA-32, VCAM-1 (clone 429), and CD45. Rat monoclonal reactive for CD4 (clone GK1.5) was obtained from R&D Systems, Minneapolis, MN). Hamster monoclonal antibodies used included CD31 (clone 2H8) from Abcam (Cambridge, MA) and ICAM-1 (clone 3E2) from BD Pharmingen. The mouse monoclonal antibody (4H-8) against the anti-laminin α2

subunit was obtained from Sigma (St. Louis, MO). Rabbit polyclonal antibodies reactive for the following proteins were also used: occludin and ZO-1 (all from Invitrogen, Carlsbad, CA), fibrinogen (Millipore, Temecula, CA), and pan-laminin (Sigma, St. Louis, MO). In addition, the rabbit polyclonal against the anti-laminin $\alpha 1$ subunit was a kind gift from Dr. Takako Sasaki (Oita University, Japan). The goat antibody reactive for collagen IV was obtained from Millipore. Fluoromyelin-red was obtained from Invitrogen. Secondary antibodies used included Cy3-conjugated anti-rat, anti-rabbit, anti-goat and anti-mouse and Cy5-conjugated anti-rabbit from Jackson Immunoresearch, (West Grove, PA) and Alexa Fluor 488-conjugated anti-rat, anti-hamster and anti-rabbit from Invitrogen (Carlsbad, CA).

Image analysis

Images were taken using a 2×, 10× or 20× objective on a Keyence 710 fluorescent microscope. All analysis was performed in the lumbar spinal cord. For each antigen, images of three randomly selected areas were taken at 10× or 20× magnification and three sections per spinal cord analyzed to calculate the mean for each subject. For each antigen in each experiment, exposure time was set to convey the maximum amount of information without saturating the image. Exposure time was maintained constant for each antigen across the different experimental groups. To quantify the degree of CD45+ or CD4+ leukocyte infiltration, fibrinogen leakage, vascular expression of ICAM-1 and VCAM-1, the tight junction proteins ZO-1 and occludin, and expression of laminins and collagen IV within blood vessels, NIH Image J software was used to measure the total fluorescent signal per field of view (FOV). Each experiment was performed with 6 different animals per condition, and the results expressed as the mean ± SEM. Statistical significance was assessed using one-way analysis of variance (ANOVA) followed by Tukey's multiple comparison post-hoc test, in which $p < 0.05$ was defined as statistically significant.

Results

Hypoxic pre-conditioning reduces the severity of EAE both clinically and histopathologically

Previous studies have shown that hypoxic pre-conditioning delays the time of onset of the chronic progressive form of EAE [8, 15]. In the current study we chose to examine the influence of hypoxic pre-conditioning in the relapsing-remitting form of EAE for two reasons. First, the relapsing-remitting form of MS constitutes more than 85% of patients, so this model has strong translational relevance [4]. Second, in contrast to the chronic progressive model, in which mice reach peak disease and then only partially recover, in the relapsing-remitting model, mice reach peak

disease before making significant recovery, but then follow a cyclical relapsing-remitting course [32, 33]. Ten weeks old female SJL/J mice were immunized with PLP$_{139-151}$ and maintained under normoxic conditions or exposed to chronic mild hypoxia (CMH) at 10% O_2 for the duration of the experiment. As shown in Fig. 1a, CMH markedly reduced clinical score both at the peak of disease activity and at all time-points thereafter for the duration of the experiment (7 weeks), resulting in a marked and sustained reduction in long-term clinical score. Histopathological assessment of spinal cord tissue with the pan-leukocyte marker CD45 and the myelin stain fluoromyelin (CD45/fluoromyelin dual-IF) revealed that compared to normoxic EAE mice, CMH-treated EAE mice showed marked reduction in the level of CD45+ leukocyte infiltration into the spinal cord (Fig. 1b). Quantification revealed that CMH significantly reduced CD45+ leukocyte infiltration (7.37 ± 1.72 vs. $19.40 \pm 3.06\%$ total CD45+ area/FOV under normoxic conditions, $p < 0.01$) (Fig. 1c) and this was associated with preservation of myelin (93.67 ± 2.11 vs. $73.74 \pm 4.15\%$ of fluoromyelin area/FOV under normoxic conditions, $p < 0.01$) (Fig. 1d). In addition, CD4 IF staining revealed that while CD4+ T cells were widely distributed in the spinal cord of EAE-normoxic mice, in EAE-CMH mice, they were tightly clustered and largely contained within perivascular aggregates (Fig. 1f-g). Compared to normoxic conditions, CMH markedly reduced CD4+ leukocyte infiltration into the spinal cord (0.96 ± 0.12 fluorescent units/FOV vs. 1.99 ± 0.29, $p < 0.01$). This demonstrates that CMH markedly suppressed EAE progression, both at the clinical and histopathological levels.

Interestingly, we noticed that the distribution of CD45+ leukocytes within the spinal cords of normoxic and CMH-treated mice differed in two respects. First, under normoxic conditions, the greatest accumulation of leukocytes was in the ventral spinal cord, while under CMH conditions, most were found in the dorsal region (Fig. 1b). Second, closer inspection of high power images (Fig. 1e) revealed that while in the normoxic spinal cord, inflammatory CD45+ leukocytes were dispersed throughout the spinal cord white and gray matter, in CMH-treated mice they were mostly organized in large perivascular aggregates and leukocyte dispersal was limited. Based on this observation, we wondered if CMH might be protecting against EAE by restricting the ability of leukocytes to cross the blood-spinal cord barrier (BSCB). To examine this process more deeply, specifically to define how CMH influences vascular integrity, we performed dual-IF with the endothelial cell marker CD31 and fibrinogen, using fibrinogen leakage as a marker of vascular breakdown (Fig. 2a-c). This revealed that while spinal cords of EAE-normoxic mice had extensive fibrinogen leakage, most notably in white matter, and strongly localized with inflammatory infiltrates, tissue from EAE-CMH mice

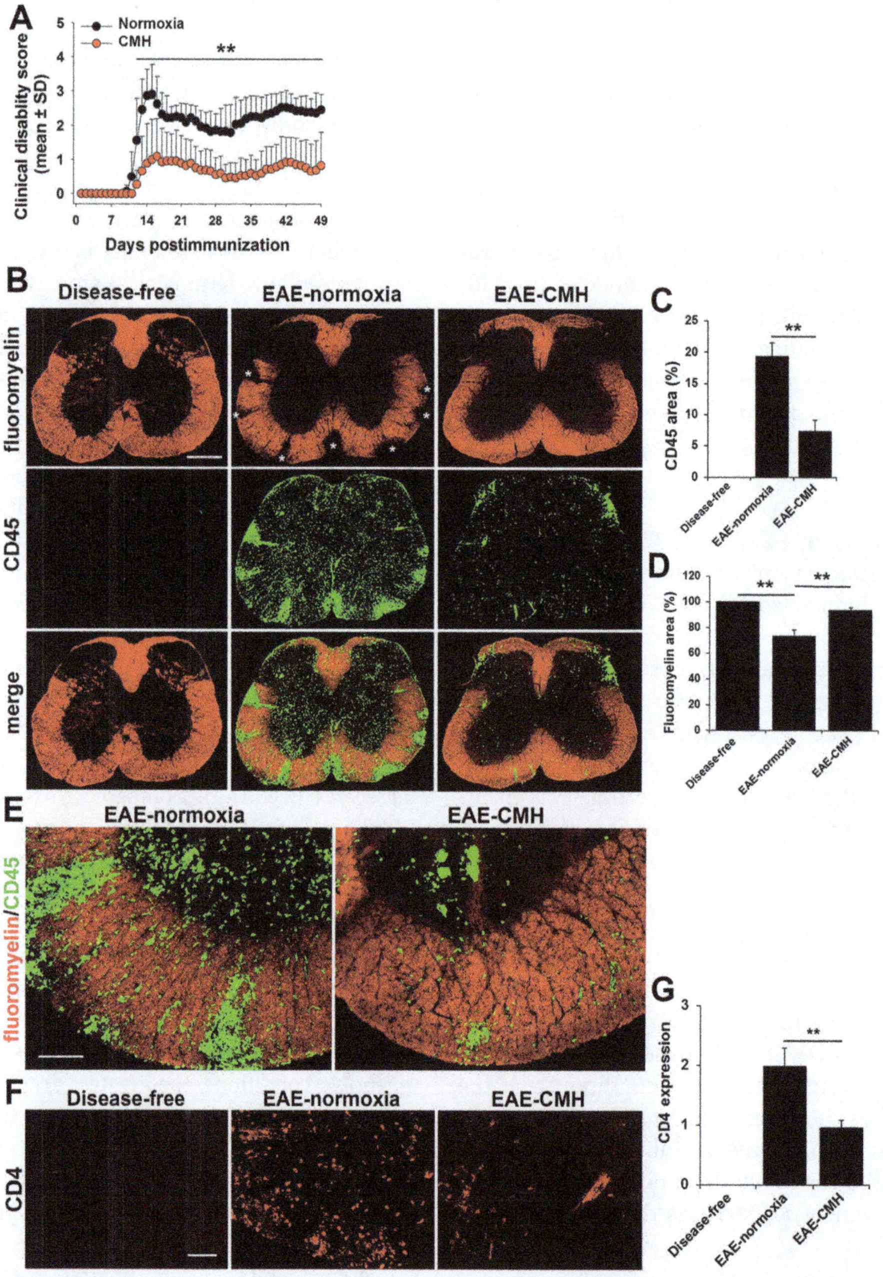

Fig. 1 Hypoxic pre-conditioning reduces the severity of EAE both clinically and histopathologically. **a.** The impact of chronic mild hypoxia (CMH) on clinical severity in EAE. The progression of EAE in mice maintained under normoxic (control) or CMH conditions was evaluated by measuring clinical score at daily intervals. All points represent the mean ± SD ($n = 15$ mice per group, representative of 4 separate experiments). Note that compared to normoxic mice, CMH markedly reduced clinical score both at the peak of disease activity and at all time-points thereafter for the duration of the experiment (7 weeks), resulting in a marked and sustained reduction in long-term clinical score. **b, e** and **f.** Frozen sections of lumbar spinal cord taken from disease-free, EAE-normoxia or EAE-CMH mice at the peak symptomatic phase of EAE (14–15 days post-immunization) were stained for the inflammatory leukocyte marker CD45 (AlexaFluor-488) and fluoromyelin-red (FM) in panels B (scale bar = 500 μm) and E (scale bar = 100 μm) or CD4 in panel F (scale bar = 100 μm). Quantification of CD45 (**c**), fluoromyelin (**d**) and CD4 (**g**) fluorescent signal at peak phase of EAE. Results are expressed as the mean ± SEM ($n = 6$ mice/group). Note that CMH markedly suppressed CD45+ and CD4+ leukocyte infiltration and protected against demyelination. In panel B asterisks mark the zones of demyelination. ** $p < 0.01$

showed significantly reduced levels of fibrinogen leak (4.71 ± 1.32 compared to 15.17 ± 1.95% total fibrinogen area/FOV under normoxic conditions, $p < 0.01$) (Fig. 2b).

In an alternative approach to examine whether blood vessels in CMH-treated mice have altered barrier properties, we also analyzed expression of MECA-32, a marker that is

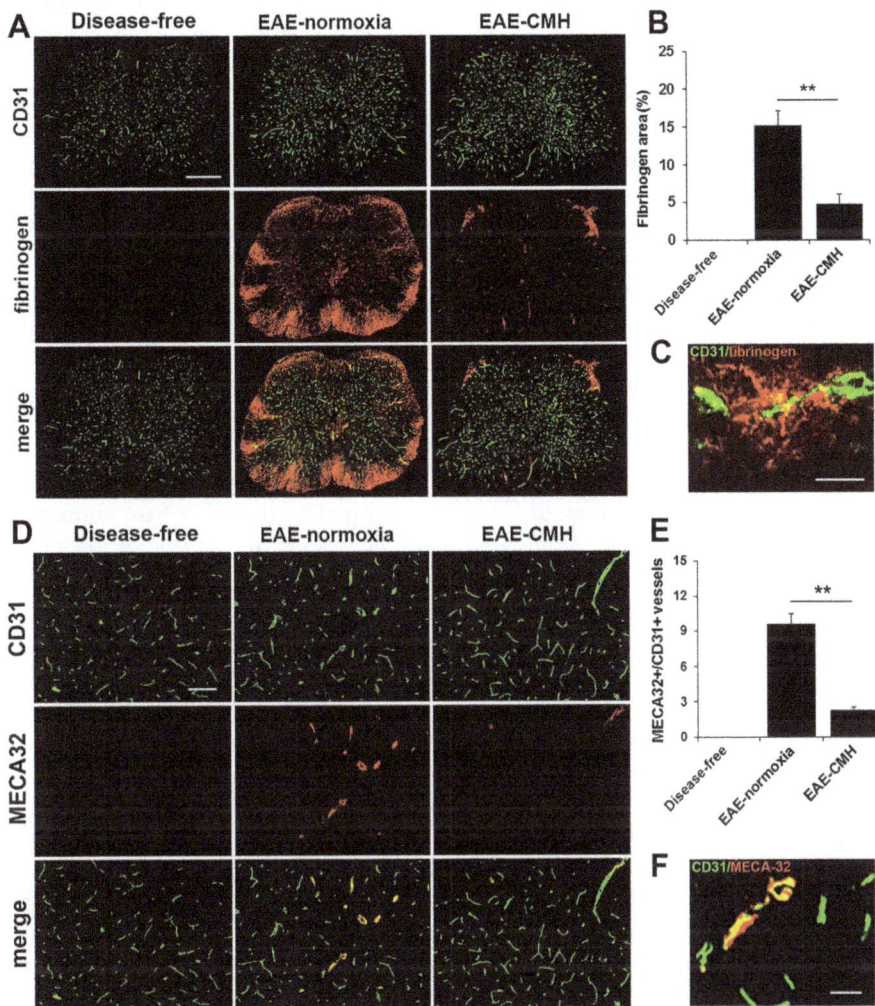

Fig. 2 CMH protects against loss of vascular integrity during EAE progression. **a** and **d**. Frozen sections of lumbar spinal cord taken from disease-free, EAE-normoxia or EAE-CMH mice at the peak symptomatic phase of EAE were stained for CD31 (AlexaFluor-488) and fibrinogen (Fbg) (Cy-3) in panel A (Scale bar = 500 μm) or CD31 (AlexaFluor-488) and MECA-32 (Cy-3) in panel D (Scale bar = 100 μm). **b** and **e**. Quantification of fibrinogen leakage (**b**) and MECA-32 expression (**e**). Results are expressed as the mean ± SEM (n = 6 mice/group). **c** and **f**. High power images of CD31/fibrinogen (**c**) and CD31/MECA-32 (**f**). Scale bar = 25 μm. Note that CMH markedly suppressed fibrinogen leakage as well as expression of MECA-32. ** p < 0.01

expressed at high levels on endothelial cells in the developing CNS, but then disappears as CNS endothelium matures [22]. Previous studies have shown that MECA-32 is re-expressed in adult CNS blood vessels during inflammatory, hypoxic or ischemic conditions [11, 29, 42], suggesting that MECA-32 can be used to identify CNS blood vessels with compromised vascular integrity. Our analysis showed that while no MECA-32 staining could be detected in disease-free spinal cord, significant vascular staining for MECA-32 was detected in EAE mice maintained under normoxic conditions (Fig. 2d-f). Importantly, blood vessels in EAE mice maintained under CMH conditions showed significantly less MECA-32 signal than those maintained under normoxic conditions (2.28 ± 0.23 compared to 9.61 ± 0.87 MECA-32+ vessels/FOV, p < 0.01). Taken together, these findings demonstrate that CNS

blood vessels in CMH-treated mice show less vascular breakdown, thus suppressing leukocyte infiltration and the progression of EAE.

CMH suppresses endothelial expression of VCAM-1 and ICAM-1 during EAE

An important clue suggesting how hypoxic pre-conditioning might be attenuating neuroinflammation was presented by the finding that CMH reduces the adhesion of circulating leukocytes to the endothelium of cerebral blood vessels in mouse models of MS and ischemic stroke [8, 43]. To transmigrate across the blood vessel wall, infiltrating leukocytes use integrin adhesion molecules (predominantly α4β1 and αLβ2 and αMβ2 integrins) to bind to counter-receptors (vascular cell adhesion molecule-1 (VCAM-1) and intercellular adhesion molecule-1 (ICAM-1)) expressed on the luminal side of endothelial cells lining blood vessels [28]. Under normal resting conditions, endothelial expression of VCAM-1 and ICAM-1 are barely detectable, but following endothelial activation, their expression is strongly induced [28]. To examine whether CMH might be inhibiting leukocyte adhesion to blood vessel walls by suppressing endothelial VCAM-1 and ICAM-1 expression, we performed dual-IF with VCAM-1/CD31 and ICAM-1/CD31 on spinal cord tissue obtained from mice that were either disease-free or had EAE, maintained under normoxic or CMH conditions. This revealed that VCAM-1 expression was strongly upregulated on spinal cord blood vessels in EAE mice maintained under normoxic conditions (from 0.03 ± 0.02 fluorescent units/FOV under disease-free conditions to 1.38 ± 0.17 at the peak stage of EAE under normoxic conditions, $p < 0.01$), but these levels were markedly suppressed in CMH-treated mice (0.53 ± 0.13 fluorescent units/FOV vs. 1.38 ± 0.17, $p < 0.01$) (Fig. 3a-b). ICAM-1 is expressed not only by activated endothelial cells but also by inflammatory leukocytes, making interpretation more difficult. However, Fig. 3c clearly shows that while ICAM-1 is absent in the spinal cords of disease-free mice, EAE-normoxic mice show strong upregulation of ICAM-1 both on infiltrating leukocytes and on activated blood vessels. Importantly, by examining areas of the spinal cord lacking leukocyte infiltration (see insets in Fig. 3c), we observed that ICAM-1 was strongly upregulated on spinal cord blood vessels in normoxic-EAE mice (from 0.03 ± 0.01 fluorescent units/FOV under disease-free conditions to 6.62 ± 1.21 at the peak stage of EAE under normoxic conditions, $p < 0.01$), but this expression was markedly suppressed in CMH-treated EAE mice (2.33 ± 0.26 fluorescent units/FOV vs. 6.62 ± 1.21, $p < 0.01$) (Fig. 3c-d). Thus in the EAE model, CMH suppresses endothelial expression of the activation molecules VCAM-1 and ICAM-1.

CMH protects against loss of the endothelial tight junction proteins ZO-1 and occludin during EAE

The vascular integrity of CNS blood vessels is highly dependent on endothelial expression of tight junction proteins such as ZO-1 and occludin, which form tight connections between neighboring endothelial cells [1, 23, 45]. Two reasons suggest this may be relevant to CMH-mediated protection against EAE. First, expression of tight junction proteins at endothelial cell-cell borders is known to be disrupted both in MS and in EAE [2, 14, 25]. Second, we previously demonstrated that CMH triggers strong upregulation of tight junction proteins on CNS blood vessels, both in the brain and spinal cord [3, 20, 30]. Therefore, to examine how CMH treatment influences endothelial expression of tight junction proteins

in the EAE model, we performed dual-IF of CD31/ZO-1 or CD31/occludin on spinal cord sections taken from CMH or normoxic mice at the peak stage of EAE. As expected, under disease-free conditions, ZO-1 and occludin co-localized tightly with the endothelial cell marker CD31 on all blood vessels (Fig. 4). However, during the peak stage of EAE in normoxic mice, vascular expression levels of ZO-1 and occludin were significantly reduced compared to disease-free control levels (Fig. 4). In contrast, blood vessels in CMH-treated EAE mice retained significant expression of ZO-1 and occludin. Quantification revealed that vascular ZO-1 levels were reduced from 2.28 ± 0.12 fluorescent units/FOV under disease-free conditions to 0.19 ± 0.07 at the peak stage of EAE under normoxic conditions ($p < 0.01$) but at the same time-point, ZO-1 levels in CMH-treated EAE mice were significantly higher than normoxic EAE mice (1.14 ± 0.2 fluorescent units/FOV vs. 0.19 ± 0.07, $p < 0.01$). In a similar manner, vascular occludin levels were reduced from 1.81 ± 0.08 fluorescent units/FOV under disease-free conditions to 0.61 ± 0.06 at the peak stage of EAE under normoxic conditions ($p < 0.01$) but at the same time-point, occludin levels in CMH-treated EAE mice were significantly higher than normoxic EAE mice (1.05 ± 0.07 fluorescent units/FOV vs. 0.61 ± 0.06, $p < 0.01$). These data demonstrate that CMH protects against loss of the endothelial tight junction proteins ZO-1 and occludin during EAE pathogenesis.

CMH enhances laminin-111 expression in the parenchymal vascular basement membrane in EAE

The basement membranes of CNS blood vessels comprise several ECM proteins including laminins, type IV collagen, and fibronectin. In the CNS, vascular basement membranes have two layers, an inner layer contributed by endothelial cells, and an outer parenchymal layer which is contributed by astrocytes and leptomeningeal cells [41]. In the normal CNS, the inner and outer membranes are indistinguishable by light microscopy and appear as one membrane, but during EAE progression, CD45+ leukocytes accumulate in the perivascular space between the two membranes and push them apart, making them clearly distinguishable when stained with a pan-laminin antibody (which recognizes all laminin isoforms; Fig. 5a). Dual-IF with the endothelial marker CD31 and a pan-laminin antibody shows the inner CD31-positive endothelial layer co-staining with laminin, but also highlights the presence of an additional outer laminin-positive layer only when leukocyte perivascular cuffing is present (Fig. 5b).

The laminins are a family of closely related heterotrimeric proteins composed of α, β and γ chains, of which there are 5 α, 3 β and 3 γ chains currently reported, that can combine to form up to 12 different isoforms of

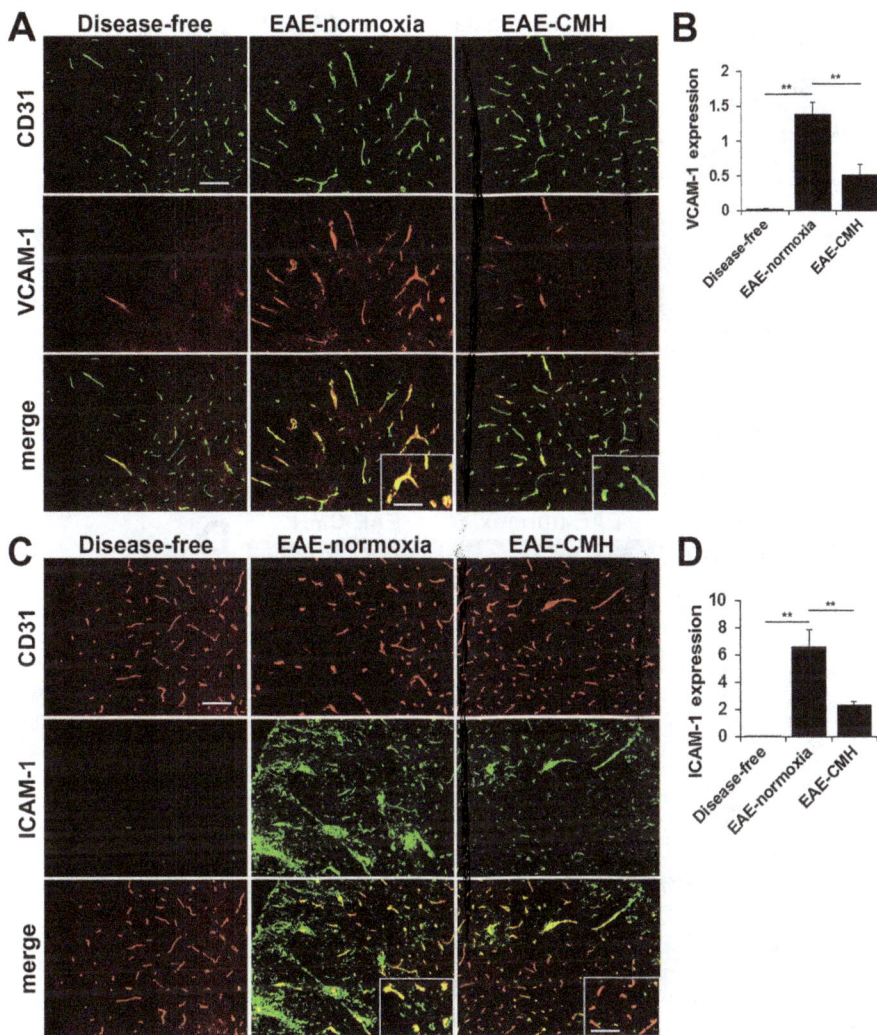

Fig. 3 CMH suppresses endothelial VCAM-1 and ICAM-1 expression during EAE. **a** and **c**. Frozen sections of lumbar spinal cord taken from disease-free, EAE-normoxia or EAE-CMH mice at the peak symptomatic phase of EAE were stained for CD31 (AlexaFluor-488) and VCAM-1 (Cy-3) in panel A or CD31 (Cy-3) and ICAM-1 (AlexaFluor-488) in panel C. Scale bar = 100 μm (inset, scale bar = 50 μm). **b** and **d**. Quantification of VCAM-1 (**b**) and ICAM-1 expression (**d**). Results are expressed as the mean ± SEM (n = 6 mice/group). Note that CMH markedly suppressed vascular expression of VCAM-1 and ICAM-1. ** $p < 0.01$

laminin [12, 13, 41]. An elegant study performed by the Sorokin lab showed that the two different basement membranes within CNS blood vessels contain different laminin isoforms, with endothelial basement membranes containing laminin-411 ($\alpha4\beta1\gamma1$) and 511 ($\alpha5\beta1\gamma1$), previously known as laminins 8 and 10 respectively, while the parenchymal basement membranes contain laminins-111 ($\alpha1\beta1\gamma1$) and 211 ($\alpha2\beta1\gamma1$), previously known as laminins 1 and 2 respectively [41]. As our initial staining indicated that CD45+ leukocytes appeared to be restrained within perivascular cuffs to a greater extent in CMH-treated mice, we performed dual-IF with CD45 and the pan-laminin antibody to examine this in greater detail. This revealed that while leukocytes in normoxic mice appeared to be initially held back within the

perivascular space, over time, leukocytes cross through the parenchymal basement membrane and enter the CNS parenchyma to migrate widely throughout the tissue (Fig. 5c). In contrast, at the same time-point, CMH-treated mice showed much greater leukocyte containment within perivascular cuffs, resulting in far less dispersal into the CNS parenchyma. In addition, while the parenchymal basement membrane in normoxic mice appeared stretched thin and discontinuous in places, in CMH-treated mice it was thick and continuous and showed a much higher level of laminin expression (Fig. 5c). Quantification revealed that while vascular expression of laminin was not changed at the peak stage of EAE under normoxic conditions relative to disease-free controls, levels in EAE-CMH mice at the same

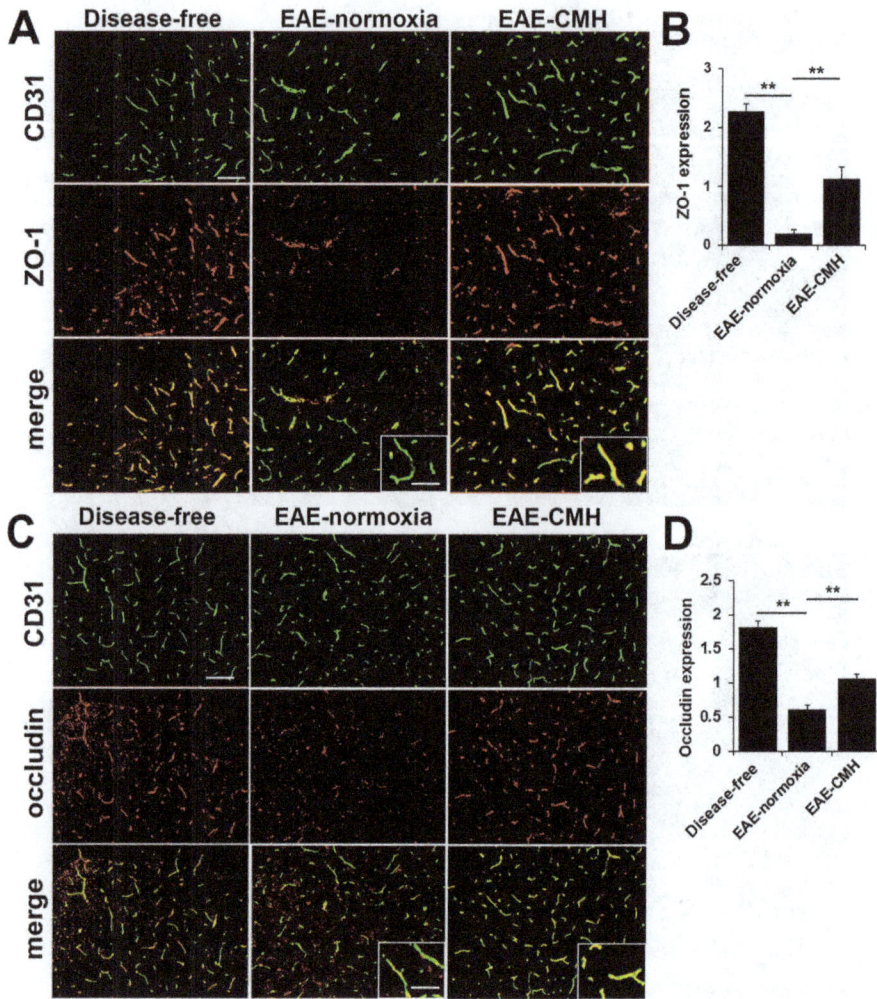

Fig. 4 CMH protects against loss of the endothelial tight junction proteins ZO-1 and occludin during EAE. **a** and **c**. Frozen sections of lumbar spinal cord taken from disease-free, EAE-normoxia or EAE-CMH mice at the peak symptomatic phase of EAE were stained for CD31 (AlexaFluor-488) and ZO-1 (Cy-3) in panel A or CD31 (AlexaFluor-488) and occludin (Cy-3) in panel C. Scale bar = 100 μm (inset, scale bar = 50 μm). **b** and **d**. Quantification of ZO-1 (**b**) and occludin expression (**d**). Results are expressed as the mean ± SEM (n = 6 mice/group). Note that CMH protected against loss of ZO-1 and occludin. ** p < 0.01

time-point were significantly higher compared to disease-free conditions (7.98 ± 0.35 fluorescent units/ FOV vs. 6.28 ± 0.17, p < 0.01) or EAE-normoxic conditions (7.98 ± 0.35 fluorescent units/FOV vs. 6.10 ± 0.19, p < 0.01) (Fig. 5d).

As parenchymal vascular basement membranes contain the specific laminins-111 and 211 [41], we next performed dual-IF with antibodies against the pan-leukocyte marker CD45 and antibodies specific for the laminin α1 chain or α2 chain to determine which specific laminin isoform accounts for the CMH-induced upregulation of laminin detected with the pan-laminin antibody. As shown in Fig. 6, this revealed that CMH induced strong upregulation of the laminin α1 chain but not α2, corresponding to elevated levels of laminin-111 in the parenchymal basement membrane. Quantification revealed that vascular

expression of the laminin α1 chain in EAE-CMH mice was significantly higher than disease-free conditions (2.81 ± 0.16 vs. 1.24 ± 0.05, p < 0.01) and EAE-normoxic conditions (2.81 ± 0.16 vs. 1.77 ± 0.07, p < 0.01) (Fig. 6b). By contrast, vascular expression of the laminin α2 chain was not appreciably different between EAE-normoxic and EAE-CMH conditions. When we examined the expression of collagen IV, another ECM protein abundantly expressed in vascular basement membranes, we found that expression was predominantly localized to the endothelial layer of the vascular basement membrane (Fig. 6d) and furthermore that CMH did not appreciably alter collagen IV expression levels in the vascular basement membrane. Triple-IF (CD31/CD45/laminin-111) of EAE spinal cord revealed that compared to EAE under normoxic conditions, the parenchymal vascular basement membrane in

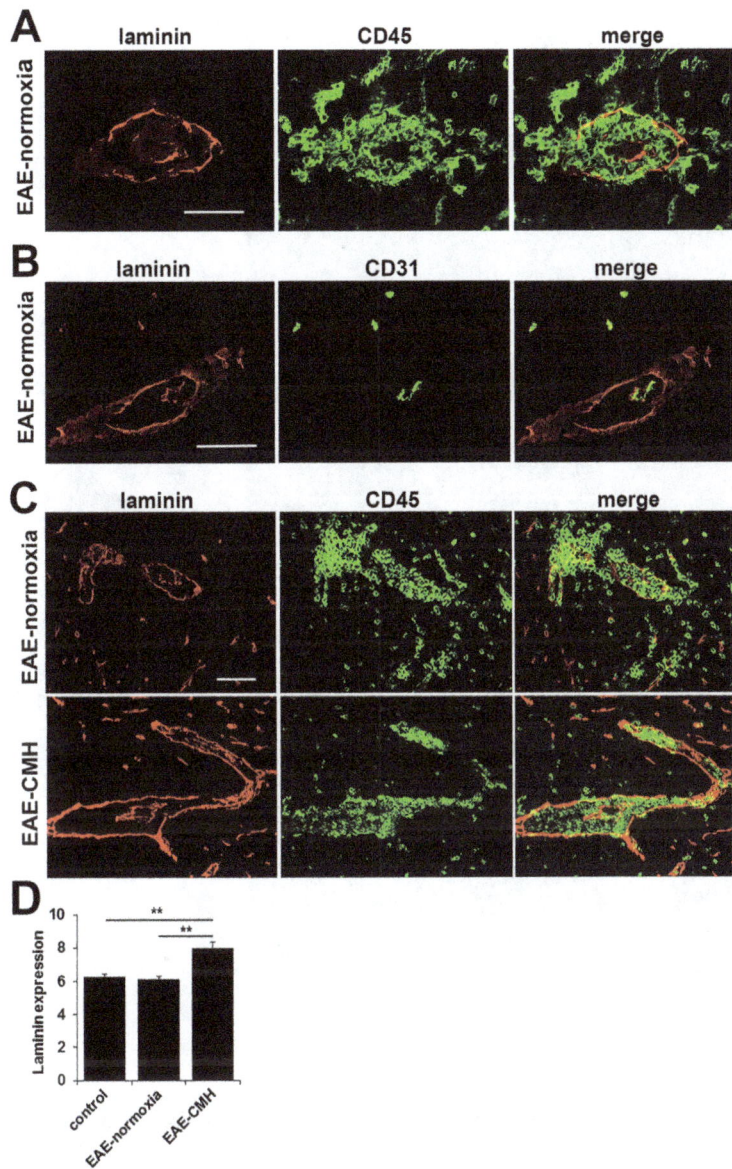

Fig. 5 CMH promotes increased laminin expression in the vascular basement membrane. **a-c.** Frozen sections of lumbar spinal cord taken from EAE-normoxia or EAE-CMH mice at the peak symptomatic phase of EAE were stained for CD45 (AlexaFluor-488) and laminin (Cy-3) in panel A, CD31 (AlexaFluor-488) and laminin (Cy-3) in panel B or CD45 (AlexaFluor-488) and laminin (Cy-3) in panel C. Scale bar = 50 μm. Note that in EAE, infiltrating leukocytes accumulate in the perivascular space between the endothelial and parenchymal layers of the vascular basement membrane, causing them to separate (**a**). In B note that only the inner layer of basement membrane co-localizes with CD31. In C note that while in the normoxic EAE spinal cord, leukocytes break through the basement membrane to migrate freely into the CNS parenchyma, CMH-treated mice showed a thicker stronger expression of laminin in the basement membrane, resulting in greater containment of leukocytes within perivascular cuffs. **d.** Quantification of vascular laminin expression. Results are expressed as the mean ± SEM ($n = 6$ mice/group). Note that CMH enhanced laminin expression within the parenchymal basement membrane. ** $p < 0.01$

CMH-treated mice contains higher levels of laminin-111, which closely correlates with reduced transmigration of CD45+ leukocytes out of the perivascular space and into the CNS parenchyma (Fig. 6e). Taken with the previous finding that of all laminin isoforms, laminin-111 is the most inhibitory substrate for T cell adhesion [41], our observations suggest that CMH-induced upregulation of the inhibitory protein laminin-111 in the parenchymal

basement membrane keeps leukocytes tightly corralled within the perivascular space, thus preventing their transmigration into the CNS parenchyma.

Discussion

The goals of this study were to examine the protective potential of hypoxic pre-conditioning in a relapsing-remitting EAE model of MS and then determine how chronic mild

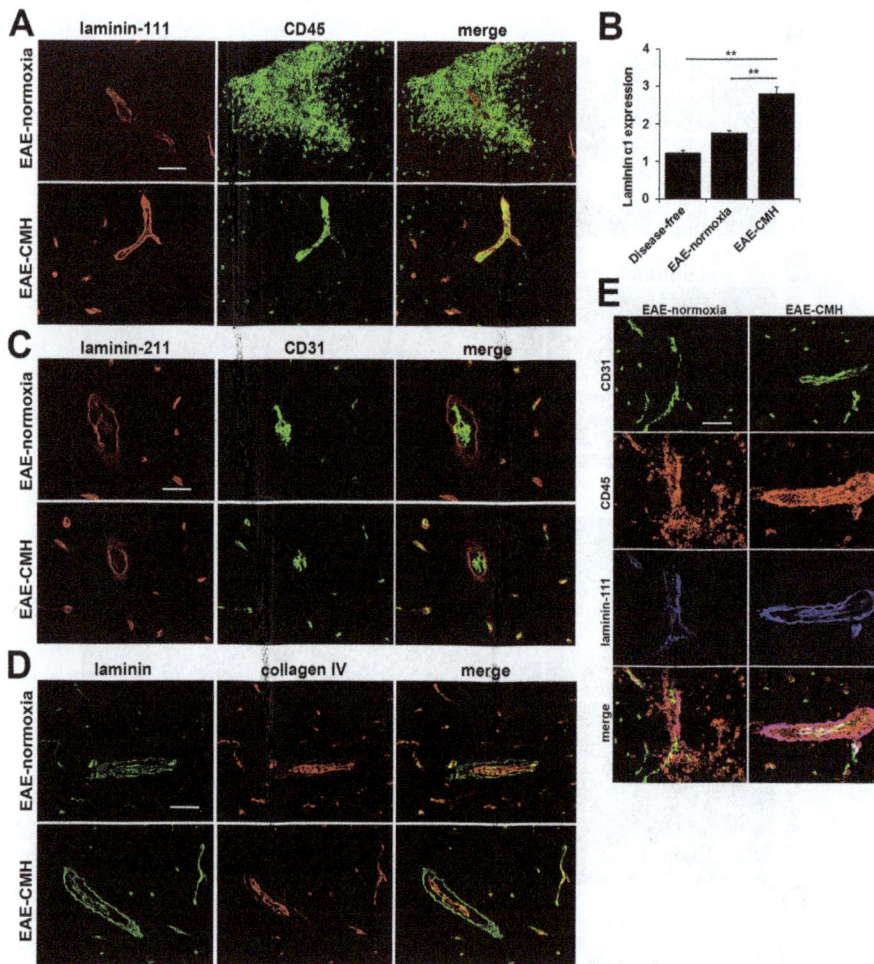

Fig. 6 CMH specifically upregulates the laminin isoform-111 in the parenchymal layer of the vascular basement membrane. Frozen sections of lumbar spinal cord taken from EAE-normoxia or EAE-CMH mice at the peak symptomatic phase of EAE were stained for CD45 (AlexaFluor-488) and the laminin α1 subunit (Cy-3) in panel A, CD31 (AlexaFluor-488) and the laminin α2 subunit (Cy-3) in panel C, or type IV collagen (Cy-3) and laminin (AlexaFluor-488) in panel D. Scale bar = 100 μm. **b**. Quantification of vascular laminin α1 subunit expression. Results are expressed as the mean ± SEM ($n = 6$ mice/group). Note that CMH enhanced laminin α1 expression within the parenchymal basement membrane but had no observable effect on laminin α2 expression. Also note that collagen IV is expressed only within the endothelial layer of the vascular basement membrane and expression is not altered by CMH (**d**). ** $p < 0.01$. **e**. CD31/CD45/laminin α1 triple-IF staining of EAE spinal cord under normoxic or CMH conditions. Note that compared to normoxic conditions, the parenchymal vascular basement membrane in CMH-treated mice contains higher levels of laminin-111 and is more effective at restricting the transmigration of CD45+ leukocytes

hypoxia (CMH) influences vascular integrity and the different cellular and molecular components underlying this integrity. We found that mice exposed to 10% O_2 (CMH) at the same time as EAE induction, were strongly protected against the development of EAE progression, as assessed both at the clinical and histopathological levels. At the mechanistic level, our studies indicate that CMH protection is mediated at least in part, by enhancing several different properties of blood vessels that contribute to vascular integrity, including (i) reduced expression of the endothelial activation molecules VCAM-1 and ICAM-1, (ii) maintained expression of the endothelial tight junction proteins ZO-1 and occludin, and (iii) enhanced expression of the leukocyte inhibitory protein laminin-111 in the parenchymal layer of

the vascular basement membrane. Taken together, these data suggest that hypoxic pre-conditioning protects against EAE by enhancing the integrity of CNS blood vessels at multiple levels.

The impact of CMH on EAE progression

The data presented here extend previous observations that chronic exposure to mild hypoxia delays the progression of EAE [8, 15]. Our study differs from those reports in that we performed our analysis in the relapsing-remitting form of EAE, in which mice reach peak disease before making significant recovery, and then follow a relapsing-remitting course [32, 33], which more closely resembles the most common form of MS in human patients. With the different models in mind, it is important to note that in the relapsing-remitting model used in our studies, CMH did not just delay EAE progression in the short term, it strongly reduced clinical score both at the peak of disease activity and at all time-points examined thereafter for the duration of the experiment (7 weeks), resulting in a marked and significant reduction in long-term clinical score. This neuroprotective effect of hypoxic pre-conditioning is consistent with a growing number of studies in animal models of ischemic stroke, whereby exposure to mild hypoxia dramatically reduces the size of ischemic infarct [10, 34, 43]. Interestingly, recent studies have highlighted the therapeutic potential of intermittent hypoxic training (IHT) in a number of other experimental neuropathologies, including Alzheimer's disease, spinal cord injury, epilepsy and ethanol withdrawal-induced stress, raising the notion of therapeutic potential for IHT [17, 19, 24, 31, 48]. While our studies demonstrate protection if hypoxic treatment is started before EAE disease occurs, to our knowledge, no-one has yet examined the impact of CMH on established EAE. In fact, considering that oxygen therapy has been shown to ameliorate clinical disease in rats with established EAE, this suggests that hypoxia applied at this time-point might actually worsen clinical disease [6]. To answer this important question, in future experiments, we plan to investigate the impact of CMH applied at different time-points leading up to peak disease, as well as at peak disease itself and during the remission phase of disease, to more completely define how the timing of application of hypoxic conditioning protects against disease relapse. Regardless of the outcome of our planned studies, it is important to recognize that our demonstration of a strong protective effect of hypoxic pre-conditioning has clear translational significance because it also underlines the importance of using CMH as a biological tool to identify the molecular mechanisms underlying this protection. Using this approach, we have determined that CMH enhances the integrity of CNS blood vessels at multiple levels, including reduced expression of the endothelial activation molecules VCAM-1 and ICAM-1, maintained expression of the endothelial tight junction proteins ZO-1 and occludin, and increased expression of the leukocyte inhibitory ECM protein laminin-111 in the vascular basement membrane.

Recent work suggested that CMH protects against EAE, at least in part, by exerting an immuno-modulatory effect, such that the spinal cords of CMH-treated mice contained reduced levels of Th17+ T cells but increased levels of regulatory T cells (Tregs), thereby promoting an anti-inflammatory milleu in the spinal cord [15]. Our findings extend this data by demonstrating that CMH likely promotes an anti-inflammatory state within CNS blood vessels via a two-pronged attack, first, by exerting an immuno-suppressive effect in the spinal cord, and second by reinforcing the vascular barrier that keeps the immune cells from entering the CNS. While it is possible that the vasculo-protective influence of CMH could be secondary to the immuno-suppressive effect, this seems highly unlikely for the simple reason that even in the absence of immune cell activation (i.e.; no EAE), CMH induces the same marked changes in vascular barrier properties as we observed in our EAE studies, namely enhanced endothelial expression of tight junction proteins and increased laminin-111 expression in the vascular basement membrane [3, 20, 21, 30]. Conversely, turning the question on its head, is it possible that the creation of an immuno-suppressed state in the spinal cord occurs secondary to changes in vascular integrity or endothelial activation state? Recent studies indicate that CMH does not directly influence immune cell activation in EAE as T cell sensitization to the myelin antigen is not altered but rather the number of Th17+ T cells that infiltrates the spinal cord is reduced [15]. This suggests that the most important determinant of the inflammatory state within the spinal cord is the manner in which blood vessels regulate the transit of the different T cell populations across the BBB. Our finding that CMH suppresses endothelial expression of the key activation molecules VCAM-1 and ICAM-1 strongly suggests that CMH reduces endothelial activation state, which together with enhanced barrier integrity due to increased expression of tight junction proteins and laminin-111 in the basement membrane, acts to reduce the influx of pro-inflammatory Th17+ T cells. Taken together, this implies that the pivotal mechanism underlying CMH protection from EAE resides at the level of enhanced BBB integrity and reduced endothelial activation state.

The influence of CMH on vascular expression of tight junction proteins during EAE

Tight junction proteins are a major determinant of the BBB [1, 23, 38]. As previous studies have shown that expression of some tight junction proteins is lost in MS and EAE lesions [2, 14, 25], but upregulated in response to CMH [3, 20, 30], this suggested that CMH might be conferring protection via influencing tight junction protein expression. Significantly, while our studies revealed that both ZO-1 and occludin are universally downregulated on all spinal cord blood vessels at the peak stage of EAE, mice treated with CMH were protected against loss of these two tight junction proteins. Interestingly, a recent study suggested a direct connection between vascular laminin and tight protein expression by showing that deletion of astrocyte laminin resulted in decreased expression of tight junction proteins at the BBB [47]. This implies that regulation of the three different components of the BBB we have described here may not be working independently of each other, but more likely are coordinated in a synchronous manner to achieve the same goal.

The influence of CMH on laminin expression in vascular basement membranes during EAE

Our data show that CMH stimulates upregulation of laminin-111 in the parenchymal basement membrane, and that this correlates with containment of infiltrating leukocytes within the perivascular space, resulting in less migration into the CNS parenchyma. The Sorokin lab has performed extensive studies to examine the roles of basement membrane laminins in restricting leukocyte infiltration across blood vessels during EAE pathogenesis. In particular, they focused on the laminins-411 and 511 that are expressed specifically within the endothelial layer of the vascular basement membrane, and found that while leukocytes migrate freely across laminin-411, they migrate less well across points in the vessel where laminin-511 is expressed, suggesting that laminin-511 may inhibit leukocyte migration [41]. This idea was later reinforced by the finding that mice deficient in laminin-411, which show laminin-511 expression distributed throughout all vessels, show reduced levels of EAE and leukocyte infiltration [46]. Our findings extend these studies by showing that not only are endothelial laminins important in regulating the passage of infiltrating leukocytes, but that laminins present in the parenchymal basement membrane, particularly laminin-111, may also play an important role. Indeed, as leukocytes appear to cross the endothelial layer relatively easily during EAE, but then get held up by the parenchymal basement membrane in the perivascular space as a result of hypoxic pre-conditioning, our findings suggest that the parenchymal basement membrane may actually be the critical gatekeeper regulating leukocyte entry into the CNS. Consistent with this idea, of all the different laminins, in vitro studies have shown that laminin-111 is the least permissive for leukocyte adhesion [41], suggesting that this specific laminin represents a robust barrier to leukocyte transmigration. Indeed, it is noteworthy that laminins-111 and 211 are only expressed in vascular basement membranes in CNS blood vessels and not detected in other vascular beds, implying that the CNS may have evolved this unique mechanism to enhance vascular integrity as a way of limiting leukocyte infiltration into the CNS.

In conclusion, in this study we have shown that CMH strongly protects against the development of EAE progression, as assessed both at the clinical and histopathological levels. Our mechanistic studies reveal that CMH protection tightly correlates with enhancement of several different properties of blood vessels that contribute to vascular integrity, including reduced endothelial expression of the activation molecules VCAM-1 and ICAM-1, enhanced endothelial expression of the tight junction proteins ZO-1 and occludin, and increased expression of the leukocyte inhibitory protein laminin-111 in the parenchymal layer of the vascular basement membrane. Together, these data suggest that hypoxic pre-conditioning protects against EAE by enhancing the integrity of CNS blood vessels at multiple different levels.

Abbreviations
BBB: Blood-brain barrier; BSCB: Blood-spinal cord barrier; CNS: Central nervous system; Dual-IF: Dual-immunofluorescence; EAE: Experimental autoimmune encephalomyelitis; ECM: Extracellular matrix; FOV: Field of view; MS: Multiple sclerosis; PLP: Proteolipid protein; SEM: Standard error of the mean; ZO-1: Zonula occludens-1

Funding
This work was supported by the NIH R56 grant NS095753. This is manuscript number 29725 from the Scripps Research Institute.

Authors' contributions
SKH and RK performed the EAE studies and analyzed the clinical progression. SKH performed the histological analysis. RM conceived of the study and drafted the manuscript. All authors read and approved the final manuscript.

Competing interests
The authors declare that they have no competing interests.

References
1. Ballabh P, Braun A, Nedergaard M (2004) The blood-brain barrier: an overview. Structure, regulation and clinical implications. Neurobiol Dis 16:1–13.
2. Bennett J, Basivreddy J, Kollar A, Biron KE, Reickmann P, Jefferies WA, McQuaid S (2010) Blood-brain barrier disruption and enhanced vascular permeability in the multiple sclerosis model EAE. J Neuroimmunol 229:180–191.
3. Boroujerdi A, Milner R (2015) Defining the critical hypoxic threshold that promotes vascular remodeling in the brain. Exp Neurol 263:132–140.
4. Brownlee WJ, Hardy TA, Fazekas F, Miller DH (2017) Diagnosis of multiple sclerosis: progress and challenges. Lancet 389:1336–1346.
5. Daneman R, Zhou L, Kebede AA, Barres BA (2010) Pericytes are required for blood-brain barrier integrity during embryogenesis. Nature 468:562–566.
6. Davies AL, Desai RA, Bloomfield PS, McIntosh PR, Chapple KJ, Linington C, Fairless R, Diem R, Kasti M, Murphy MP, Smith KJ (2013) Neurological deficits caused by tissue hypoxia in neuroinflammatory disease. Ann Neurol 74:815–825.
7. del Zoppo GJ, Milner R (2006) Integrin-matrix interactions in the cerebral microvasculature. Arterioscler Thromb Vasc Biol 26:1966–1975.
8. Dore-Duffy P, Wencel M, Katyshev V, Cleary K (2011) Chronic mild hypoxia ameliorates chronic inflammatory activity in myelin oligodendrocyte glycoprotein (MOG) peptide induced experimental autoimmune encephalomyelitis (EAE). Adv Exp Med Biol 701:165–173.
9. Doshi A, Chataway J (2017) Multiple sclerosis, a treatable disease. Clin Med 17:530–536.
10. Dowden J, Corbett D (1999) Ischemic preconditioning in 18- to 20-month-old gerbils: long-term survival with functional outcome measures. Stroke 30:1240–1246.
11. Engelhardt B, Conley FK, Butcher EC (1994) Cell adhesion molecules on vessels during neuroinflammation in the mouse central nervous system. J Neuroimmunol 51:199–208.

12. Engvall E (1993) Laminin variants: why, where and when? Kidney Int 43:2–6.

13. Engvall E, Wewer UM (1996) Domains of laminin. J Cell Biochem 61:493–501.

14. Errede M, Girolamo F, Ferrara G, Stripploi M, Morando S, Boldrin V, Rizzi V, Uccelli A, Perris R, Bendotti C et al (2012) Blood-brain barrier alterations in the cerebral cortex in experimental autoimmune encephalomyelitis. J Neuropathol Exp Neurol 71:840–854.

15. Esen N, Katyshev V, Serkin Z, Katysheva S, Dore-Duffy P (2016) Endogenous adaptation to low oxygen modulates T-cell regulatory pathways in EAE. J Neuroinflammation 13:13.

16. ffrench-Constant C (1994) Pathogenesis of multiple sclerosis. Lancet 343: 271–275.

17. Fuller DD, Johnson SM, Olson EBJ, Mitchell GS (2003) Synaptic pathways to phrenic motorneurons are enhanced by chronic intermittent hypoxia after cervical spinal cord injury. J Neurosci 23:2993–3000.

18. Gay D, Esiri M (1991) Blood-brain barrier damage in acute multiple sclerosis plaques. Brain 114:557–572.

19. Golder FJ, Mitchell GS (2005) Spinal synaptic enhancement with acute intermittent hypoxia imrpoves respiratory function after chronic cervical spinal cord injury. J Neurosci 25:2925–2932.

20. Halder SK, Kant R, Milner R (2018) Chronic mild hypoxia promotes profound vascular remodeling in spinal cord blood vessels, preferentially in white matter, via an α5β1 integrin-mediated mechanism. Angiogenesis 21:251–266.

21. Halder SK, Kant R, Milner R (2018) Chronic mild hypoxia increases expression of laminins 111 and 411 and the laminin receptor α6β1 integrin at the blood-brain barrier. Brain Res 1700:78–85.

22. Hallman R, Mayer DN, Berg EL, Broermann R, Butcher EC (1995) Novel mouse endothelial cell surface marker is suppressed during differentiation of the blood brain barrier. Dev Dyn 202:325–332.

23. Huber JD, Egleton RD, Davis TP (2001) Molecular physiology and pathophysiology of tight junctions in the blood-brain barrier. Trends Neourosci 24:719–725.

24. Ju X, Mallet RT, Metzger DB, Jung ME (2012) Intermittent hypoxia conditioning protects mitochondrial cytochrome c oxidase of rat cerebellum from ethanol withdrawal stress. J Appl Physiol 112:1706–1714.

25. Kirk J, Plumb J, Mirakhur M, McQuaid S (2003) Tight junction abnormality in multiple sclerosis white matter affects all calibres of vessel and is associated with blood-brain barrier leakage and active demyelination. J Pathol 201:319–327.

26. LaManna JC, Chavez JC, Pichiule P (2004) Structural and functional adaptation to hypoxia in the rat brain. J Exp Biol 207:3163–3169.

27. Lassmann H (1998) Multiple sclerosis pathology. In: Compston A (ed) McAlpine's multiple sclerosis, 3rd edn. London: Churchill Livingstone, pp 323–358.

28. Lee SJ, Benveniste EN (1999) Adhesion molecule expression and regulation on cells of the central nervous system. J Neuroimmunol 98:77–88.

29. Li L, Liu F, Welser-Alves JV, McCullough LD, Milner R (2012) Upregulation of fibronectin and the α5β1 and αvβ3 integrins on blood vessels within the cerebral ischemic penumbra. Exp Neurol 233:283–291.

30. Li L, Welser JV, Dore-Duffy P, Del Zoppo GJ, LaManna JC, Milner R (2010) In the hypoxic central nervous system, endothelial cell proliferation is followed by astrocyte activation, proliferation, and increased expression of the α6β4 integrin and dystroglycan. Glia 58:1157–1167.

31. Manukhina EB, Goryacheva AV, Barskov IV, Viktorov IV, Guseva AA, Pshennikova MG, Khomenko IP, Mashina SY, Pokidyshev DA, Malyschev IY (2010) Prevention of neurodegnerative damage to the brain in rats in experimental Alzheimer's disease by adaptation to hypoxia. Neurosci Behav Physiol 40:737–743.

32. McRae BL, Kennedy MK, Tan LJ, Dal Canto MC, Picha KS, Miller SD (1992) Induction of active and adoptive relapsing experimental autoimmune encephalomyelitis (EAE) using an encephalitogenic epitope of proteolipid protein. J Neuroimmunol 38:229–240.

33. McRae BL, Vanderlugt CL, Dal Canto MC, Miller SD (1995) Functional evidence for epitope spreading in the relapsing pathology of experimental autoimmune encephalomyelitis. J Exp Med 182:75–85.

34. Miller BA, Perez RS, Shah AR, Gonzales ER, Park TS, Gidday JM (2001) Cerebral protection by hypoxic preconditioning in a murine model of focal ischemia-reperfusion. Neuroreport 12:1663–1669.

35. Milner R, Campbell IL (2002) Developmental regulation of β1 integrins during angiogenesis in the central nervous system. Mol Cell Neurosci 20: 616–626.

36. Milner R, Hung S, Erokwu B, Dore-Duffy P, LaManna JC, del Zoppo GJ (2008) Increased expression of fibronectin and the α5β1 integrin in angiogenic cerebral blood vessels of mice subject to hypobaric hypoxia. Mol Cell Neurosci 38:43–52.

37. Osada T, Gu Y-H, Kanazawa M, Tsubota Y, Hawkins BT, Spatz M, Milner R, del Zoppo GJ (2011) Interendothelial claudin-5 expression depends on cerebral endothelial cell-matrix adhesion by β1 integrins. J Cereb Blood Flow Metab 31:1972–1985.

38. Pardridge WM (2003) Blood-brain barrier drug targetting: the future of brain drug development. Mol Med 3:90–105.

39. Roscoe WA, Welsh ME, Carter DE, Karlik SJ (2009) VEGF and angiogenesis in acute and chronic MOG (35-55) peptide induced EAE. J Neuroimmunol 209:6–15.

40. Seabrook TJ, Littlewood-Evans A, Brinkmann V, Pollinger B, Schnell C, Hiestand PC (2010) Angiogenesis is present in experimental autoimmune encephalomyelitis and pro-angiogenic factors are increased in multiple sclerosis lesions. J Neuroinflammation 7:95.

41. Sixt M, Engelhardt B, Pausch F, Hallmann R, Wendler O, Sorokin L (2001) Endothelial cell laminin isoforms, laminins 8 and 10, play decisive roles in T cell recruitment across the blood-brain barrier in experimental autoimmune encephalomyelitis. J Cell Biol 153:933–945.

42. Sparks DL, Kuo YM, Roher A, Martin T, Lukas RJ (2000) Alterations of Alzheimer's disease in the cholesterol-fed rabbit, including vascular inflammation. Preliminary observations. Ann N Y Acad Sci 903:335–344.

43. Stowe AM, Altay T, Freie AB, Gidday JM (2011) Repetitive hypoxia extends endogenous neurovascular protection for stroke. Ann Neurol 69:975–985.

44. Wingerchuk DM, Carter JL (2014) Multiple sclerosis: current and emerging disease-modifying therapies and treatment strategies. Mayo Clin Proc 89: 225–240.

45. Wolburg H, Lippoldt A (2002) Tight junctions of the blood-brain barrier; development, composition and regulation. Vasc Pharmacol 38:323–337.

46. Wu C, Ivars F, Anderson P, Hallmann R, Vestweber D, Nilsson P, Robenek H, Tryggvason K, Song J, Korpos E et al (2009) Endothelial basement membrane laminin α5 selectively inhibits T lymphocyte extravasation into the brain. Nat Med 15:519–527.

47. Yao Y, Chen Z-L, Norris EH, Strickland S (2014) Astrocytic laminin regulates pericyte differentiation and maintains blood brain barrier integrity. Nat Commun 5:3413.

48. Zhen J, Wang W, Zhou J, Qu Z, Fang H, Zhao R, Lu Y, Wang H, Zang H (2014) Chronic intermittent hypoxic preconditioning suppresses pilocarpine-induced seizures and associated hippocampal neurodegeneration. Brain Res 1563:122–130.

17

Mutant UBQLN2^{P497H} in motor neurons leads to ALS-like phenotypes and defective autophagy in rats

Tianhong Chen[1†], Bo Huang[2,3†], Xinglong Shi[1], Limo Gao[4] and Cao Huang[1*]

Abstract

Mutations in ubiquilin2 (UBQLN2) have been linked to abnormal protein aggregation in amyotrophic lateral sclerosis (ALS). The mechanisms underlying UBQLN2-related neurodegenerative diseases remain unclear. Using a tetracycline-regulated gene expression system, the ALS-linked UBQLN2^{P497H} mutant was selectively expressed in either the spinal motor neurons or astrocytes in rats. We found that selectively expressing mutant UBQLN2^{P497H} in the spinal motor neurons caused several core features of ALS, including the progressive degeneration of motor neurons, the denervation atrophy of skeletal muscles, and the abnormal protein accumulation. Furthermore, mutant UBQLN2^{P497H} accumulation was associated with an age-dependent decrease in several core autophagy-related proteins. ALS-like phenotypes were not observed when mutant UBQLN2^{P497H} was overexpressed in the astrocytes, however, even though the expression of the mutant UBQLN2^{P497H} protein was higher in these rats. Our results suggest that selectively expressing mutant UBQLN2^{P497H} in motor neurons is sufficient to trigger the development of ALS in rats. Our results further indicate that the compromised autophagy-lysosomal pathway plays a critical role in the pathogenesis of UBQLN2-related neurodegenerative diseases.

Keywords: Amyotrophic lateral sclerosis, ALS, UBQLN2, P62, Motor neuron degeneration, Autophagy, Rats, Protein aggregation

Introduction

Amyotrophic lateral sclerosis (ALS) is a fatal neurodegenerative disease characterized by the degeneration of motor neurons, progressive muscle wasting, and reduced mobility [25, 55]. Genetic studies have linked mutations in ubiquilin2 (UBQLN2) to both ALS and frontotemporal lobar degeneration (FTLD) [8, 10, 48]. How UBQLN2 mutations cause neuronal death remains to be determined.

A prominent feature of Ubqln2-linked diseases is protein aggregation [8], which is well reproduced in transgenic rats and mice overexpressing mutant Ubqln2 [10, 25, 52]. Both TDP-43 pathology and ubiquitination are common features in a variety of neurological diseases, including ALS, FTLD, and Alzheimer's disease (AD) [31, 37]. Ubqln2-positive inclusions exist not just in patients harboring a Ubqln2 mutation but also in chromosome 9 open reading frame 72 (C9ORF72)-linked cases [5, 8]. Ubqln2 is an X-linked gene that consists of an ubiquitin-like domain (UBL) at the N-terminus and an ubiquitin-associated domain (UBA) at the C-terminus [20]. UBQLN2 shuttles between the nucleus and cytoplasm to perform functions related to protein degradation via proteasomes and autophagy [36, 41]. UBQLN2 inclusion is a well reproduced feature in in vivo models of ALS [10, 14, 25, 52]. Another ALS-linked gene, p62/SQSTM1, co-localizes with abnormal UBQLN2 inclusions [8, 10, 14, 52], suggesting a synergistic effect of UBQLN2 and p62 during neurodegenerative disease progression. Thus, accumulating evidence in both patients and rodent models suggests that Ubqln2-positive inclusions play an important role in proteinopathy in neurodegenerative disorders.

Although both mutant SOD1 and mutant TDP-43 reproduce typical ALS features in rodent models, overexpression of mutant SOD1 in spinal motor neurons does

---

* Correspondence: cao.huang@jefferson.edu
†Tianhong Chen and Bo Huang contributed equally to this work.
[1]Department of Pathology, Anatomy & Cell Biology, Thomas Jefferson University, 1020 Locust Street, Philadelphia, PA 19107, USA
Full list of author information is available at the end of the article

not lead to motor neuron death [29, 39], whereas select-ive expression of mutant TDP-43 in motor neurons causes substantial motor neuron death [16] in rats. These findings suggest different contributions of mutant SOD1 and mutant TDP43 to ALS. Previous studies have shown that mutant UBQLN2^{P497H} transgenic rat or mouse models as well as a UBQLN2^{P520T} knock-in mouse model harboring the equivalent human P506T mutation exhibited memory deficits but did not develop any phenotypes of motor neuron disease [10, 13]. It has also been shown that selective expression of either wild-type or ALS–FTLD mutant UBQLN2^{P497S} or UBQLN2^{P506T} in the motor neurons of mice leads to both memory deficits and abnormal motor phenotypes [25]. However, the influence of selectively expressing ALS-linked mutant UBQLN2 in the spinal motor neu-rons remains unknown.

As the most abundant glial cells in the central nervous system (CNS), astrocytes play an important role during central nervous system (CNS) development [32]. Astro-cytes also serve as mediators of inflammatory responses in the CNS [45]. Recent studies suggest, however, that reactive astrocytes cause detrimental effects in neurons in several neurological disorders [2, 19, 26, 27, 35]. The contribution of astrocytes to the pathogenesis of ALS re-mains controversial.

Here, we show that the selective overexpression of mutant UBQLN2^{P497H} in the spinal motor neurons led to age-dependent impairment of motor functions in ChATtTA/UBQLN2^{P497H} rats, including motor neuron degeneration, skeletal muscle atrophy, progressive im-pairment of motor function, TDP-43 pathology, ubiquiti-nation and glial reactions, and abnormal protein accumulation. In contrast, selective overexpression of mutant UBQLN2^{P497H} in astrocytes was not associated with motor impairment. The accumulation of p62 and ubiquitin was increased, however, in the spinal cord as-trocytes of GFAPtTA/UBQLN2^{P497H} rats.

Materials and methods
Generation of transgenic rats
ChATtTA-9 transgenic rats [16] were crossed with TRE-UBQLN^{P497H} transgenic rats [52] to generate ChATtTA/UBQLN^{P497H} bigenic rats expressing mutant UBQLN^{P497H} in motor neurons. All rats were maintained on a Sprague-Dawley background. Similarly, GFAPtTA-line-2 transgenic rats [49] were chosen to generate GFAPtTA/UBQLN^{P497H} bigenic rats that overexpress mu-tant UBQLN^{P497H} in astrocytes. Multiple sets of primers were used for identifying transgenic rats: ChATtTA (5'-TGAGTTCCAGGCAAACCAAG-3' and 5'-TCCAAGGC AGAGTTGATGAC-3'), GFAPtTA (5'-TGAGTGAGA TAATGCCTGGG-3' and 5'-ACCCTCTCTCTAGGAAGG TG-3'), and TRE-UBQLN^{P497H} (5'- AGGATCATAATCA

GCCATACCAC-3' and 5'- CTGCACCTAGTGAAACCA CGA -3'). To suppress transgene expression in bigenic rats, breeding rats were fed DOX (50 μg/ml) in their drinking water during embryonic development. DOX was with-drawn from the drinking water at birth to induce the ex-pression of mutant UBQLN^{P497H} transgene [52].

Animal behavior tests
Mobility was tested via open-field and accelerating rotarod (Med Associates, Inc. VT, USA) tests. The total distance that a rat traveled in the open field within 10 min was recorded. The latency to fall from the accel-erating rotarod (0–40 rpm) was recorded over 5 trials for 2 min per trial.

Cresyl violet staining and cell counting
The transverse sections of the rat spinal cord (L3-L5) were dissected as previously reported [16], and stained with cresyl violet for cell counting. Using ImageJ soft-ware (NIH; Bethesda, MD, USA), both sides of every 10th section (30 μm) were counted for motor neurons larger than 300 μm^2 (i.e., 15–20 sections per rat).

Toluidine blue and silver staining
Rat tissues were fixed in 4% paraformaldehyde. The L3 roots of the spinal cords were dissected for toluidine blue staining. Transverse sections (5 μm) were stained in 1% toluidine blue. Using ImageJ software, the motor axons of the entire ventral roots were counted. A modi-fied Bielschowsky's silver stain kit (American Master-Tech; Lodi, CA, USA) was used according to the manufacturer's instructions to detect degenerating neu-rons. Transverse sections (10 μm) were cut by a Leica CM1950 cryostat for the staining. The degenerating neu-rons were stained as grey to black and normal neurons were stained as yellow to gold.

Immunoblotting and fluorescence staining in the spinal cord
Total proteins of rat tissues were extracted with RIPA buf-fer and separated via SDS-PAGE for immunoblotting as described previously [16]. The resolved proteins were transferred onto nitrocellulose membranes and detected with the following targeted primary antibodies: rabbit anti-ATG7 (Cell Signaling Technology; Danvers, MA, USA), rabbit anti-LAMP2a (Abcam; Cambridge, UK), mouse anti-GFAP (Millipore; Burlington, MA, USA), mouse anti-P62 (Novus Biologicals; Littleton, CO, USA), and mouse anti-GAPDH (Abcam). The spinal cords of rats were fixed in 4% PFA and then cryopreserved in 30% sucrose for sections on the cryostat. The tissues were sec-tioned transversely (20 μm) and stained for the following antibodies: mouse anti-Ubqln2 (Abnova; Taipei, Taiwan), goat anti-ChAT (Millipore), rabbit anti-LC3 (Proteintech;

Rosemont, IL, USA), rabbit anti-GFAP (DAKO; Lexington, MA, USA), rabbit anti-P62 (Proteintech), chicken anti-ubiquitin (Sigma; St. Louis, MO, USA) and rabbit anti-TDP-43 (Proteintech). The tissues were then incubated with the following secondary antibodies: donkey anti-rabbit IgG Alexa Fluor 488 (ThermoFisher; Waltham, MA, USA), donkey anti-mouse IgG Alexa Fluor 594 (ThermoFisher), goat anti-chicken IgY Alexa Fluor 488 (ThermoFisher), and donkey anti-goat IgG Alexa Fluor® 488 (Jackson ImmunoResearch; West Grove, PA, USA). The images were captured by a Nikon digital camera, and single layer photos were scanned with a Nikon A1R microscope confocal system (Imaging Facility of Kimmel Cancer Center at Jefferson).

Histology and fluorescence staining for skeletal muscles

Fresh gastrocnemius muscles were snap-frozen in liquid nitrogen and cut into 10-μm thick sections on a cryostat. As previously described [16], H&E staining, nonspecific esterase, and ATPas staining were used to examine structures in the gastrocnemius muscles. Using the α-napthyl acetate protocol, nonspecific esterase activity was detected. The red-brown color revealed denervated muscle fibers, whereas yellow-to-brown color revealed normal fibers. Myosin ATPase staining pH 4.6, which revealed type 1, 2b, and 2c, and pH 10.45, which revealed type 2a and 2b, were used to detect the four types of skeletal muscle fibers. Specific mouse antibodies against myosin from the Developmental Studies Hybridoma Bank (DSHB; Iowa City, Iowa) were stained for gastrocnemius muscles along with DMD (Dystrophin, a plasma membrane marker). The images were captured by a Nikon digital camera. To reveal the integrity of the neuromuscular junctions (NMJ), 40-μm thick transverse sections of gastrocnemius muscles fixed in 4% PFA were stained for α-bungarotoxin conjugated with Alexa Fluor 594 (ThermoFisher), mouse monoclonal antibodies to neurofilament (ThermoFisher), and synaptophysin (ThermoFisher). These sections were then incubated with the secondary antibody donkey anti-mouse IgG Alexa Fluor 488 (ThermoFisher). The projected images of the NMJs were captured with a Nikon A1R microscope confocal system.

Statistics

The numbers of motor neurons in the spinal cord or motor axons in the L3 ventral roots of the spinal cords were compared among rats using paired t tests. $P < 0.05$ was considered statistically significant.

Results

Expressing the ALS-linked UBQLN2^{P497H} mutation in motor neurons of rats

Tetracycline-controlled transcriptional activation is a commonly used method for inducible gene expression

[54]. A tetracycline-regulated expression system has proven to be a highly efficient way to regulate transgene expression in our rat models [15, 16]. As we have previously reported, expression of the ALS-linked UBQLN2 mutation (P497H substitution) in the forebrain causes progressive neuron death and learning deficits in rats [52]. We have also shown that the mouse ChAT promoter region drives the selective expression of the human TDP-43 transgene in the spinal motor neurons of rats [16], and the human GFAP promoter also works well to restrict transgene expression to the astrocytes in rats [49]. To study the effect of mutant UBQLN2^{P497H} on motor neurons, we crossed TRE-UBQLN2^{P497H} rats with the ChATtTA-9 line to produce ChATtTA/UBQLN2^{P497H} double transgenic rats that selectively express mutant UBQLN2^{P497H} in the spinal motor neurons (Fig. 1). This finding is consistent with our previous study, in which more than 70% of spinal motor neurons expressed the LacZ transgene or human TDP-43 in the ChATtTA-9 line [16].

Fifty micrograms (μg) of doxycycline (DOX) was added to the drinking water to prevent transgene expression during the prenatal stages (Fig. 1a). To induce the expression of the transgene UBQLN2^{P497H}, the transgenic rats were deprived of DOX after birth. UBQLN2 is an X-linked gene [8]; therefore, we conducted Western blots independently on male and female rats, which revealed that only ChATtTA/UBQLN2^{P497H} double transgenic rats exhibited human UBQLN2 expression in the spinal cord at 30 days old. In addition, both female and male rats had similar expression levels of human UBQLN2 compared to endogenous UBQLN2, and there also was no differentiated expression of endogenous UBQLN2 between male and female rats (Fig 1b, c).

To verify whether endogenous UBQLN2 has similar expression in both male and female adult rats, different tissues were examined in non-transgenic rats at 90 days old via immunoblotting Additional file 1: Figure S1. There was no statistical difference in the expression levels of endogenous UBQLN2 between male and female adult rats at 90 days old Additional file 1: Figure S1. As described previously in ChATtTA/TDP-43 rats [16], immunofluorescence staining revealed that more than 70% of spinal motor neurons in ChATtTA/UBQLN2^{P497H} rats expressed human UBQLN2 at 12 months old compared to only 20% at 1 month old (Fig. 1d), but no accumulation of UBQLN2 in ChATtTA rats (Fig. 1e). In addition, compared to ChATtTA single transgenic rats, UBQLN2 accumulated in both the nuclei and neurites in ChATtTA/UBQLN2^{P497H} bigenic rats at 30 days old (Fig. 1f-i). In contrast, no accumulation in choline acetyltransferase (ChAT, a marker of motor neurons) was observed (Fig. 1f-g). Thereafter, ChAT was accumulated in both the nuclei and neurites of most spinal motor

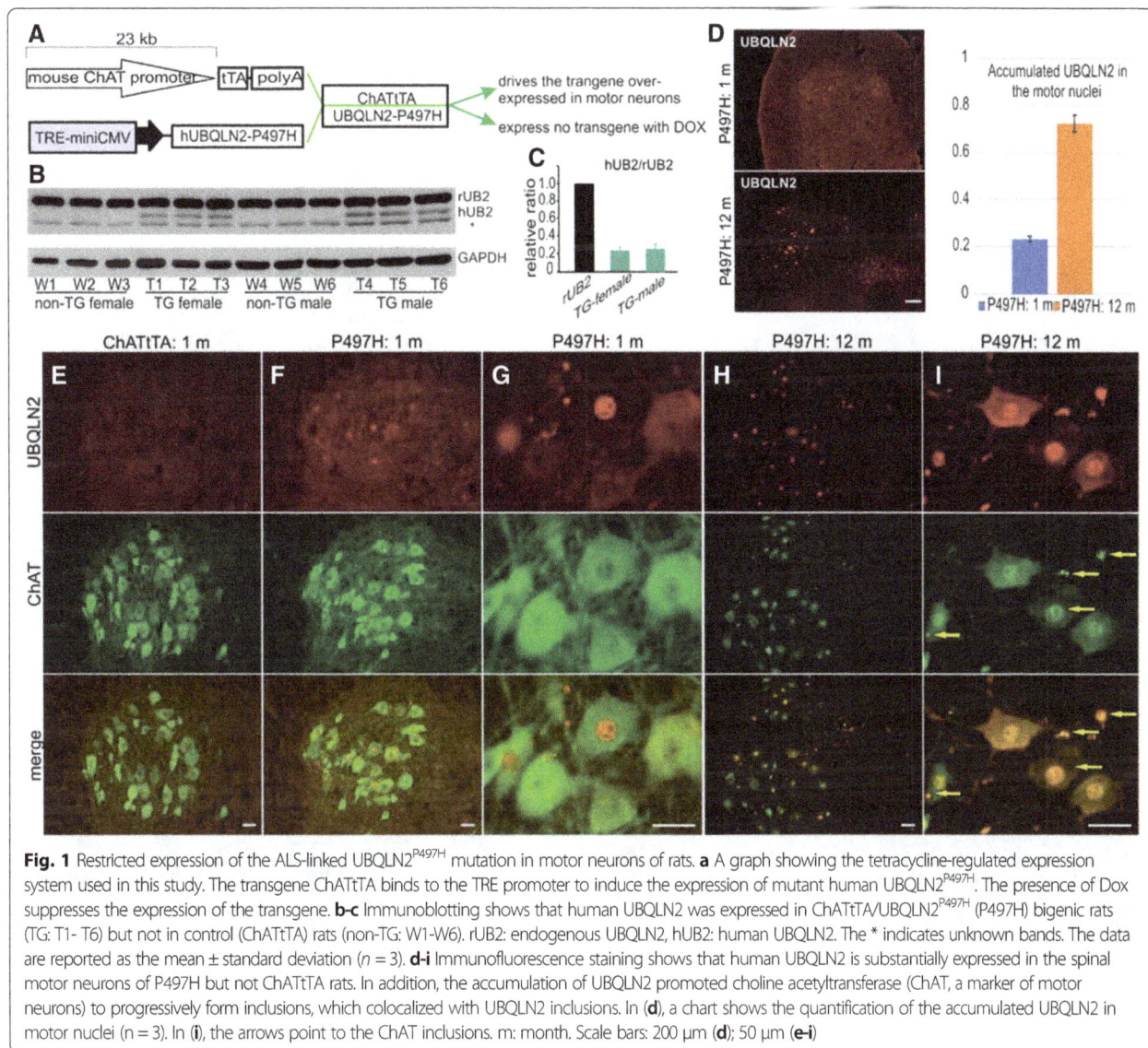

Fig. 1 Restricted expression of the ALS-linked UBQLN2^{P497H} mutation in motor neurons of rats. **a** A graph showing the tetracycline-regulated expression system used in this study. The transgene ChATtTA binds to the TRE promoter to induce the expression of mutant human UBQLN2^{P497H}. The presence of Dox suppresses the expression of the transgene. **b-c** Immunoblotting shows that human UBQLN2 was expressed in ChATtTA/UBQLN2^{P497H} (P497H) bigenic rats (TG: T1- T6) but not in control (ChATtTA) rats (non-TG: W1-W6). rUB2: endogenous UBQLN2, hUB2: human UBQLN2. The * indicates unknown bands. The data are reported as the mean ± standard deviation ($n = 3$). **d-i** Immunofluorescence staining shows that human UBQLN2 is substantially expressed in the spinal motor neurons of P497H but not ChATtTA rats. In addition, the accumulation of UBQLN2 promoted choline acetyltransferase (ChAT, a marker of motor neurons) to progressively form inclusions, which colocalized with UBQLN2 inclusions. In (**d**), a chart shows the quantification of the accumulated UBQLN2 in motor nuclei (n = 3). In (**i**), the arrows point to the ChAT inclusions. m: month. Scale bars: 200 μm (**d**); 50 μm (**e-i**)

neurons at 12 months old, and colocalized with UBQLN2 inclusions (Fig. 1h-i). These results suggest that selectively expressing mutant UBQLN2^{P497H} in motor neurons leads to a predominance accumulation of UBQLN2 inclusions, resulting in abnormal ChAT accumulation.

Mutant UBQLN2^{P497H} in motor neurons results in ALS-like phenotypes in rats

DOX was withdrawn at birth to induce mutant UBQLN2^{P497H} protein expression in rats. Substantial expression of mutant UBQLN2 in the spinal cord of ChATtTA/UBQLN2^{P497H} rats was observed via immunoblotting (Fig. 1). To investigate the effect of mutant UBQLN2 on motor neurons in rats, the L3-L5 regions of the spinal cord were stained with 0.5% cresyl violet (Fig. 2a-d). Neurons larger than 300 μm^2 were

counted with ImageJ software. There was a decrease in large neurons compared to ChATtTA single transgenic rats (Fig. 2e), indicating a loss of motor neurons in ChATtTA/UBQLN2^{P497H} rats. Consistent with the loss of motor neurons, there also was a substantial degeneration of motor neurons as determined via Bielschowsky's silver staining (Fig. 2f-i). The motor axons at the L3 ventral roots were stained with 1% toluidine solution and quantified, which further revealed a dramatic loss of large axons larger than 80 μm^2 in ChATtTA/UBQLN2^{P497H} rats at 12 months old (Fig. 2j-l).

Muscle weakness and decreased mobility are two key features of ALS [4, 28, 55]. As described in a TDP-43 rat model of ALS [16, 49], both muscular atrophy and loss of mobility occur as the disease progresses. Body weight was monitored and behavioral testing was conducted to investigate the role of mutant UBQLN2 in rats. As

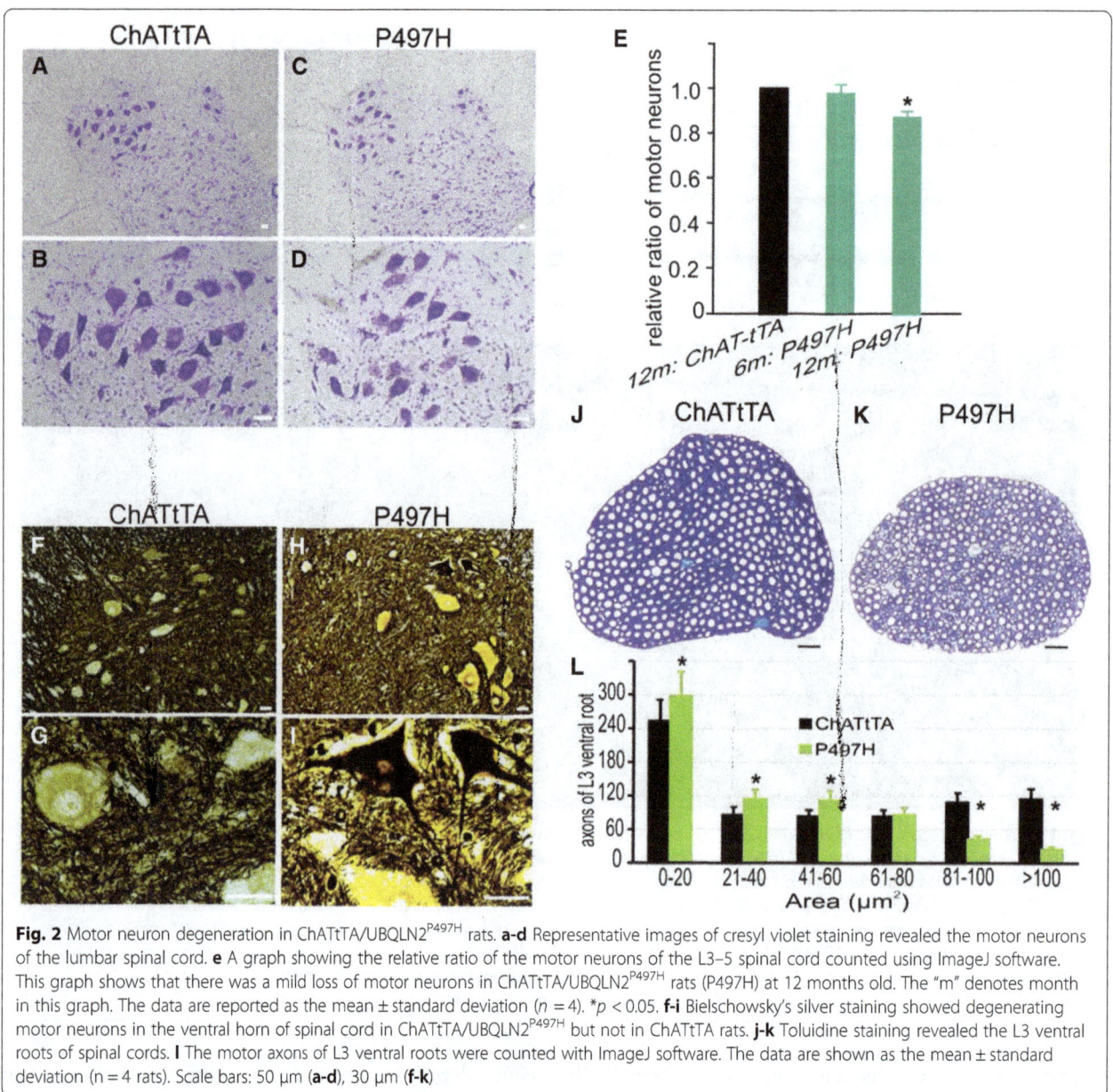

Fig. 2 Motor neuron degeneration in ChATtTA/UBQLN2^{P497H} rats. **a-d** Representative images of cresyl violet staining revealed the motor neurons of the lumbar spinal cord. **e** A graph showing the relative ratio of the motor neurons of the L3–5 spinal cord counted using ImageJ software. This graph shows that there was a mild loss of motor neurons in ChATtTA/UBQLN2^{P497H} rats (P497H) at 12 months old. The "m" denotes month in this graph. The data are reported as the mean ± standard deviation ($n = 4$). *$p < 0.05$. **f-i** Bielschowsky's silver staining showed degenerating motor neurons in the ventral horn of spinal cord in ChATtTA/UBQLN2^{P497H} but not in ChATtTA rats. **j-k** Toluidine staining revealed the L3 ventral roots of spinal cords. **l** The motor axons of L3 ventral roots were counted with ImageJ software. The data are shown as the mean ± standard deviation (n = 4 rats). Scale bars: 50 μm (**a-d**), 30 μm (**f-k**)

shown in Fig. 3, rats with mutant UBQLN2^{P497H} exhibited atrophic hind limbs (Fig. 3a) compared with ChATtTA rats (Fig. 3b), decreased body weight (Fig. 3d), reduced distance traveled in an open-field test (Fig. 3e), and reduced latency to fall from an accelerating rotarod device (Fig. 3f) compared to ChATtTA single transgenic rats. Severe muscle wasting (about 50%) in the gastrocnemius muscles was observed in mutant UBQLN2^{P497H} rats at 12 months old (Fig. 3c), whereas no significant alterations in either the tibialis or gastrocnemius muscles were observed at 1 month old (Additional file 1: Figure S2A-B). In addition, only mild weight loss (about 20%) was observed at 12 months old. Taken together, these findings indicate that overexpressing mutant UBQLN2^{P497H} in

motor neurons cause the degeneration of both motor neurons and motor axons, progressive deficits in performance on both open-field and rotarod tests, and reductions in both body weight and gastrocnemius muscle weight.

We next examined whether mutant UBQLN2 affects muscle architecture via histology and immunostaining of the gastrocnemius muscles. H&E staining and histochemistry for nonspecific esterase revealed groups of muscle atrophy in the gastrocnemius muscles of ChATtTA/UBQLN2^{P497H} rats. No muscle atrophy was observed in ChATtTA single transgenic rats (Fig. 4a-h). H&E staining revealed that a substantial proportion of the nuclei were located internally in mutant UBQLN2^{P497H} rats compared to ChATtTA single transgenic rats. Both pH 4.6 and

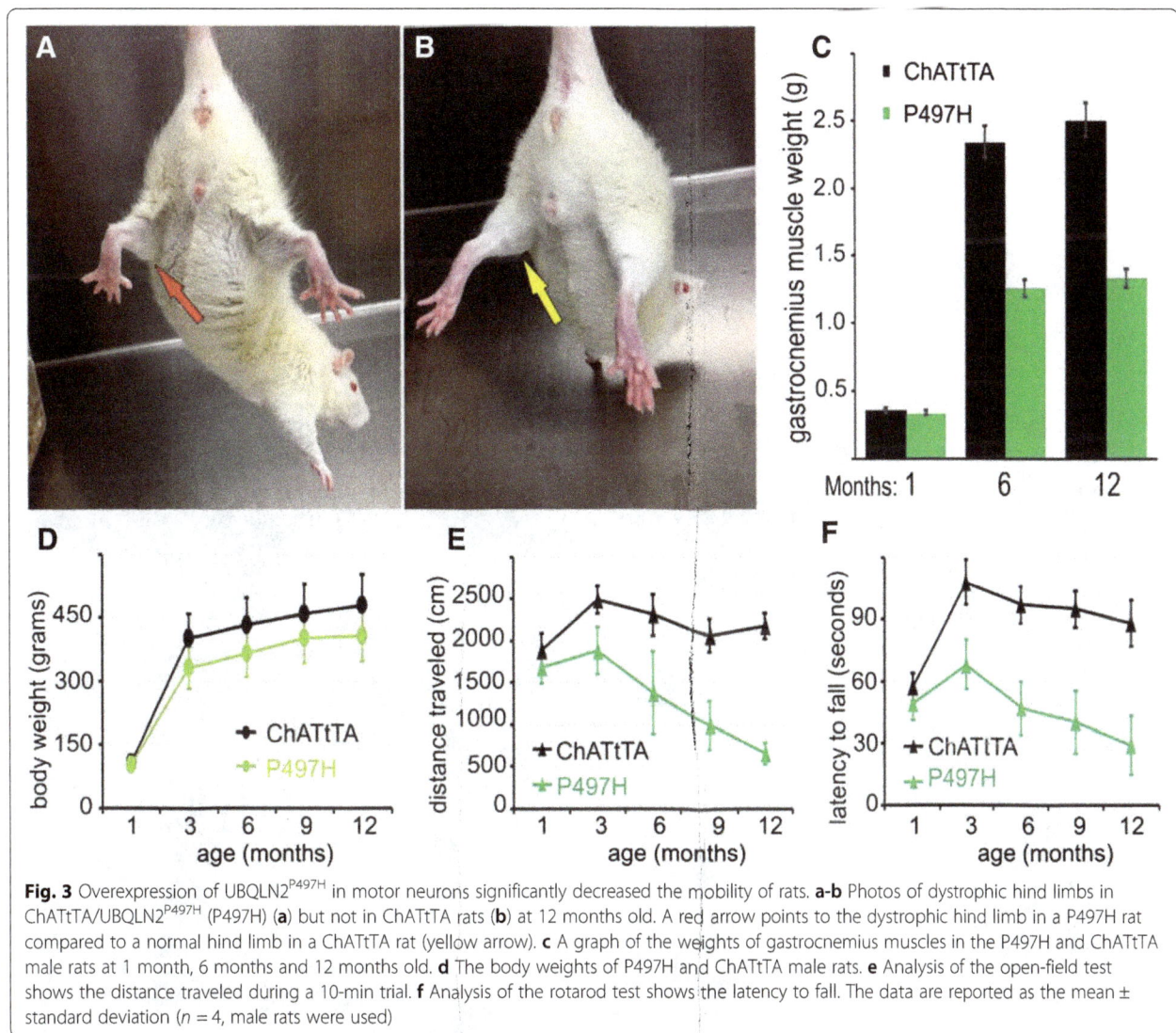

Fig. 3 Overexpression of UBQLN2^{P497H} in motor neurons significantly decreased the mobility of rats. **a-b** Photos of dystrophic hind limbs in ChATtTA/UBQLN2^{P497H} (P497H) (**a**) but not in ChATtTA rats (**b**) at 12 months old. A red arrow points to the dystrophic hind limb in a P497H rat compared to a normal hind limb in a ChATtTA rat (yellow arrow). **c** A graph of the weights of gastrocnemius muscles in the P497H and ChATtTA male rats at 1 month, 6 months and 12 months old. **d** The body weights of P497H and ChATtTA male rats. **e** Analysis of the open-field test shows the distance traveled during a 10-min trial. **f** Analysis of the rotarod test shows the latency to fall. The data are reported as the mean ± standard deviation (*n* = 4, male rats were used)

pH 10.4 ATPase staining also showed groups of atrophic muscle fibers, including type 1 and type 2 muscle fibers (Additional file 1: Figure S3, A and B). Immunofluorescence revealed that dystrophic myofibers were accumulated in the gastrocnemius muscles (Additional file 1: Figure S3, C-F), which further suggests that abnormal protein inclusion is a prominent feature of UBQLN2-related diseases [8, 10, 25].

Impairment of neuromuscular junctions is one of the earliest features to emerge in rodent models of ALS, and occurs at the presynaptic stage of the disease [33]. Longitudinal sections of gastrocnemius muscles were labeled with α-bungarotoxin (to label the motor end-plate) together with neurofilament and synaptophysin (to label the neuromuscular synapses). Confocal images showed a significant amount of denervated neuromuscular junctions (NMJ) in ChATtTA/UBQLN2^{P497H} rats as early as 3 months old but not in ChATtTA single transgenic rats

(Fig. 4i-l), and a substantially increased number of the denervated NMJs with age (Additional file 1: Figure S2C), indicating that the neuromuscular synapses are more vulnerable than the motor neurons in rats that selectively express mutant UBQLN2^{P497H} in the spinal motor neurons.

Collectively, our results suggest that overexpression of mutant UBQLN2^{P497H} in the spinal motor neurons leads to motor neuron degeneration, impaired mobility, denervation atrophy of the skeletal muscles, and accumulation of myofibers in rats.

Age-dependent reduction of autophagy-related proteins in UBQLN2^{P497H} rats

UBQLN2 plays a role in both the ubiquitin-proteasome and autophagy-lysosome systems [12, 24, 41]. To detect whether mutant UBQLN2^{P497H} affected the autophagy pathway, we examined two autophagy substrates, p62 and

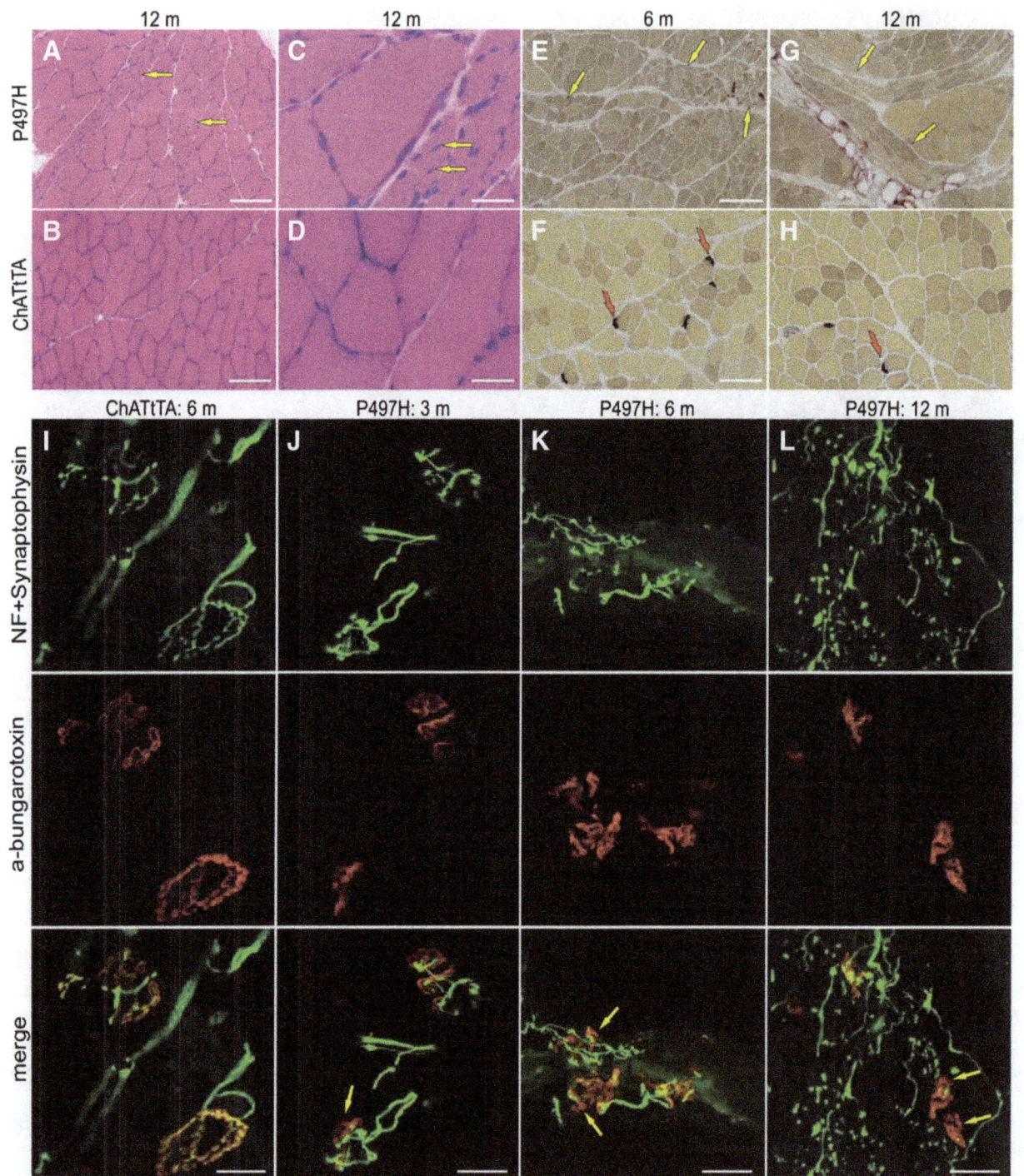

Fig. 4 Denervation atrophy of skeletal muscles in ChATtTA/UBQLN2^P497H rats. **a-d** H&E staining shows groups of atrophic muscle fibers (**a,** arrows) and ectopic nuclei (**c,** arrows) in the gastrocnemius muscles of ChATtTA/UBQLN2^P497H (P497H) but not in ChATtTA single transgenic (ChATtTA) rats at 12 months old. **e-h** nonspecific esterase staining shows the grouped muscle atrophy (**e, g,** arrows) in the gastrocnemius muscles of P497H rats, and which are more severe atrophy in 12-month old rats than 6 months, but not in ChATtTA rats. The red arrows point to the neuromuscular junctions (NMJ). **i-l** The projection of confocal images reveals the innervation of NMJs in gastrocnemius muscles. The arrows (**j-l:** P497H) show that the motor end-plates are poorly innervated in P497H rats compared to ChATtTA rats (**I**), and the neurofilaments progressively form inclusions accompanied with the denervation of NMJ in P497H rats from 3 months to 12 months old. Scale bars: 100 μm (**a-b, e-h**), 30 μm (**c, d**), 20 μm (**i-l**)

LC3, in the spinal cord of rats. Fluorescence staining revealed that the signals of diffused p62 and LC3 in the cytoplasm were weaker in the ventral horns in ChATtTA/UBQLN2^{P497H} rats compared to ChATtTA single transgenic rats (Fig. 5a, b). Furthermore, most cytoplasmic p62 was depleted at 12 months old (Fig. 5a). Concomitantly,

p62 predominantly accumulated in the nucleus in ChATtTA/UBQLN2^{P497H} rats, which also colocalized with UBQLN2 inclusions (Fig. 5a) or ChAT inclusions (Additional file 1: Figure S4). We further confirmed these findings in the spinal cord lysates via immunoblotting (Fig. 5c, d). Interestingly, age-related reductions in LC3-I, LC3-II, and the ratio

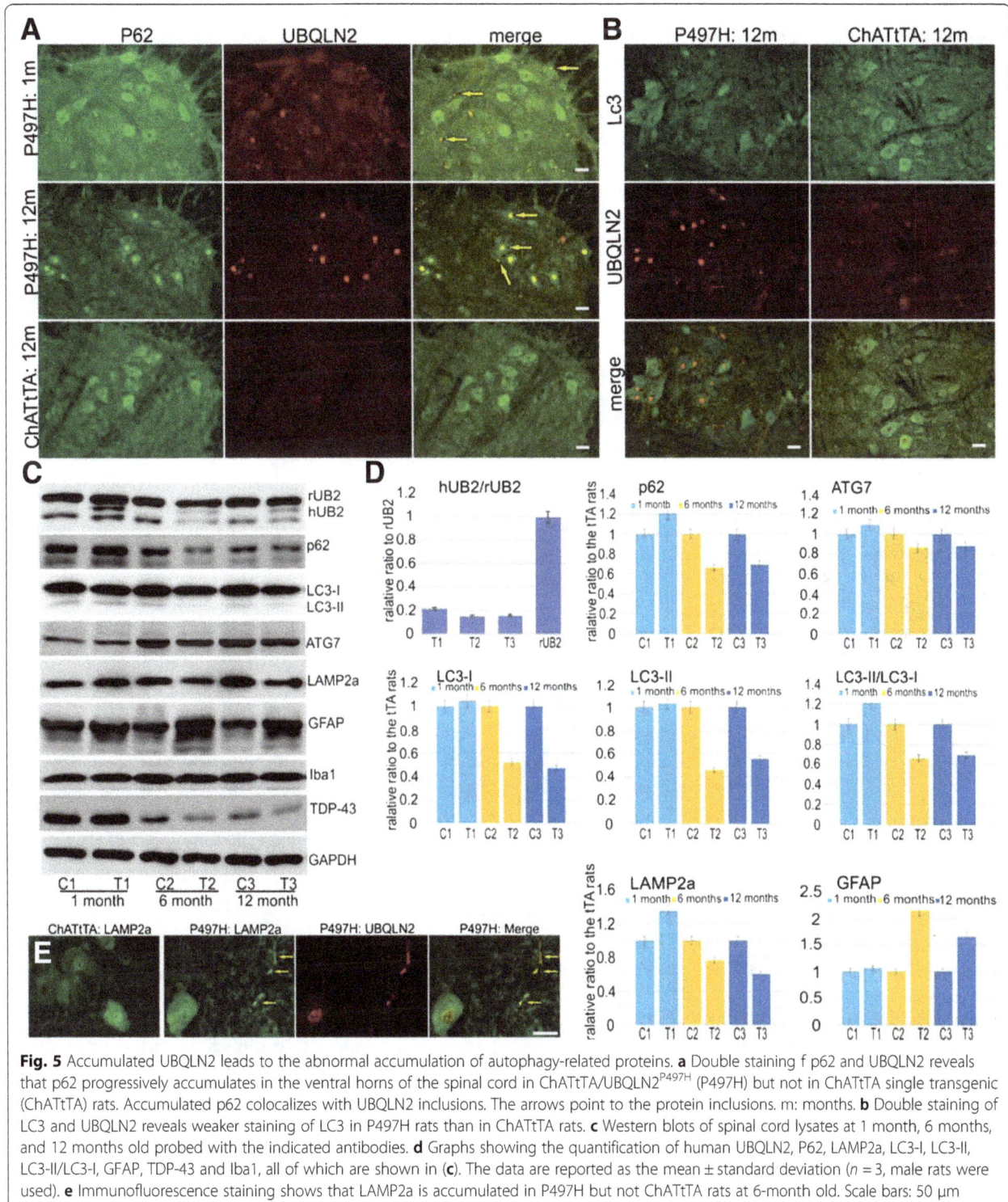

Fig. 5 Accumulated UBQLN2 leads to the abnormal accumulation of autophagy-related proteins. a Double staining f p62 and UBQLN2 reveals that p62 progressively accumulates in the ventral horns of the spinal cord in ChATtTA/UBQLN2^{P497H} (P497H) but not in ChATtTA single transgenic (ChATtTA) rats. Accumulated p62 colocalizes with UBQLN2 inclusions. The arrows point to the protein inclusions. m: months. b Double staining of LC3 and UBQLN2 reveals weaker staining of LC3 in P497H rats than in ChATtTA rats. c Western blots of spinal cord lysates at 1 month, 6 months, and 12 months old probed with the indicated antibodies. d Graphs showing the quantification of human UBQLN2, P62, LAMP2a, LC3-I, LC3-II, LC3-II/LC3-I, GFAP, TDP-43 and Iba1, all of which are shown in (c). The data are reported as the mean ± standard deviation ($n = 3$, male rats were used). e Immunofluorescence staining shows that LAMP2a is accumulated in P497H but not ChATtTA rats at 6-month old. Scale bars: 50 μm

of LC3-II to LC3-I as well as in p62 were detected. Suppression of LC3-II and Beclin1 expression reflects impaired autophagy, and LC3-II levels are correlated with the extent of autophagosome formation [18]. In addition, in patients with AD, the reduction of functional p62 causes autophagy failure, which accelerates the development of AD [44, 51]. Our results are consistent with these findings and indicate that mutant UBQLN2 impairs autophagy in rats.

We also found reduced expression of another autophagy protein, ATG7, and a lysosomal protein, LAMP2a, which acts as a receptor in the lysosomal membrane for substrate proteins of chaperone-mediated autophagy [7]. LAMP2a was accumulated in the spinal cord sections of ChATtTA/UBQLN2^{P497H} rats and colocalized with UBQLN2 inclusions (Fig. 5e). Taken together, our findings suggest that mutant UBQLN2^{P497H} compromises the autophagy-lysosomal pathway in rats.

TDP-43 pathology and ubiquitination in ChATtTA/UBQLN2^{P497H} rats

Previous reports have shown that UBQLN2 inclusions co-exist with TDP-43 inclusions in patients with ALS [8, 41]. UBQLN2 also binds to the C-terminal region of TDP-43 [6]. Furthermore, pathologic TDP-43 is also hyper-phosphorylated [37]. We stained the coronal sections of spinal cord with phosphorylated TDP-43 antibody (S403-TDP-43), and found that phosphorylated TDP-43 was accumulated in ChATtTA/UBQLN2^{P497H} rats but did not colocalize with UBQLN2-positive inclusions (Fig. 6a). We did not detect any obvious reduction of nuclear TDP-43 by fluorescence staining (data not shown), but the total TDP-43 was decreased with age in ChATtTA/UBQLN2^{P497H} rats by immunoblot (Fig. 5c).

UBQLN2 binds to ubiquitin via its C-terminal ubiquitin associated domain [9, 21]. We therefore examined whether UBQLN2 inclusions promoted the accumulation of ubiquitin in ChATtTA/UBQLN2^{P497H} rats. Double immunofluorescence staining revealed that only minimal ubiquitin accumulation in the spinal cord of ChATtTA/UBQLN2^{P497H} rats occurred. In contrast, no accumulation was observed in ChATtTA rats (Fig. 6b). Accumulated ubiquitin colocalized with UBQLN2 inclusions, as shown by confocal single-scan images (Fig. 6b). Substantially increased GFAP expression was observed in the spinal cord lysates of ChATtTA/UBQLN2^{P497H} rats compared to ChATtTA rats (Fig. 5c, d), but there were no obvious alterations in microglia via immunoblotting with IBa1. Thus, our findings suggest that both the phosphorylation of TDP-43 and the ubiquitin inclusions that are observed in ALS patients could be replicated in our rat model.

Mutant UBQLN2^{P497H} in astrocytes does not cause motor deficits in rats

To test whether mutant UBQLN2 expressed in astrocytes induces motor neuron death, we crossed TRE-UBQLN2^{P497H} rats with the GFAPtTA$^{\#}$2 line (Fig. 7a). As previously reported [49], the GFAPtTA$^{\#}$2 line is driven by a 21-kb human GFAP promoter, which induces restricted transgene expression in the astrocytes of spinal cord and brain. As in the ChATtTA/UBQLN2^{P497H} experiments, GFAPtTA/UBQLN2^{P497H} rats were deprived of DOX at birth. One month after DOX deprivation, immunoblotting revealed a substantial expression of human UBQLN2 in the spinal cord, which was similar in level to the expression of endogenous UBQLN2 (Fig. 7b, c). Compared to ChATtTA/UBQLN2^{P497H} rats, in which expression of human UBQLN2 accounted for about 20% of endogenous UBQLN2 expression, GFAPtTA/UBQLN2^{P497H} rats expressed higher amounts of transgene in the spinal cord. Immunofluorescence staining revealed accumulated UBQLN2 in the spinal cord astrocytes of GFAPtTA/UBQLN2^{P497H} but not in GFAPtTA rats at 6 months old (Fig. 7d-e).

To examine their mobility, GFAPtTA/UBQLN2^{P497H} rats were subjected to monthly open-field and rotarod tests. No significant behavioral differences between GFAPtTA/UBQLN2^{P497H} rats and GFAPtTA rats were observed. In contrast to the rats that expressed mutant UBQLN2^{P497H} in motor neurons, no reduction in mobility, no motor neuron loss, no muscular atrophy, and no obvious denervation of neuromuscular junctions were observed in GFAPtTA/UBQLN2^{P497H} rats at 6 months old (Fig. 8). In addition to UBQLN2, however, both p62 and ubiquitin also were accumulated in the spinal cord astrocytes of GFAPtTA/UBQLN2^{P497H} but not GFAPtTA rats (Additional file 1: Figure S5). And we did not detect any pathological alterations in phosphorylated TDP-43, LC3, Lamp2a, and ATG7 (data not shown). These findings suggest that mutant UBQLN2 expression in astrocytes does not lead to motor phenotypes in 6-month old rats.

Discussion

Mutations in UBQLN2 have been linked to ALS-FLTD, and the abnormal accumulation of UBQLN2 inclusions is a remarkable feature of pathological alterations linked to the UBQLN2 mutation [8, 46]. Several groups have recapitulated this specific pathological change in rodent models [10, 13, 25, 52]. No studies to date, however, have shown the effect of expressing mutant UBQLN2 either in the motor neurons or in the astrocytes to test whether mutant UBQLN2 expression leads to motor neuron degeneration in a cell-autonomous manner. To test this hypothesis, therefore, we created novel transgenic models

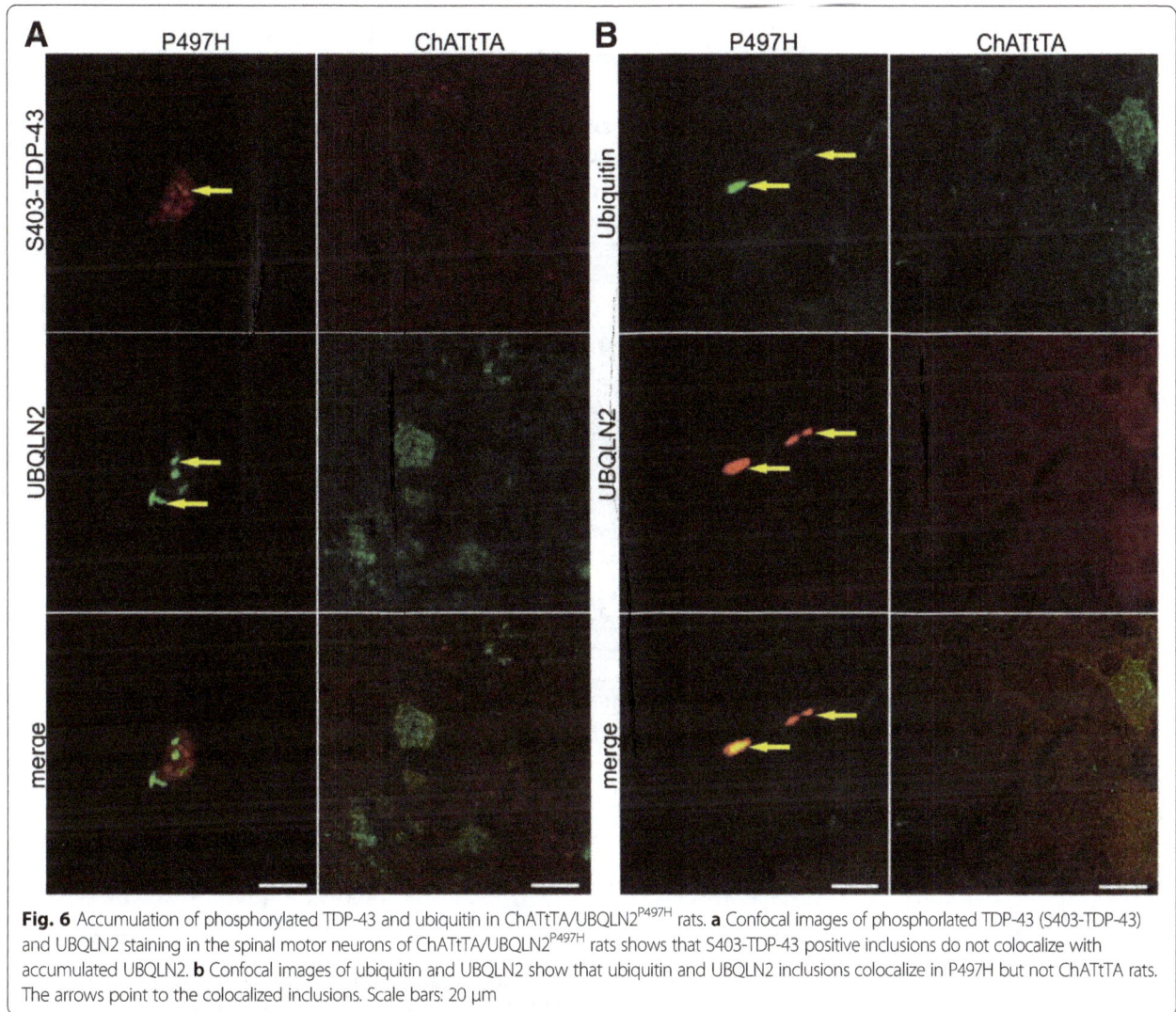

Fig. 6 Accumulation of phosphorylated TDP-43 and ubiquitin in ChATtTA/UBQLN2^{P497H} rats. **a** Confocal images of phosphorlated TDP-43 (S403-TDP-43) and UBQLN2 staining in the spinal motor neurons of ChATtTA/UBQLN2^{P497H} rats shows that S403-TDP-43 positive inclusions do not colocalize with accumulated UBQLN2. **b** Confocal images of ubiquitin and UBQLN2 show that ubiquitin and UBQLN2 inclusions colocalize in P497H but not ChATtTA rats. The arrows point to the colocalized inclusions. Scale bars: 20 μm

expressing mutant UBQLN2^{P497H} in the spinal motor neurons or astrocytes in rats.

One recent report showed that transgenic mice expressing either the UBQLN2 P497S or P506T mutation developed both cognitive deficits and motor phenotypes, including progressive reduction of mobility, progressive loss of motor neurons in the spinal cord, and denervation of skeletal muscles as well as abnormal accumulation of UBQLN2 inclusions [25]. Similar motor phenotypes were observed in our novel ChATtTA/TRE-UBQLN2^{P497H} transgenic rats. In particular, denervation atrophy of the gastrocnemius muscles was observed as early as 3 months old, but loss of motor neurons was not detected at that age. The motor phenotypes, however, appeared for even low levels of mutant UBQLN2 (about 20% of the endogenous levels). In contrast, disease did not develop in SOD1^{G93A} mice until the levels of mutant SOD1 were three times that of endogenous SOD1 protein [11]. Moreover, both Gorrie et

al. [10] and Hjerpe et al. [13] reported progressive accumulation of UBQLN2 inclusions and progressive cognitive deficits in mice expressing either the UBQLN2 P497H or P506T mutation. All these findings indicate that mutant UBQLN2 leads to neuron degeneration in rodent models. Furthermore, the abnormal accumulation of UBQLN2 inclusions is a remarkable pathological feature of UBQLN2-related diseases.

Similar findings have been reported in transgenic rats expressing mutant TDP43 (M337 V substitution) in the spinal motor neurons, which causes rapid degeneration of motor neurons and paralysis [16]. In contrast, transgenic mice expressing mutant SOD1 in the motor neurons do not develop motor phenotypes [29, 50]. The causes of these differences remain unknown. One possible reason for these differences is that different disease mechanisms may underlie UBQLN2, TDP-43, and SOD1 genes. For example, UBQLN2 involves protein degradation via both autophagy and the ubiquitin-proteasome

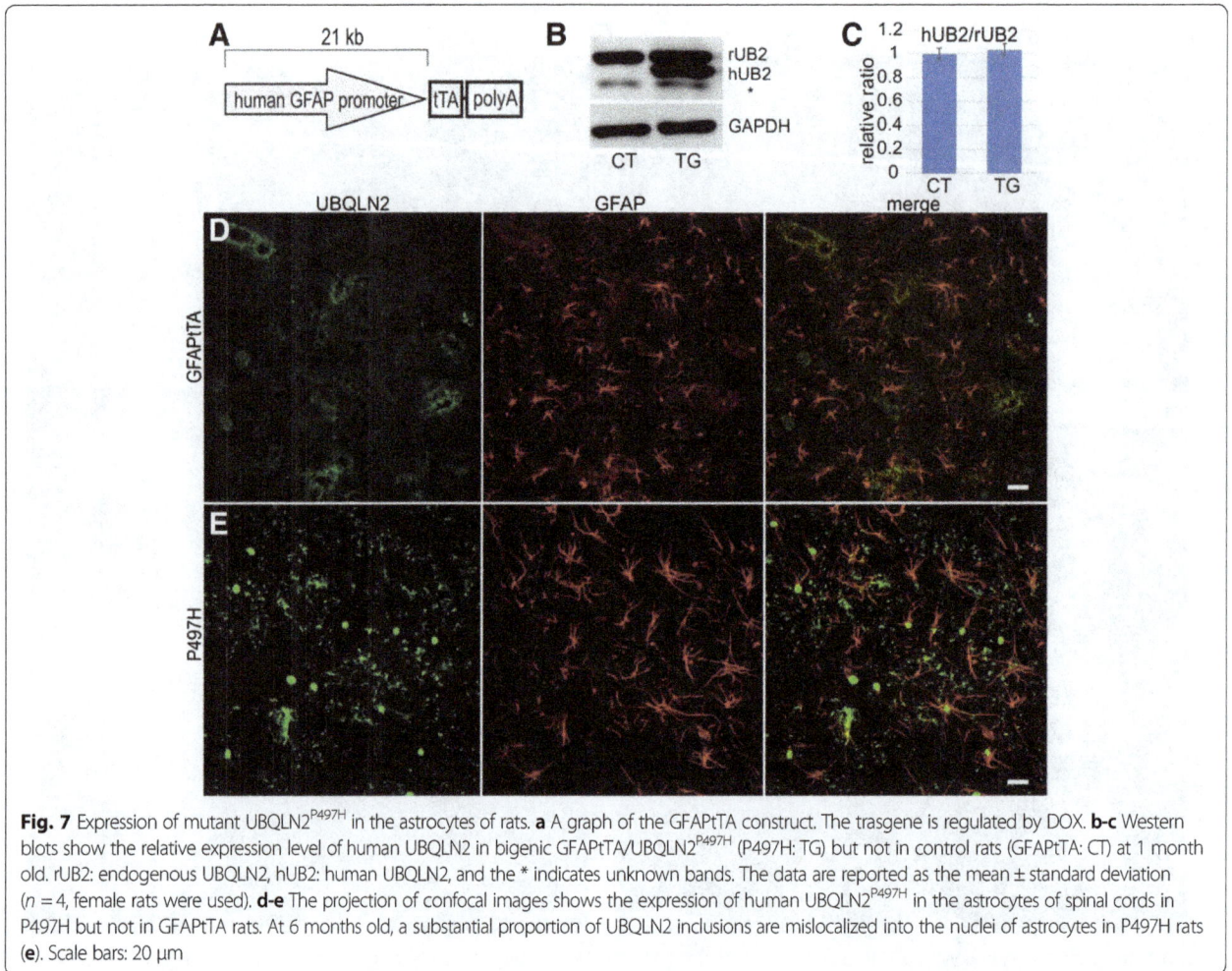

Fig. 7 Expression of mutant UBQLN2[P497H] in the astrocytes of rats. **a** A graph of the GFAPtTA construct. The trasgene is regulated by DOX. **b-c** Western blots show the relative expression level of human UBQLN2 in bigenic GFAPtTA/UBQLN2[P497H] (P497H: TG) but not in control rats (GFAPtTA: CT) at 1 month old. rUB2: endogenous UBQLN2, hUB2: human UBQLN2, and the * indicates unknown bands. The data are reported as the mean ± standard deviation ($n = 4$, female rats were used). **d-e** The projection of confocal images shows the expression of human UBQLN2[P497H] in the astrocytes of spinal cords in P497H but not in GFAPtTA rats. At 6 months old, a substantial proportion of UBQLN2 inclusions are mislocalized into the nuclei of astrocytes in P497H rats (**e**). Scale bars: 20 μm

pathway [9, 13, 36, 41, 53]. The overexpression of UBQLN2[P497H] in the spinal motor neurons caused the autophagy substrate p62 to progressively accumulate as well as colocalize with both UBQLN2 and ChAT inclusions in the ventral horn of spinal cord in ChATtTA/UBQLN2[P497H] rats, which is similar to the results from transgenic rats expressing UBQLN2 in forebrain neurons [14, 52]. At 12 months old, p62 accumulated predominantly in the nucleus and cytoplasmic p62 was mostly depleted. Under physiological conditions, however, p62 is commonly considered a cytoplasmic protein. p62 contains two nuclear localization signals (NLS) and a nuclear export signal, however, and it has been confirmed that p62 also shuttles between the nucleus and cytoplasm, a process that is regulated by the phosphorylation of NLS [38]. The mislocalization of p62, as observed in our study, may be the underlying cause of the abnormal functions observed in our ChATtTA/UBQLN2[P497H] rats. Total p62 was increased in ChATtTA/UBQLN2[P497H] rats at 1 month old, which is similar to the findings in rats expressing mutant UBQLN2 in the forebrain [52]. As an autophagy substrate, p62 is essential to neurons

[22], and mutations in p62 have been linked to ALS and FTLD [42]. In mouse models, loss of p62 leads to neurodegeneration [40]. Our finding that accumulated p62 colocalizes with UBQLN2 inclusions is similar to our previous reports in other rat models [14, 52]. These findings imply that the two disease genes may share similar mechanisms underlying neurodegeneration. Specifically, mutant UBQLN2[P497H] may compromise the functions of autophagy, leading to abnormal protein accumulations of UBQLN2, p62, and others.

Although p62 has been used as one indicator of autophagy [3, 30, 43], autophagic flux should be measured by an LC3 turnover assay in addition to p62. LC3-II is one isoform of LC3, and is widely used to measure the autophagic process [22, 47]. The suppression of LC3-II expression reflects impaired autophagy, and the amount of LC3-II is correlated with the extent of autophagosome formation [18]. ATG7 is another autophagy component that is essential for autophagosome formation. The loss of ATG7 leads to the reduction of autophagy in mice [23]. In our ChATtTA/UBQLN2[P497H] rats, both LC3 and ATG7 were accumulated at 1 month old but

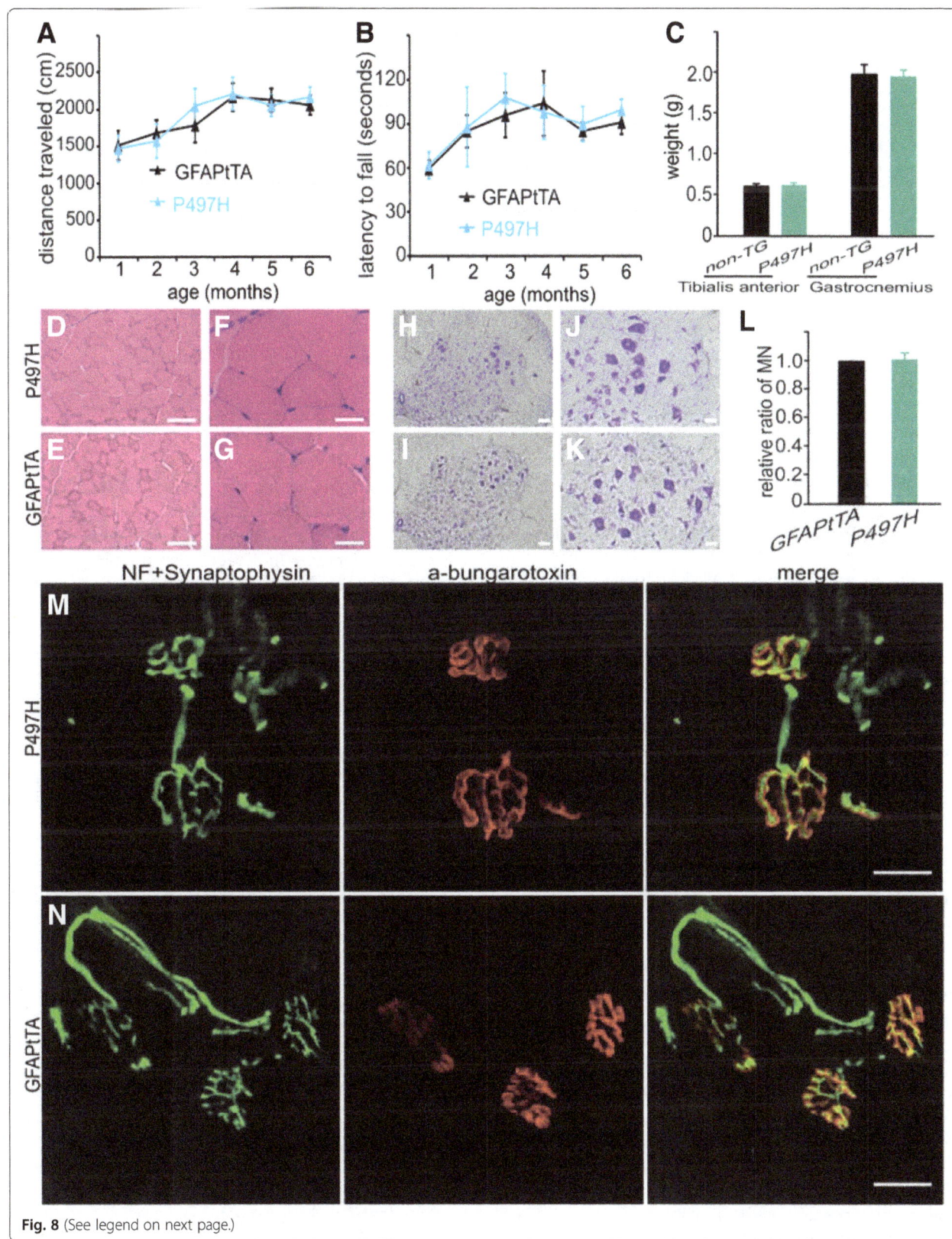

Fig. 8 (See legend on next page.)

(See figure on previous page.)
Fig. 8 No motor phenotypes in GFAPtTA/UBQLN2^{P497H} rats. **a-b** Results of beavioral tests in GFAPtTA/UBQLN2^{P497H} bigenic (P497H) and GFAPtTA single transgenic rats. **c** The weights of tibialis anterior and gastrocnemius muscles at 6 months old in P497H and GFAPtTA female rats. The data are reported as the mean ± standard deviation (n = 4). **d-g** H&E staining shows the structures of gastrocnemius muscle in both P497H and GFAPtTA rats; **h-l** Cresyl violet staining shows the motor neurons in the ventral horn of the spinal cord. The quantification of motor neurons in the L3–5 spinal cord shows that there is no statistical difference between P497H and GFAPtTA rats (n = 4). **m-n** Confocal images show the structures of neuromuscular junctions (NMJ) in gastrocnemius muscles. The sections were stained with the presynaptic neuronal marker neurofilament (NF) and synaptophysin together with α-bungarotoxin to show the post-synaptic structures. Scale bars: 100 μm (**d**, **e**, **h**, **i**), 50 μm (**j**, **k**), 30 μm (**f**, **g**), 20 μm (**m**, **n**)

decreased substantially after 6-month old. Similarly, the lysosomal membrane protein LAMP2a also was accumulated and colocalized with UBQLN2 inclusions in 12-month old ChATtTA/UBQLN2^{P497H} rats. Consistent with these findings, the selective loss of LAMP2A protein directly correlated with increased levels of α-synuclein in early Parkinson's disease [34]. All these results suggest that mutant UBQLN2^{P497H} compromises autophagy-lysosomal pathways in an age-dependent manner. Moreover, the decrease of several core ATG proteins suggests that mutant UBQLN2^{P497H} is more likely to suppress autophagy at upstream stages.

The hyperphosphorylated form of TDP-43 has been identified as a core component of cytosolic inclusions in sporadic ALS [1, 37]. In ChATtTA/UBQLN2^{P497H} rats, relatively little phosphorylated TDP-43 was detected in the spinal cord and did not colocalize with UBQLN2 inclusions. In contrast, accumulated ubiquitin was colocalized with UBQLN2 inclusions. Ubiquitin accumulation is one of the key pathological alterations in neurodegenerative diseases, and ubiquitin accumulation may correlate with neurodegeneration in our rats. In contrast, the expression of the astrocyte marker GFAP was elevated in our rats, but no significant changes in IBa1, a marker of microglia, were observed. These findings are different from those of other rodent models, in which increased expression in both astrocytes and microglia have been observed [16, 17, 25, 52]. This difference may be due to the slow progression of the disease and a mild loss of motor neurons in ChATtTA/UBQLN2^{P497H} rats compared to other rat models, indicating that astrocytes are more sensitive to stress conditions than microglia in our mutant UBQLN2^{P497H} rats.

We did not observe any motor deficits at 6-month old GFAPtTA/UBQLN2^{P497H} rats, which is not consistent with the motor phenotypes observed in mutant TDP-43 or mutant SOD1 rodent models [26, 35, 49]. Mutant UBQLN2 protein expression was higher in the spinal cord of GFAPtTA/UBQLN2^{P497H} rats compared to ChATtTA/UBQLN2^{P497H} rats. These findings suggest that phenotypes caused by mutant UBQLN2^{P497H} are not dependent solely on the expression level of mutant proteins in motor neurons and astrocytes in rats. It would be important to investigate whether any disease phenotypes can be induced in older rats (up to

18 months old) expressing mutant UBQLN2^{P497H} in astrocytes. In addition, future studies are needed to examine whether mutant UBQLN2 will initiate motor neuron degeneration in a non-cell autonomous manner when overexpressing mutant UBQLN2 in other non-neuronal cells, such as microglia or oligodendrocytes.

Conclusions

Our results showed that mutant UBQLN2^{P497H} selectively expressed in motor neurons other than astrocytes leads to several key features of motor neuron disease in rats, including abnormal accumulation of UBQLN2, p62, and ChAT; mobility impairment; motor neuron degeneration; and reductions in several core autophagy-related proteins. This study indicates that expressing mutant UBQLN2 in motor neurons leads to progressive motor deficits and impairment of the autophagy-lysosomal pathway, but that overexpression of mutant UBQLN2 in astrocytes alone is not sufficient to develop motor phenotypes or defective autophagy.

Additional file

Additional file 1: Figure S1. Similar expression of UBQLN2 in male and female non-transgenic rats. Western blotting showed the endogenous UBQLN2 (rUB2) had no differential expression between male and female non-transgenic rats at the age of 90 days. The upper graph showed the relative ratios of endogenous UBQLN2 between female and male among different tissues. (M: male, F: female. "*" denotes non-specific band). Data are shown as mean ± s.d. (n = 3). **Figure S2.** Muscle structures in rats. (**A-B**), H&E staining showed no alteration was observed in both tibialis anterior and gastrocnemius muscles of ChATtTA/UBQLN2P497H rats (P497H) compared with ChATtTA single transgenic rats (ChATtTA) at 1 month old. Panel A: 4x objective, and Panel B: 10x objective. Scale bars: A (250 μm), B (100 μm). (**C**), Quantification of the impaired neuromuscular junctions in P497H rats at indicated ages, which are the same rats shown in Fig. 4i-l. (> 20 NMJs were counted randomly for each rats). **Figure S3.** Accumulation of myofibers in ChATtTA/UBQLN2P497H rats. (**A-B**), Both pH 4.6 and pH 10.4 ATPase staining revealed groups of atrophic muscle fibers in gastrocnemius muscles of ChATtTA/UBQLN2P497H rats (P497H) at 12 months old, not in the age-matched ChATtTA single transgenic rats (ChATtTA). (**C-F**), Immunofluorescent staining of myofibers (MYH-S and MYH-1) and DMD (a plasma membrane protein) showed the atrophic myofibers accumulated in gastrocnemius muscles of P497H rats, not in ChATtTA rats. Arrows point to groups of myofiber atrophy. Scale bars: 100 μm. **Figure S4.** The colocalization of the accumulated ChAT and p62 in rats. (**A-C**), Double staining of p62 and ChAT revealed the accumulation of p62 in ChATtTA/UBQLN2P497H rats (P497H, arrows point to the accumulations), not in ChATtTA single transgenic rats (ChATtTA). At 12 months old, a substantial proportion of ChAT mislocalized into nuclei and also colocalized with the p62 inclusions (**C**). Scale bars: 100 μm. **Figure S5.** Accumulations of P62 and ubiquitin in

GFAPtTA/UBQLN2P497H rats. (**A**), Double staining of P62 and GFAP revealed the accumulations of P62 were colocalized with astrocytes in GFAPtTA/UBQLN2P497H rats (P497H, arrows point to the colocalizations of inclusions), not in GFAPtTA single transgenic rats (GFAPtTA). (**B**), The projected confocal images of ubiquitin and GFAP showed the colocalization of the accumulated ubiquitin and astrocytes in P497H rats (arrows point to the colocalizations), not in GFAPtTA rats. Scale bars: 30 μm (**A**), 20 μm (**B**). (PDF 1240 kb)

Abbreviations

AD: Alzheimer's disease; ALS: Amyotrophic lateral sclerosis; C9ORF72: Chromosome 9 open reading frame 72; CHAT: Choline acetyltransferase; CNS: Central nervous system; dox: Doxycycline; FTLD: Frontotemporal lobar degeneration; UBA: Ubiquitin associated domain; UBL: Ubiquitin-like domain; UBQLN2: Ubiquilin2

Acknowledgements

The authors would like to thank Dr. Stephen Peiper's guidance on this study, and Dr. Jay Schneider's useful comments on the manuscript.

Funding

This work was supported by grants from the National Institutes of Health (NS095972 to C. H.) and the Health Planning Commission foundation of Shanxi Province (2017016 to B.H.). The content is the responsibility of the authors and does not necessarily represent the official view of the NIH.

Authors' contributions

THC, BH, and CH conceived and designed the experiments. THC, BH, XLS and CH performed the experiments. THC, BH, LMG and CH analyzed the data and wrote the paper. CTH and B.H. contributed equally to this work. All authors read and approved the final manuscript.

Competing interests

The authors declare that they have no competing interests.

Author details

[1]Department of Pathology, Anatomy & Cell Biology, Thomas Jefferson University, 1020 Locust Street, Philadelphia, PA 19107, USA. [2]Laboratory Animal Center, Shanxi Provincial People's Hospital, Taiyuan, Shanxi 030012, People's Republic of China. [3]Animal Laboratory of Nephrology, Shanxi Provincial People's Hospital, Taiyuan, Shanxi 030012, People's Republic of China. [4]Department of Ophthalmology, The Third Xiangya Hospital of Central South University, Changsha, Hunan 410013, People's Republic of China.

References

1. Arai T, Hasegawa M, Akiyama H, Ikeda K, Nonaka T, Mori H et al (2006) TDP-43 is a component of ubiquitin-positive tau-negative inclusions in frontotemporal lobar degeneration and amyotrophic lateral sclerosis. Biochem Biophys Res Commun 351:602–611
2. Bi F, Huang C, Tong J, Qiu G, Huang B, Wu Q et al (2013) Reactive astrocytes secrete lcn2 to promote neuron death. Proc Natl Acad Sci U S A 110:4069–4074
3. Bjorkoy G, Lamark T, Brech A, Outzen H, Perander M, Overvatn A et al (2005) p62/SQSTM1 forms protein aggregates degraded by autophagy and has a protective effect on huntingtin-induced cell death. J Cell Biol 171:603–614
4. Boillee S, Yamanaka K, Lobsiger CS, Copeland NG, Jenkins NA, Kassiotis G et al (2006) Onset and progression in inherited ALS determined by motor neurons and microglia. Science 312:1389–1392
5. Brettschneider J, Van Deerlin VM, Robinson JL, Kwong L, Lee EB, Ali YO et al (2012) Pattern of ubiquilin pathology in ALS and FTLD indicates presence of C9ORF72 hexanucleotide expansion. Acta Neuropathol 123:825–839
6. Cassel JA, Reitz AB (2013) Ubiquilin-2 (UBQLN2) binds with high affinity to the C-terminal region of TDP-43 and modulates TDP-43 levels in H4 cells: characterization of inhibition by nucleic acids and 4-aminoquinolines. Biochim Biophys Acta 1834:964–971
7. Cuervo AM, Dice JF (2000) Unique properties of lamp2a compared to other lamp2 isoforms. J Cell Sci 24:4441–4450
8. Deng HX, Chen W, Hong ST, Boycott KM, Gorrie GH, Siddique N et al (2011) Mutations in UBQLN2 cause dominant X-linked juvenile and adult-onset ALS and ALS/dementia. Nature 477:211–215
9. Gao L, Tu H, Shi ST, Lee KJ, Asanaka M, Hwang SB et al (2003) Interaction with a ubiquitin-like protein enhances the ubiquitination and degradation of hepatitis C virus RNA-dependent RNA polymerase. J Virol 77:4149–4159
10. Gorrie GH, Fecto F, Radzicki D, Weiss C, Shi Y, Dong H et al (2014) Dendritic spinopathy in transgenic mice expressing ALS/dementia-linked mutant UBQLN2. Proc Natl Acad Sci U S A 111:14524–14529
11. Gurney ME, Pu H, Chiu AY, Dal Canto MC, Polchow CY, Alexander DD et al (1994) Motor neuron degeneration in mice that express a human Cu, Zn superoxide dismutase mutation. Science 264:1772–1775
12. He C, Klionsky DJ (2009) Regulation mechanisms and signaling pathways of autophagy. Annu Rev Genet 43:67–93
13. Hjerpe R, Bett JS, Keuss MJ, Solovyova A, McWilliams TG, Johnson C et al (2016) UBQLN2 mediates autophagy-independent protein aggregate clearance by the proteasome. Cell 166:935–949
14. Huang B, Wu Q, Zhou H, Huang C, Xia XG (2016) Increased Ubqln2 expression causes neuron death in transgenic rats. J Neurochem 139:285–293
15. Huang C, Tong J, Bi F, Wu Q, Huang B, Zhou H et al (2012) Entorhinal cortical neurons are the primary targets of FUS mislocalization and ubiquitin aggregation in FUS transgenic rats. Hum Mol Genet 21:4602–4614
16. Huang C, Tong J, Bi F, Zhou H, Xia XG (2012) Mutant TDP-43 in motor neurons promotes the onset and progression of ALS in rats. J Clin Invest 122:107–118
17. Huang C, Zhou H, Tong J, Chen H, Wang D et al (2011) FUS transgenic rats develop the phenotypes of amyotrophic lateral sclerosis and frontotemporal lobar degeneration. PLoS Genet 7:e1002011
18. Kabeya Y, Mizushima N, Ueno T, Yamamoto A, Kirisako T, Noda T et al (2000) LC3, a mammalian homologue of yeast Apg8p, is localized in autophagosome membranes after processing. EMBO J 19:5720–5728
19. Kia A, McAvoy K, Krishnamurthy K, Trotti D, Pasinelli P (2018) Astrocytes expressing ALS-linked mutant FUS induce motor neuron death through release of tumor necrosis factor-alpha. Glia 66:1016–1033
20. Kleijnen MF, Shih AH, Zhou P, Kumar S, Soccio RE, Kedersha NL et al (2000) The hPLIC proteins may provide a link between the ubiquitination machinery and the proteasome. Mol Cell 6:409–419
21. Ko HS, Uehara T, Tsuruma K, Nomura Y (2004) Ubiquilin interacts with ubiquitylated proteins and proteasome through its ubiquitin-associated and ubiquitin-like domains. FEBS Lett 566:110–114
22. Komatsu M, Waguri S, Koike M, Sou YS, Ueno T, Hara T et al (2007) Homeostatic levels of p62 control cytoplasmic inclusion body formation in autophagy-deficient mice. Cell 131:1149–1163
23. Komatsu M, Waguri S, Ueno T, Iwata J, Murata S, Tanida I et al (2005) Impairment of starvation-induced and constitutive autophagy in Atg7-deficient mice. J Cell Biol 169:425–434
24. Korolchuk VI, Mansilla A, Menzies FM, Rubinsztein DC (2009) Autophagy inhibition compromises degradation of ubiquitin-proteasome pathway substrates. Mol Cell 33:517–527
25. Le NT, Chang L, Kovlyagina I, Georgiou P, Safren N, Braunstein KE et al (2016) Motor neuron disease, TDP-43 pathology, and memory deficits in mice expressing ALS-FTD-linked UBQLN2 mutations. Proc Natl Acad Sci U S A 113:E7580–E7589
26. Levine JB, Kong J, Nadler M, Xu Z (1999) Astrocytes interact intimately with degenerating motor neurons in mouse amyotrophic lateral sclerosis (ALS). Glia 28:215–224

27. Liddelow SA, Guttenplan KA, Clarke LE, Bennett FC, Bohlen CJ, Schirmer L et al (2017) Neurotoxic reactive astrocytes are induced by activated microglia. Nature 541:481–487

28. Lim MA, Selak MA, Xiang Z, Krainc D, Neve RL, Kraemer BC et al (2012) Reduced activity of AMP-activated protein kinase protects against genetic models of motor neuron disease. J Neurosci 32:1123–1141

29. Lino MM, Schneider C, Caroni P (2002) Accumulation of SOD1 mutants in postnatal motoneurons does not cause motoneuron pathology or motoneuron disease. J Neurosci 22:4825–4832

30. Liu WJ, Ye L, Huang WF, Guo LJ, Xu ZG, Wu HL et al (2016) p62 links the autophagy pathway and the ubiqutin-proteasome system upon ubiquitinated protein degradation. Cell Mol Biol Lett 21:29

31. Mackenzie IR, Bigio EH, Ince PG, Geser F, Neumann M, Cairns NJ et al (2007) Pathological TDP-43 distinguishes sporadic amyotrophic lateral sclerosis from amyotrophic lateral sclerosis with SOD1 mutations. Ann Neurol 61:427–434

32. Molofsky AV, Deneen B (2015) Astrocyte development: a guide for the perplexed. Glia 63:1320–1329

33. Moloney EB, de Winter F, Verhaagen J (2014) ALS as a distal axonopathy: molecular mechanisms affecting neuromuscular junction stability in the presymptomatic stages of the disease. Front Neurosci 8:252

34. Murphy KE, Gysbers AM, Abbott SK, Spiro AS, Furuta A, Cooper A et al (2015) Lysosomal-associated membrane protein 2 isoforms are differentially affected in early Parkinson's disease. Mov Disord 30:1639–1647

35. Nagai M, Re DB, Nagata T, Chalazonitis A, Jessell TM, Wichterle H et al (2007) Astrocytes expressing ALS-linked mutated SOD1 release factors selectively toxic to motor neurons. Nat Neurosci 10:615–622

36. N'Diaye EN, Kajihara KK, Hsieh I, Morisaki H, Debnath J, Brown EJ (2009) PLIC proteins or ubiquilins regulate autophagy-dependent cell survival during nutrient starvation. EMBO Rep 10:173–179

37. Neumann M, Sampathu DM, Kwong LK, Truax AC, Micsenyi MC, Chou TT et al (2006) Ubiquitinated TDP-43 in frontotemporal lobar degeneration and amyotrophic lateral sclerosis. Science 314:130–133

38. Pankiv S, Lamark T, Bruun JA, Overvatn A, Bjorkoy G, Johansen T (2010) Nucleocytoplasmic shuttling of p62/SQSTM1 and its role in recruitment of nuclear polyubiquitinated proteins to promyelocytic leukemia bodies. J Biol Chem 285:5941–5953

39. Pramatarova A, Laganiere J, Roussel J, Brisebois K, Rouleau GA (2001) Neuron-specific expression of mutant superoxide dismutase 1 in transgenic mice does not lead to motor impairment. J Neurosci 21:3369–3374

40. Ramesh Babu J, Lamar Seibenhener M, Peng J, Strom AL, Kemppainen R, Cox N et al (2008) Genetic inactivation of p62 leads to accumulation of hyperphosphorylated tau and neurodegeneration. J Neurochem 106:107–120

41. Rothenberg C, Srinivasan D, Mah L, Kaushik S, Peterhoff CM, Ugolino J et al (2010) Ubiquilin functions in autophagy and is degraded by chaperone-mediated autophagy. Hum Mol Genet 19:3219–3232

42. Rubino E, Rainero I, Chio A, Rogaeva E, Galimberti D, Fenoglio P et al (2012) SQSTM1 mutations in frontotemporal lobar degeneration and amyotrophic lateral sclerosis. Neurology 79:1556–1562

43. Sahani MH, Itakura E, Mizushima N (2014) Expression of the autophagy substrate SQSTM1/p62 is restored during prolonged starvation depending on transcriptional upregulation and autophagy-derived amino acids. Autophagy 10:431–441

44. Salminen A, Kaarniranta K, Haapasalo A, Hiltunen M, Soininen H, Alafuzoff I (2012) Emerging role of p62/sequestosome-1 in the pathogenesis of Alzheimer's disease. Prog Neurobiol 96:87–95

45. Sofroniew MV (2015) Astrocyte barriers to neurotoxic inflammation. Nat Rev Neurosci 16:249–263

46. Synofzik M, Maetzler W, Grehl T, Prudlo J, Vom Hagen JM, Haack T et al (2012) Screening in ALS and FTD patients reveals 3 novel UBQLN2 mutations outside the PXX domain and a pure FTD phenotype. Neurobiol Aging 33(2949):e13–e17

47. Tanida I, Minematsu-Ikeguchi N, Ueno T, Kominami E (2005) Lysosomal turnover, but not a cellular level, of endogenous LC3 is a marker for autophagy. Autophagy 1:84–91

48. Teyssou E, Chartier L, Amador MD, Lam R, Lautrette G, Nicol M et al (2017) Novel UBQLN2 mutations linked to amyotrophic lateral sclerosis and atypical hereditary spastic paraplegia phenotype through defective HSP70-mediated proteolysis. Neurobiol Aging 58:239 e211–2239 e20

49. Tong J, Huang C, Bi F, Wu Q, Huang B, Liu X et al (2013) Expression of ALS-linked TDP-43 mutant in astrocytes causes non-cell-autonomous motor neuron death in rats. EMBO J 32:1917–1926

50. Wang L, Sharma K, Deng HX, Siddique T, Grisotti G, Liu E et al (2008) Restricted expression of mutant SOD1 in spinal motor neurons and interneurons induces motor neuron pathology. Neurobiol Dis 29:400–408

51. Wooten MW, Geetha T, Babu JR, Seibenhener ML, Peng J, Cox N et al (2008) Essential role of sequestosome 1/p62 in regulating accumulation of Lys63-ubiquitinated proteins. J Biol Chem 283:6783–6789

52. Wu Q, Liu M, Huang C, Liu X, Huang B, Li N et al (2015) Pathogenic Ubqln2 gains toxic properties to induce neuron death. Acta Neuropathol 129:417–428

53. Wu S, Mikhailov A, Kallo-Hosein H, Hara K, Yonezawa K, Avruch J (2002) Characterization of ubiquitin 1, an mTOR-interacting protein. Biochim Biophys Acta 1542:41–56

54. Yamamoto A, Hen R, Dauer WT (2001) The ons and offs of inducible transgenic technology: a review. Neurobiol Dis 8:923–932

55. Yamanaka K, Boillee S, Roberts EA, Garcia ML, McAlonis-Downes M, Mikse OR et al (2008) Mutant SOD1 in cell types other than motor neurons and oligodendrocytes accelerates onset of disease in ALS mice. Proc Natl Acad Sci 105:7594–7599

18

Stable transgenic C9orf72 zebrafish model key aspects of the ALS/FTD phenotype and reveal novel pathological features

Matthew P. Shaw[1], Adrian Higginbottom[1], Alexander McGown[1], Lydia M. Castelli[1], Evlyn James[1], Guillaume M. Hautbergue[1], Pamela J. Shaw[1†] and Tennore M. Ramesh[1,2*†] 🆔

Abstract

A hexanucleotide repeat expansion (HRE) within the chromosome 9 open reading frame 72 (C9orf72) gene is the most prevalent cause of amyotrophic lateral sclerosis/fronto-temporal dementia (ALS/FTD). Current evidence suggests HREs induce neurodegeneration through accumulation of RNA foci and/or dipeptide repeat proteins (DPR). C9orf72 patients are known to have transactive response DNA binding protein 43 kDa (TDP-43) proteinopathy, but whether there is further cross over between C9orf72 pathology and the pathology of other ALS sub-types has yet to be revealed.

To address this, we generated and characterised two zebrafish lines expressing C9orf72 HREs. We also characterised pathology in human C9orf72-ALS cases. In addition, we utilised a reporter construct that expresses DsRed under the control of a heat shock promoter, to screen for potential therapeutic compounds.

Both zebrafish lines showed accumulation of RNA foci and DPR. Our C9-ALS/FTD zebrafish model is the first to recapitulate the motor deficits, cognitive impairment, muscle atrophy, motor neuron loss and mortality in early adulthood observed in human C9orf72-ALS/FTD. Furthermore, we identified that in zebrafish, human cell lines and human post-mortem tissue, C9orf72 expansions activate the heat shock response (HSR). Additionally, HSR activation correlated with disease progression in our C9-ALS/FTD zebrafish model. Lastly, we identified that the compound ivermectin, as well as riluzole, reduced HSR activation in both C9-ALS/FTD and SOD1 zebrafish models.

Thus, our C9-ALS/FTD zebrafish model is a stable transgenic model which recapitulates key features of human C9orf72-ALS/FTD, and represents a powerful drug-discovery tool.

Keywords: Amyotrophic lateral sclerosis, C9orf72, SOD1, TDP-43, Zebrafish, Drug-screening

Introduction

Amyotrophic lateral sclerosis (ALS) is a neurodegenerative disorder characterised by motor neuron loss, leading to progressive muscle weakness and eventual death, primarily due to respiratory failure. Approximately 10% of ALS is inherited in an autosomal dominant fashion, this is known as familial-ALS (fALS). The remaining 90% of ALS cases are caused by complex genetic and environmental interactions which are currently not well understood, this is known as sporadic-ALS (sALS). Mutations in multiple genetic loci have been identified as causes of ALS including the SOD1 and TARDBP loci. See Amyotrophic Lateral Sclerosis Online Genetics Database for comprehensive information (http://alsod.iop.kcl.ac.uk/). The most common known genetic cause of ALS and frontotemporal dementia (FTD) is a hexanucleotide expansion within the first intron of the C9orf72 gene [11, 32]. Carriers of the C9orf72 hexanucleotide expansion may show symptoms of ALS or FTD exclusively, but can also present with symptoms of both diseases concurrently.

Concerning pathology in C9orf72 patients, there are three major, non-mutually exclusive routes of toxicity which have

* Correspondence: t.ramesh@sheffield.ac.uk
†Pamela J. Shaw and Tennore Ramesh contributed equally to this work.
[1]Sheffield Institute for Translational Neuroscience, University of Sheffield, 385a Glossop Road, Sheffield S10 2HQ, UK
[2]The Bateson Centre, Firth Court, The University of Sheffield, Western Bank, Sheffield S10 2TN, UK

been proposed to arise from the *C9orf72* expansion: **1)** Sense and antisense RNA foci which sequester RNA binding proteins causing dysregulation of RNA processing [7, 11]. **2)** Dipeptide repeat proteins (DPRs) produced via non-canonical repeat associated non-ATG (RAN) translation, form insoluble aggregates in the nucleus and cytoplasm [42]. **3)** Hexanucleotide expansion mediated haploinsufficiency may cause dysregulation of endogenous C9orf72 pathways such as autophagy [12, 39].

To date, several models have been generated to help dissect out the mechanisms of *C9orf72* expansion mediated toxicity. Most drosophila and zebrafish models support an RNA/DPR mediated gain of toxic function hypothesis [18, 26, 28, 37]. In addition, transgenic mouse models have been generated containing the human patient *C9orf72* gene (complete with G_4C_2 expansion and flanking regions). Two transgenic mouse models demonstrate the reduced survival, neuronal loss and motor deficits observed in human C9-ALS/FTD [14, 20]. However, a further two independently generated *C9orf72* transgenic models showed no signs of neuronal loss or reduced survival. [29, 30]. This highlights the wide variability observed in *C9orf72* expansion in vivo models. *C9orf72* knockdown in the zebrafish causes mild motor defects [6]. However, early reports from *C9orf72* knockout zebrafish do not recapitulate the knockdown motor phenotypes ([34]; Schmid, Hruscha, Haass, unpublished). Additionally, four independently generated *C9orf72* knockout mice did not demonstrate any neurodegenerative phenotype [1, 13, 17, 35].

Whilst mouse models are a useful tool for understanding the pathobiology of *C9orf72*-related ALS, they are not amenable to high throughput drug screening. Genetic modifier screens have been carried out in drosophila, but their CNS is much simpler compared to the human CNS and findings in this invertebrate model are less likely to translate to the clinic [3, 15]. Zebrafish are vertebrates with a more complex CNS, and therefore represent a practical compromise for assessing the efficacy of therapeutic compounds.

Here we present a novel transgenic zebrafish model which stably expresses *C9orf72* expansions. These zebrafish recapitulate the behavioural deficits, cognitive abnormalities, motor decline and early mortality observed in C9-ALS patients. Additionally we show that *C9orf72* expansions activate the heat shock response in human cell lines, post-mortem ALS tissue and our model zebrafish. Using these *C9orf72* zebrafish and our previously reported *SOD1* zebrafish in tandem [31], we show that riluzole and a newly identified compound, ivermectin, are able to reduce cellular stress in both *C9orf72* and *SOD1* in vivo models. We therefore propose that our *C9orf72* zebrafish model effectively bridges the gap between drosophila and mouse models by providing an efficient tool for high-throughput in vivo drug screening assays.

Materials and methods

Generating and maintenance of transgenic zebrafish

Zebrafish embryos were injected with a DNA construct containing 89 C9orf72 hexanucleotide repeats driven by a zebrafish ubiquitin promotor (Fig. 1a, Additional file 1). Creation and identification of transgenic zebrafish was performed as previously described [31] and maintained using established practices [40].

In situ hybridisation and immunofluorescence

In situ hybridization of paraffin embedded tissue sections to detect CCCCGG (C_4G_2) foci was performed on 5dpf embryos using methods described previously [8]. For immunofluorescence staining, paraffin embedded tissue was dewaxed, antigen retrieved and stained as previously described [9].

Western blotting

Ethical approval for use of human cerebellum samples was obtained by the Sheffield Brain Tissue Bank Management Board, and approval to release tissue under REC 08/MRE00/103 was granted. Human cerebellum samples and adult zebrafish tissue, brain, spinal cord and whole zebrafish embryos were snap frozen in liquid nitrogen and processed for western blotting. Laemmli buffer was added in the ratio of 10 µl:1 mg of tissue and sonicated. SDS-PAGE and immunoblotting were performed as previously described [39]. Antibodies used were Rb-anti-PR (gift from Dieter Edbauer), Rb-anti-Dsred (Clontech 632,496), Ms-anti-tubulin (Abcam). Species specific HRP conjugated secondary antibodies were used and imaged by chemiluminescence using G-Box.

Embryonic behaviour

For spontaneous locomotor activity, 5 dpf zebrafish were placed into individual wells of a 96well plate and habituated in the dark for 10 min before a light stimulus was turned on. 10 min of light was followed by 10 min dark and repeated once more. Recordings were carried out using ZebraBox software (ViewPoint Behaviour Technologies), movement thresholds used were slow (x < 5 mm/sec), intermediate (5 < x < 15 mm/sec) and fast (x > 15 mm/sec).

For centre avoidance behaviour, 5 dpf zebrafish were placed into a 6 well plate at a density of 30 zebrafish per well. After a 30 min habituation period with the lights on, the lights were turned off for 5 min then on for 5 min for 6 cycles. Frame grab was performed at 30 s for every minute in the lights on condition using the Image-grab tool, and this was repeated for each of the 6 lights on periods. Using ImageJ, circles of the same size were placed around the outside of every well so that only the

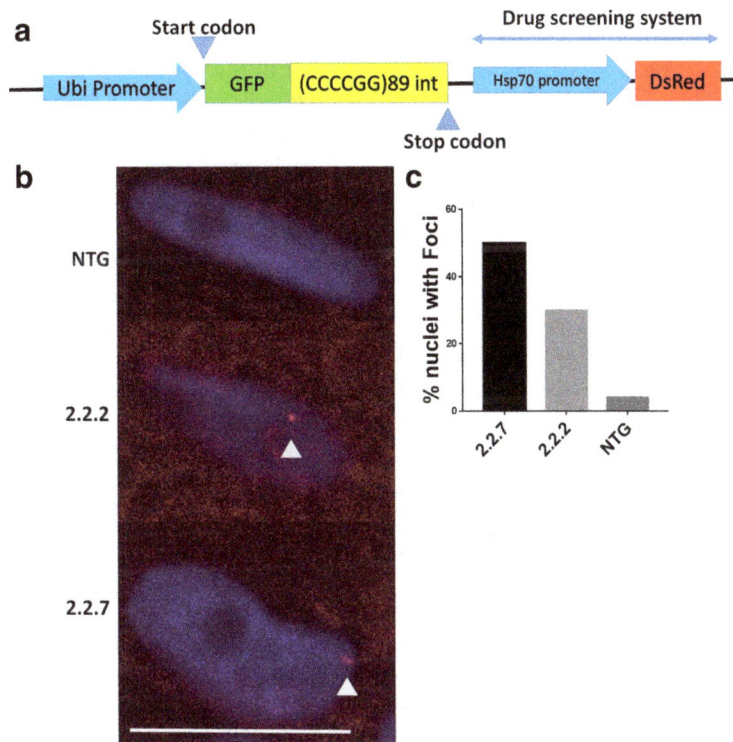

Fig. 1 *C9orf72* model zebrafish display RNA foci in the nucleus. (**a**) Schematic representation of the transgene inserted into 2.2 zebrafish. A zebrafish ubiquitin promotor drives GFP-DPR expression. An *hsp70* promotor then drives DsRed production as a read out of cellular stress. (**b**) In situ hybridisation of paraffin embedded sections of 10dpf 2.2–7 zebrafish using a Cy3-conjugated (red) GC probe (GGGGCC)X4 showed that RNA foci are present in the nuclei of muscle cells. Arrow heads denote RNA foci. Scale bar = 10 µm. (**c**) Quantification of RNA foci showed Immunofluorescence labelling of adult zebrafish muscle tissue showed that poly-GP DPR protein localises to the nucleus in 2.2–2 and 2.2–7 transgenic zebrafish

centre of the well was visible, the % of zebrafish present in the centre of the well was then blind counted for every image and the average per well was calculated.

Adult locomotor behaviour

Zebrafish swimming ability was tested using a swim tunnel with an intial flow-rate of 2 L/min, increasing in 2 L/min increments every 5 min until the maximum flow rate of 11.6 L/min was achieved. Data were analysed as previously described [31]. 5 min post-testing, the spontaneous swimming behaviour of the fish was measured for 30 min using a camera linked to ZebraLab software (ViewPoint Behaviour Technologies). Speed thresholds used were slow (x < 60 mm/sec), intermediate (60 < x < 120 mm/sec) and fast (x > 120 mm/sec).

Motor neuron counts and myotome measurements

Spinal motor neurons were counted from paraffin embedded adult zebrafish segments cut anterior to the pelvic fin, sectioned at 10 µm and stained with haematoxylin and eosin. Cells with a soma size $>75\mu m^2$ and within $25,000\mu m^2$ proximity of the central canal were designated as motor neurons. Three sections/per animal

were analysed by two independent blinded investigators and averaged. The areas of individual myotomes were measured by a blinded investigator from 6 images per animal. All muscle images were obtained from the epaxial muscle region just lateral to the dorsal spinal bone. Any myotome which was incomplete due to being partially out of frame was not included in the analysis.

Cell culture and transfections

Cells were maintained in a 37 °C incubator with 5% CO2. HEK293T cells were cultured in Dulbecco's Modified Eagle Medium (Sigma) supplemented with 10% foetal bovine serum (FBS) (Gibco) and 5 U ml^{-1} Penstrep (Lonza). Neuro-2a(N2A) (ATCC) cells were cultured in Dulbecco's Modified Eagle Medium (Sigma) supplemented with 10% FBS (Gibco), 5 U ml^{-1} Penstrep (Lonza) and 5 mM sodium pyruvate.

HEK293T and N2A cells were transfected with 700 ng of plasmid using 3.5 µg PEI/ml media and one tenth media volume of OptiMEM in a 24 well format. Approximately, 50,000 HEK293T cells were seeded / well and 75,000 N2A cells were seeded per well of the 24 well plate. *Proteins were extracted 72 h post-transfection. Cells were washed in* *ice cold phosphate buffered saline (PBS) and subsequently lysed in ice cold lysis buffer (*50 mM Hepes pH 7.5, 150 mM NaCl, 10% glycerol, 0.5% Triton X-100, 1 mM EDTA, 1 mM DTT, protease inhibitor cocktail (Sigma)) for 10 min on ice. Extracts were then centrifuged at 17,000 g for 5 min at 4 °C. Extracts were quantified using Bradford Reagent (BioRAD), resolved by SDS-PAGE, electroblotted onto nitrocellulose membrane and probed to the relevant primary antibodies.

Heat shock cell stress drug screening assay
At 2 dpf, transgenic zebrafish were placed into a 96 well plate in 200 μl of drug or DMSO containing E3 zebrafish media. At 5 dpf zebrafish were sonicated in the well for 10 s each and then centrifuged in a plate spinner at 3000 rpm for 10 min. From each well, 20 μl of supernatant was transferred into a 385 well plate, and the DsRed levels in each individual lysate were quantified using a FLUOstar Omega fluorescence plate reader (BMG labtech).

Quantification and statistical analysis
Data were analysed by one way ANOVA with Tukey's post hoc test or two way ANOVA with Sidak's post hoc test for multiple comparisons, t-test or Kaplan Meier analysis as indicated in the appropriate figure legend. Significance is denoted as * $P < 0.05$, ** $P < 0.01$, *** $P < 0.001$ and **** $P < 0.0001$. Individual myotome size data were counted into bins with a 0.5mm^2 size range. The frequency distribution of each genotype was then compared using a chi-squared test for trend.

Results
Generation of transgenic zebrafish
To better understand ALS/FTD pathogenesis and screen potential therapeutic agents, we generated a *C9orf72* zebrafish model. At the single cell stage zebrafish embryos were injected with a DNA construct containing 89 C9orf72 hexanucleotide repeats (Fig. 1a, Additional file 1). Of the 3 zebrafish lines generated, one was extremely toxic, resulting in death within 7 days of fertilisation (dpf). Therefore, only the 2 remaining lines were maintained to breeding age and established for further characterisation. These two transgenic zebrafish lines which were established to adulthood will henceforth be known as line 2.2–2 and line 2.2–7, or collectively as 2.2-zebrafish lines. Both 2.2-zebrafish lines give rise to 1:1 ratios of transgenic:NTG offspring when outbred, suggesting a single site of transgene insertion.

C9orf72 zebrafish lines express RNA foci and DPR
The hallmark features of *C9orf72* pathology are expression of RNA foci and DPR species. Using in situ hybridisation and immunofluorescence, we identified expression of

RNA foci and DPR species in both 2.2-zebrafish lines. Antisense RNA foci (CCCCGG, the same orientation with respect to the construct) can be detected in the nuclei of muscle cells in both 2.2-zebrafish lines (Fig. 1b), no more than one focus is observed per nucleus, and no cytoplasmic foci were detected. 50% (11/22) of nuclei in 2.2.7 line showed RNA nuclear foci while fewer foci (30%, 6/20) were observed in 2.2.2 line. Non-transgenics showed 4% (1/25) foci like staining but failed to show colocalisation in the nuclei (Fig. 1c). It is presumed, that the single focus observed in the NTG zebrafish was due to non-specific binding of the in situ probe. To determine whether repeat RNA was translated into DPR proteins, antibodies specific to antisense DPR species poly-GP, PA and PR were used. All three antisense DPR species were detected in the nuclei of muscle cells from both 2.2-zebrafish lines (Fig. 2a,c,e) with over 50% of the nuclei expressing the DPRs (Fig. 2b,d,f).

C9orf72 zebrafish produce multiple distinct DPR species
The various DPR species are known to have differential toxicity, with arginine rich species being considered the most toxic. To investigate whether there is a relationship between molecular weight (MW) and species toxicity, western blotting was performed on zebrafish lysates. The transgene construct expressed in both 2.2-zebrafish lines causes the production of GFP tagged DPR proteins via canonical ATG (start codon) dependent translation. The full length GFP fusion protein is predicted to be 48 kDa while any truncation 3′ of any C4G2 repeats would result in the production of GFP alone (28KDa). The schematic of the GFP-DPR fusion protein is shown (Fig. 3a). GFP tagged DPRs are produced from C_4G_2 transcripts and can be detected at 5 dpf (Fig. 3b, left most panel). Interestingly, multiple GFP bands are detected in both the 2.2–2 and 2.2–7 zebrafish lines, and these bands were often unique to one zebrafish line or the other, and were consistent over > 10 clutches. The differential expression of DPRs between 2.2–2 and 2.2–7 zebrafish also holds true when probing for the DPR proteins directly (Fig. 3b, 3 right panels). The full length GFP-DPR fusion at 48 kDa was expressed but at low levels (Fig. 3b, 48 kDa band). Probing antibodies against DPR proteins also revealed that some DPR bands detected did not co-localise with any of the ATG-dependent translation bands detected using the GFP antibody, suggesting that these bands are likely to be produced via non-canonical RAN translation (Fig. 3b, three right panels marked with asterix).

In addition to the poly-PA, PR and GP DPRs produced from the (C_4G_2) RNA transcripts, we were also able to detect poly(GA) DPR produced from the (G_4C_2) RNA transcript, however poly(GA) was only detected in the 2.2–7

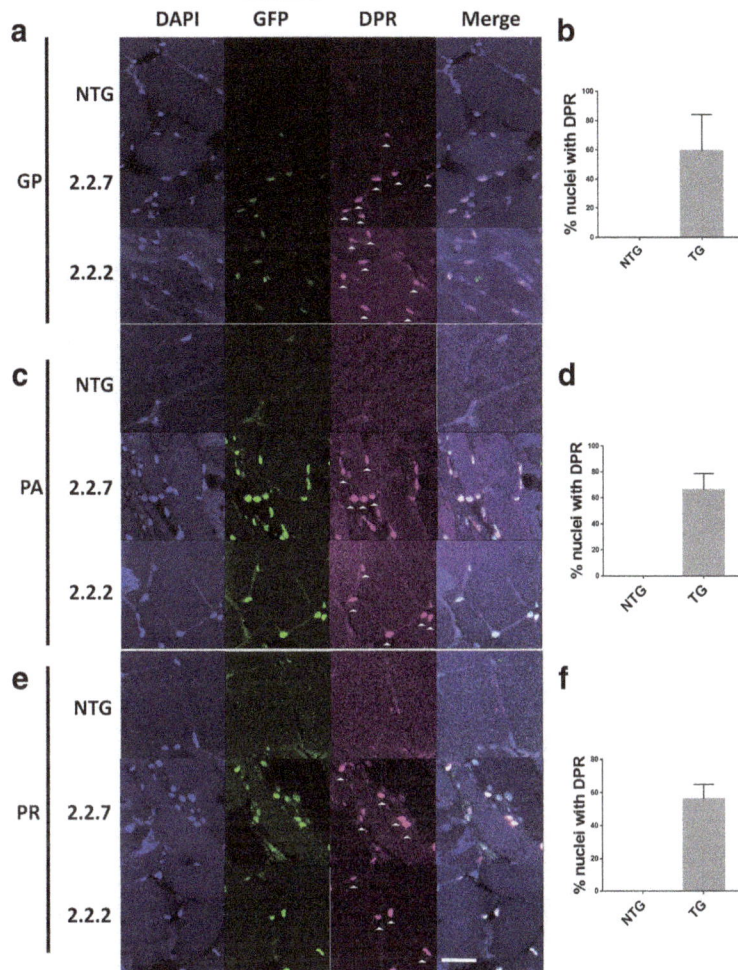

Fig. 2 C9orf72 model zebrafish display DPR expression in the nucleus. (**a,b**) Immunofluorescence labelling of adult zebrafish muscle tissue showed that poly-GP DPR protein localises to the nucleus in 2.2–2 and 2.2–7 transgenic zebrafish. (**c,d**) Immunofluorescence labelling of adult zebrafish muscle tissue showed that poly-PA DPR protein localises to the nucleus in 2.2–2 and 2.2–7 transgenic zebrafish. (**e,f**) Immunofluorescence labelling of adult zebrafish muscle tissue showed that poly-PA DPR protein localises to the nucleus in 2.2–2 and 2.2–7 transgenic zebrafish. For all DPR images nuclei are stained with Hoechst (blue), GFP is stained with GFP antibody (green) and DPR proteins are stained with the relevant DPR antibody (purple), white arrow heads denote DPR positive staining. Scale bar = 25 µm for all DPR images

zebrafish line (Fig. 3c). The detection of poly(GA) indicates that bidirectional transcription of the GC rich region is occurring in the presence of our transgene. As the transcription of the RNA transcript containing the (G_4C_2) expansion is not driven by a conventional promotor region, this strongly indicates that poly(GA) protein is indeed produced via RAN translation.

In human ALS, *C9orf72* associated toxicity occurs primarily in cells of the CNS, and so it is essential to ascertain whether DPR species are also produced within the CNS of this *C9orf72* model zebrafish. In adult brain and spinal cord of both 2.2-zebrafish lines, GFP-tagged DPR species and DPR species which were not immunoreactive with GFP antibodies (RAN translation bands), could be detected (Fig. 4). This suggests

that both ATG-dependent translation and RAN translation of DPR species occurs within the CNS of the 2.2-zebrafish.

In summary, both 2.2-zebrafish lines exhibit DPR species generated by conventional ATG-dependent translation and RAN translation in the muscle and the CNS. In addition, the 2.2–7 zebrafish line shows bi-directional transcription, producing DPR species from both G_4C_2 and C_4G_2 RNA transcripts. In both 2.2-zebrafish lines, the band pattern of DPRs detected largely remains constant from 5 dpf until adulthood, although higher MW (>50KDa) poly(PR) positive bands are more abundant in adult tissue. Of all the DPR species examined here, poly(PR) generally has the highest propensity to form high MW RAN-translation mediated bands.

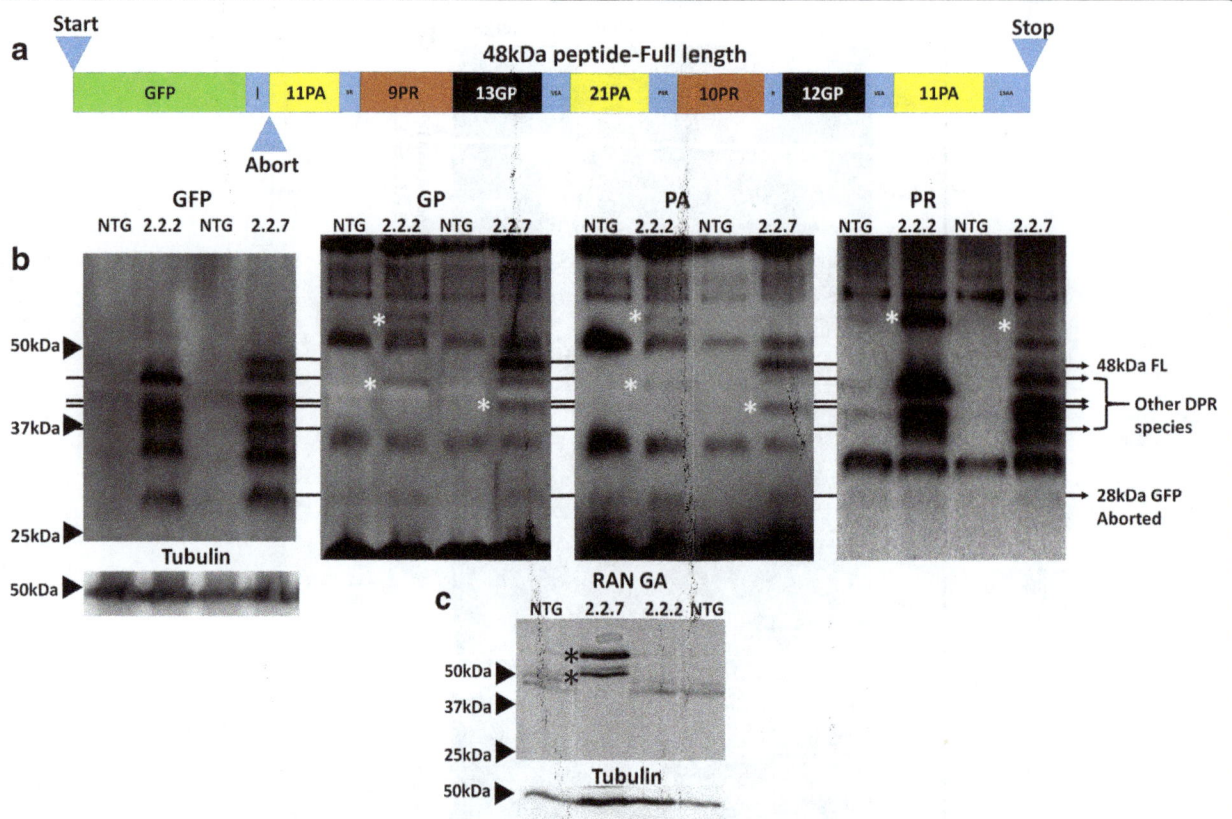

Fig. 3 *C9orf72* model zebrafish produce multiple species of DPRs from sense and anti-sense transcripts (**a**) Schematic of the GFP-DPR fusion protein produced by AUG driven translation. (**b**) Anti-sense DPRs (predominately ATG-driven) containing full length-GFP-DPR fusion, intermediate GFP-DPR fusion and GFP alone bands are detected in 5dpf embryonic lysates. Non-AUG driven GFP deficient RAN translation DPR are also detected in both 2.2.2 and 2.2.7 transgenic lines (Asterix) (**C**) Sense Poly(GA) DPRs (exclusively RAN-translation driven) detected in 5dpf embryonic lysates

Early mortality, altered swimming behaviour and reduced weight gain in transgenic *C9orf72* zebrafish

Neither 2.2-zebrafish lines showed any overt morphological abnormalities during embryonic development (0–5 dpf). At 5 dpf zebrafish begin to express a wider repertoire of behaviours, including more frequent swimming and independent feeding. For this reason, rigorous evaluation was performed on 5 dpf zebrafish to test for underlying motor and behavioural deficits. In order to test the spontaneous locomotor activity of embryonic zebrafish, we monitored 5 dpf zebrafish in 96 well plates using the Viewpoint behaviour monitoring setup. No significant difference was observed between the groups in the proportion of times transitioning occurred into slow or medium movements (Fig. 5a). However, a significant reduction in the proportion of transitions into fast movement was detected in 2.2–7 zebrafish, when compared to either NTG or 2.2–2 zebrafish (Fig. 5a).

As *C9orf72* expansions in human ALS cause a spectrum of both motor and cognitive deficits, we examined whether normal zebrafish behaviour was affected in

2.2–7 zebrafish at 5 dpf. Centre avoidance behaviour assays are a validated means of measuring willingness to explore in zebrafish [33], and are comparable to the open field test performed in mice. It was determined that 2.2–7 zebrafish were significantly less likely to venture into the centre of the well when compared to their NTG clutchmates (Fig. 5b+c).

To determine if the early embryonic expression of RNA foci and DPR impacted upon the viability of the *C9orf72* zebrafish, we carried out early (1–15 dpf) survival analysis. Heterozygous 2.2–2 zebrafish do not show any change in survival within 15 dpf as compared to NTG zebrafish (data from NTG clutchmates of all genotypes are pooled; Fig. 5d). However, heterozygous 2.2–7 zebrafish did show a significant decrease in survival within 15 dpf as compared to NTG zebrafish (Fig. 5d), but not in comparison to 2.2–2 zebrafish.

It was noted that during early development, the 2.2–7 zebrafish appeared smaller than their NTG clutchmates. At 30 dpf there was a significant decrease in total body weight of 2.2–7 zebrafish compared to their NTG

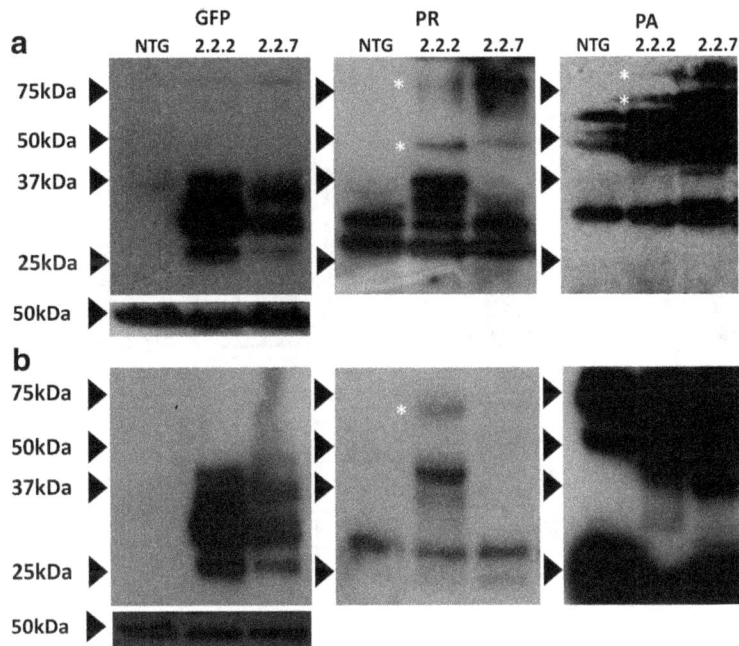

Fig. 4 *C9orf72* model zebrafish produce multiple species of DPRs in the adult CNS. (**a**) Anti-sense DPRs (predominately ATG-driven) detected in adult brain lysates. (**b**) Anti-sense DPRs (predominately ATG-driven) detected in adult spinal cord lysates. Asterix (*) denotes protein bands which are proposed to have been produced via RAN-translation

clutchmates (Fig. 5e). However, 2.2–2 zebrafish did not show a significant difference in body weight as compared to their own clutchmates at the same age (Fig. 5f).

In summary, 2.2–7 zebrafish but not 2.2–2 zebrafish, show significant reduction in survival at 15 dpf, and reduction in bodyweight at 30 dpf. At 5 dpf, 2.2–7 zebrafish also show defects in swimming activity and displayed signs of atypical behaviour. Behaviour of the phenotypically more severe 2.2–7 zebrafish was also studied through adulthood.

C9orf72 zebrafish display adult onset ALS-like behavioural phenotypes

To assess the neuro-muscular integrity of the 2.2–7 transgenic zebrafish, swimming endurance was tested using a swim tunnel, the aquatic equivalent to a treadmill [31]. At 9 months of age more 2.2–7 transgenic zebrafish failed to maintain swimming at the maximum flow rate as compared with their NTG clutchmates (Fig. 6a). Despite decreased body mass during early development, body mass and body size were not significantly different between adult transgenic and NTG groups from 9 months of age (Additional file 2: Figure S1). Spontaneous swimming was observed immediately following swim tunnel testing, but no difference was observed between the two groups (Fig. 6d). The swim tunnel test was repeated with the same cohort of zebrafish at 12 months of age, and the ability to swim at maximum speed continued to decrease in the 2.2–7 zebrafish (Fig. 6b). Interestingly, at 12 months

2.2–7 zebrafish now showed defects in spontaneous swimming behaviour following the swim tunnel testing. 12-month-old zebrafish showed an increase in the proportion of times transitioned into slow speed movements and a concomitant decrease in the proportion of times transitioned into fast speed movement, as compared to NTG clutchmates at the first-time point following swim tunnel testing (Fig. 6e).

Adult survival was also monitored from 8 months post-fertilisation onwards. By 17 months post-fertilisation, survival rates of the 2.2–7 transgenic zebrafish were significantly reduced in comparison to their NTG clutchmates (44% vs 100% survival respectively; Fig. 6c). A zebrafish was defined as having reached end-stage once it had lost the ability to maintain normal swimming (showing signs of paralysis) to the extent where it was no longer able to obtain food. End-stage 2.2–7 zebrafish displayed severe wasting in the body muscle region and had very poor locomotor skills (Additional file 3: video 1, no NTG zebrafish displayed this wasting phenotype.

Muscle atrophy and motor neuron loss in C9orf72 zebrafish

Progressive muscle atrophy is observed in all ALS patients. Similarly, end-stage 2.2–7 zebrafish muscle displayed widespread severe atrophy, muscle fibres were disorganised, and a large increase in nuclei was observed (Fig. 7a). The muscle of 2.2–2 zebrafish displayed more subtle changes, with myotomes being significantly smaller

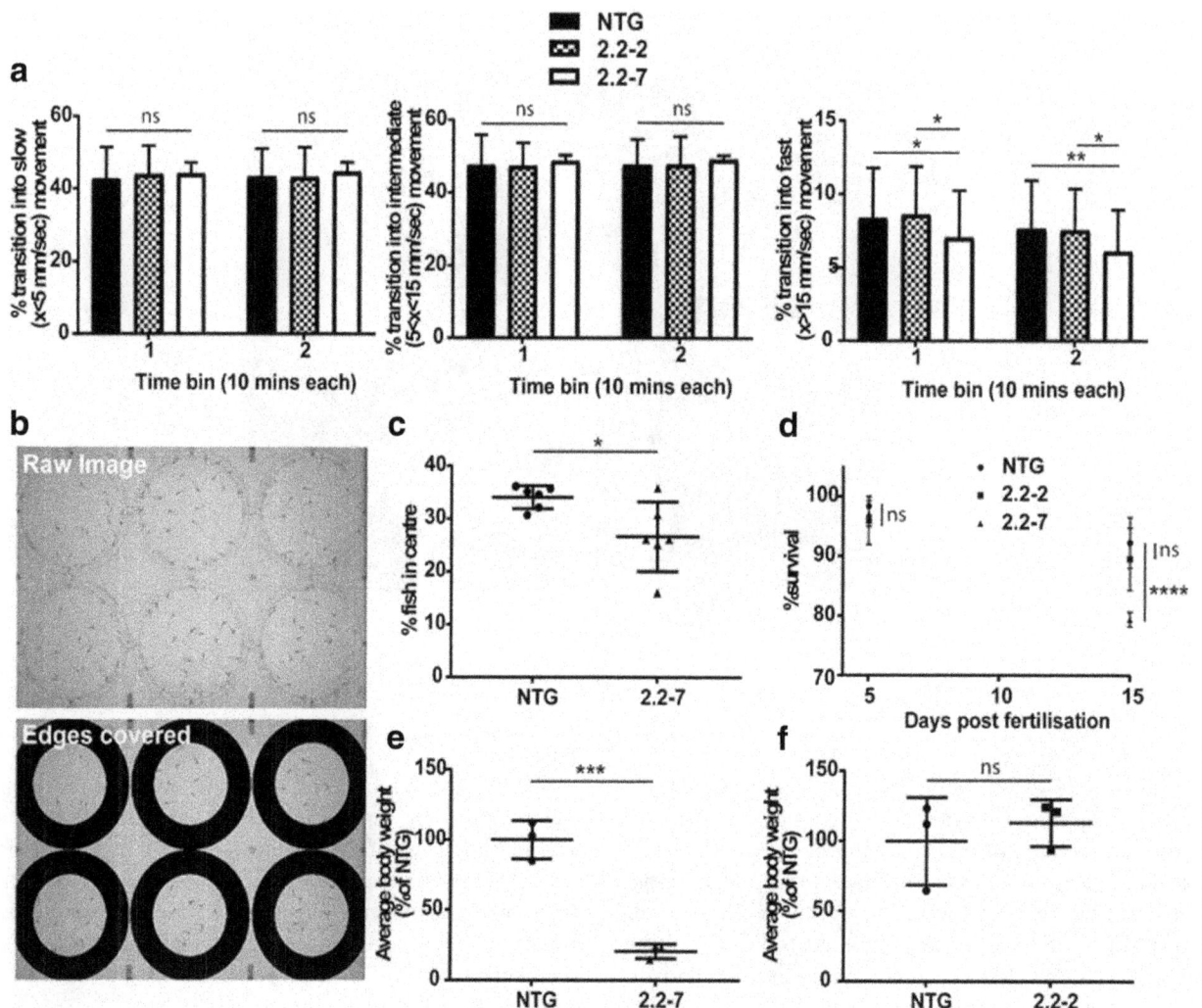

Fig. 5 *C9orf72* model zebrafish show early motor deficits, behavioural defects and reduced viability. (**a**) When kept under dark conditions, no difference is observed in the proportion of times fish transition into a slow movement (left) or intermediate movement (middle). However, the proportion of transitions into fast movements is significantly reduced in 2.2–7 zebrafish. $N = 60$ individual fish per genotype, from 3 different clutches. (**b**) Representative images of the plate set-up used to monitor centre avoidance behaviour in zebrafish. 30 fish were placed in each well and one image every minute was analysed. Image shown as recorded (top) and then following removal of the region around the edge of the plate for analysis (bottom). In these images 2.2–7 are placed across the top 3 wells and NTG across the bottom 3 wells. (**c**) Quantification of centre avoidance behaviour showing 2.2–7 zebrafish are significantly less often found in the plate centre. $N = 6$ clutches per genotype. (**d**) Survival of zebrafish did not change by 5dpf, however by 15dpf survival of the 2.2–7 line was significantly reduced compared to NTG. $N = 4$ clutches per genotype. (**e**) At 30dpf 2.2–7 zebrafish have reduced average body weight in comparison to their NTG clutch mates. $N = 3$ clutches per genotype. (**f**) At 30dpf there was no difference in average body weight between 2.2–2 zebrafish and their NTG clutch mates. $N = 3$ clutches per genotype. All data are shown as mean +/− standard deviation; $*P < 0.05$, $**P < 0.01$, $***P < 0.001$ and $****P < 0.0001$

and more numerous as compared to NTG muscle (Fig. 7a +b). We did not quantify end-stage 2.2–7 zebrafish muscle fibre size, as their myofibres were too disorganised to discern individual myotomes.

In ALS patients, the underlying molecular pathology ultimately leads to motor neuron death. Similarly, significant loss of ventral horn motor neurons was observed in end-stage 2.2–7 zebrafish as compared with NTG controls (Fig. 7c+d). A small, non-significant reduction in motor neurons was observed in 2.2–2 zebrafish as compared with NTG controls.

Heat shock stress response is activated by *C9orf72* expansions

Heat shock proteins are upregulated in response to the presence of aberrant cellular proteins [4, 10]. We hypothesised that the low-complexity structure of DPR proteins might drive activation of the heat shock response (HSR).

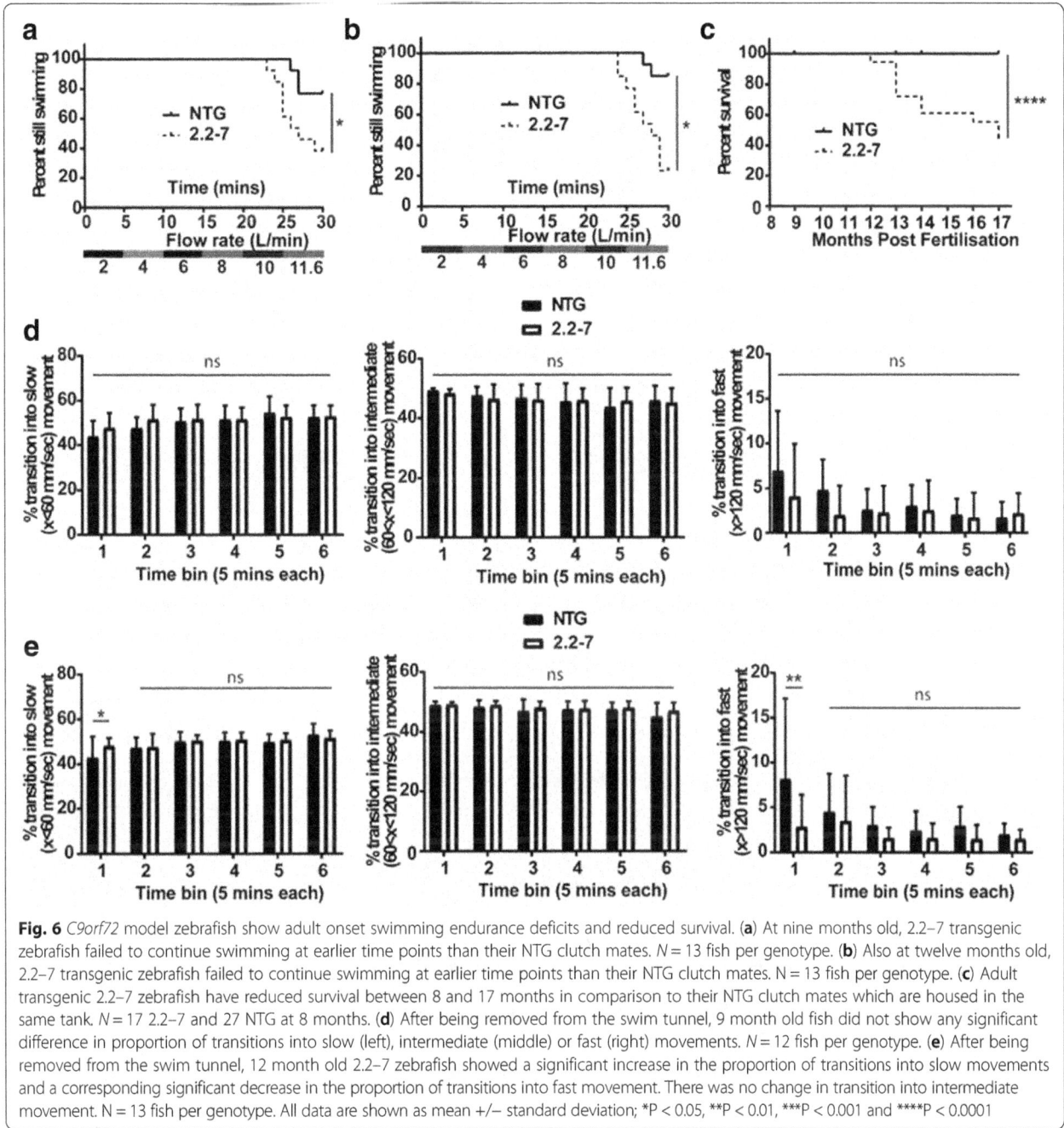

Fig. 6 *C9orf72* model zebrafish show adult onset swimming endurance deficits and reduced survival. (**a**) At nine months old, 2.2–7 transgenic zebrafish failed to continue swimming at earlier time points than their NTG clutch mates. N = 13 fish per genotype. (**b**) Also at twelve months old, 2.2–7 transgenic zebrafish failed to continue swimming at earlier time points than their NTG clutch mates. N = 13 fish per genotype. (**c**) Adult transgenic 2.2–7 zebrafish have reduced survival between 8 and 17 months in comparison to their NTG clutch mates which are housed in the same tank. N = 17 2.2–7 and 27 NTG at 8 months. (**d**) After being removed from the swim tunnel, 9 month old fish did not show any significant difference in proportion of transitions into slow (left), intermediate (middle) or fast (right) movements. N = 12 fish per genotype. (**e**) After being removed from the swim tunnel, 12 month old 2.2–7 zebrafish showed a significant increase in the proportion of transitions into slow movements and a corresponding significant decrease in the proportion of transitions into fast movement. There was no change in transition into intermediate movement. N = 13 fish per genotype. All data are shown as mean +/− standard deviation; *P < 0.05, **P < 0.01, ***P < 0.001 and ****P < 0.0001

To test this, we transfected both HEK 293 T and N2A cells with *C9orf72* expansion containing pure HRE and interrupted HRE constructs. The repeats were expressed in tandem with a *hsp70* promotor driving a DsRed gene, as a readout of heat shock response activation. As DsRed is more stable than hsp70, it allows more sensitive detection of small but chronic HSR activation [24]. In both HEK and N2A cells, cells transfected with 39 C_4G_2 pure repeats (left two panels) or 89 interrupted repeats (right sided panel) showed strong RAN-translated V5-tagged DPR or ATG driven PR-tagged DPR production and

markedly higher DsRed production (Fig. 8a). In contrast, cells transfected with only 2 C_4G_2 repeats displayed no RAN-translated DPRs and less or undectable DsRed production. As expected cells transfected with 39 C_4G_2 repeats but no *hsp70:DsRed* heat shock readout, produced abundant RAN-translated DPRs but no DsRed protein.

To assess differences in HSR activation in the more phenotypically severe 2.2–7 zebrafish vs the less severe 2.2–2 zebrafish, we screened 5 dpf zebrafish for DsRed (produced via *hsp70* promotor activation). The more severe 2.2–7 zebrafish showed significantly increased DsRed

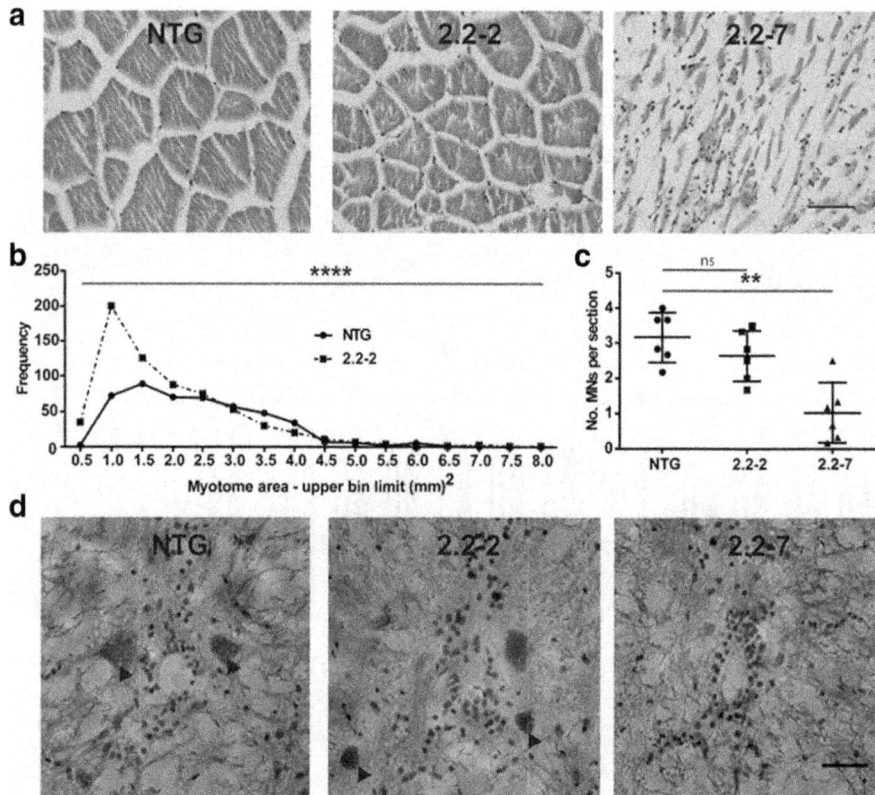

Fig. 7 *C9orf72* model zebrafish display muscle atrophy and motor neuron loss. (**a**) Representative H&E staining of zebrafish epaxial muscle (body muscle) myotomes. Scale bar = 50 μm. (**b**) Frequency distribution of 2.2–2 and NTG myotome sizes. N = 6 individual zebrafish per genotype. (**c**) Motor neuron counts show that 2.2–7 zebrafish have significant motor neuron loss compared to NTG. N = 6 individual fish per genotype. (**d**) Representative H&E staining of zebrafish spinal cord sections, motor neurons are denoted by arrowheads. Scale bar = 25 μm. Myotome size data are shown as the frequency of myotome sizes binned into defined ranges, motor neuron count data are mean +/− standard deviation; *P < 0.05, **P < 0.01, ***P < 0.001 and ****P < 0.0001

fluorescence in comparison to 2.2–2 zebrafish at 5dpf (Fig. 8b). Importantly, GFP fluorescence (from GFP-tagged DPRs) was not significantly different between 2.2–7 and 2.2–2 zebrafish (Fig. 8c).

To assess how HSR activation changes as phenotypic severity increases, we examined GFP and DsRed production in adult zebrafish brains, from 3 end-stage 2.2–7 zebrafish (ages 15, 15 and 19 months), 3 pre-symptomatic 2.2–7 zebrafish (all aged 7 months) and 3 NTG zebrafish (age matched to end-stage). Pre-symptomatic was defined as fish which did not show any overt swimming or muscle abnormalities. GFP tagged DPRs were increased in the brains of end-stage zebrafish in comparison to the brains of pre-symptomatic zebrafish (Fig. 8d+e). Similarly, DsRed also increased in the brains of end-stage zebrafish in comparison to the brains of pre-symptomatic zebrafish (Fig. 8d+f), thus suggesting an association between DPR production and HSR induction.

Finally, we examined whether HSR activation could occur in the presence of the DPR proteins in cerebellar post-mortem tissue from *C9orf72* ALS patients.

Cerebellum tissue was selected to study the effect of DPRs on HSR, as previous reports indicate cerebellum tissue consistently shows a high DPR load [2, 9, 21, 22]. Firstly, we confirmed that DPR species are expressed in the cerebellum of these C9-ALS patients (Additional file 4: Figure S2. Next, HSP70 protein levels in human cerebellum were assessed using western blotting. C9-ALS patients had significantly higher cerebellar levels of HSP70 as compared with non-neurological-disease controls (Fig. 8g+h). Taken together, our data demonstrate that *C9orf72* expansions activate the heat shock response.

Both *C9orf72* and *SOD1* ALS zebrafish models express a *hsp70* promotor which drives DsRed protein production. Cell stress from a variety of insults increases the drive on the *hsp70* promotor, and upregulation of the HSP70 protein has been reported in neurodegenerative disorders such as multiple sclerosis and, in the present study, ALS [19, 23, 27]. Therefore, in our ALS zebrafish models, the abundance of DsRed produced via hsp70 promotor activation is used as a

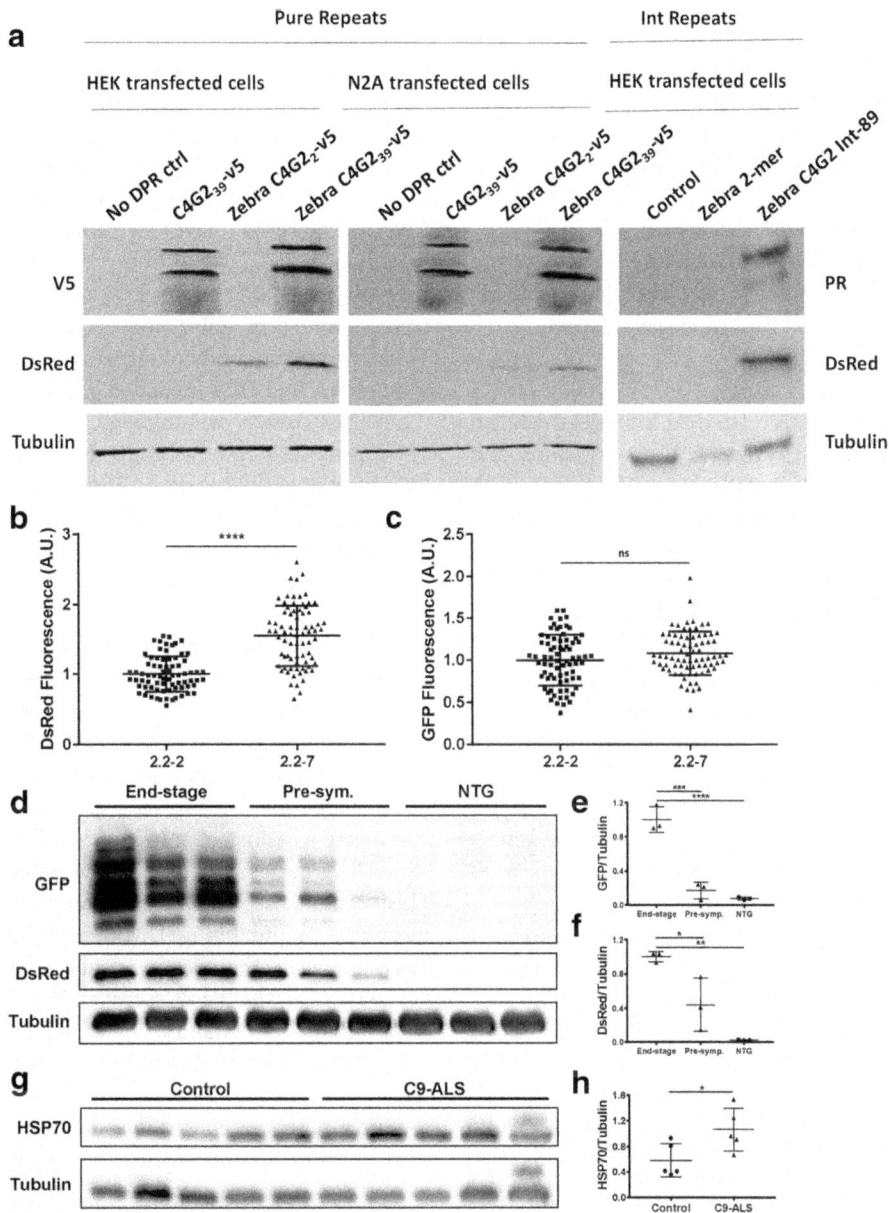

Fig. 8 Heat shock stress response activation is induced by *C9orf72* expansions. (**a**) In lysates from both HEK 293 T and N2A cell lines, DsRed levels are higher in cells transfected with 39 C4G2 pure repeats (Left and middle panel) or 89 C4G2 interrupted repeats (Right panel) compared with those transfected with only 2 C4G2 repeats. (**b**) At 5dpf, 2.2-7 zebrafish show significantly higher DsRed fluorescence than 2.2-2 zebrafish. N = 75 2.2-2 and 76 2.2-7 individual zebrafish. (**c**) At 5dpf, GFP fluorescence is not significantly different between 2.2-7 and 2.2-2 zebrafish. N = 75 2.2-2 and 76 2.2-7 individual zebrafish. (**d**) In end-stage 2.2-7 zebrafish brains, levels of GFP tagged DPR and DsRed proteins are increased compared with pre-symptomatic 2.2-7 and NTG. (**e**) Quantification of GFP tagged DPR protein normalised to tubulin in adult zebrafish brains. N = 3 adult brains per condition. (**f**) Quantification of DsRed protein normalised to tubulin in adult zebrafish brains. N = 3 adult brains per condition. (**g**) In human cerebellum samples, HSP70 protein levels are higher in C9-ALS patients as compared to non-neurological-disease controls. N = 5 samples per group. (**h**) Quantification of HSP70 protein levels normalised to tubulin in human cerebellum. All data are shown as mean +/− standard deviation; *$P < 0.05$, **$P < 0.01$, ***$P < 0.001$ and ****$P < 0.0001$

readout of cellular stress. Drugs which reduce cellular stress, and thereby reduce *hsp70* promotor mediated DsRed production can be identified by treating zebrafish with the drug from 2 to 5 dpf, and then measuring DsRed levels in a fluorescence plate reader [25]. To

date, thousands of compounds have been tested using this drug screening paradigm in *SOD1*-ALS zebrafish models (current authors, data not shown). Ivermectin is a compound which was identified as one of the most efficacious drugs in the *SOD1* zebrafish screen. In *SOD1* zebrafish ivermectin treatment reduced the level of HSR activation (as measured by DsRed fluorescence) to a similar degree as riluzole (the only disease modifying treatment currently prescribed for ALS; Fig. 9a). Thus, in C9orf72 zebrafish ivermectin treatment also resulted in a significant reduction of HSR activation, and compared with the SOD1 zebrafish screen, the efficacy of ivermectin was comparable to that of riluzole (Fig. 9b). Therefore, these data suggest that cross over between SOD1 and C9orf72 pathology may allow for a single treatment to be efficacious in both disease forms.

Discussion

We have generated C9orf72-related ALS model zebrafish which stably express interrupted C_4G_2 expansions and exhibit RNA foci and DPR pathology. These zebrafish accurately recapitulate key aspects of the behavioural, cognitive, motor defects and reduced survival associated with C9-ALS/FTD. Additionally, these zebrafish have been utilised to identify that poly(PR) DPRs form higher molecular weight species. Furthermore, these C9orf72 zebrafish were used in conjunction with human cell lines and human post-mortem tissue to identify that C9orf72 expansions activate the HSR. Finally, we identified that ivermectin treatment reduces cell stress HSR activation in both SOD1 and C9orf72 zebrafish models. The novel aspects of the C9orf72 zebrafish model we have generated here are compared and contrasted to other C9orf72 in vivo models in Table 1.

The zebrafish model presented here lends support to a gain of function as the toxic mechanism underlying C9orf72 ALS/FTD. Our data are consistent with several other studies in animal models showing toxicity mediated by RNA foci and DPRs [5, 20, 26, 38], including two independently generated C9orf72 zebrafish models [18, 28]. Furthermore, our data are consistent with four independently generated C9orf72 knock-out mice and one

knockout zebrafish model, none of which display any motor or neurodegenerative changes, arguing against haploinsufficiency as a major contributor to C9orf72 ALS/FTD [1, 13, 17, 35], (Schmid, Hruscha, Haass, unpublished). In contrast, decreased C9orf72 transcript levels have been reported in the CNS of G_4C_2 expansion bearing patients, and morpholino mediated knockdown of C9orf72 transcripts have been linked with motor deficits in zebrafish [6, 11]. However, morpholinos notoriously have off-target effects and may fail to mimic the phenotypes observed in stable knockout mutant zebrafish [16]. Thus, the current body of evidence is heavily weighted towards RNA foci/DPR mediated gain of function toxicity in C9orf72 expansion pathobiology.

Western blotting of zebrafish lysates revealed that multiple lengths of GFP-tagged DPRs are produced (including the predicted 48KDa full length peptide) producing a laddered appearance. Both sense and antisense DPR were detected and were produced by both conventional and RAN-translation. Detection of species of varying MW has also been reported during RAN-translation of CAG repeats [42], and during RAN-translation of GGGGCC in C9-ALS patients [43]. More RAN-translation mediated bands were detected in 2.2–7 zebrafish compared to 2.2–2. Interestingly, poly(PR) species were detected at higher MWs than other DPR species, and it will be important to investigate whether the tendency of poly(PR)s to form high MW species is related to the potent in vivo toxicity. This suggests that RAN-translation blocking agents aimed specifically at inhibiting HMW poly(PR) formation may be an important therapeutic avenue to pursue.

The more severe 2.2–7 zebrafish line showed embryonic onset motor defects and evidence of cognitive abnormalities, thus suggesting that DPR/RNA foci pathology is adversely affecting not only the motor unit, but also cognitive function; consistent with the spectrum of ALS/FTD in C9orf72 patients. Assessment of centre avoidance

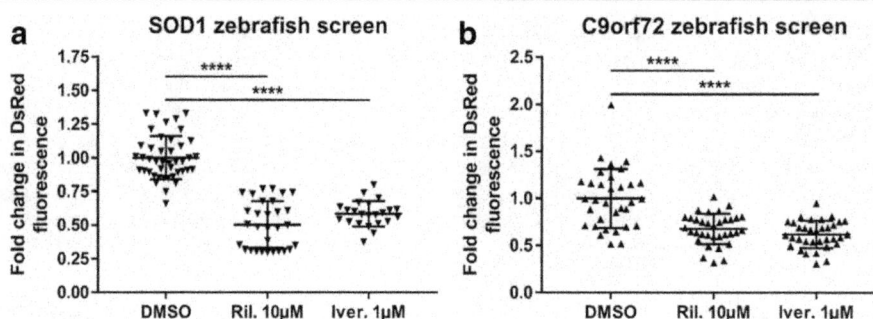

Fig. 9 Riluzole and Ivermectin modulate HSR in sod1 and C9orf72 zebrafish. (a) Treatment with either 10 µM riluzole or 1 µM ivermectin from 2 to 5 dpf resulted in a significant reduction in DsRed fluorescence in sod1 zebrafish, as compared to DMSO treatment. N = 30 riluzole treated, 23 ivermectin treated and 43 DMSO treated individual zebrafish. (b) Treatment with either 10 µM riluzole or 1 µM ivermectin from 2 to 5 dpf resulted in a significant reduction in DsRed fluorescence in C9orf72 zebrafish (2.2–7 line), as compared to DMSO treatment. N = 34 riluzole treated, 34 ivermectin treated and 33 DMSO treated individual zebrafish. All data are shown as mean +/− standard deviation; *P < 0.05, **P < 0.01, ***P < 0.001 and ****P < 0.0001

Table 1 Comparison of Stable *C9orf72* stable mouse and zebrafish mutants showing the distinct phenotype and utility of each model

DNA Construct	Species	RNA Foci	Sense RAN DPR	Antisense RAN DPR	ALS phenotype	FTD like phenotype	Stable or Transient	Phenotype amenable to drug screen	Efficacy of riluzole	Reference
BAC HRE	Mouse	Yes	Yes	No	Yes	Yes	Stable	No	Not tested	[14]
BAC HRE	Mouse	Yes	Yes	No	Yes	Yes	Stable	No	Not tested	[20]
BAC HRE	Mouse	Yes	Yes	No	No	No	Stable	No	Not tested	[29]
BAC HRE	Mouse	Yes	Yes	No	No	No	Stable	No	Not tested	[30]
C9 K/O	Mouse	NA	NA	NA	No	No	Stable	No	NA	[1, 13, 17, 35]
C9 K/D	Zebrafish	NA	NA	NA	Axonal growth defect	No	Transient	No	Not tested	[6]
C9 K/O	Zebrafish	NA	NA	NA	No	No	Stable	No	NA	[34]; (Schmid, Hruscha, Haass, unpublished)
C9 HRE	Zebrafish	Yes	No	No	No (Mild cardiac phenotype)	No	Stable	No	Not tested	[28]
C9-ATG GA	Zebrafish	Yes	No	No	No (Severe cardiac phenotype)	No	Stable	No (lethal)	Not tested	[28]
C9 -ATG HRE	Zebrafish	Yes	Yes	Yes	Yes	Yes	Stable	Yes	Yes	Current manuscript

NA Not applicable, *K/O* Knockout, *K/D* Knockdown, Grey boxes represents the features that represent similarity to human ALS/FTD or utility in the high throughput screening of novel therapeutics

behaviour indicated that 2.2–7 zebrafish showed an unwillingness to explore, similar to *C9orf72* mice assayed with the open field paradigm [20]. Early mortality is also observed in the more severe 2.2–7 zebrafish, indicating that motor and cognitive defects detectable at the embryonic stage later become severe enough to impact upon survival. Reduction in body weight was observed in 2.2–7 zebrafish at the larval stage, however this later recovered by adulthood, suggesting that the reduction was due to retardation of the growth process rather than tissue degeneration. Indeed, it is possible that slowed growth during early development of the 2.2–7 line may be due to the observed motor defects reducing access to food.

Swim tunnel performance of the 2.2–7 zebrafish was significantly poorer than that of their NTG clutchmates at both 9 and 12 months. Swim tunnel performance is mainly indicative of the neuromuscular integrity of zebrafish body muscle, however cardiovascular involvement cannot be ruled out. Small differences in spontaneous swimming behaviour observed at 9 months became significantly different at 12 months, indicating progression of phenotypic severity. Disease progression was also confirmed when the same 2.2–7 swim tunnel tested zebrafish displayed clear signs of muscular atrophy and became unable to swim, necessitating culling. None of the NTG clutchmates showed this progressive atrophic phenotype. By 17 months of age over 50% of the 2.2–7 zebrafish required to be culled, however most of the remaining zebrafish appeared healthy. This indicates a heterogeneity in progression of phenotype in the 2.2–7 zebrafish, and suggests that genetic, epigenetic or other

factors may modulate the disease phenotype. Indeed, this phenomenon may explain why the 2.2–2 zebrafish model present a less severe phenotype. Similar variability in phenotypic severity has previously been reported in BAC mice expressing the *C9orf72* gene [20].

Abnormal muscle histology was observed in both 2.2–2 and 2.2–7 zebrafish. Generally muscle fibres were smaller and more numerous in the transgenic zebrafish, consistent with atrophy and attempted regeneration. Significant motor neuron loss was also observed in 2.2–7 zebrafish and a trend in the same direction was observed in the 2.2–2 zebrafish. At this point it is not possible to determine whether the degeneration of the neuromuscular unit was neurogenic or myogenic in origin, and given that it is now known that DPR may transmit from cell to cell there may well be a contribution to toxicity from both tissues [41].

Previous transient RNA-injection zebrafish models suggest that G_4C_2 RNA is sufficient to cause activation of apoptosis and motor axonopathy [18, 36]. It is important to note that transient RNA-injection models express RNA in much higher concentrations than would be observed in stable animal models, therefore the observed pathology is less likely to be reflective of pathology under physiological conditions. The RNA-injection zebrafish were not characterised longitudinally as the transgene is only expressed transiently (typically for 1–3 days). Additionally, an independently generated stable zebrafish model has previously shown that 80 X (G_4C_2) RNA or poly(GA) DPR expression leads to pericardial oedema related toxicity at 4 dpf, but no neurological or motor phenotype was reported at any time point [28]. In contrast, over a comparable time period (5 dpf), the zebrafish presented here showed both motor and cognitive dysfunction. Additionally, our zebrafish model survived to adulthood and displayed adult-onset motor defects which eventually lead to motor neuron loss and death, thus recapitulating key features of human ALS/FTD over multiple time points. If model organisms are to be reliable in terms of the mechanistic insights or the therapeutic targets they generate, then they must reflect disease features accurately. Future models should include as many disease relevant features as possible until the exact mechanisms of *C9orf72* expansion toxicity are better understood.

HSP70 protein levels were found to be increased in C9-ALS patient cerebellar tissue. Consistent with previous reports, these cerebellum samples were found to have a substantial DPR load, thus DPRs may mediate cerebellar HSR activation [2, 9, 21, 22]. Activation of the HSR as measured by DsRed protein expression under the control of the *hsp70* promotor, was found to be higher in cells transfected with 39 C_4G_2 repeats compared to cells transfected with only 2 C_4G_2 repeats, thus indicating that *C9orf72* expansions of a pathological length are required for activation of the *hsp70* promotor. Additionally, activation of the HSR as measured by DsRed protein expression, was higher in 2.2–7 zebrafish compared with 2.2–2 zebrafish. However, in the same fish GFP fluorescence was not significantly different, indicating that the total amount of DPR in each of the 2.2-zebrafish lines is equivalent. The reason for a greater activation of HSR in 2.2–7 could be due to the differential pattern of DPR expression between the two zebrafish lines. Variability in transgene copy number is unlikely to underlie the difference in DsRed production between the 2.2–7 and 2.2–2 zebrafish, as GFP levels between the two are not significantly different. DsRed and GFP tagged DPRs also progressively increased in the brains of end-stage zebrafish, indicating that DsRed production positively correlates with both DPR production and disease severity.

Furthermore, *C9orf72* and *SOD1* ALS zebrafish models were both validated as good quality drug screening models by demonstrating reduced cell stress HSR activation following treatment with riluzole. More importantly, *SOD1* zebrafish identified the compound ivermectin as reducing cell stress HSR activation, and this finding was then mirrored in *C9orf72* zebrafish, further suggesting that there is cross over between *SOD1* and *C9orf72* pathology.

Conclusion

The stable transgenic *C9orf72* zebrafish model we have generated exhibits RAN-translation of DPRs, motor neuron loss, muscle atrophy, motor impairment, cognitive abnormalities and reduced adult survival. Thus, our zebrafish model accurately recapitulates the more complex aspects of human C9-ALS/FTD pathobiology, which is essential for studying the underlying mechanisms of ALS/FTD. In addition to all previous in vivo models of any species, our zebrafish model offers the unique benefit of being validated for screening of therapeutic compounds. Using this *C9orf72* zebrafish model we have identified novel insights into the pathogenesis of C9-ALS/FTD. Specifically, we identified that poly(PR) DPRs are RAN-translated into higher molecular weight species compared to other DPRs, which may explain the greater in vivo toxicity of this DPR species. Blocking formation of HMW poly(PR) proteins may therefore represent a novel therapeutic avenue. Additionally, we identified that the heat shock response is activated by *C9orf72* expansions, indicating that protein chaperone machinery may modify the disease course through a role in attempted preservation of protein homeostasis. Finally, by tandem drug screening with *sod1* and *C9orf72* zebrafish we identified that ivermectin may hold therapeutic potential in both of these forms of ALS. Rapid drug screening and validation of hits in zebrafish models of multiple ALS disease genes will be a powerful drug-discovery tool going forward.

Additional files

Additional file 1: Sequence of transgene injected to create C9-HRE transgenic zebrafish. (PDF 120 kb)

Additional file 2: Figure S1. Body mass and body length were not significantly different at the time of swim tunnel testing. (**a**) At 9 months old, body mass of the 2.2–7 and NTG zebrafish tested in the swim tunnel was not significantly different. $N = 12$ zebrafish per genotype. (**b**) At 9 months old, body length of the 2.2–7 and NTG zebrafish tested in the swim tunnel was not significantly different. N = 12 zebrafish per genotype. (**c**) At 12 months old, body mass of the 2.2–7 and NTG zebrafish tested in the swim tunnel was not significantly different. $N = 13$ zebrafish per genotype. (**d**) At 12 months old, body length of the 2.2–7 and NTG zebrafish tested in the swim tunnel was not significantly different. N = 13 zebrafish per genotype. All measurements were carried out ~40 min after removal from the swim tunnel (5 min rest, 30 min spontaneous behaviour recording and another 5 min of rest). (TIF 360 kb)

Additional file 3: End-stage 2.2–7 zebrafish video. (MP4 15919 kb)

Additional file 4: Figure S2. Poly(GA) and poly(GP) DPR proteins are produced in cerebellum of C9orf72 patients. (**a**) Dot blots of grey matter cerebellum samples from $n = 5$ control, sALS and C9orf72 patients each. Immunoblotting with an antibody against tubulin reveals mostly even loading amongst the numerous samples. Immunoblotting with an antibody against poly(GA) reveals that C9orf72 patients express abundant poly(GA) DPRs, whereas control and sALS samples do not. And immunoblotting with an antibody against poly(GP) reveals that C9orf72 patients express abundant poly(GP) DPRs, whereas control and sALS samples do not. (**b**) Quantification showing that in cerebellum grey matter, significantly higher poly(GA) signal is detected in C9-ALS samples in comparison to control samples, when normalised to tubulin. (**c**) Quantification showing that in cerebellum grey matter, significantly higher poly(GP) signal is detected in C9-ALS samples in comparison to control samples, when normalised to tubulin. Con: Control, sALS: sporadic-ALS, C9: C9orf72-ALS. (TIF 485 kb)

Acknowledgements

We thank Dr. Henry Roehl for providing the plasmid for Ubi cloning, and the staff at the Bateson Centre Zebrafish Facility for the maintenance of zebrafish. This work was supported by a Motor Neurone Disease Association (MNDA) Prize Studentship grant (Ramesh/Shaw/Oct14/875-792). PJS is supported as an NIHR Senior Investigator and by the Sheffield NIHR Biomedical Research Centre for Translational Neuroscience.

Declarations

Raw images and data of the figures and data represented in this manuscript is stored on hard-drives for permanent storage and additionally also stored on the cloud. These data will be available on request.

Authors' contributions

TR initiated and designed the project, TR, PJS and AH supervised and advised on the project, MPS, AH, AM, LMC, EJ, GMH and TR performed studies and analysed the data. MS wrote the manuscript and TR, AH and PJS edited the manuscript. All authors read and approved the final manuscript.

Competing interest

The authors declare that they have no competing interest.

References

1. Atanasio A, Decman V, White D, Ramos M, Ikiz B, Lee HC, Siao CJ, Brydges S, LaRosa E, Bai Y, Fury W, Burfeind P, Zamfirova R, Warshaw G, Orengo J, Oyejide A, Fralish M, Auerbach W, Poueymirou W, Freudenberg J, Gong G, Zambrowicz B, Valenzuela D, Yancopoulos G, Murphy A, Thurston G, Lai KM (2016) C9orf72 ablation causes immune dysregulation characterized by leukocyte expansion, autoantibody production, and glomerulonephropathy in mice. Sci Rep 6:23204. https://doi.org/10.1038/srep23204
2. Baborie A, Griffiths TD, Jaros E, Perry R, McKeith IG, Burn DJ, Masuda-Suzukake M, Hasegawa M, Rollinson S, Pickering-Brown S, Robinson AC, Davidson YS, Mann DM (2015) Accumulation of dipeptide repeat proteins predates that of TDP-43 in frontotemporal lobar degeneration associated with hexanucleotide repeat expansions in C9ORF72 gene. Neuropathol Appl Neurobiol 41:601–612. https://doi.org/10.1111/nan.12178
3. Boeynaems S, Bogaert E, Michiels E, Gijselinck I, Sieben A, Jovicic A, De Baets G, Scheveneels W, Steyaert J, Cuijt I, Verstrepen KJ, Callaerts P, Rousseau F, Schymkowitz J, Cruts M, Van Broeckhoven C, Van Damme P, Gitler AD, Robbrecht W, Van Den Bosch L (2016) Drosophila screen connects nuclear transport genes to DPR pathology in c9ALS/FTD. Sci Rep 6:20877. https://doi.org/10.1038/srep20877
4. Bukau B, Weissman J, Horwich A (2006) Molecular chaperones and protein quality control. Cell 125:443–451. https://doi.org/10.1016/j.cell.2006.04.014
5. Chew J, Gendron TF, Prudencio M, Sasaguri H, Zhang YJ, Castanedes-Casey M, Lee CW, Jansen-West K, Kurti A, Murray ME, Bieniek KF, Bauer PO, Whitelaw EC, Rousseau L, Stankowski JN, Stetler C, Daughrity LM, Perkerson EA, Desaro P, Johnston A, Overstreet K, Edbauer D, Rademakers R, Boylan KB, Dickson DW, Fryer JD, Petrucelli L (2015) Neurodegeneration. C9ORF72 repeat expansions in mice cause TDP-43 pathology, neuronal loss, and behavioral deficits. Science (New York, NY) 348:1151–1154. doi:https://doi.org/10.1126/science.aaa9344
6. Ciura S, Lattante S, Le Ber I, Latouche M, Tostivint H, Brice A, Kabashi E (2013) Loss of function of C9orf72 causes motor deficits in a zebrafish model of amyotrophic lateral sclerosis. Ann Neurol 74:180–187. https://doi.org/10.1002/ana.23946
7. Cooper-Knock J, Bury JJ, Heath PR, Wyles M, Higginbottom A, Gelsthorpe C, Highley JR, Hautbergue G, Rattray M, Kirby J, Shaw PJ (2015) C9ORF72 GGGGCC expanded repeats produce splicing dysregulation which correlates with disease severity in amyotrophic lateral sclerosis. PLoS One 10:e0127376. https://doi.org/10.1371/journal.pone.0127376
8. Cooper-Knock J, Walsh MJ, Higginbottom A, Robin Highley J, Dickman MJ, Edbauer D, Ince PG, Wharton SB, Wilson SA, Kirby J, Hautbergue GM, Shaw PJ (2014) Sequestration of multiple RNA recognition motif-containing proteins by C9orf72 repeat expansions. Brain : a journal of neurology 137: 2040–2051. https://doi.org/10.1093/brain/awu120
9. Davidson Y, Robinson AC, Liu X, Wu D, Troakes C, Rollinson S, Masuda-Suzukake M, Suzuki G, Nonaka T, Shi J, Tian J, Hamdalla H, Ealing J, Richardson A, Jones M, Pickering-Brown S, Snowden JS, Hasegawa M, Mann DM (2016) Neurodegeneration in frontotemporal lobar degeneration and motor neurone disease associated with expansions in C9orf72 is linked to TDP-43 pathology and not associated with aggregated forms of dipeptide repeat proteins. Neuropathol Appl Neurobiol 42:242–254. https://doi.org/10.1111/nan.12292
10. Dedmon MM, Christodoulou J, Wilson MR, Dobson CM (2005) Heat shock protein 70 inhibits alpha-synuclein fibril formation via preferential binding to prefibrillar species. J Biol Chem 280:14733–14740. https://doi.org/10.1074/jbc.M413024200
11. DeJesus-Hernandez M, Mackenzie IR, Boeve BF, Boxer AL, Baker M, Rutherford NJ, Nicholson AM, Finch NA, Flynn H, Adamson J, Kouri N, Wojtas A, Sengdy P, Hsiung GY, Karydas A, Seeley WW, Josephs KA, Coppola G, Geschwind DH, Wszolek ZK, Feldman H, Knopman DS, Petersen RC, Miller BL, Dickson DW, Boylan KB, Graff-Radford NR, Rademakers R (2011) Expanded GGGGCC hexanucleotide repeat in noncoding region of C9ORF72 causes chromosome 9p-linked FTD and ALS. Neuron 72:245–256. https://doi.org/10.1016/j.neuron.2011.09.011
12. Gijselinck I, Van Langenhove T, van der Zee J, Sleegers K, Philtjens S, Kleinberger G, Janssens J, Bettens K, Van Cauwenberghe C, Pereson S, Engelborghs S, Sieben A, De Jonghe P, Vandenberghe R, Santens P, De Bleecker J, Maes G, Baumer V, Dillen L, Joris G, Cuijt I, Corsmit E, Elinck E, Van Dongen J, Vermeulen S, Van den Broeck M, Vaerenberg C, Mattheijssens M, Peeters K, Robberecht W, Cras P, Martin JJ, De Deyn PP, Cruts M, Van Broeckhoven C (2012) A C9orf72 promoter repeat expansion in a Flanders-Belgian cohort with disorders of the frontotemporal lobar degeneration-amyotrophic lateral sclerosis spectrum: a gene identification study. The Lancet Neurology 11:54–65. https://doi.org/10.1016/s1474-4422(11)70261-7
13. Ji Y, Ugolino J, Brady NR, Hamacher-Brady A, Wang J (2017) Systemic deregulation of autophagy upon loss of ALS- and FTD-linked C9orf72. Autophagy 0. https://doi.org/10.1080/15548627.2017.1299312
14. Jiang J, Zhu Q, Gendron TF, Saberi S, McAlonis-Downes M, Seelman A, Stauffer JE, Jafar-Nejad P, Drenner K, Schulte D, Chun S, Sun S, Ling SC, Myers B, Engelhardt J, Katz M, Baughn M, Platoshyn O, Marsala M, Watt A, Heyser CJ, Ard MC, De Muynck L, Daughrity LM, Swing DA, Tessarollo L, Jung CJ, Delpoux A, Utzschneider DT, Hedrick SM, de Jong PJ, Edbauer D, Van Damme P, Petrucelli L, Shaw CE, Bennett CF, Da Cruz S, Ravits J, Rigo F, Cleveland DW, Lagier-Tourenne C (2016) Gain of toxicity from ALS/FTD-linked repeat expansions in C9ORF72 is alleviated by antisense oligonucleotides targeting GGGGCC-containing RNAs. Neuron 90:535–550. https://doi.org/10.1016/j.neuron.2016.04.006
15. Jovicic A, Mertens J, Boeynaems S, Bogaert E, Chai N, Yamada SB, Paul JW 3rd, Sun S, Herdy JR, Bieri G, Kramer NJ, Gage FH, Van Den Bosch L, Robberecht W, Gitler AD (2015) Modifiers of C9orf72 dipeptide repeat toxicity connect nucleocytoplasmic transport defects to FTD/ALS. Nat Neurosci 18:1226–1229. https://doi.org/10.1038/nn.4085
16. Kok FO, Shin M, Ni CW, Gupta A, Grosse AS, van Impel A, Kirchmaier BC, Peterson-Maduro J, Kourkoulis G, Male I, DeSantis DF, Sheppard-Tindell S, Ebarasi L, Betsholtz C, Schulte-Merker S, Wolfe SA, Lawson ND (2015) Reverse genetic screening reveals poor correlation between morpholino-induced and mutant phenotypes in zebrafish. Dev Cell 32:97–108. https://doi.org/10.1016/j.devcel.2014.11.018
17. Koppers M, Blokhuis AM, Westeneng HJ, Terpstra ML, Zundel CA, Vieira de Sa R, Schellevis RD, Waite AJ, Blake DJ, Veldink JH, van den Berg LH, Pasterkamp RJ (2015) C9orf72 ablation in mice does not cause motor neuron degeneration or motor deficits. Ann Neurol 78:426–438. https://doi.org/10.1002/ana.24453
18. Lee YB, Chen HJ, Peres JN, Gomez-Deza J, Attig J, Stalekar M, Troakes C, Nishimura AL, Scotter EL, Vance C, Adachi Y, Sardone V, Miller JW, Smith BN, Gallo JM, Ule J, Hirth F, Rogelj B, Houart C, Shaw CE (2013) Hexanucleotide repeats in ALS/FTD form length-dependent RNA foci, sequester RNA

binding proteins, and are neurotoxic. Cell Rep 5:1178–1186. https://doi.org/10.1016/j.celrep.2013.10.049

19. Lee YJ, Corry PM (1998) Metabolic oxidative stress-induced HSP70 gene expression is mediated through SAPK pathway. Role of Bcl-2 and c-Jun NH2-terminal kinase. J Biol Chem 273:29857–29863

20. Liu Y, Pattamatta A, Zu T, Reid T, Bardhi O, Borchelt DR, Yachnis AT, Ranum LP (2016) C9orf72 BAC mouse model with motor deficits and neurodegenerative features of ALS/FTD. Neuron 90:521–534. https://doi.org/10.1016/j.neuron.2016.04.005

21. Mackenzie IR, Arzberger T, Kremmer E, Troost D, Lorenzl S, Mori K, Weng SM, Haass C, Kretzschmar HA, Edbauer D, Neumann M (2013) Dipeptide repeat protein pathology in C9ORF72 mutation cases: clinico-pathological correlations. Acta Neuropathol 126:859–879. https://doi.org/10.1007/s00401-013-1181-y

22. Mann DM, Rollinson S, Robinson A, Bennion Callister J, Thompson JC, Snowden JS, Gendron T, Petrucelli L, Masuda-Suzukake M, Hasegawa M, Davidson Y, Pickering-Brown S (2013) Dipeptide repeat proteins are present in the p62 positive inclusions in patients with frontotemporal lobar degeneration and motor neurone disease associated with expansions in C9ORF72. Acta Neuropathol Commun 1:68. https://doi.org/10.1186/2051-5960-1-68

23. Mansilla MJ, Comabella M, Rio J, Castillo J, Castillo M, Martin R, Montalban X, Espejo C (2014) Up-regulation of inducible heat shock protein-70 expression in multiple sclerosis patients. Autoimmunity 47:127–133. https://doi.org/10.3109/08916934.2013.866104

24. McGown A, McDearmid JR, Panagiotaki N, Tong H, Al Mashhadi S, Redhead N, Lyon AN, Beattie CE, Shaw PJ, Ramesh TM (2013) Early interneuron dysfunction in ALS: insights from a mutant sod1 zebrafish model. Ann Neurol 73:246–258. https://doi.org/10.1002/ana.23780

25. McGown A, Shaw DP, Ramesh T (2016) ZNStress: a high-throughput drug screening protocol for identification of compounds modulating neuronal stress in the transgenic mutant sod1G93R zebrafish model of amyotrophic lateral sclerosis. Mol Neurodegener 11:56. https://doi.org/10.1186/s13024-016-0122-3

26. Mizielinska S, Gronke S, Niccoli T, Ridler CE, Clayton EL, Devoy A, Moens T, Norona FE, Woollacott IOC, Pietrzyk J, Cleverley K, Nicoll AJ, Pickering-Brown S, Dols J, Cabecinha M, Hendrich O, Fratta P, Fisher EMC, Partridge L, Isaacs AM (2014) C9orf72 repeat expansions cause neurodegeneration in drosophila through arginine-rich proteins. Science (New York, NY) 345:1192–1194. https://doi.org/10.1126/science.1256800

27. Mosser DD, Caron AW, Bourget L, Denis-Larose C, Massie B (1997) Role of the human heat shock protein hsp70 in protection against stress-induced apoptosis. Mol Cell Biol 17:5317–5327

28. Ohki Y, Wenninger-Weinzierl A, Hruscha A, Asakawa K, Kawakami K, Haass C, Edbauer D, Schmid B (2017) Glycine-alanine dipeptide repeat protein contributes to toxicity in a zebrafish model of C9orf72 associated neurodegeneration. Mol Neurodegener 12:6. https://doi.org/10.1186/s13024-016-0146-8

29. O'Rourke JG, Bogdanik L, Muhammad AK, Gendron TF, Kim KJ, Austin A, Cady J, Liu EY, Zarrow J, Grant S, Ho R, Bell S, Carmona S, Simpkinson M, Lall D, Wu K, Daughrity L, Dickson DW, Harms MB, Petrucelli L, Lee EB, Lutz CM, Baloh RH (2015) C9orf72 BAC transgenic mice display typical pathologic features of ALS/FTD. Neuron 88:892–901. https://doi.org/10.1016/j.neuron.2015.10.027

30. Peters OM, Cabrera GT, Tran H, Gendron TF, McKeon JE, Metterville J, Weiss A, Wightman N, Salameh J, Kim J, Sun H, Boylan KB, Dickson D, Kennedy Z, Lin Z, Zhang YJ, Daughrity L, Jung C, Gao FB, Sapp PC, Horvitz HR, Bosco DA, Brown SP, de Jong P, Petrucelli L, Mueller C, Brown RH, Jr. (2015) Human C9ORF72 Hexanucleotide expansion reproduces RNA foci and dipeptide repeat proteins but not neurodegeneration in BAC transgenic mice. Neuron 88:902–909. doi:https://doi.org/10.1016/j.neuron.2015.11.018

31. Ramesh T, Lyon AN, Pineda RH, Wang C, Janssen PM, Canan BD, Burghes AH, Beattie CE (2010) A genetic model of amyotrophic lateral sclerosis in zebrafish displays phenotypic hallmarks of motoneuron disease. Dis Model Mech 3:652–662. https://doi.org/10.1242/dmm.005538

32. Renton AE, Majounie E, Waite A, Simon-Sanchez J, Rollinson S, Gibbs JR, Schymick JC, Laaksovirta H, van Swieten JC, Myllykangas L, Kalimo H, Paetau A, Abramzon Y, Remes AM, Kaganovich A, Scholz SW, Duckworth J, Ding J, Harmer DW, Hernandez DG, Johnson JO, Mok K, Ryten M, Trabzuni D, Guerreiro RJ, Orrell RW, Neal J, Murray A, Pearson J, Jansen IE, Sondervan D, Seelaar H, Blake D, Young K, Halliwell N, Callister JB, Toulson G, Richardson

A, Gerhard A, Snowden J, Mann D, Neary D, Nalls MA, Peuralinna T, Jansson L, Isoviita VM, Kaivorinne AL, Holtta-Vuori M, Ikonen E, Sulkava R, Benatar M, Wuu J, Chio A, Restagno G, Borghero G, Sabatelli M, Heckerman D, Rogaeva E, Zinman L, Rothstein JD, Sendtner M, Drepper C, Eichler EE, Alkan C, Abdullaev Z, Pack SD, Dutra A, Pak E, Hardy J, Singleton A, Williams NM, Heutink P, Pickering-Brown S, Morris HR, Tienari PJ, Traynor BJ (2011) A hexanucleotide repeat expansion in C9ORF72 is the cause of chromosome 9p21-linked ALS-FTD. Neuron 72:257–268. https://doi.org/10.1016/j.neuron.2011.09.010

33. Schnorr SJ, Steenbergen PJ, Richardson MK, Champagne DL (2012) Measuring thigmotaxis in larval zebrafish. Behav Brain Res 228:367–374. https://doi.org/10.1016/j.bbr.2011.12.016

34. Stepto A1, Gallo JM, Shaw CE, Hirth F (2014) Modelling C9ORF72 hexanucleotide repeat expansion in amyotrophic lateral sclerosis and frontotemporal dementia. Acta Neuropathol. 127(3):377–89.

35. Sudria-Lopez E, Koppers M, de Wit M, van der Meer C, Westeneng HJ, Zundel CA, Youssef SA, Harkema L, de Bruin A, Veldink JH, van den Berg LH, Pasterkamp RJ (2016) Full ablation of C9orf72 in mice causes immune system-related pathology and neoplastic events but no motor neuron defects. Acta Neuropathol. https://doi.org/10.1007/s00401-016-1581-x

36. Swinnen B, Bento-Abreu A, Gendron TF, Boeynaems S, Bogaert E, Nuyts R, Timmers M, Scheveneels W, Hersmus N, Wang J, Mizielinska S, Isaacs AM, Petrucelli L, Lemmens R, Van Damme P, Van Den Bosch L, Robberecht W (2018) A zebrafish model for C9orf72 ALS reveals RNA toxicity as a pathogenic mechanism. Acta Neuropathol. https://doi.org/10.1007/s00401-017-1796-5

37. Tran H, Almeida S, Moore J, Gendron TF, Chalasani U, Lu Y, Du X, Nickerson JA, Petrucelli L, Weng Z, Gao FB (2015) Differential toxicity of nuclear RNA foci versus dipeptide repeat proteins in a drosophila model of C9ORF72 FTD/ALS. Neuron 87:1207–1214. https://doi.org/10.1016/j.neuron.2015.09.015

38. Walker C, Herranz-Martin S, Karyka E, Liao C, Lewis K, Elsayed W, Lukashchuk V, Chiang SC, Ray S, Mulcahy PJ, Jurga M, Tsagakis I, Iannitti T, Chandran J, Coldicott I, De Vos KJ, Hassan MK, Higginbottom A, Shaw PJ, Hautbergue GM, Azzouz M, El-Khamisy SF (2017) C9orf72 expansion disrupts ATM-mediated chromosomal break repair. Nat Neurosci 20:1225–1235. https://doi.org/10.1038/nn.4604

39. Webster CP, Smith EF, Bauer CS, Moller A, Hautbergue GM, Ferraiuolo L, Myszczynska MA, Higginbottom A, Walsh MJ, Whitworth AJ, Kaspar BK, Meyer K, Shaw PJ, Grierson AJ, De Vos KJ (2016) The C9orf72 protein interacts with Rab1a and the ULK1 complex to regulate initiation of autophagy. EMBO J 35:1656–1676. https://doi.org/10.15252/embj.201694401

40. Westerfield M (2000) The zebrafish book. In: A guide for the laboratory use of zebrafish (Danio rerio), 4th edn. Univ. of Oregon Press, Eugene

41. Westergard T, Jensen BK, Wen X, Cai J, Kropf E, Iacovitti L, Pasinelli P, Trotti D (2016) Cell-to-cell transmission of dipeptide repeat proteins linked to C9orf72-ALS/FTD. Cell Rep 17:645–652. https://doi.org/10.1016/j.celrep.2016.09.032

42. Zu T, Gibbens B, Doty NS, Gomes-Pereira M, Huguet A, Stone MD, Margolis J, Peterson M, Markowski TW, Ingram MA, Nan Z, Forster C, Low WC, Schoser B, Somia NV, Clark HB, Schmechel S, Bitterman PB, Gourdon G, Swanson MS, Moseley M, Ranum LP (2011) Non-ATG-initiated translation directed by microsatellite expansions. Proc Natl Acad Sci U S A 108:260–265. https://doi.org/10.1073/pnas.1013343108

43. Zu T, Liu Y, Banez-Coronel M, Reid T, Pletnikova O, Lewis J, Miller TM, Harms MB, Falchook AE, Subramony SH, Ostrow LW, Rothstein JD, Troncoso JC, Ranum LP (2013) RAN proteins and RNA foci from antisense transcripts in C9ORF72 ALS and frontotemporal dementia. Proc Natl Acad Sci U S A 110:E4968–E4977. https://doi.org/10.1073/pnas.1315438110

19

The physiology of foamy phagocytes in multiple sclerosis

Elien Grajchen, Jerome J. A. Hendriks[†] and Jeroen F. J. Bogie[*][†]ⓘ

Abstract

Multiple sclerosis (MS) is a chronic disease of the central nervous system characterized by massive infiltration of immune cells, demyelination, and axonal loss. Active MS lesions mainly consist of macrophages and microglia containing abundant intracellular myelin remnants. Initial studies showed that these foamy phagocytes primarily promote MS disease progression by internalizing myelin debris, presenting brain-derived autoantigens, and adopting an inflammatory phenotype. However, more recent studies indicate that phagocytes can also adopt a beneficial phenotype upon myelin internalization. In this review, we summarize and discuss the current knowledge on the spatiotemporal physiology of foamy phagocytes in MS lesions, and elaborate on extrinsic and intrinsic factors regulating their behavior. In addition, we discuss and link the physiology of myelin-containing phagocytes to that of foamy macrophages in other disorders such atherosclerosis.

Keywords: Macrophage, Microglia, Polarization, Neuroinflammation, Remyelination, Multiple sclerosis

Introduction

Macrophages are mononuclear phagocytes that reside in every tissue of the body in which they play a crucial role in maintaining tissue homeostasis. They fulfill this task by interacting with microorganisms, remodeling tissue, and dealing with injury. Alongside their role in protective immunity and homeostasis, they also contribute to the pathology of numerous disorders. Hence, there is considerable interest in harnessing phagocyte function for therapeutic benefit, either by suppressing the activity of disease-promoting phagocytes or enhancing the mobilization of phagocyte subtypes that are advantageous. Such interventions require a thorough understanding of the spatiotemporal phenotypes that phagocytes display during disease progression.

Multiple sclerosis (MS) is an inflammatory and neurodegenerative disease of the central nervous system (CNS) with unknown etiology. While initially regarded to be a lymphocyte-driven disorder, increasing evidence indicates that phagocytes, such as infiltrated monocyte-derived macrophages, CNS border-associated macrophages, and microglia, play an essential role in the pathogenesis of MS [14, 141]. Until recently, phagocytes were regarded to primarily cause lesion progression by releasing inflammatory and toxic mediators that negatively impact neuronal and oligodendrocyte integrity [152, 188], internalizing the intact myelin sheath [214], and presenting brain antigens to autoreactive T cells [68, 129]. However, this unambiguous concept has been challenged and it is now thought that phagocytes also have beneficial properties in MS. For example, clearance of damaged myelin is essential to facilitate CNS repair [137, 168]. Moreover, phagocytes release anti-inflammatory and neurotrophic mediators in CNS lesions and can suppress the disease-promoting activity of astrocytes and autoaggressive effector T cells [13, 18, 81, 167]. Of particular interest are myelin-containing foamy phagocytes as they make up the bulk of immune cells within active and the rim of chronic active MS lesions (Fig. 1 and [111]). Recent evidence has shed light on the many roles that these cells play in promoting and suppressing MS lesion progression, as well as the cellular mechanisms that drive their functional properties.

In this review we summarize and discuss 1) the mechanisms involved in the uptake and cellular handling of myelin, 2) the spatiotemporal phenotypes that foamy phagocytes adopt in MS patients, and 3) the intrinsic and extrinsic factors that impact the physiology of foamy

* Correspondence: Jeroen.bogie@uhasselt.be
[†]Jerome J. A. Hendriks and Jeroen F. J. Bogie contributed equally to this work.
Biomedical Research Institute, Hasselt University, Diepenbeek, Belgium/ School of Life Sciences, Transnationale Universiteit Limburg, Diepenbeek, Belgium

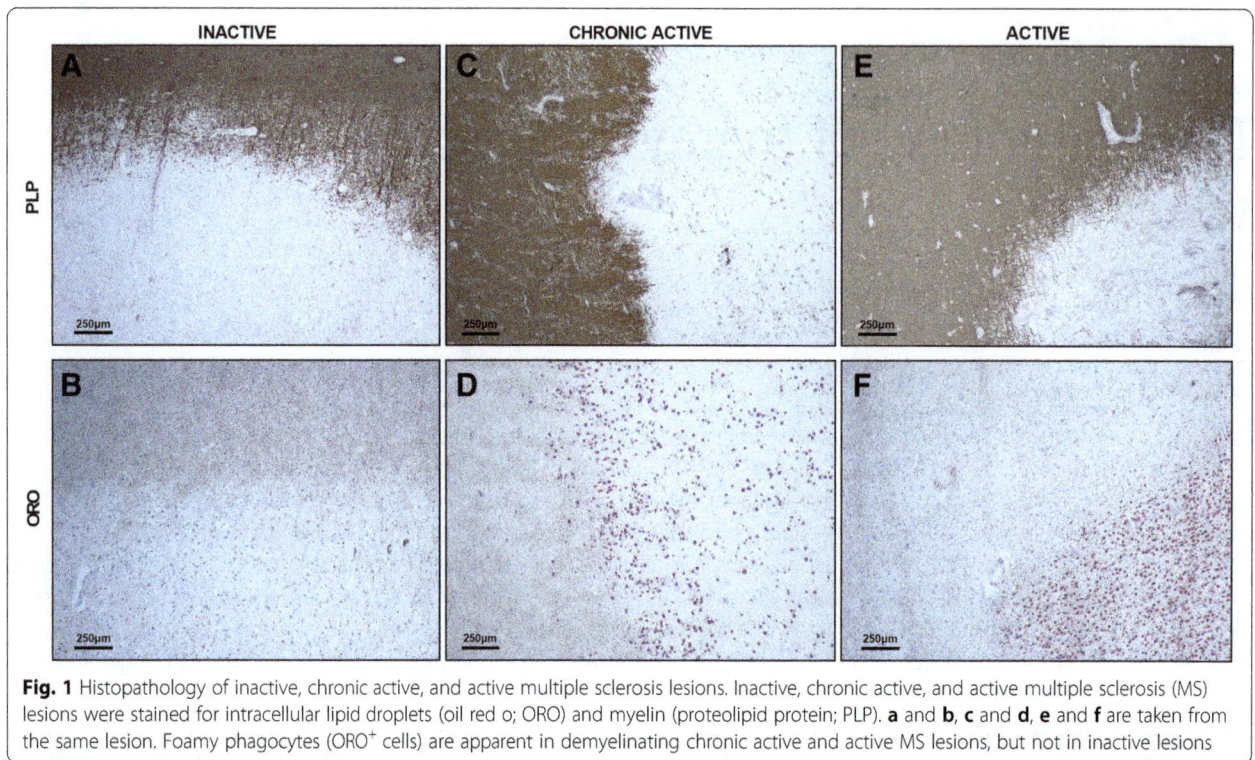

Fig. 1 Histopathology of inactive, chronic active, and active multiple sclerosis lesions. Inactive, chronic active, and active multiple sclerosis (MS) lesions were stained for intracellular lipid droplets (oil red o; ORO) and myelin (proteolipid protein; PLP). **a** and **b**, **c** and **d**, **e** and **f** are taken from the same lesion. Foamy phagocytes (ORO⁺ cells) are apparent in demyelinating chronic active and active MS lesions, but not in inactive lesions

phagocytes. In addition, we link the physiology of foamy phagocytes in MS to that of lipid-laden foamy macrophages in other disease such as atherosclerosis. Increasing evidence indicates that many parallels can be drawn between phagocyte subsets in various disorders.

To accomplish their functionally distinct roles in health and disease, tissue macrophages and monocyte-derived macrophages can differentiate into a spectrum of phenotypes [208]. The *ex vivo* induced M1 and M2 phenotypes represent two extremes. However, the phenotypes found *in vivo* substantially differ from these extremes. To designate the functional properties of phagocytes, we will utilize the term "M1-like" or "disease-promoting" for phagocytes that express pro-inflammatory mediators and promote MS lesion progression, and "M2-like" or "disease-resolving" for those that release anti-inflammatory and neurotrophic mediators.

Myelin internalization

The uptake of myelin by phagocytes is a pathological hallmark of MS lesions and other neurodegenerative disorders. The presence of foamy phagocytes is even used as an index of MS lesion activity [160]. Initial evidence that myelin internalization largely depends on receptor-mediated endocytosis came from the observation that myelin lamellae are attached to coated pits on the macrophage surface in an animal model for MS, experimental autoimmune encephalomyelitis (EAE) [47]. Clathrin-coated pits are sites where ligand-receptor complexes cluster

prior to internalization [66]. Since the discovery of receptor-mediated endocytosis of myelin, researchers have attempted to identify the culprit receptors involved in the uptake of myelin. To date, numerous receptors such as Fc, complement, and scavenger receptors are reported to drive myelin internalization. In this part of review, we elaborate on these receptors and touch upon cell extrinsic and intrinsic factors that influence myelin uptake by phagocytes (Fig. 2).

Fc receptors

The discovery of immunoglobulin G (IgG) capping on the surface of phagocytes located amongst myelinated nerve cells in active MS lesions was the first evidence for the involvement of antibody opsonization and Fc receptors in the internalization of myelin [162]. In line with this initial discovery, a follow-up study showed that parenchymal and perivascular phagocytes in demyelinating MS lesions display a strong expression of Fc receptor I (FcRI), FcRII, and FcRIII, while microglia in the normal-appearing white matter (NAWM) barely express these receptors [192]. Subsequent *in vitro* studies confirmed the contribution of Fc receptors to the internalization of myelin by showing that opsonization of myelin with anti-myelin or galactocerebroside antibodies profoundly augments the uptake of myelin by macrophages and microglia [140, 170, 177, 179, 190]. The amount of internalized myelin was further found to depend on the degree of opsonization and the myelin epitope

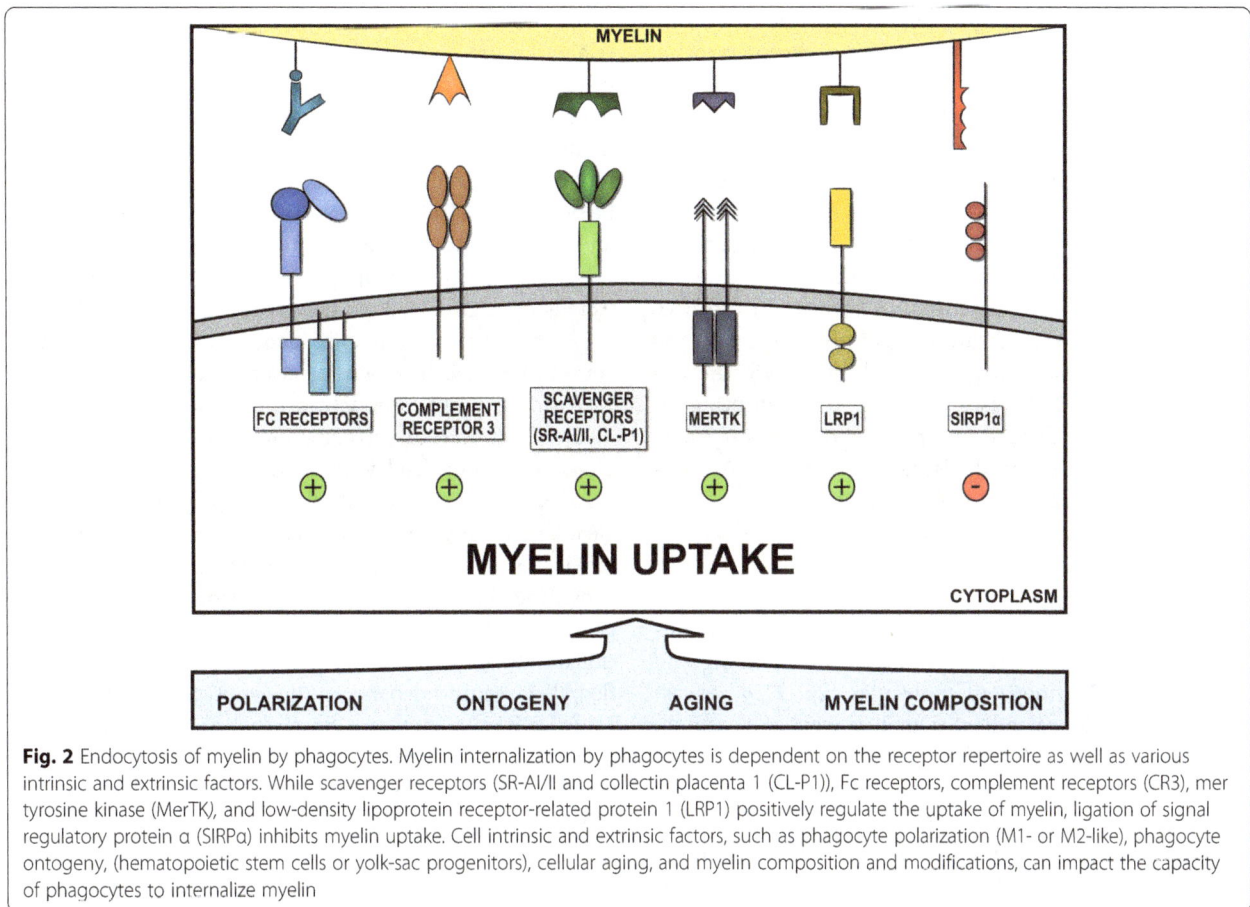

Fig. 2 Endocytosis of myelin by phagocytes. Myelin internalization by phagocytes is dependent on the receptor repertoire as well as various intrinsic and extrinsic factors. While scavenger receptors (SR-AI/II and collectin placenta 1 (CL-P1)), Fc receptors, complement receptors (CR3), mer tyrosine kinase (MerTK), and low-density lipoprotein receptor-related protein 1 (LRP1) positively regulate the uptake of myelin, ligation of signal regulatory protein α (SIRPα) inhibits myelin uptake. Cell intrinsic and extrinsic factors, such as phagocyte polarization (M1- or M2-like), phagocyte ontogeny, (hematopoietic stem cells or yolk-sac progenitors), cellular aging, and myelin composition and modifications, can impact the capacity of phagocytes to internalize myelin

recognized by the antibodies [64]. However, while anti-myelin antibodies are present in the circulation of MS patients [205], serum of MS patients does not opsonize more than that of healthy controls [65]. This can be explained by the existence of anti-myelin antibodies in the sera of healthy controls, as their presence is not limited to MS patients [205]. To date, the opsonic properties of the cerebrospinal fluid (CSF) of MS patients have not been determined yet. The presence of B cell-rich meningeal follicles in the CNS of MS patients argues for the presence of a local, more concentrated, source of myelin-directed immunoglobulins in the CSF [31]. Of interest, the microenvironment also affects Fc receptor-mediated uptake of myelin. While Ig treatment was found to increase Fc receptor-mediated uptake of myelin by macrophages in a sciatic nerve model, it did not increase myelin internalization by microglia in an optic nerve model, even after addition of macrophages [112]. Follow-up studies should define if the Fc receptor expression profile on phagocytes differs in these models. In contrast to FcRI, FcRIIa, and FcRIII, FcRIIb contains an immunoreceptor tyrosine-based inhibitory motif embedded in its intracellular domain [189], which might negatively impact myelin internalization after being activated. Collectively, these studies stress the importance of Fc receptors in the uptake of myelin but also indicate that Fc receptor-mediated uptake is fundamentally different in the central and peripheral nervous system.

Complement receptors

In addition to Fc receptors, ample evidence indicates that complement receptors are involved in the uptake of myelin by phagocytes. For instance, damaged myelin in areas of active myelin breakdown and within phagocytes colocalizes with complement components in MS lesions [2, 20, 21]. Similar, an increased density of phagocytes expressing complement receptors is observed in MS lesions [124, 204]. In particular, early studies found that the complement receptor 3 (CR3) tightly controls myelin internalization [23, 140, 164, 165, 178]. CR3 contributes to the uptake of myelin for up to 80% in the presence of active complement, while it was involved for 55-60% in the absence of active complement [164]. Counterintuitively, myelin clearance by macrophages from CR3-KO mice is not impaired [182]. A possible explanation for this discrepancy is that CR3 can both induce and reduce myelin phagocytosis at the same time. CR3 can reduce uptake of myelin by phagocytes through the activation of spleen tyrosine kinase (Syk), a non-receptor tyrosine kinase that phagocytic receptors recruit upon activation [70]. This Syk-mediated feedback mechanism was suggested to protect phagocytes from excessive intracellular accumulation of myelin. Collectively, these studies provide evidence that CR3-mediated uptake of myelin is more complex than initially regarded, being both inhibitory and stimulatory. Despite the latter studies, anti-CR3 antibodies reduce disease severity in the EAE model [85]. CR3 neutralization was found to reduce the recruitment of macrophages towards the CNS, thereby ameliorating EAE disease severity. It is tempting to speculate that a diminished phagocytic capacity may also underlie the reduced disease severity in EAE animals treated with anti-CR3 antibodies.

Scavenger receptors
Scavenger receptors are a large family of structurally diverse proteins, which are implicated in the binding and uptake of a wide range of molecules [26, 219]. A vast amount of evidence indicates that scavenger receptors mediate the uptake of myelin. By using an organ culture model of peripheral nerves and a monoclonal blocking antibody, the scavenger receptors class AI/II (SR-AI/II) were initially found to mediate the uptake of myelin by rat macrophages [36]. At high antibody concentrations, macrophage invasion of the nerves was completely abolished, emphasizing that SR-AI/II also regulates macrophage adhesion and migration [54, 176], similar to CR3 [54, 85, 176]. Follow-up studies further defined that SR-AI/AII blocking or knockout decreases myelin uptake by mouse macrophages and microglia [49, 164, 178], and that SR-A$^{-/-}$ mice show reduced demyelination and disease severity in the EAE model [115]. In MS lesions, SR-AI/II is highly expressed by foamy phagocytes in the rim and by ramified microglia around chronic active MS lesions [76]. This expression profile argues for the involvement of SR-AI/II in the uptake of myelin by phagocytes in MS lesions, and SR-AI/II being involved in early uptake of myelin by microglia. Aside from SR-AI/II, we recently showed that collectin placenta 1 (CL-P1), a novel class A scavenger receptor [26], also contributes to the uptake of myelin by phagocytes. In active demyelinating MS lesions, CL-P1 immunoreactivity colocalizes primarily with perivascular and parenchymal myelin-laden phagocytes. Finally, while evidence concerning its role in myelin clearance is still lacking, expression of lectin-like oxidized low-density lipoprotein receptor 1 (LOX1) is elevated at sites of active demyelination in MS lesions [76]. Future studies should define whether blockage of this class E scavenger receptor impacts myelin internalization by phagocytes.

Other receptors
Alongside scavenger, Fc, and complement receptors, several other receptors are implicated in the endocytosis of myelin. Recently, the mer tyrosine kinase (MerTK) was found to be a functional regulator of myelin uptake by human monocyte-derived macrophages and microglia [74]. MerTK belongs to the Tyro3, Axl, and Mer (TAM) receptor family and has a hand in the internalization of apoptotic cells [114, 158]. Of interest, apoptotic cell engulfment engages a vicious cycle that leads to enhanced expression of MerTK [142, 145]. This vicious cycle depends on the intracellular activation of the lipid-sensing liver X receptor (LXR) and peroxisome proliferator-activated receptor (PPAR). Previously, we showed that myelin-containing phagocytes (myephagocytes) also display active LXR and PPARβ signaling [11, 15, 126]. This suggests that myelin promotes its own clearance through an LXR- and PPAR-dependent increase of MerTK. The significance of MerTK in MS pathogenesis is evidenced by the fact that polymorphisms in the MerTK gene are linked to MS susceptibility [87]. While the functional outcome of these polymorphisms remain to be clarified, they seem to depend on the genotype of individuals at HLA-DRB1 [9], another MS risk gene [135]. In addition to MerTK, the low-density lipoprotein receptor-related protein 1 (LRP1) is an essential receptor for myelin phagocytosis by microglia in vitro [58]. In EAE and MS lesions, the LRP1 protein is highly expressed by phagocytes, providing evidence for involvement of LRP1 in MS pathogenesis [30, 58]. By using conditional knockout models, LRP1 deficiency in microglia but not macrophages was found to worsen EAE severity [30]. Increased EAE disease severity was associated with robust demyelination and increased infiltration of immune cells. While the authors provide evidence that microglia lacking LRP1 have a pro-inflammatory signature due to increased NF-kβ signaling, reduced microglial clearance of inhibitory myelin debris may also explain the observed effects. Collectively, these studies stress the importance of MerTK and LRP1 in the uptake of myelin by phagocytes.

The inhibitory SIRPα-CD47 axis
Aside from receptors that stimulate myelin internalization, phagocytes also express receptors that inhibit the uptake of particles. These receptors likely evolved to limit the uptake of 'self' antigens or as a feedback mechanism to inhibit excessive uptake of particles. With respect to myelin internalization, signal regulatory protein α (SIRPα), a membrane glycoprotein expressed primarily by phagocytes, represents such a inhibitory receptor. Interaction of SIRPα with the "don't eat me" protein CD47 on myelin decreases the uptake of myelin by macrophages and microglia [61, 73]. Of interest, serum also promotes an SIRPα-dependent decrease in myelin uptake irrespective of CD47 expressed on myelin [61]. A

potential mechanism could be the transactivation of SIRPα by soluble SIRPα ligands present in serum. In follow-up studies, SIRPα was demonstrated to inhibit myelin internalization by remodeling of F-actin and thereby cytoskeleton function [60]. Inactivation of the paxillin-cofilin signaling axis upon SIRPα activation underlies the impact of SIRPα on cytoskeleton function and myelin uptake. Of interest, the paxillin-cofilin signaling axis also positively regulates the uptake of myelin by the scavenger, complement and Fc receptors [60, 70]. These findings place paxillin and cofilin centrally in the process of myelin internalization.

Clearance of myelin debris

Whereas internalization of the intact myelin sheath fuels demyelination, ample evidence indicates that removal of damaged myelin debris at the lesion site promotes CNS repair. Early studies already showed that myelin contains growth inhibitory molecules such as Nogo A, which exhibit strong inhibitory effects on neurite growth and axonal regeneration [67]. Kotter et al. extended these findings by showing that myelin debris removal by phagocytes is a critical step for efficient remyelination [106]. Myelin debris was found to exert potent inhibitory effects on the ability of oligodendrocyte progenitor cells to differentiate into mature remyelinating oligodendrocytes [107, 159]. In concordance, by using the cuprizone- and lysolecithin-induced demyelination models, reduced uptake of myelin debris by macrophages and microglia resulted in inefficient axonal remyelination characterized with aberrant myelin patterns in vivo [113, 147, 168]. Collectively, these studies stress that clearance of myelin debris is mandatory for efficient CNS repair to progress or even initiate. Interestingly, a recent study defined that blood-derived macrophages and resident microglia have functionally divergent roles in myelin internalization. Macrophages were found to associate with nodes of Ranvier and initiate demyelination in the EAE model, whereas microglia appeared to primarily clear debris [214]. To date, the mechanisms underlying this difference remain elusive. Once identified they hold great promise for future therapeutics aimed at improving CNS repair in MS.

Cell intrinsic and extrinsic factors influencing myelin internalization

Phagocytosis is a dynamic process involving both structural rearrangements, complex signaling events, and a plethora of phagocytic receptors. Not surprisingly, diverse intrinsic and extrinsic factors are associated with alterations in the phagocytic capacity of macrophages and microglia. For example, ample evidence indicates that the polarization status of phagocytes drives their phagocytic capacity. With respect to the latter, phagocytosis of apoptotic cells, bioparticles, and oxidized low-density lipoproteins (oxLDL) is more robust in M-CSF, IL-4/IL-10, or M-CSF/IL-10 stimulated M2-like phagocytes as compared to GM-CSF, IFNγ, or LPS stimulated M1-like phagocytes [99, 196, 222]. The uptake of myelin also matches the phenotype of macrophages and microglia. Phagocytes stimulated with the anti-inflammatory cytokines TGFβ, IL-4/IL13, IFNβ, or IL-4/IL-13/IL-10 display a higher phagocytic capacity than naïve or LPS/IFNγ stimulated M1-like phagocytes [44, 74]. These studies indicate that cytokines in the microenvironment of MS lesions, and in particular the presence of those cytokines that drive phagocyte polarization such as TGFβ, IFNγ, IL-10, and IL-4, regulate the phagocytic features of phagocytes.

A number of studies further indicate that peripheral macrophages and CNS-derived microglia differ in their capacity to internalize myelin [44, 74, 112, 140, 178]. Microglia generally show a higher capacity to internalize myelin as compared to peripheral macrophage subsets [44, 74, 140]. Differences in macrophage and microglia ontogeny, being derived from hematopoietic stem cells or yolk-sac progenitors respectively, might well explain discrepancies in their receptor expression profile and phagocytic capacity [101, 173]. On that note, both the basal and inducible expression of MerTK and myelin phagocytosis are higher in microglia as compared to monocyte-derived macrophages [74]. Likewise, we recently showed that myelin uptake increases the cell surface expression of the phagocytic receptor CL-P1 by mouse and human macrophages, but not by primary mouse microglia in vitro [12]. Finally, in contrast to peripheral macrophages, immunoglobulin treatment increases Fc receptor density on microglia [112]. Collectively, these studies suggest that differences in the density of phagocytic receptors and/or activity of signaling pathways involved in driving the expression of these receptors underlie discrepancies in the phagocytic properties of macrophages and microglia. It is also noteworthy to mention that blood-derived macrophages associate with nodes of Ranvier and initiate demyelination, whereas microglia mainly clear myelin debris [214]. This study suggests that differences in myelin uptake might also rely on the presence of receptors that recognize cryptic myelin epitopes that are not exposed on intact myelin. As phagocytosis experiments are generally carried out using myelin debris, differences in the recognition of cryptic myelin epitopes by macrophages and microglia remain to be determined.

Another factor that impacts the physiology of phagocytes is aging. Several studies indicate that aged macrophages less efficiently internalize apoptotic cells [102, 212], bacteria [75], latex beads, and opsonized sheep erythrocytes [183]. By using toxin-induced focal demyelination in the mouse spinal cord, together with heterochronic parabiosis, Ruckh et al. demonstrated that aged blood-derived macrophages also clear myelin debris less efficiently as compared to young macrophages [168]. *In vitro* experiments using mouse macrophages and microglia and human monocyte-derived macrophages confirmed that aging impairs myelin debris clearance by these phagocytes [147]. The authors further show that reduced activity of the retinoid X receptor (RXR) signaling pathway partially accounts for the observed difference in myelin uptake between young and old phagocytes. Via which pathways RXR signaling decreases the uptake of myelin by aged phagocytes remains to be clarified. While loss of RXR can directly impact the expression of phagocytic receptors such as MerTK, impaired phagocytosis can also be a mere consequence of an inability to adopt an M2-like phenotype [100]. In a follow-up study, it was demonstrated that MS-derived monocytes show a reduced uptake of myelin irrespective of the patients' age [148]. This finding suggests that the disease state influences the phagocytic features of phagocytes in MS. It is tempting to speculate that premature innate immunosenescence, possibly due to chronic inflammation ("inflammaging"), impacts phagocyte physiology in MS patients. Increasing evidence indicates that premature aging of the immune system is apparent in MS patients [16]. Interestingly, in contrast to macrophages, aged human microglia do not show a reduction in myelin uptake compared to their younger counterparts [77]. This finding suggests that aging impact macrophages and microglia differently, and endorses the previously discussed phagocytic divergence between peripheral macrophages and CNS-derived microglia.

In addition to the polarization status, ontogeny, and aging, changes in myelin itself are reported to impact its uptake by phagocytes. Myelin isolated from MS patients is more efficiently internalized by THP-1 cells, a human monocytic cell line, and primary human microglia as compared to myelin isolated from healthy donors [77]. Enhanced uptake of myelin was not due to differences in the oxidation status of myelin. Further studies are warranted to define which modifications or changes in composition underlie the increased uptake of MS-derived myelin.

Collectively, these studies stress the complexity of myelin uptake by phagocytes, being dependent on the receptor repertoire as well as various intrinsic and extrinsic factors. Even more, while one should keep in mind that uptake of myelin debris is advantageous for CNS repair, uptake of intact myelin causes demyelination. Hence, *in vitro* studies using myelin debris should always be interpreted with caution before extrapolating to the *in vivo* situation.

Phenotype of myelin-containing phagocytes

Ample evidence indicates that myelin uptake changes the functional properties of macrophages and microglia. Some studies reported an M2-like phenotype of phagocytes upon internalization of myelin, whereas others described no effect at all, or even an M1-like activation status. In this section, we elaborate on the phenotypes of mye-phagocytes as well as the signaling pathways directing these phenotypes (Fig. 3).

The abundant presence of foamy phagocytes in MS lesions sparked interest at the end of the 20th century into defining the phenotypes of these cells. In line with the prevailing dogma at that time that phagocytes merely promote lesion progression, uptake of myelin was initially demonstrated to promote the release of substantial amounts of TNFα and nitric oxide (NO) by macrophages [194]. In agreement, myelin engulfment by adult human-derived microglia induced the oxidative burst and the release of IL-1, TNFα, and IL-6 [210]. Furthermore, exposure of M-CSF stimulated M2-like macrophages to myelin debris led to a significant decrease in the expression of M2 markers and increase in the expression of markers characteristic for M1-like macrophages [203]. These studies indicate that naïve as well as pre-differentiated M2-like phagocytes adopt an inflammatory phenotype after uptake of myelin *in vitro*. Also in *in vivo* models and MS lesions, several studies defined the presence of M1-like mye-phagocytes. In the spinal cord injury (SCI) model, the accumulation of M1-like phagocytes closely correlates with the intracellular presence of myelin-derived lipids [110, 203]. Kroner and colleagues extended these findings by showing that TNFα and iron are important determinants in inducing this inflammatory phenotype of mye-phagocytes as they prevent the conversion of M1- to M2-like cells [110]. Also within MS lesions, numerous studies have demonstrated the presence of disease-promoting phagocytes in actively demyelinating lesions [14]. Interestingly, in yet another study, myelin was found to modulate microglia differentiation with a biphasic temporal pattern. Especially during the first 6h after myelin uptake, microglia display an inflammatory M1-like phenotype. However, prolonged uptake of myelin (6-24h) quenches this initial inflammatory profile of mye-microglia [121]. The speed by which myelin induces the inflammatory phenotype suggests that it ensues after rapid activation of receptor-mediated signaling pathways, instead of relying on uptake and intracellular processing of myelin. In support of this hypothesis, the myelin-induced release of inflammatory cytokines by macrophages depends on CR3 and subsequent activation of the FAK/PI3K/Akt/NF-κB signaling pathway [182]. As scavenger and Fc receptors are also closely associated with inflammatory signaling cascades [117, 219], their involvement in skewing mye-phagocytes towards a more

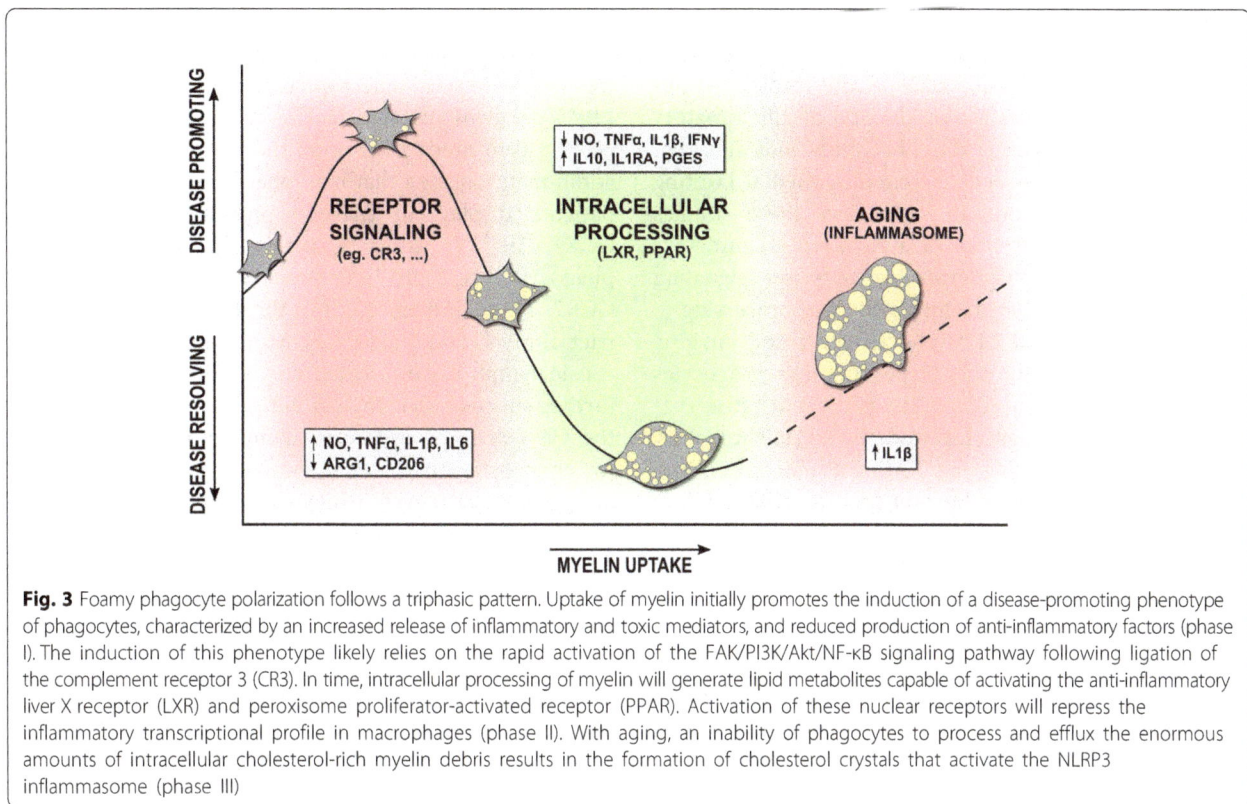

Fig. 3 Foamy phagocyte polarization follows a triphasic pattern. Uptake of myelin initially promotes the induction of a disease-promoting phenotype of phagocytes, characterized by an increased release of inflammatory and toxic mediators, and reduced production of anti-inflammatory factors (phase I). The induction of this phenotype likely relies on the rapid activation of the FAK/PI3K/Akt/NF-κB signaling pathway following ligation of the complement receptor 3 (CR3). In time, intracellular processing of myelin will generate lipid metabolites capable of activating the anti-inflammatory liver X receptor (LXR) and peroxisome proliferator-activated receptor (PPAR). Activation of these nuclear receptors will repress the inflammatory transcriptional profile in macrophages (phase II). With aging, an inability of phagocytes to process and efflux the enormous amounts of intracellular cholesterol-rich myelin debris results in the formation of cholesterol crystals that activate the NLRP3 inflammasome (phase III)

inflammatory phenotype merits further investigation. In summary, these studies stress that, at least for a certain period of time, mye-phagocytes display an M1-like phenotype.

While early studies predominantly defined inflammatory features of mye-phagocytes, more recent studies indicate that mye-phagocytes can also acquire anti-inflammatory and wound-healing properties. Mye-phagocytes in the center of MS lesions and in *in vitro* cultures express a series of anti-inflammatory molecules while lacking pro-inflammatory cytokines [18, 220], suggesting that myelin uptake polarizes phagocytes towards an M2-like phenotype. In agreement, exposure of macrophages to sciatic or optic nerves leads to the formation of mye-macrophages that display an unique M2-like phenotype [195]. Moreover, we and others demonstrated that mye-phagocytes show a less-inflammatory phenotype in response to prototypical inflammatory stimuli, suppress autoreactive T cell proliferation, and inhibit Th1 cell polarization [11, 13, 15, 110, 121, 198]. By using adult dorsal root ganglia neurons, conditioned medium of mye-macrophages even enhanced neuron survival and neurite regeneration [81], suggesting that myelin uptake also increases the neurotrophic features of phagocytes. While studying the phenotype of mye-phagocytes, care should be taken to prevent endotoxin contamination in myelin isolates. In one study, endotoxin contamination was found to induce insensitivity to LPS in foamy

macrophages [63]. Collectively, these studies indicate that myelin uptake can direct phagocytes towards an M2-like phenotype. This phenotype is shared by foamy phagocytes in other disorders, as discussed in the next sections.

Based on the assumption that myelin modulates phagocyte differentiation with a biphasic temporal pattern [121], the delayed anti-inflammatory phenotype switch of mye-phagocytes likely relies on intracellular processing of myelin-derived constituents. In line with this finding, we found that activation of the nuclear receptor LXR after myelin uptake and processing directs the less-inflammatory phenotype that mye-phagocytes display [15]. LXRs are well-known to repress an inflammatory transcriptional profile in macrophages. Moreover, LXRs are endogenously activated by cholesterol metabolites, which are abundantly present in myelin or can be formed after engulfment and processing of myelin-derived cholesterol [126]. Of interest, the deactivated phenotype of cholesterol-loaded macrophages in atherosclerotic lesions also depends in part on the LXR signaling pathway [180]. In addition to LXRs, we also showed that myelin-derived phosphatidylserine activates the fatty acid-sensing PPARβ/δ, thereby reducing the release of inflammatory mediators such as NO [11]. Similar to LXRs, PPARs can repress inflammatory responses mediated by NF-kβ in phagocytes. Active LXR and PPAR signaling in lesional phagocytes further emphasizes the key role that these nuclear receptors play in directing the phenotype of foamy phagocytes in MS lesions [11, 126]. Yet another study demonstrated that the p47–PHOX-mediated production of ROS after prolonged uptake of myelin represses the production of inflammatory mediators by microglia [121]. This study indicates that ROS drives a negative-feedback-circuit aimed at limiting microglia inflammation. In summary, these studies strongly suggest that the delayed anti-inflammatory phenotype of mye-phagocytes depends on signaling pathways activated after myelin uptake and processing.

Similar to the uptake of myelin, extrinsic and intrinsic factors can influence the phenotypes that mye-phagocytes adopt. For instance, a recent study demonstrated that aging skews mye-phagocytes towards an inflammatory phenotype [27]. By using the EAE and cuprizone- and lysolecithin-induced demyelination models, inflammatory foam cells harbouring large amounts of lysosomal free cholesterol were observed in old mice. An inability of aged phagocytes to process and efflux the high amounts of intracellular cholesterol-rich myelin debris appeared to underlie the accumulation of lysosomal cholesterol. In time, the accumulation of free cholesterol resulted in the formation of cholesterol crystals, which induced lysosomal rupture and activated the NLRP3 inflammasome. This study suggests that the phenotypes that foamy phagocytes display in aged individuals might even be triphasic. In addition to aging, spatiotemporal-dependent differences in the presence of cytokines are likely to impact the phenotype of mye-phagocytes differently. Future studies should define the precise cytokine milieu in active and chronic active MS lesions and determine the impact of the most abundantly expressed cytokines on the functional properties of mye-phagocytes. Finally, while both macrophages and microglia change their phenotype in a similar fashion upon myelin internalization, ontogenic differences may impact the degree of expression of the characteristic M1 and M2 markers. With respect to the latter, subtle differences have been noted in the polarization of both cell types in response to LPS, IFNγ, IL-4, and IL-13 in vitro [44, 59]. In depth genomic and proteomic profiling experiments may unravel differences in the phenotypes that macrophages and microglia adopt upon myelin internalization.

Myelin-containing phagocytes in secondary lymphoid organs

While abundantly present in MS lesions, few studies demonstrated the presence of mye-phagocytes in the CNS-draining lymphoid organs of MS patients and EAE animals. De Vos et al. observed a redistribution of myelin antigens from brain lesions to cervical lymph nodes (CLNs) in primate EAE models and MS patients [38]. Antigens were found in phagocytic cells expressing MHC class II and costimulatory molecules, which were

located directly juxtaposed to T cells. Likewise, by using ultrasound guided fine needle aspiration biopsy to extract cells in vivo, macrophages containing MBP and PLP were demonstrated in CLN of MS patients [51]. A more recent study confirmed the latter two studies and additionally showed that mye-phagocytes in CLNs of MS patients display an M2-like phenotype and express CCR7 [197]. In contrast, neuronal antigen-containing phagocytes were pro-inflammatory and did not express CCR7. These findings confirm the anti-inflammatory impact of myelin on phagocytes. Moreover, as CCR7 is crucial in lymph node-directed chemotaxis [32], this study further suggests that myelin antigens are transported to the CNS-draining secondary lymph nodes after uptake by phagocytes that subsequently migrate to CLNs by chemotaxis. However, while the increase in CCR7 on mye-phagocytes was functional in vitro [199], CCR7 deficiency did not alter the number of myelin-containing cells in CLNs of EAE mice compared to WT mice [197]. This implies that other chemokine receptors are involved or that myelin antigens are transported to CNS-draining lymph nodes as soluble antigens. Of interest, the recently described lymphatic vasculature in the CNS, which is connected to the deep CLNs, may lend myelin or mye-phagocytes easy access to CNS-draining lymph nodes [123]. With respect to the latter, myelin antigens and mye-phagocytes are apparent in the CSF of MS patients [105, 153], which is drained by the lymphatic vessels lining the dural sinuses [123]. Finally, after selective killing of oligodendrocytes in an in vivo animal model, a significant increase in intracellular lipids was found in deep CLNs, evidenced by increased Oil Red O (ORO) reactivity [122]. ORO reactivity represented intracellular myelin, as the authors also detected increased MBP and MOG levels in lumbar lymph nodes. Altogether these studies indicate that CNS demyelination coincides with the accumulation of mye-phagocytes within CNS-draining lymph nodes. How myelin antigens gain excess to these lymphoid organs, either after uptake by phagocytes that migrate by chemotaxis or as soluble particles, remains to be clarified.

To date, the pathological impact of mye-phagocytes in CNS-draining lymph nodes remains ambiguous. Mye-phagocytes in secondary lymphoid organs may present myelin antigens to autoreactive T cells, thereby driving epitope spreading and MS disease progression or even initiation [181]. Especially considering that they are located directly juxtaposed to T cells and express MHC class II and costimulatory molecules [18, 38, 50, 198]. Moreover, cervical lymphadenectomy reduces the level of brain lesions in cryolesion-enhanced EAE in rats [157]. This argues for a key role of CLNs in the induction of EAE, possibly as a site for T cell priming. In support of an immunostimulatory role of mye-phagocytes, human mye-macrophages were found to promote CD4$^+$ and CD8$^+$ T cell proliferation in an allogeneic mixed lymphocyte reaction and a recall response against influenza virus [198]. Macrophages treated with oxidized LDL and LDL did not impact lymphocyte proliferation, suggesting that the immunostimulatory impact is specific for myelin and not merely a hallmark of foam cells in general. Interestingly, the authors also show that mouse mye-phagocytes reduce the release of IFNγ by Th1 cells and that MOG-pulsed mye-macrophages suppress EAE severity. The latter indicates that mye-phagocytes in CLNs are not only aggressors in MS pathogenesis but can also dampen T cell-induced autoimmunity in MS. Supportive of this notion, CLNs are reported to be instrumental in the induction of intranasally induced immunological tolerance [211]. We further showed that mye-macrophages inhibit TCR-triggered lymphocyte proliferation in an antigen-independent manner in vitro [13]. Inhibition of T cell proliferation depended on direct contact between both cell types and the release of NO by mye-phagocytes. Interestingly, while mye-phagocytes reduced proliferation of non-myelin reactive T cells in vivo, they increased myelin-reactive T cell proliferation and worsened EAE severity. These findings suggest that mye-macrophages can both limit and promote T cell-induced neuroinflammation, depending on the TCR-specificity of surrounding T cells. Of note, lymph node resident CD169$^+$ macrophages activate invariant natural killer T (iNKT) cells by presenting lipid antigens in a CD1d-dependent manner [3]. CD1d-restricted iNKT cells and lipid-reactive non-invariant T cells reduce neuroinflammation [39, 90]. As myelin is rich in lipids, the capacity of mye-phagocytes to activate these immune cells merits further investigation. Collectively, these studies highlight the pleiotropic impact that mye-phagocytes in CNS-draining lymph nodes may have on T cell-mediated autoimmunity in MS.

To what extent extrinsic and intrinsic factors influence the accumulation and antigen presenting capacity of mye-phagocytes in CNS lymph nodes remains to be determined. Interestingly, aging negatively impacts phagocyte migration and their antigen presenting capacity [37, 80], and therefore might well alter the ability of mye-phagocytes to home to secondary lymph nodes and present myelin-derived antigens [37]. In addition, motility seems to be differently regulated in macrophages and microglia [132], suggesting that ontogenic differences might also be involved. On that note, while both macrophages and microglia express CCR7 [42, 199], differences in the expression of other chemokine receptors such as CX3CR1 and CCR2 are reported between microglia and specific peripheral monocyte subsets [14]. Interestingly, the transmembrane chemokine CX3CL1 is induced in inflamed lymphatic endothelium and dendritic cell-specific deletion

of CX3CR1 markedly delays lymphatic trafficking [94]. These findings suggest that CX3CR1^{hi} microglia are more prone to home to secondary lymph nodes in MS than CX3CR1^{lo} monocyte subsets. However, more research is warranted to certify the abovementioned claims.

Parallels with foamy macrophages in other disorders

Myelin-containing phagocytes are a pathological hallmark of CNS disorders such as MS. However, foamy macrophages packed with lipid bodies are also abundantly present in many peripheral pathologies associated with chronic inflammation, such as atherosclerosis and non-alcoholic steatohepatitis (NASH), and following infections with persistent pathogens like *Mycobacterium tuberculosis* (Mtb), *Chlamydia pneumoniae*, and *Toxoplasma gondii* [98, 139, 161, 169, 213]. Especially in atherosclerosis, foamy macrophage physiology has been thoroughly investigated. In atherosclerotic lesions, macrophages acquire a foamy appearance through the uptake and degradation of native and modified lipoproteins, such as oxLDL. Generally, macrophages are well equipped to cope with minor intracellular increases of LDL. However, sustained intracellular accumulation of LDL-derived lipids leads to disturbances in pathways that mediate the degradation, storage, and efflux of these lipids. As a consequence, macrophages become engorged with lipids and obtain a disease-promoting phenotype. In this section, we discuss and link the malfunctioning of these pathways to the development and physiology of phagocytes that internalized the lipid-rich myelin sheath (Fig. 4).

Uncontrolled internalization of myelin

In atherosclerosis, the swift removal of modified LDL from the intima provides protection against its cytotoxic and damaging effects. However, continuous uptake of modified LDL by macrophages also promotes the formation of inflammatory, lipid-engorged, foamy macrophages, which eventually may be an even more harmful event. Diverse studies suggest that feedback regulation of receptors involved in the uptake of modified LDL goes awry in atherosclerosis. For example, the expression of receptors involved in the uptake of modified LDL, such as CD36 and SR-A, remains high throughout lesion development in atherosclerosis [138]. Similar to atherosclerosis, uptake of myelin may also be a continuous process in neurodegenerative disorders. This is supported by the finding that the expression of receptors involved in the uptake of myelin, such as FcRIII, SR-AI/II, and MerTK, is elevated in active MS lesions [76, 206]. We further demonstrated that myelin uptake results in the activation of LXRs and PPARβ/δ [11, 15, 126]. Both nuclear receptors induce the expression of MerTK and

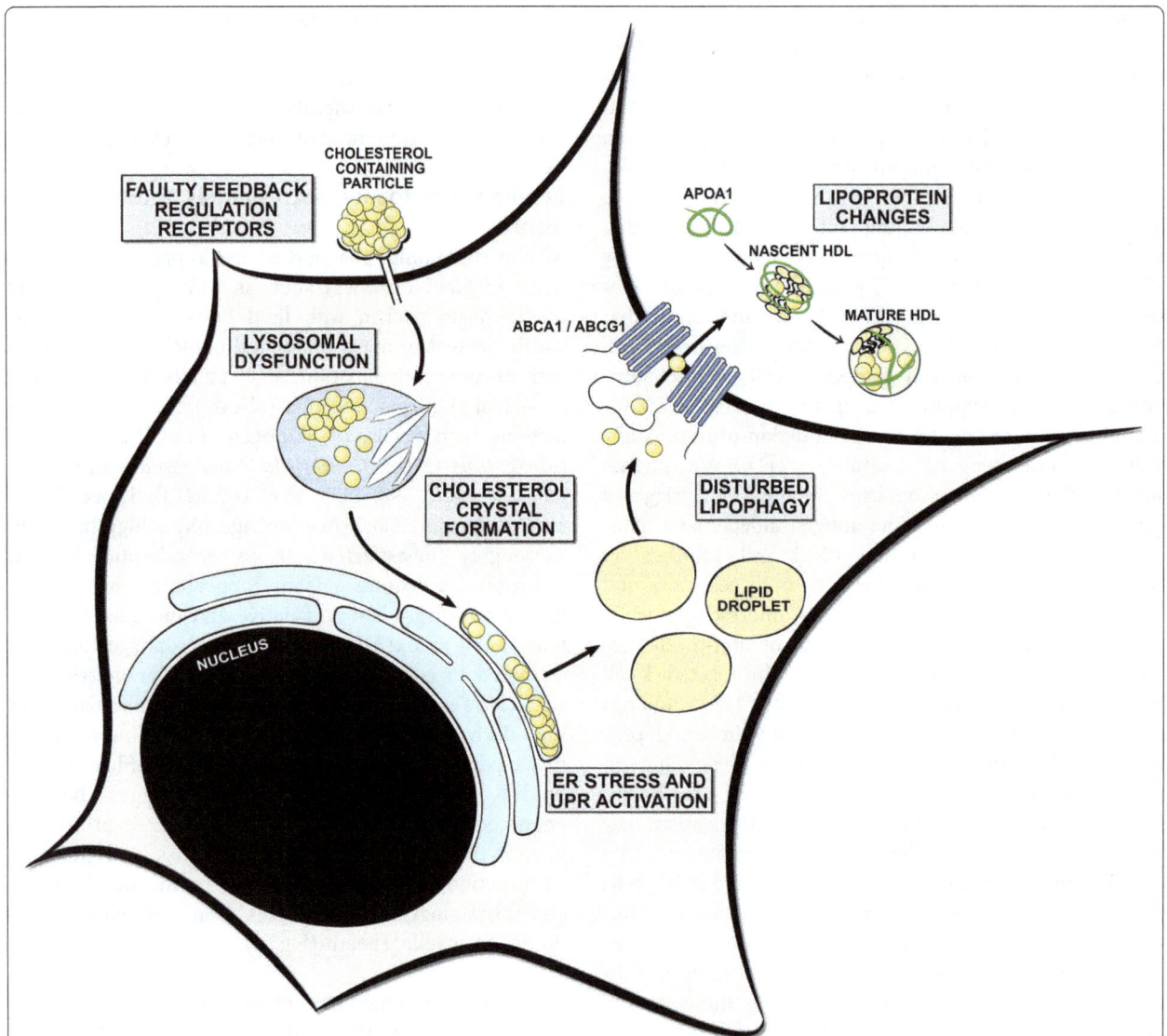

Fig. 4 Homeostatic and dysfunctional processing of cholesterol-containing lipid particles. During homeostasis, phagocytes are well equipped to cope with relatively minor increases of cholesterol. However, sustained intracellular accumulation of cholesterol, as observed in in many peripheral pathologies and following infections with persistent pathogens, can lead to disturbances in pathways that mediate the degradation, storage, or efflux of cholesterol. First, faulty feedback regulation of phagocytic receptors may result in an uncontrolled uptake of cholesterol-containing lipid particles. Second, lysosomal cholesterol accumulation can result in lysosomal dysfunction by reducing lysosomal acidification and causing lysosomal leakiness. In addition, sustained accumulation of cholesterol can lead to the formation of cholesterol crystals that activate the caspase-1-activating NLRP3 inflammasome. Third, persistent cholesterol trafficking to ER membranes can trigger ER stress and the unfolded protein response (UPR). Fourth, dysfunctional lipophagy machinery can hamper the capacity of foamy phagocytes to process cholesterol within lipid droplets, thereby impeding the cells' capacity to dispose of intracellular cholesterol. Finally, quantitative and qualitative changes in lipoproteins can impact the capacity of foamy phagocytes to efflux cholesterol. Altogether, disturbances in the abovementioned pathways are well-known to promote the induction of a disease-promoting phenotype of foamy phagocytes and eventually even cause apoptosis. While ample evidence suggests that faulty regulation of these pathways also occurs in myelin-containing phagocytes, more research is warranted to define to what extent they impact their inflammatory features

opsonins, such as C1qa, and C1qb [142, 145]. This increase in expression may augment the internalization of myelin by phagocytes in demyelinating disorders. Of interest, continuous activation of PPARγ by modified oxLDL may promote a similar vicious cycle of LDL uptake in oxLDL-loaded macrophages by inducing the expression of CD36 [89, 146]. Furthermore, we demonstrated that oxidized myelin more potently increases the expression of the phagocytic scavenger receptor CL-P1 compared to unmodified myelin [12]. More importantly, while CL-P1 surface expression gradually decreases on macrophages treated with unmodified myelin, macrophages exposed to oxidized myelin retain a high expression of CL-P1 over time. These findings indicate that unmodified and oxidized myelin impact macrophage function differently, similar to native and oxLDL. In addition, they suggest faulty feedback regulation of CL-P1 when phagocytes are exposed to oxidized forms of myelin. While counter regulatory processes that inhibit myelin internalization such as the CD47/SIRPα axis exist [61], CD47 was found to be decreased at the mRNA level and expressed at low abundance on protein level in MS lesions [73]. Even more, microRNA profiling of MS lesions identified modulators of the regulatory protein CD47 [96, 187]. Reduced signaling through this inhibitory CD47/SIRPαinhibitory pathway may further boost myelin uptake and demyelination. Collectively, these studies stress that faulty regulation of phagocytic and inhibitory receptors in MS lesions can lead to the uncontrolled internalization of myelin by phagocytes.

Lysosomal dysfunction

Ample evidence indicates that lysosomal dysfunction is a critical step in the formation of M1-like foam cells and disease progression in atherosclerosis and NASH [78]. The sequestration of LDL-derived free cholesterol within lysosomes is regarded to underlie lysosomal dysfunction and the induction of M1-like macrophages in these disorders [7, 33, 46, 92, 116, 191, 218]. In MS patients, an increase in several lysosomal enzymes is apparent in plaques, periplaque areas, NAWM, and CSF samples [35, 45, 72], which indicates active breakdown of lipids and other macromolecules in the CNS. Strikingly, while active MS lesions are packed with metabolically active mye-phagocytes, lysosomal function or dysfunction within these cells remains largely uninvestigated. Free cholesterol is the predominant form of cholesterol in myelin. Hence, continuous uptake of myelin by phagocytes is likely to result in lysosomal accumulation of free cholesterol and consequently lead to lysosomal and phagocyte dysfunction. Interestingly, an early study using the EAE model demonstrated that abnormalities in lysosomal permeability are apparent before the development of clinical and histological changes [56]. Similar, cerebral lysosomes seem to be more fragile in MS white matter compared to white matter of healthy controls [128]. Lysosomal abnormalities equally affected the plaque, periplaque, and NAWM in MS patients. These studies suggest that lysosomes in the CNS of MS patients are more prone to become dysfunctional. A more recent study showed that aged mye-phagocytes have a tendency to accumulate large amounts of lysosomal cholesterol [27]. Lysosomal accumulation of myelin-derived cholesterol led to the activation of NLRP3 inflammasome. Despite these studies, it remains unclear to what extent lysosomal dysfunction occurs in foamy phagocytes in MS

lesions, and what the impact of lysosomal accumulation of myelin-derived cholesterol is on lysosomal integrity.

LDL loading is reported to downregulate the expression of Niemann Pick Disease type C1 and C2 (NPC1 an NPC2) in macrophages. NPC1 and NP2 are membrane proteins that facilitate the transfer of free cholesterol from lysosomes to the endoplasmic reticulum (ER) for further processing [91]. Hence, a reduced expression of NPC1 and NPC2 can augment lysosomal free cholesterol sequestration and lysosomal dysfunction. While no studies defined changes in the expression of NPC1 and NPC2 in phagocytes upon myelin uptake, fingolimod (FTY720), which is currently used for treatment of MS, increases the expression of NPC1 and NPC2 on both mRNA and protein level in NPC mutant fibroblasts [150]. Likewise, FTY720 increases the expression of NPC1 in human macrophages and improves their survival after sustained lipid uptake [10]. This increase in NPC expression may boost the trafficking of free cholesterol to the ER in mye-phagocytes, thereby counteracting the accumulation of free cholesterol in lysosomes and preventing lysosomal dysfunction. Thus, apart from blocking the egress of leukocytes from secondary lymph nodes [22], FTY720 can suppress MS lesion progression by restoring or retaining lysosomal function in mye-phagocytes.

Whereas it is generally assumed that lysosomal dysfunction is a secondary event in the pathophysiology of atherosclerosis and NASH, a genome-wide association study identified polymorphisms in the gene encoding the lysosomal enzyme galactocerebrosidase (GALC) in MS patients [87]. This argues for lysosomal dysfunction being a potential primary pathological event in MS. In Krabbe disease, lack of GALC activity results in lysosomal accumulation of galactosylcerebrosides and galactosphingosine in phagocytes and oligodendrocytes, leading to severe demyelination [103]. Haematopoietic stem cell transplantation corrects the metabolic defect in Krabbe disease, which indicates the importance of dysfunctional GALC in leukocytes in disease pathogenesis [109]. To what extent polymorphisms in the GALC gene impact lysosomal function and lipid accumulation in phagocytes in MS upon myelin uptake remains to be clarified. In summary, several studies suggest that lysosomal dysfunction can occur in mye-phagocytes in MS lesions. However, more in-depth studies examining the abovementioned lysosomal parameters in *in vitro* cultured mye-phagocytes and within MS lesions are warranted to certitude this claim.

Formation of cholesterol crystals and inflammasome activation

Sustained accumulation of cholesterol within foamy macrophages in atherosclerosis, NASH, and following Mtb infections results in the formation of cholesterol crystals [6, 25, 88]. Several studies indicate that choles-terol crystals destabilize lysosomes, thereby activating the caspase-1-activating NLRP3 inflammasome and pro-moting the release of IL-1β [43, 55, 82, 119]. Similar to foamy phagocytes in these disorders, phagocytes accumu-late copious amounts of cholesterol *in vitro* and *in vivo* following uptake of myelin [12, 126]. Moreover, several studies demonstrated the presence of cholesterol crystal-like structures in mye-phagocytes [8, 27, 113]. By using electron microscopy imaging, numerous mono-nuclear cells containing degenerated myelin were found to accumulate needle-shaped cholesterol structures in late stages of Wallerian degeneration [8]. Cholesterol crystals are also apparent in IBA1+ mye-microglia in the corpus callosum of cuprizone-treated animals [113]. Finally, a more recent study showed that aging results in the accu-mulation of cholesterol crystals in mye-phagocytes, lead-ing to NLRP3 inflammasome activation [27]. To date, it remains unclear whether cholesterol crystals are also formed in foamy phagocytes within MS lesions, and to what extent inflammasome activation in these cells im-pacts MS lesion progression. With respect to the latter, inflammasome activation is apparent in the CNS and per-ipheral cells in several neurodegenerative disorders [79, 83, 136, 156]. Furthermore, mice lacking NLRP3, caspase-1, or IL-18 exhibit reduced neuroinflammation, demyelination, and neurodegeneration [69, 79, 86, 93, 125, 215, 216], which underscores the pathogenic role for the inflammasome in neurodegenerative disorders. Notably, predominantly macrophages and microglia produce IL-1β in EAE and MS lesions [24, 193], arguing for phagocytes being the culprit cells involved in the abovementioned knockout models. Of particular interest, the scavenger re-ceptor CD36 is closely associated with the *de novo* forma-tion of intracellular cholesterol crystals and NLRP3 inflammasome activation in oxLDL-loaded macrophages [175]. Hence, CD36 may well fulfill a similar function in mye-phagocytes [49]. More in-depth studies are needed to define if *de novo* formation of cholesterol crystals under-lies inflammasome activation within mye-phagocytes or if lysosomal destabilization due to the free cholesterol accu-mulation causes inflammasome activation.

ER stress and the unfolded protein response
The ER plays a key role in the biosynthesis, processing, and trafficking of proteins. Environmental factors or ele-vated protein synthesis can lead to the accumulation of misfolded or unfolded proteins in the ER, also called ER stress. ER stress triggers the unfolded protein response (UPR), which attempts to restore ER homeostasis by attenuating global protein synthesis and degrading un-folded proteins. If the UPR fails to restore ER homeosta-sis, apoptotic signaling pathways are activated to remove stressed cells [202].

ER stress and UPR activation are known to occur in oxLDL-loaded macrophages *in vitro* and macrophages in human atherosclerotic lesions and apoE-knockout mice [144, 217, 221]. Moreover, cholesterol trafficking to ER membranes in cholesterol-loaded macrophages results in UPR activation and promotes phagocyte apoptosis [41, 53]. Similar to atherosclerosis, ER stress and UPR activa-tion is apparent in MS and EAE lesions. An increased mRNA and protein expression of activating transcription factor 4, CCAAT-enhancer-binding protein homologous protein, calreticulin, X-box-binding protein 1, and immunoglobulin-heavy-chain-binding protein was found in NAWM and demyelinating lesions of MS patients [34, 71, 130, 134, 143, 151]. Interestingly, calreticulin co-localizes with ORO+ phagocytes in MS lesions, which points towards ER stress and UPR activation in mye-phagocytes [151]. Likewise, foamy phagocytes in ac-tive MS lesions show an increased expression of the mitochondria-associated membrane protein Rab32, which is closely associated with the UPR [71]. Active UPR signaling is also observed in phagocytes, T cells, as-trocytes, and oligodendrocytes during the course of EAE [28, 40, 131, 151]. Importantly, inhibition of the UPR using crocin reduces ER stress and the inflammatory burden in EAE animals. The reduced EAE disease severity was paralleled with preserved myelination and axonal density, and reduced immune cell infiltration and phagocyte activation [40]. This study underscores the detrimental impact of ER stress and the UPR on neuro-inflammation and neurodegeneration. Remarkably, des-pite ER stress and UPR activation, no studies have reported the presence of apoptotic and necrotic foamy phagocytes in active demyelinating MS lesions yet. Phagocyte apoptosis might be difficult to detect histolog-ically, owing to the fact that dying cells are rapidly cleared by neighboring phagocytes through efferocytosis [209]. Thus, while studies point towards a role for ER stress and UPR activation in MS pathology, more re-search is warranted to define the underlying mecha-nisms, culprit cell types, and functional outcome.

Disturbed autophagy/lipophagy
Autophagy is a catabolic process essential for cellular and tissue homeostasis. While it is crucial for the deg-radation of dysfunctional and unwanted proteins and or-ganelles, increasing evidence indicates that it also controls lipid degradation, a process called lipophagy [120]. Ouimet et al. defined that lipophagy plays a key role in cholesterol efflux from lipid-laden macrophages [154]. During lipophagy, autophagosomes and lysosomes fuse with lipid droplets after which esterified cholesterol is hydrolyzed by specific enzymes, such as lysosomal acid lipase, into free cholesterols. Unlike esterified chol-esterol, free cholesterol is a substrate for ABCA1 and

ABCG1-mediated efflux to apoA-I or HDL, respectively. Hence, active lipophagy represents a way to dispose intracellular cholesterol, thereby preventing their intracellular accumulation.

Autophagy is tightly linked to the pathogenesis of MS. However, the precise role that autophagy plays in the pathogenesis of MS and to what extent the autophagy machinery is dysfunctional is poorly understood. To date, the majority of studies have focused on the impact of autophagy on lymphocyte survival and homeostasis in MS [1, 48, 108]. However, autophagy likely also impacts foamy phagocyte function in MS lesions. As autophagy regulates the antigen presenting capacity of dendritic cells [5], future studies should define whether is it also involved in the presentation of myelin antigens by foamy phagocytes locally in the CNS and secondary lymphoid organs. Similar, the influence of autophagy/lipophagy on lipid efflux by foamy phagocytes merits further investigation, in particular with respect to aging. Recently, aging was reported to hamper the efflux efficacy of mye-phagocytes in diverse animal models for demyelination [27]. Malfunction of the lipophagy machinery may underlie the age-related discrepancy in the capacity of foamy phagocytes to dispose of intracellular cholesterol. Of interest, increasing evidence suggests that dysfunctional autophagy is apparent in foamy macrophages in atherosclerosis, and contributes to lipid accumulation, apoptosis, and inflammasome hyperactivation in these cells [118, 163]. As autophagy regulates phagocytosis by modulating the expression of phagocytic receptors [17], defining the impact of autophagy on the uptake of myelin also deserves further attention. Thus, while increasingly being acknowledged to impact MS disease progression, more research is warranted to define the role that autophagy plays in directing the functional properties of foamy phagocytes, and elucidate whether the autophagy machinery becomes dysfunctional in phagocytes engorged with myelin-derived lipids.

Lipoprotein alterations and modifications

While we focused in the previous sections on intracellular processes going awry in cholesterol-loaded foamy phagocytes, extracellular factors such as lipoproteins can also impact lipid processing, thereby directing the physiology of these foamy macrophages [172]. Generally, high levels of LDL, and in particular modified forms of LDL, drive the inflammatory activation of macrophages after sustained uptake, thereby promoting lesion formation and progression in atherosclerosis, as described in the previous sections. In contrast, high-density lipoproteins (HDL) have anti-atherogenic properties, which are attributed to their crucial role in reverse cholesterol transport [166]. Ample evidence suggests that lipoprotein levels, subclasses, and function are also altered in MS patients and associated with disease activity. For

instance, disability in MS patients is positively correlated to plasma LDL, apoB, and total cholesterol levels [127, 186, 207]. Furthermore, MS patients display elevated oxLDL levels in plasma and the CNS [149, 155], and an increase in plasma auto-antibodies directed against oxLDL [4]. In contrast to LDL, controversy exists regarding HDL levels in MS patients. Whereas some studies demonstrated a decrease [133], other showed no change or even an increase in HDL levels [4, 62, 171]. Of note, we recently reported that distinguishing between different HDL subclasses is of importance when investigating HDL levels [95]. Irrespective of these studies, higher serum HDL levels correlate with reduced blood-brain barrier injury and a decreased infiltration of immune cells into the CSF of MS patients [52]. We recently identified an altered lipoprotein profile in relapsing-remitting MS (RR-MS) patients, especially in low-BMI RR-MS patients, with modified and dysfunctional HDL [95]. By using LC-MS/MS, we demonstrated that HDL is modified at its ApoA-I tyrosine and tryptophan residues. Such modifications are increasingly being acknowledged to alter HDL function [104, 166, 174]. Specifically, the Trp50 and Trp72 domains are responsible for the initiation of lipid binding to ApoA-I [84, 201]. This suggests that in in low-BMI RR-MS patients, cholesterol efflux may be dysfunctional, potentially leading to the inflammatory accumulation of myelin-derived lipids in mye-phagocytes. In line with this hypothesis, serum HDL of RR-MS patients less efficiently accepts cholesterol via the ABCG1 transporter compared to serum HDL of healthy controls [95]. To what extent tyrosine and tryptophan modifications underlie changes in HDL functionality in RR-MS patients remains to be clarified. Altogether, these studies strongly suggest that quantitative and qualitative changes in lipoproteins are apparent in MS and can impact phagocyte lipid load and physiology. In particular, the function of phagocytes containing abundant myelin-derived lipids can potentially be severely compromised by these changes in LDL and HDL.

Protective foamy macrophages

Similar to MS, increasing evidence indicates that the phenotype of lesional macrophages in atherosclerosis is more complex than previously thought [184]. For a long time, sustained cholesterol uptake and consequent disturbances in metabolic pathways were believed to promote the induction of inflammatory, pro-atherogenic macrophages, as discussed in the previous paragraphs. However, a regulated accumulation of desmosterol following cholesterol loading also suppresses the inflammatory activation of foamy phagocytes in the absence of overt inflammation [180]. Of interest, desmosterol was found to mediate its effects on the macrophage phenotype by activating LXRs.

Likewise, another study demonstrated that oxLDL loading increases the expression of the typical M2 marker arginase I in a PPAR-dependent manner [57]. These findings suggest that LDL accumulation can also suppress inflammation and may limit lesion progression when the inflammatory burden in atherosclerotic lesions is low. In line with these studies, considerable phenotypic variation of macrophages is apparent in atherosclerotic lesions [19, 29, 97, 185]. Strikingly, similar to oxLDL-loaded macrophages, we found that myelin-derived lipids skew phagocytes towards a less inflammatory phenotype in LXR- and PPAR-dependent manner upon uptake of myelin [11, 15]. Also, within MS lesions considerable phenotypic variation is observed [18, 200]. Boven et al. demonstrated that foamy phagocytes in the lesion center display a more anti-inflammatory phenotype compared to foamy phagocytes in the lesion rim [18]. Vogel extended these findings by showing the majority of foam cells within MS lesions have an intermediate activation status, expressing markers that are characteristic for both inflammatory and anti-inflammatory phagocytes [200]. Collectively, these findings indicate that foamy macrophages showing an M2-like phenotype are apparent in both MS and atherosclerotic lesions, and that alike nuclear receptor signaling pathways drive the formation of these cells. Hence, identifying ways to specifically target these pathways in phagocytes will open therapeutic avenues for both MS and atherosclerosis.

Conclusions and future perspectives

Our understanding of the role of foamy phagocytes in the pathophysiology of MS has increased tremendously over the last few years. It is becoming clear that the uptake of myelin by phagocytes is not merely a disease-promoting process but also a prerequisite for CNS repair. By simply inhibiting the uptake of myelin or reducing the number of lesional phagocytes, one will suppress the clearance of inhibitory myelin and counteract the protective phenotype that phagocytes adopt upon myelin internalization. To illustrate, the majority of therapeutics for MS are based on the assumption that prevention of immune cell infiltration into the CNS or elimination of them altogether is key to stop MS disease progression. While these therapeutics effectively reduce disease severity in early disease stages, they do not prevent lesion progression or promote CNS repair. Interventions that focus on enhancing the mobilization of phagocytes subtypes that are advantageous and/or depleting those that are detrimental may be more effective. For this purpose, naturally-occurring reparative processes should be exploited as our body has designed these processes to act accordingly. The uptake of myelin debris and the protective impact that myelin internalization has on the phenotype of phagocytes represent such processes.

Despite of the presence of protective foamy phagocytes, the majority of MS lesions evolve into chronic lesions as disease progresses. To date, it remains elusive what causes failure of foamy phagocytes to stop lesion progression and promote CNS repair as disease advances. Aging impacts immune cell function and recent evidence indicates that aging drives foamy phagocytes towards an inflammatory phenotype. Although MS is generally not regarded an age-related disorder, chronic inflammation might well lead to premature innate immunosenescence in MS patients. At the same time, valuable lessons can be learned from foamy macrophages in atherosclerosis and other diseases. As delineated in this review, ample evidence indicates that checkpoints involved in lipid handling are malfunctioning in macrophages following massive lipid uptake, leading to the intracellular accumulation of inflammatory lipids. Future studies should define whether faulty regulation of these pathways also occurs in mye-phagocytes. This could lead to the identification of new targets for therapeutic interventions and may open up new avenues for therapeutics currently used to treat other disorders characterized by the presence of foamy macrophages.

Acknowledgements

This work was supported by grants of the Belgian Charcot Foundation, Research Foundation Flanders (FWO), and the Transnational University Limburg.

Authors' contributions

EG and JB designed and drafted the review. JH revised critically for important intellectual content. EG, JH, and JB approved the final manuscript to be published. All authors read and approved the final manuscript.

Competing interests

The authors declare that they have no competing interests.

References

1. Alirezaei M, Fox HS, Flynn CT, Moore CS, Hebb AL, Frausto RF, Bhan V, Kiosses WB, Whitton JL, Robertson GS, Crocker SJ (2009) Elevated ATG5 expression in autoimmune demyelination and multiple sclerosis. Autophagy 5:152–158.
2. Barnett MH, Parratt JD, Cho ES, Prineas JW (2009) Immunoglobulins and complement in postmortem multiple sclerosis tissue. Ann Neurol 65:32–46. https://doi.org/10.1002/ana.21524.
3. Barral P, Polzella P, Bruckbauer A, van Rooijen N, Besra GS, Cerundolo V, Batista FD (2010) CD169(+) macrophages present lipid antigens to mediate early activation of iNKT cells in lymph nodes. Nat Immunol 11:303–312. https://doi.org/10.1038/ni.1853.
4. Besler HT, Comoglu S (2003) Lipoprotein oxidation, plasma total antioxidant capacity and homocysteine level in patients with multiple sclerosis. Nutr Neurosci 6:189–196. https://doi.org/10.1080/1028415031000115945.
5. Bhattacharya A, Parillon X, Zeng S, Han S, Eissa NT (2014) Deficiency of autophagy in dendritic cells protects against experimental autoimmune encephalomyelitis. J Biol Chem 289:26525–26532. https://doi.org/10.1074/jbc.M114.575860.

6. Bieghs V, Hendrikx T, van Gorp PJ, Verheyen F, Guichot YD, Walenbergh SM, Jeurissen ML, Gijbels M, Rensen SS, Bast A, Plat J, Kalhan SC, Koek GH, Leitersdorf E, Hofker MH, Lutjohann D, Shiri-Sverdlov R (2013) The cholesterol derivative 27-hydroxycholesterol reduces steatohepatitis in mice. Gastroenterol 144(167-178):e161. https://doi.org/10.1053/j.gastro.2012.09.062.

7. Bieghs V, Walenbergh SM, Hendrikx T, van Gorp PJ, Verheyen F, Olde Damink SW, Masclee AA, Koek GH, Hofker MH, Binder CJ, Shiri-Sverdlov R (2013) Trapping of oxidized LDL in lysosomes of Kupffer cells is a trigger for hepatic inflammation. Liver Int 33:1056–1061. https://doi.org/10.1111/liv.12170.

8. Bignami A, Ralston HJ 3rd (1969) The cellular reaction to Wallerian degeneration in the central nervous system of the cat. Brain Res 13:444–461.

9. Binder MD, Fox AD, Merlo D, Johnson LJ, Giuffrida L, Calvert SE, Akkermann R, Ma GZ, Anzgene PAA, Gresle MM, Laverick L, Foo G, Fabis-Pedrini MJ, Spelman T, Jordan MA, Baxter AG, Foote S, Butzkueven H, Kilpatrick TJ, Field J (2016) Common and Low Frequency Variants in MERTK Are Independently Associated with Multiple Sclerosis Susceptibility with Discordant Association Dependent upon HLA-DRB1*15:01 Status. PLoS Genet 12:e1005853. https://doi.org/10.1371/journal.pgen.1005853.

10. Blom T, Back N, Mutka AL, Bittman R, Li Z, de Lera A, Kovanen PT, Diczfalusy U, Ikonen E (2010) FTY720 stimulates 27-hydroxycholesterol production and confers atheroprotective effects in human primary macrophages. Circ Res 106:720–729. https://doi.org/10.1161/CIRCRESAHA.109.204396.

11. Bogie JF, Jorissen W, Mailleux J, Nijland PG, Zelcer N, Vanmierlo T, Van Horssen J, Stinissen P, Hellings N, Hendriks JJ (2013) Myelin alters the inflammatory phenotype of macrophages by activating PPARs. Acta Neuropathol Commun 1:43. https://doi.org/10.1186/2051-5960-1-43.

12. Bogie JF, Mailleux J, Wouters E, Jorissen W, Grajchen E, Vanmol J, Wouters K, Hellings N, Van Horsen J, Vanmierlo T, Hendriks JJ (2017) Scavenger receptor collectin placenta 1 is a novel receptor involved in the uptake of myelin by phagocytes. Sci Rep 7:44794. https://doi.org/10.1038/srep44794.

13. Bogie JF, Stinissen P, Hellings N, Hendriks JJ (2011) Myelin-phagocytosing macrophages modulate autoreactive T cell proliferation. J Neuroinflammation 8:85. https://doi.org/10.1186/1742-2094-8-85.

14. Bogie JF, Stinissen P, Hendriks JJ (2014) Macrophage subsets and microglia in multiple sclerosis. Acta Neuropathol 128:191–213. https://doi.org/10.1007/s00401-014-1310-2.

15. Bogie JF, Timmermans S, Huynh-Thu VA, Irrthum A, Smeets HJ, Gustafsson JA, Steffensen KR, Mulder M, Stinissen P, Hellings N, Hendriks JJ (2012) Myelin-derived lipids modulate macrophage activity by liver X receptor activation. PLoS One 7:e44998. https://doi.org/10.1371/journal.pone.0044998.

16. Bolton C, Smith PA (2018) The influence and impact of ageing and immunosenescence (ISC) on adaptive immunity during multiple sclerosis (MS) and the animal counterpart experimental autoimmune encephalomyelitis (EAE). Ageing Res Rev 41:64–81. https://doi.org/10.1016/j.arr.2017.10.005.

17. Bonilla DL, Bhattacharya A, Sha Y, Xu Y, Xiang Q, Kan A, Jagannath C, Komatsu M, Eissa NT (2013) Autophagy regulates phagocytosis by modulating the expression of scavenger receptors. Immunity 39:537–547. https://doi.org/10.1016/j.immuni.2013.08.026.

18. Boven LA, Van Meurs M, Van Zwam M, Wierenga-Wolf A, Hintzen RQ, Boot RG, Aerts JM, Amor S, Nieuwenhuis EE, Laman JD (2006) Myelin-laden macrophages are anti-inflammatory, consistent with foam cells in multiple sclerosis. Brain 129:517–526. https://doi.org/10.1093/brain/awh707.

19. Boyle JJ, Harrington HA, Piper E, Elderfield K, Stark J, Landis RC, Haskard DO (2009) Coronary intraplaque hemorrhage evokes a novel atheroprotective macrophage phenotype. Am J Pathol 174:1097–1108. https://doi.org/10.2353/ajpath.2009.080431.

20. Breij EC, Brink BP, Veerhuis R, van den Berg C, Vloet R, Yan R, Dijkstra CD, van der Valk P, Bo L (2008) Homogeneity of active demyelinating lesions in established multiple sclerosis. Ann Neurol 63:16–25. https://doi.org/10.1002/ana.21311.

21. Brink BP, Veerhuis R, Breij EC, van der Valk P, Dijkstra CD, Bo L (2005) The pathology of multiple sclerosis is location-dependent: no significant complement activation is detected in purely cortical lesions. J Neuropathol Exp Neurol 64:147–155.

22. Brinkmann V, Billich A, Baumruker T, Heining P, Schmouder R, Francis G, Aradhye S, Burtin P (2010) Fingolimod (FTY720): discovery and development of an oral drug to treat multiple sclerosis. Nat Rev Drug Discov 9:883–897. https://doi.org/10.1038/nrd3248.

23. Bruck W, Friede RL (1990) Anti-macrophage CR3 antibody blocks myelin phagocytosis by macrophages in vitro. Acta Neuropathol 80:415–418.

24. Burm SM, Peferoen LA, Zuiderwijk-Sick EA, Haanstra KG, t Hart BA, van der Valk P, Amor S, Bauer J, Bajramovic JJ (2016) Expression of IL-1beta in rhesus EAE and MS lesions is mainly induced in the CNS itself. J Neuroinflammation 13:138. https://doi.org/10.1186/s12974-016-0605-8.

25. Caceres N, Tapia G, Ojanguren I, Altare F, Gil O, Pinto S, Vilaplana C, Cardona PJ (2009) Evolution of foamy macrophages in the pulmonary granulomas of experimental tuberculosis models. Tuberculosis (Edinb) 89:175–182. https://doi.org/10.1016/j.tube.2008.11.001.

26. Canton J, Neculai D, Grinstein S (2013) Scavenger receptors in homeostasis and immunity. Nat Rev Immunol 13:621–634. https://doi.org/10.1038/nri3515.

27. Cantuti-Castelvetri L, Fitzner D, Bosch-Queralt M, Weil MT, Su M, Sen P, Ruhwedel T, Mitkovski M, Trendelenburg G, Lutjohann D, Mobius W, Simons M (2018) Defective cholesterol clearance limits remyelination in the aged central nervous system. Science 359:684–688. https://doi.org/10.1126/science.aan4183.

28. Chakrabarty A, Danley MM, LeVine SM (2004) Immunohistochemical localization of phosphorylated protein kinase R and phosphorylated eukaryotic initiation factor-2 alpha in the central nervous system of SJL mice with experimental allergic encephalomyelitis. J Neurosci Res 76:822–833. https://doi.org/10.1002/jnr.20125.

29. Chinetti-Gbaguidi G, Colin S, Staels B (2015) Macrophage subsets in atherosclerosis. Nat Rev Cardiol 12:10–17. https://doi.org/10.1038/nrcardio.2014.173.

30. Chuang TY, Guo Y, Seki SM, Rosen AM, Johanson DM, Mandell JW, Lucchinetti CF, Gaultier A (2016) LRP1 expression in microglia is protective during CNS autoimmunity. Acta Neuropathol Commun 4:68. https://doi.org/10.1186/s40478-016-0343-2.

31. Claes N, Fraussen J, Stinissen P, Hupperts R, Somers V (2015) B Cells Are Multifunctional Players in Multiple Sclerosis Pathogenesis: Insights from Therapeutic Interventions. Front Immunol 6:642. https://doi.org/10.3389/fimmu.2015.00642.

32. Comerford I, Harata-Lee Y, Bunting MD, Gregor C, Kara EE, McColl SR (2013) A myriad of functions and complex regulation of the CCR7/CCL19/CCL21 chemokine axis in the adaptive immune system. Cytokine Growth Factor Rev 24:269–283. https://doi.org/10.1016/j.cytogfr.2013.03.001.

33. Cox BE, Griffin EE, Ullery JC, Jerome WG (2007) Effects of cellular cholesterol loading on macrophage foam cell lysosome acidification. J Lipid Res 48:1012–1021. https://doi.org/10.1194/jlr.M600390-JLR200.

34. Cunnea P, Mhaille AN, McQuaid S, Farrell M, McMahon J, FitzGerald U (2011) Expression profiles of endoplasmic reticulum stress-related molecules in demyelinating lesions and multiple sclerosis. Multiple Scler 17:808–818. https://doi.org/10.1177/1352458511399114.

35. Cuzner ML, Davison AN (1973) Changes in cerebral lysosomal enzyme activity and lipids in multiple sclerosis. J Neurol Sci 19:29–36.

36. da Costa CC, van der Laan LJ, Dijkstra CD, Bruck W (1997) The role of the mouse macrophage scavenger receptor in myelin phagocytosis. Eur J Neurosci 9:2650–2657.

37. Damani MR, Zhao L, Fontainhas AM, Amaral J, Fariss RN, Wong WT (2011) Age-related alterations in the dynamic behavior of microglia. Aging cell 10:263–276. https://doi.org/10.1111/j.1474-9726.2010.00660.x.

38. de Vos AF, van Meurs M, Brok HP, Boven LA, Hintzen RQ, van der Valk P, Ravid R, Rensing S, Boon L, t Hart BA, Laman JD (2002) Transfer of central nervous system autoantigens and presentation in secondary lymphoid organs. J Immunol 169:5415–5423.

39. Denney L, Kok WL, Cole SL, Sanderson S, McMichael AJ, Ho LP (2012) Activation of invariant NKT cells in early phase of experimental autoimmune encephalomyelitis results in differentiation of Ly6Chi inflammatory monocyte to M2 macrophages and improved outcome. J Immunol 189:551–557. https://doi.org/10.4049/jimmunol.1103608.

40. Deslauriers AM, Afkhami-Goli A, Paul AM, Bhat RK, Acharjee S, Ellestad KK, Noorbakhsh F, Michalak M, Power C (2011) Neuroinflammation and endoplasmic reticulum stress are coregulated by crocin to prevent demyelination and neurodegeneration. J Immunol 187:4788–4799. https://doi.org/10.4049/jimmunol.1004111.

41. Devries-Seimon T, Li Y, Yao PM, Stone E, Wang Y, Davis RJ, Flavell R, Tabas I (2005) Cholesterol-induced macrophage apoptosis requires ER stress pathways and engagement of the type A scavenger receptor. J Cell Biol 171:61–73. https://doi.org/10.1083/jcb.200502078.

42. Dijkstra IM, de Haas AH, Brouwer N, Boddeke HW, Biber K (2006) Challenge with innate and protein antigens induces CCR7 expression by microglia in vitro and in vivo. Glia 54:861–872. https://doi.org/10.1002/glia.20426.

43. Duewell P, Kono H, Rayner KJ, Sirois CM, Vladimer G, Bauernfeind FG, Abela GS, Franchi L, Nunez G, Schnurr M, Espevik T, Lien E, Fitzgerald KA, Rock KL, Moore KJ, Wright SD, Hornung V, Latz E (2010) NLRP3 inflammasomes are required for atherogenesis and activated by cholesterol crystals. Nature 464:1357–1361. https://doi.org/10.1038/nature08938.

44. Durafourt BA, Moore CS, Zammit DA, Johnson TA, Zaguia F, Guiot MC, Bar-Or A, Antel JP (2012) Comparison of polarization properties of human adult microglia and blood-derived macrophages. Glia 60:717–727. https://doi.org/10.1002/glia.22298.

45. Einstein ER, Csejtey J, Dalal KB, Adams CW, Bayliss OB, Hallpike JF (1972) Proteolytic activity and basic protein loss in and around multiple sclerosis plaques: combined biochemical and histochemical observations. J Neurochem 19:653–662.

46. Emanuel R, Sergin I, Bhattacharya S, Turner JN, Epelman S, Settembre C, Diwan A, Ballabio A, Razani B (2014) Induction of lysosomal biogenesis in atherosclerotic macrophages can rescue lipid-induced lysosomal dysfunction and downstream sequelae. Arterioscler Thromb Vas Biol 34:1942–1952. https://doi.org/10.1161/ATVBAHA.114.303342.

47. Epstein LG, Prineas JW, Raine CS (1983) Attachment of myelin to coated pits on macrophages in experimental allergic encephalomyelitis. J Neurol Sci 61:341–348.

48. Esposito M, Ruffini F, Bellone M, Gagliani N, Battaglia M, Martino G, Furlan R (2010) Rapamycin inhibits relapsing experimental autoimmune encephalomyelitis by both effector and regulatory T cells modulation. J Neuroimmunol 220:52–63. https://doi.org/10.1016/j.jneuroim.2010.01.001.

49. Eto M, Yoshikawa H, Fujimura H, Naba I, Sumi-Akamaru H, Takayasu S, Itabe H, Sakoda S (2003) The role of CD36 in peripheral nerve remyelination after crush injury. Eur J Neurosci 17:2659–2666.

50. Fabriek BO, Van Haastert ES, Galea I, Polfliet MM, Dopp ED, Van Den Heuvel MM, Van Den Berg TK, De Groot CJ, Van Der Valk P, Dijkstra CD (2005) CD163-positive perivascular macrophages in the human CNS express molecules for antigen recognition and presentation. Glia 51:297–305. https://doi.org/10.1002/glia.20208.

51. Fabriek BO, Zwemmer JN, Teunissen CE, Dijkstra CD, Polman CH, Laman JD, Castelijns JA (2005) In vivo detection of myelin proteins in cervical lymph nodes of MS patients using ultrasound-guided fine-needle aspiration cytology. J Neuroimmunol 161:190–194. https://doi.org/10.1016/j.jneuroim.2004.12.018.

52. Fellows K, Uher T, Browne RW, Weinstock-Guttman B, Horakova D, Posova H, Vaneckova M, Seidl Z, Krasensky J, Tyblova M, Havrdova E, Zivadinov R, Ramanathan M (2015) Protective associations of HDL with blood-brain barrier injury in multiple sclerosis patients. J Lipid Res 56:2010–2018. https://doi.org/10.1194/jlr.M060970.

53. Feng B, Yao PM, Li Y, Devlin CM, Zhang D, Harding HP, Sweeney M, Rong JX, Kuriakose G, Fisher EA, Marks AR, Ron D, Tabas I (2003) The endoplasmic reticulum is the site of cholesterol-induced cytotoxicity in macrophages. Nat Cell Biol 5:781–792. https://doi.org/10.1038/ncb1035.

54. Fraser I, Hughes D, Gordon S (1993) Divalent cation-independent macrophage adhesion inhibited by monoclonal antibody to murine scavenger receptor. Nature 364:343–346. https://doi.org/10.1038/364343a0.

55. Freigang S, Ampenberger F, Spohn G, Heer S, Shamshiev AT, Kisielow J, Hersberger M, Yamamoto M, Bachmann MF, Kopf M (2011) Nrf2 is essential for cholesterol crystal-induced inflammasome activation and exacerbation of atherosclerosis. Eur J Immunol 41:2040–2051. https://doi.org/10.1002/eji.201041316.

56. Gabrielescu E (1969) Contributions to enzyme histochemistry of the experimental demyelination. Revue roumaine de physiologie 6:45–54.

57. Gallardo-Soler A, Gomez-Nieto C, Campo ML, Marathe C, Tontonoz P, Castrillo A, Corraliza I (2008) Arginase I induction by modified lipoproteins in macrophages: a peroxisome proliferator-activated receptor-gamma/delta-mediated effect that links lipid metabolism and immunity. Mol Endocrinol 22:1394–1402. https://doi.org/10.1210/me.2007-0525.

58. Gaultier A, Wu X, Le Moan N, Takimoto S, Mukandala G, Akassoglou K, Campana WM, Gonias SL (2009) Low-density lipoprotein receptor-related protein 1 is an essential receptor for myelin phagocytosis. J Cell Sci 122:1155–1162. https://doi.org/10.1242/jcs.040717.

59. Girard S, Brough D, Lopez-Castejon G, Giles J, Rothwell NJ, Allan SM (2013) Microglia and macrophages differentially modulate cell death after brain injury caused by oxygen-glucose deprivation in organotypic brain slices. Glia 61:813–824. https://doi.org/10.1002/glia.22478.

60. Gitik M, Kleinhaus R, Hadas S, Reichert F, Rotshenker S (2014) Phagocytic receptors activate and immune inhibitory receptor SIRPalpha inhibits phagocytosis through paxillin and cofilin. Front Cell Neurosci 8:104. https://doi.org/10.3389/fncel.2014.00104.

61. Gitik M, Liraz-Zaltsman S, Oldenborg PA, Reichert F, Rotshenker S (2011) Myelin down-regulates myelin phagocytosis by microglia and macrophages through interactions between CD47 on myelin and SIRPalpha (signal regulatory protein-alpha) on phagocytes. J Neuroinflammation 8:24. https://doi.org/10.1186/1742-2094-8-24.

62. Giubilei F, Antonini G, Di Legge S, Sormani MP, Pantano P, Antonini R, Sepe-Monti M, Caramia F, Pozzilli C (2002) Blood cholesterol and MRI activity in first clinical episode suggestive of multiple sclerosis. Acta Neurol Scand 106:109–112.

63. Glim JE, Vereyken EJ, Heijnen DA, Garcia Vallejo JJ, Dijkstra CD (2010) The release of cytokines by macrophages is not affected by myelin ingestion. Glia 58:1928–1936. https://doi.org/10.1002/glia.21062.

64. Van der Goes A, Kortekaas M, Hoekstra K, Dijkstra CD, Amor S (1999) The role of anti-myelin (auto)-antibodies in the phagocytosis of myelin by macrophages. J Neuroimmunol 101:61–67.

65. Goldenberg PZ, Troiano RA, Kwon EE, Prineas JW (1990) Sera from MS patients and normal controls opsonize myelin. Neurosci lett 109:353–356.

66. Goldstein JL, Anderson RG, Brown MS (1979) Coated pits, coated vesicles, and receptor-mediated endocytosis. Nature 279:679–685.

67. GrandPre T, Nakamura F, Vartanian T, Strittmatter SM (2000) Identification of the Nogo inhibitor of axon regeneration as a Reticulon protein. Nature 403:439–444. https://doi.org/10.1038/35000226.

68. Grau-Lopez L, Raich D, Ramo-Tello C, Naranjo-Gomez M, Davalos A, Pujol-Borrell R, Borras FE, Martinez-Caceres E (2009) Myelin peptides in multiple sclerosis. Autoimmun Rev 8:650–653. https://doi.org/10.1016/j.autrev.2009.02.013.

69. Gris D, Ye Z, Iocca HA, Wen H, Craven RR, Gris P, Huang M, Schneider M, Miller SD, Ting JP (2010) NLRP3 plays a critical role in the development of experimental autoimmune encephalomyelitis by mediating Th1 and Th17 responses. J Immunol 185:974–981. https://doi.org/10.4049/jimmunol.0904145.

70. Hadas S, Spira M, Hanisch UK, Reichert F, Rotshenker S (2012) Complement receptor-3 negatively regulates the phagocytosis of degenerated myelin through tyrosine kinase Syk and cofilin. J Neuroinflammation 9:166. https://doi.org/10.1186/1742-2094-9-166.

71. Haile Y, Deng X, Ortiz-Sandoval C, Tahbaz N, Janowicz A, Lu JQ, Kerr BJ, Gutowski NJ, Holley JE, Eggleton P, Giuliani F, Simmen T (2017) Rab32 connects ER stress to mitochondrial defects in multiple sclerosis. J Neuroinflammation 14:19. https://doi.org/10.1186/s12974-016-0788-z.

72. Halonen T, Kilpelainen H, Pitkanen A, Riekkinen PJ (1987) Lysosomal hydrolases in cerebrospinal fluid of multiple sclerosis patients. A follow-up study. J Neurol Sci 79:267–274.

73. Han MH, Lundgren DH, Jaiswal S, Chao M, Graham KL, Garris CS, Axtell RC, Ho PP, Lock CB, Woodard JI, Brownell SE, Zoudilova M, Hunt JF, Baranzini SE, Butcher EC, Raine CS, Sobel RA, Han DK, Weissman I, Steinman L (2012) Janus-like opposing roles of CD47 in autoimmune brain inflammation in humans and mice. J Exp Med 209:1325–1334. https://doi.org/10.1084/jem.20101974.

74. Healy LM, Perron G, Won SY, Michell-Robinson MA, Rezk A, Ludwin SK, Moore CS, Hall JA, Bar-Or A, Antel JP (2016) MerTK Is a Functional Regulator of Myelin Phagocytosis by Human Myeloid Cells. J Immunol 196:3375–3384. https://doi.org/10.4049/jimmunol.1502562.

75. Hearps AC, Martin GE, Angelovich TA, Cheng WJ, Maisa A, Landay AL, Jaworowski A, Crowe SM (2012) Aging is associated with chronic innate immune activation and dysregulation of monocyte phenotype and function. Aging cell 11:867–875. https://doi.org/10.1111/j.1474-9726.2012.00851.x.

76. Hendrickx DA, Koning N, Schuurman KG, van Strien ME, van Eden CG, Hamann J, Huitinga I (2013) Selective upregulation of scavenger receptors in and around demyelinating areas in multiple sclerosis. J Neuropathol Exp Neurol 72:106–118. https://doi.org/10.1097/NEN.0b013e31827fd9e8.

77. Hendrickx DA, Schuurman KG, van Draanen M, Hamann J, Huitinga I (2014) Enhanced uptake of multiple sclerosis-derived myelin by THP-1 macrophages and primary human microglia. J Neuroinflammation 11:64. https://doi.org/10.1186/1742-2094-11-64.

78. Hendrikx T, Walenbergh SM, Hofker MH, Shiri-Sverdlov R (2014) Lysosomal cholesterol accumulation: driver on the road to inflammation during atherosclerosis and non-alcoholic steatohepatitis. Obes Rev 15:424–433. https://doi.org/10.1111/obr.12159.

79. Heneka MT, Kummer MP, Stutz A, Delekate A, Schwartz S, Vieira-Saecker A, Griep A, Axt D, Remus A, Tzeng TC, Gelpi E, Halle A, Korte M, Latz E, Golenbock DT (2013) NLRP3 is activated in Alzheimer's disease and contributes to pathology in APP/PS1 mice. Nature 493:674–678. https://doi.org/10.1038/nature11729.

80. Herrero C, Marques L, Lloberas J, Celada A (2001) IFN-gamma-dependent transcription of MHC class II IA is impaired in macrophages from aged mice. J Clin Invest 107:485–493. https://doi.org/10.1172/JCI11696.

81. Hikawa N, Takenaka T (1996) Myelin-stimulated macrophages release neurotrophic factors for adult dorsal root ganglion neurons in culture. Cell Mol Neurobiol 16:517–528.

82. Hornung V, Bauernfeind F, Halle A, Samstad EO, Kono H, Rock KL, Fitzgerald KA, Latz E (2008) Silica crystals and aluminum salts activate the NALP3 inflammasome through phagosomal destabilization. Nat Immunol 9:847–856. https://doi.org/10.1038/ni.1631.

83. Huang WX, Huang P, Hillert J (2004) Increased expression of caspase-1 and interleukin-18 in peripheral blood mononuclear cells in patients with multiple sclerosis. Multiple Scler 10:482–487.

84. Huang Y, DiDonato JA, Levison BS, Schmitt D, Li L, Wu Y, Buffa J, Kim T, Gerstenecker GS, Gu X, Kadiyala CS, Wang Z, Culley MK, Hazen JE, Didonato AJ, Fu X, Berisha SZ, Peng D, Nguyen TT, Liang S, Chuang CC, Cho L, Plow EF, Fox PL, Gogonea V, Tang WH, Parks JS, Fisher EA, Smith JD, Hazen SL (2014) An abundant dysfunctional apolipoprotein A1 in human atheroma. Nature Med 20:193–203. https://doi.org/10.1038/nm.3459.

85. Huitinga I, Damoiseaux JG, Dopp EA, Dijkstra CD (1993) Treatment with anti-CR3 antibodies ED7 and ED8 suppresses experimental allergic encephalomyelitis in Lewis rats. Eur J Immunol 23:709–715. https://doi.org/10.1002/eji.1830230321.

86. Inoue M, Williams KL, Gunn MD, Shinohara ML (2012) NLRP3 inflammasome induces chemotactic immune cell migration to the CNS in experimental autoimmune encephalomyelitis. Proc Natl Acad Sci U S A 109:10480–10485. https://doi.org/10.1073/pnas.1201836109.

87. International Multiple Sclerosis Genetics C, Wellcome Trust Case Control C, Sawcer S, Hellenthal G, Pirinen M, Spencer CC, Patsopoulos NA, Moutsianas L, Dilthey A, Su Z, Freeman C, Hunt SE, Edkins S, Gray E, Booth DR, Potter SC, Goris A, Band G, Oturai AB, Strange A, Saarela J, Bellenguez C, Fontaine B, Gillman M, Hemmer B, Gwilliam R, Zipp F, Jayakumar A, Martin R, Leslie S, Hawkins S, Giannoulatou E, D'Alfonso S, Blackburn H, Martinelli Boneschi F, Liddle J, Harbo HF, Perez ML, Spurkland A, Waller MJ, Mycko MP, Ricketts M, Comabella M, Hammond N, Kockum I, McCann OT, Ban M, Whittaker P, Kemppinen A, Weston P, Hawkins C, Widaa S, Zajicek J, Dronov S, Robertson N, Bumpstead SJ, Barcellos LF, Ravindrarajah R, Abraham R, Alfredsson L, Ardlie K, Aubin C, Baker A, Baker K, Baranzini SE, Bergamaschi L, Bergamaschi R, Bernstein A, Berthele A, Boggild M, Bradfield JP, Brassat D, Broadley SA, Buck D, Butzkueven H, Capra R, Carroll WM, Cavalla P, Celius EG, Cepok S, Chiavacci R, Clerget-Darpoux F, Clysters K, Comi G, Cossburn M, Cournu-Rebeix I, Cox MB, Cozen W, Cree BA, Cross AH, Cusi D, Daly MJ, Davis E, de Bakker PI, Debouverie M, D'Hooghe MB, Dixon K, Dobosi R, Dubois B, Ellinghaus D, Elovaara I, Esposito F, Fontenille C, Foote S, Franke A, Galimberti D, Ghezzi A, Glessner J, Gomez R, Gout O, Graham C, Grant SF, Guerini FR, Hakonarson H, Hall P, Hamsten A, Hartung HP, Heard RN, Heath S, Hobart J, Hoshi M, Infante-Duarte C, Ingram G, Ingram W, Islam T, Jagodic M, Kabesch M, Kermode AG, Kilpatrick TJ, Kim C, Klopp N, Koivisto K, Larsson M, Lathrop M, Lechner-Scott JS, Leone MA, Leppa V, Liljedahl U, Bomfim IL, Lincoln RR, Link J, Liu J, Lorentzen AR, Lupoli S, Macciardi F, Mack T, Marriott M, Martinelli V, Mason D, McCauley JL, Mentch F, Mero IL, Mihalova T, Montalban X, Mottershead J, Myhr KM, Naldi P, Ollier W, Page A, Palotie A, Pelletier J, Piccio L, Pickersgill T, Piehl F, Pobywajlo S, Quach HL, Ramsay PP, Reunanen M, Reynolds R, Rioux JD, Rodegher M, Roesner S, Rubio JP, Ruckert IM, Salvetti M, Salvi E, Santaniello A, Schaefer CA, Schreiber S, Schulze C, Scott RJ, Sellebjerg F, Selmaj KW, Sexton D, Shen L, Simms-Acuna B, Skidmore S, Sleiman PM, Smestad C, Sorensen PS, Sondergaard HB, Stankovich J, Strange RC, Sulonen AM, Sundqvist E, Syvanen AC, Taddeo F, Taylor B, Blackwell JM, Tienari P, Bramon E, Tourbah A, Brown MA, Tronczynska E, Casas JP, Tubridy N, Corvin A, Vickery J, Jankowski J, Villoslada P, Markus HS, Wang K, Mathew CG, Wason J, Palmer CN, Wichmann HE, Plomin R, Willoughby E, Rautanen A, Winkelmann J, Wittig M, Trembath RC, Yaouanq J, Viswanathan AC, Zhang H, Wood NW, Zuvich R, Deloukas P, Langford C, Duncanson A, Oksenberg JR, Pericak-Vance MA, Haines JL, Olsson T, Hillert J, Ivinson AJ, De Jager PL, Peltonen L, Stewart GJ, Hafler DA, Hauser SL, McVean G, Donnelly P, Compston A (2011) Genetic risk and a primary role for cell-mediated immune mechanisms in multiple sclerosis. Nature 476:214–219. https://doi.org/10.1038/nature10251.

88. Ioannou GN, Haigh WG, Thorning D, Savard C (2013) Hepatic cholesterol crystals and crown-like structures distinguish NASH from simple steatosis. J Lipid Res 54:1326–1334. https://doi.org/10.1194/jlr.M034876.

89. Ishii T, Itoh K, Ruiz E, Leake DS, Unoki H, Yamamoto M, Mann GE (2004) Role of Nrf2 in the regulation of CD36 and stress protein expression in murine macrophages: activation by oxidatively modified LDL and 4-hydroxynonenal. Circ Res 94:609–616. https://doi.org/10.1161/01.RES.0000119171.44657.45.

90. Jahng A, Maricic I, Aguilera C, Cardell S, Halder RC, Kumar V (2004) Prevention of autoimmunity by targeting a distinct, noninvariant CD1d-reactive T cell population reactive to sulfatide. J Exp Med 199:947–957. https://doi.org/10.1084/jem.20031389.

91. Jelinek D, Patrick SM, Kitt KN, Chan T, Francis GA, Garver WS (2009) Physiological and coordinate downregulation of the NPC1 and NPC2 genes are associated with the sequestration of LDL-derived cholesterol within endocytic compartments. J Cell Biochem 108:1102–1116. https://doi.org/10.1002/jcb.22339.

92. Jerome WG, Cox BE, Griffin EE, Ullery JC (2008) Lysosomal cholesterol accumulation inhibits subsequent hydrolysis of lipoprotein cholesteryl ester. Microsc Microanal 14:138–149. https://doi.org/10.1017/S1431927608080069.

93. Jha S, Srivastava SY, Brickey WJ, Iocca H, Toews A, Morrison JP, Chen VS, Gris D, Matsushima GK, Ting JP (2010) The inflammasome sensor, NLRP3, regulates CNS inflammation and demyelination via caspase-1 and interleukin-18. J Neurosci 30:15811–15820. https://doi.org/10.1523/JNEUROSCI.4088-10.2010.

94. Johnson LA, Jackson DG (2013) The chemokine CX3CL1 promotes trafficking of dendritic cells through inflamed lymphatics. J Cell Sci 126:5259–5270. https://doi.org/10.1242/jcs.135343.

95. Jorissen W, Wouters E, Bogie JF, Vanmierlo T, Noben JP, Sviridov D, Hellings N, Somers V, Valcke R, Vanwijmeersch B, Stinissen P, Mulder MT, Remaley AT, Hendriks JJ (2017) Relapsing-remitting multiple sclerosis patients display an altered lipoprotein profile with dysfunctional HDL. Sci Rep 7:43410. https://doi.org/10.1038/srep43410.

96. Junker A, Krumbholz M, Eisele S, Mohan H, Augstein F, Bittner R, Lassmann H, Wekerle H, Hohlfeld R, Meinl E (2009) MicroRNA profiling of multiple sclerosis lesions identifies modulators of the regulatory protein CD47. Brain 132:3342–3352. https://doi.org/10.1093/brain/awp300.

97. Kadl A, Meher AK, Sharma PR, Lee MY, Doran AC, Johnstone SR, Elliott MR, Gruber F, Han J, Chen W, Kensler T, Ravichandran KS, Isakson BE, Wamhoff BR, Leitinger N (2010) Identification of a novel macrophage phenotype that develops in response to atherogenic phospholipids via Nrf2. Circ Res 107:737–746. https://doi.org/10.1161/CIRCRESAHA.109.215715.

98. Kalayoglu MV, Byrne GI (1998) Induction of macrophage foam cell formation by Chlamydia pneumoniae. J Infect Dis 177:725–729.

99. Kapellos TS, Taylor L, Lee H, Cowley SA, James WS, Iqbal AJ, Greaves DR (2016) A novel real time imaging platform to quantify macrophage phagocytosis. Biochem Pharmacol 116:107–119. https://doi.org/10.1016/j.bcp.2016.07.011.

100. Kidani Y, Bensinger SJ (2012) Liver X receptor and peroxisome proliferator-activated receptor as integrators of lipid homeostasis and immunity. Immunol Rev 249:72–83. https://doi.org/10.1111/j.1600-065X.2012.01153.x.

101. Kierdorf K, Erny D, Goldmann T, Sander V, Schulz C, Perdiguero EG, Wieghofer P, Heinrich A, Riemke P, Holscher C, Muller DN, Luckow B, Brocker T, Debowski K, Fritz G, Opdenakker G, Diefenbach A, Biber K, Heikenwalder M, Geissmann F, Rosenbauer F, Prinz M (2013) Microglia emerge from erythromyeloid precursors via Pu.1- and Irf8-dependent pathways. Nat Neurosci 16:273–280. https://doi.org/10.1038/nn.3318.

102. Kim OH, Kim H, Kang J, Yang D, Kang YH, Lee DH, Cheon GJ, Park SC, Oh BC (2017) Impaired phagocytosis of apoptotic cells causes accumulation of bone marrow-derived macrophages in aged mice. BMB Rep 50:43–48.

103. Kohlschutter A (2013) Lysosomal leukodystrophies: Krabbe disease and metachromatic leukodystrophy. Handb Clin Neurol 113:1611–1618. https://doi.org/10.1016/B978-0-444-59565-2.00029-0.

104. Kontush A, Lhomme M, Chapman MJ (2013) Unraveling the complexities of the HDL lipidome. J Lipid Res 54:2950–2963. https://doi.org/10.1194/jlr.R036095.

105. Kooi EJ, van Horssen J, Witte ME, Amor S, Bo L, Dijkstra CD, van der Valk P, Geurts JJ (2009) Abundant extracellular myelin in the meninges of patients

with multiple sclerosis. Neuropathol Appl Neurobiol 35:283–295. https://doi.org/10.1111/j.1365-2990.2008.00986.x.

106. Kotter MR, Li WW, Zhao C, Franklin RJ (2006) Myelin impairs CNS remyelination by inhibiting oligodendrocyte precursor cell differentiation. J Neurosci 26:328–332. https://doi.org/10.1523/JNEUROSCI.2615-05.2006.

107. Kotter MR, Zhao C, van Rooijen N, Franklin RJ (2005) Macrophage-depletion induced impairment of experimental CNS remyelination is associated with a reduced oligodendrocyte progenitor cell response and altered growth factor expression. Neurobiol Dis 18:166–175. https://doi.org/10.1016/j.nbd.2004.09.019.

108. Kovacs JR, Li C, Yang Q, Li G, Garcia IG, Ju S, Roodman DG, Windle JJ, Zhang X, Lu B (2012) Autophagy promotes T-cell survival through degradation of proteins of the cell death machinery. Cell Death Differ 19:144–152. https://doi.org/10.1038/cdd.2011.78.

109. Krivit W, Shapiro EG, Peters C, Wagner JE, Cornu G, Kurtzberg J, Wenger DA, Kolodny EH, Vanier MT, Loes DJ, Dusenbery K, Lockman LA (1998) Hematopoietic stem-cell transplantation in globoid-cell leukodystrophy. N Engl J Med 338:1119–1126. https://doi.org/10.1056/NEJM199804163381605.

110. Kroner A, Greenhalgh AD, Zarruk JG, Passos Dos Santos R, Gaestel M, David S (2014) TNF and increased intracellular iron alter macrophage polarization to a detrimental M1 phenotype in the injured spinal cord. Neuron 83:1098–1116. https://doi.org/10.1016/j.neuron.2014.07.027.

111. Kuhlmann T, Ludwin S, Prat A, Antel J, Bruck W, Lassmann H (2017) An updated histological classification system for multiple sclerosis lesions. Acta Neuropathol 133:13–24. https://doi.org/10.1007/s00401-016-1653-y.

112. Kuhlmann T, Wendling U, Nolte C, Zipp F, Maruschak B, Stadelmann C, Siebert H, Bruck W (2002) Differential regulation of myelin phagocytosis by macrophages/microglia, involvement of target myelin, Fc receptors and activation by intravenous immunoglobulins. J Neurosci Res 67:185–190. https://doi.org/10.1002/jnr.10104.

113. Lampron A, Larochelle A, Laflamme N, Prefontaine P, Plante MM, Sanchez MG, Yong VW, Stys PK, Tremblay ME, Rivest S (2015) Inefficient clearance of myelin debris by microglia impairs remyelinating processes. J Exp Med 212:481–495. https://doi.org/10.1084/jem.20141656.

114. Lemke G, Burstyn-Cohen T (2010) TAM receptors and the clearance of apoptotic cells. Ann N Y Acad Sci 1209:23–29. https://doi.org/10.1111/j.1749-6632.2010.05744.x.

115. Levy-Barazany H, Frenkel D (2012) Expression of scavenger receptor A on antigen presenting cells is important for CD4+ T-cells proliferation in EAE mouse model. J Neuroinflammation 9:120. https://doi.org/10.1186/1742-2094-9-120.

116. Li W, Yuan XM, Olsson AG, Brunk UT (1998) Uptake of oxidized LDL by macrophages results in partial lysosomal enzyme inactivation and relocation. Arterioscler Thromb Vasc Biol 18:177–184.

117. Li X, Kimberly RP (2014) Targeting the Fc receptor in autoimmune disease. Expert Opin Ther Targets 18:335–350. https://doi.org/10.1517/14728222.2014.877891.

118. Liao X, Sluimer JC, Wang Y, Subramanian M, Brown K, Pattison JS, Robbins J, Martinez J, Tabas I (2012) Macrophage autophagy plays a protective role in advanced atherosclerosis. Cell Metab 15:545–553. https://doi.org/10.1016/j.cmet.2012.01.022.

119. Lim RS, Suhalim JL, Miyazaki-Anzai S, Miyazaki M, Levi M, Potma EO, Tromberg BJ (2011) Identification of cholesterol crystals in plaques of atherosclerotic mice using hyperspectral CARS imaging. J Lipid Res 52:2177–2186. https://doi.org/10.1194/jlr.M018077.

120. Liu K, Czaja MJ (2013) Regulation of lipid stores and metabolism by lipophagy. Cell Death Differ 20:3–11. https://doi.org/10.1038/cdd.2012.63.

121. Liu Y, Hao W, Letiembre M, Walter S, Kulanga M, Neumann H, Fassbender K (2006) Suppression of microglial inflammatory activity by myelin phagocytosis: role of p47-PHOX-mediated generation of reactive oxygen species. J Neurosci 26:12904–12913. https://doi.org/10.1523/JNEUROSCI.2531-06.2006.

122. Locatelli G, Wortge S, Buch T, Ingold B, Frommer F, Sobottka B, Kruger M, Karram K, Buhlmann C, Bechmann I, Heppner FL, Waisman A, Becher B (2012) Primary oligodendrocyte death does not elicit anti-CNS immunity. Nature neuroscience 15:543–550. https://doi.org/10.1038/nn.3062.

123. Louveau A, Smirnov I, Keyes TJ, Eccles JD, Rouhani SJ, Peske JD, Derecki NC, Castle D, Mandell JW, Lee KS, Harris TH, Kipnis J (2015) Structural and functional features of central nervous system lymphatic vessels. Nature 523:337–341. https://doi.org/10.1038/nature14432.

124. Loveless S, Neal JW, Howell OW, Harding KE, Sarkies P, Evans R, Bevan RJ, Hakobyan S, Harris CL, Robertson NP, Morgan BP (2017) Tissue microarray methodology identifies complement pathway activation and dysregulation in progressive multiple sclerosis. Brain Pathol. https://doi.org/10.1111/bpa.12546.

125. Ma Q, Chen S, Hu Q, Feng H, Zhang JH, Tang J (2014) NLRP3 inflammasome contributes to inflammation after intracerebral hemorrhage. Ann Neurol 75:209–219. https://doi.org/10.1002/ana.24070.

126. Mailleux J, Vanmierlo T, Bogie JF, Wouters E, Lutjohann D, Hendriks JJ, van Horssen J (2018) Active liver X receptor signaling in phagocytes in multiple sclerosis lesions. Multiple Scler 24:279–289. https://doi.org/10.1177/1352458517696595.

127. Mandoj C, Renna R, Plantone D, Sperduti I, Cigliana G, Conti L, Koudriavtseva T (2015) Anti-annexin antibodies, cholesterol levels and disability in multiple sclerosis. Neurosci Lett 606:156–160. https://doi.org/10.1016/j.neulet.2015.08.054.

128. McKeown SR, Allen IV (1979) The fragility of cerebral lysosomes in multiple sclerosis. Neuropathol Appl Neurobiol 5:405–415.

129. McMahon EJ, Bailey SL, Castenada CV, Waldner H, Miller SD (2005) Epitope spreading initiates in the CNS in two mouse models of multiple sclerosis. Nature Med 11:335–339. https://doi.org/10.1038/nm1202.

130. McMahon JM, McQuaid S, Reynolds R, FitzGerald UF (2012) Increased expression of ER stress- and hypoxia-associated molecules in grey matter lesions in multiple sclerosis. Multiple Scler 18:1437–1447. https://doi.org/10.1177/1352458512438455.

131. Meares GP, Liu Y, Rajbhandari R, Qin H, Nozell SE, Mobley JA, Corbett JA, Benveniste EN (2014) PERK-dependent activation of JAK1 and STAT3 contributes to endoplasmic reticulum stress-induced inflammation. Mol Cell Biol 34:3911–3925. https://doi.org/10.1128/MCB.00980-14.

132. Meller J, Chen Z, Dudiki T, Cull RM, Murtazina R, Bal SK, Pluskota E, Stefl S, Plow EF, Trapp BD, Byzova TV (2017) Integrin-Kindlin3 requirements for microglial motility in vivo are distinct from those for macrophages. JCI Insight 2. https://doi.org/10.1172/jci.insight.93002.

133. Meyers L, Groover CJ, Douglas J, Lee S, Brand D, Levin MC, Gardner LA (2014) A role for Apolipoprotein A-I in the pathogenesis of multiple sclerosis. J Neuroimmunol 277:176–185. https://doi.org/10.1016/j.jneuroim.2014.10.010.

134. Mhaille AN, McQuaid S, Windebank A, Cunnea P, McMahon J, Samali A, FitzGerald U (2008) Increased expression of endoplasmic reticulum stress-related signaling pathway molecules in multiple sclerosis lesions. J Neuropathol Exp Neurol 67:200–211. https://doi.org/10.1097/NEN.0b013e318165b239.

135. Milo R, Kahana E (2010) Multiple sclerosis: geoepidemiology, genetics and the environment. Autoimmun Rev 9:A387–A394. https://doi.org/10.1016/j.autrev.2009.11.010.

136. Ming X, Li W, Maeda Y, Blumberg B, Raval S, Cook SD, Dowling PC (2002) Caspase-1 expression in multiple sclerosis plaques and cultured glial cells. J Neurol Sci 197:9–18.

137. Miron VE, Boyd A, Zhao JW, Yuen TJ, Ruckh JM, Shadrach JL, van Wijngaarden P, Wagers AJ, Williams A, Franklin RJ, Ffrench-Constant C (2013) M2 microglia and macrophages drive oligodendrocyte differentiation during CNS remyelination. Nature Neurosci. https://doi.org/10.1038/nn.3469.

138. Moore KJ, Freeman MW (2006) Scavenger receptors in atherosclerosis: beyond lipid uptake. Arterioscler Thromb Vasc Biol 26:1702–1711. https://doi.org/10.1161/01.ATV.0000229218.97976.43.

139. Moore KJ, Sheedy FJ, Fisher EA (2013) Macrophages in atherosclerosis: a dynamic balance. Nat Rev Immunol 13:709–721. https://doi.org/10.1038/nri3520.

140. Mosley K, Cuzner ML (1996) Receptor-mediated phagocytosis of myelin by macrophages and microglia: effect of opsonization and receptor blocking agents. Neurochem Res 21:481–487.

141. Mrdjen D, Pavlovic A, Hartmann FJ, Schreiner B, Utz SG, Leung BP, Lelios I, Heppner FL, Kipnis J, Merkler D, Greter M, Becher B (2018) High-Dimensional Single-Cell Mapping of Central Nervous System Immune Cells Reveals Distinct Myeloid Subsets in Health, Aging, and Disease. Immun 48:599. https://doi.org/10.1016/j.immuni.2018.02.014.

142. Mukundan L, Odegaard JI, Morel CR, Heredia JE, Mwangi JW, Ricardo-Gonzalez RR, Goh YP, Eagle AR, Dunn SE, Awakuni JU, Nguyen KD, Steinman L, Michie SA, Chawla A (2009) PPAR-delta senses and orchestrates clearance of apoptotic cells to promote tolerance. Nat Med 15:1266–1272. https://doi.org/10.1038/nm.2048.

143. Mycko MP, Papoian R, Boschert U, Raine CS, Selmaj KW (2004) Microarray gene expression profiling of chronic active and inactive lesions in multiple sclerosis. Clin Neurol Neurosurg 106:223–229. https://doi.org/10.1016/j.clineuro.2004.02.019.

144. Myoishi M, Hao II, Minamino T, Watanabe K, Nishihira K, Hatakeyama K, Asada Y, Okada K, Ishibashi-Ueda H, Gabbiani G, Bochaton-Piallat ML, Mochizuki N, Kitakaze M (2007) Increased endoplasmic reticulum stress in atherosclerotic plaques associated with acute coronary syndrome. Circ 116: 1226–1233. https://doi.org/10.1161/CIRCULATIONAHA.106.682054.

145. N AG, Bensinger SJ, Hong C, Beceiro S, Bradley MN, Zelcer N, Deniz J, Ramirez C, Diaz M, Gallardo G, de Galarreta CR, Salazar J, Lopez F, Edwards P, Parks J, Andujar M, Tontonoz P, Castrillo A (2009) Apoptotic cells promote their own clearance and immune tolerance through activation of the nuclear receptor LXR. Immun 31:245–258. https://doi.org/10.1016/j.immuni. 2009.06.018.

146. Nagy L, Tontonoz P, Alvarez JG, Chen H, Evans RM (1998) Oxidized LDL regulates macrophage gene expression through ligand activation of PPARgamma. Cell 93:229–240.

147. Natrajan MS, de la Fuente AG, Crawford AH, Linehan E, Nunez V, Johnson KR, Wu T, Fitzgerald DC, Ricote M, Bielekova B, Franklin RJ (2015) Retinoid X receptor activation reverses age-related deficiencies in myelin debris phagocytosis and remyelination. Brain 138:3581–3597. https://doi.org/10.1093/brain/awv289.

148. Natrajan MS, Komori M, Kosa P, Johnson KR, Wu T, Franklin RJ, Bielekova B (2015) Pioglitazone regulates myelin phagocytosis and multiple sclerosis monocytes. Ann Clin Transl Neurol 2:1071–1084. https://doi.org/10.1002/acn3.260.

149. Newcombe J, Li H, Cuzner ML (1994) Low density lipoprotein uptake by macrophages in multiple sclerosis plaques: implications for pathogenesis. Neuropathol Appl Neurobiol 20:152–162.

150. Newton J, Hait NC, Maceyka M, Colaco A, Maczis M, Wassif CA, Cougnoux A, Porter FD, Milstien S, Platt N, Platt FM, Spiegel S (2017) FTY720/fingolimod increases NPC1 and NPC2 expression and reduces cholesterol and sphingolipid accumulation in Niemann-Pick type C mutant fibroblasts. FASEB J 31:1719–1730. https://doi.org/10.1096/fj.201601041R.

151. Ni Fhlathartaigh M, McMahon J, Reynolds R, Connolly D, Higgins E, Counihan T, Fitzgerald U (2013) Calreticulin and other components of endoplasmic reticulum stress in rat and human inflammatory demyelination. Acta Neuropathol Commun 1:37. https://doi.org/10.1186/2051-5960-1-37.

152. Nikic I, Merkler D, Sorbara C, Brinkoetter M, Kreutzfeldt M, Bareyre FM, Bruck W, Bishop D, Misgeld T, Kerschensteiner M (2011) A reversible form of axon damage in experimental autoimmune encephalomyelitis and multiple sclerosis. Nat Med 17:495–499. https://doi.org/10.1038/nm.2324.

153. Ohta M, Ohta K (2002) Detection of myelin basic protein in cerebrospinal fluid. Exp Rev Mol Diagn 2:627–633. https://doi.org/10.1586/14737159.2.6.627.

154. Ouimet M, Franklin V, Mak E, Liao X, Tabas I, Marcel YL (2011) Autophagy regulates cholesterol efflux from macrophage foam cells via lysosomal acid lipase. Cell Metab 13:655–667. https://doi.org/10.1016/j.cmet.2011.03.023.

155. Palavra F, Marado D, Mascarenhas-Melo F, Sereno J, Teixeira-Lemos E, Nunes CC, Goncalves G, Teixeira F, Reis F (2013) New markers of early cardiovascular risk in multiple sclerosis patients: oxidized-LDL correlates with clinical staging. Dis Markers 34:341–348. https://doi.org/10.3233/DMA-130979.

156. Peelen E, Damoiseaux J, Muris AH, Knippenberg S, Smolders J, Hupperts R, Thewissen M (2015) Increased inflammasome related gene expression profile in PBMC may facilitate T helper 17 cell induction in multiple sclerosis. Mol Immun 63:521–529. https://doi.org/10.1016/j.molimm.2014.10.008.

157. Phillips MJ, Needham M, Weller RO (1997) Role of cervical lymph nodes in autoimmune encephalomyelitis in the Lewis rat. J Pathol 182:457–464. https://doi.org/10.1002/(SICI)1096-9896(199708)182:4<457::AID-PATH870>3.0.CO;2-Y.

158. Pittoni V, Valesini G (2002) The clearance of apoptotic cells: implications for autoimmunity. Autoimmun Rev 1:154–161.

159. Plemel JR, Manesh SB, Sparling JS, Tetzlaff W (2013) Myelin inhibits oligodendroglial maturation and regulates oligodendrocytic transcription factor expression. Glia 61:1471–1487. https://doi.org/10.1002/glia.22535.

160. Popescu BF, Pirko I, Lucchinetti CF (2013) Pathology of multiple sclerosis: where do we stand? Continuum (Minneap Minn) 19:901–921. https://doi.org/10.1212/01.CON.0000433291.23091.65.

161. Portugal LR, Fernandes LR, Pietra Pedroso VS, Santiago HC, Gazzinelli RT, Alvarez-Leite JI (2008) Influence of low-density lipoprotein (LDL) receptor on lipid composition, inflammation and parasitism during Toxoplasma gondii infection. Microbes Infect 10:276–284. https://doi.org/10.1016/j.micinf.2007.12.001.

162. Prineas JW, Graham JS (1981) Multiple sclerosis: capping of surface immunoglobulin G on macrophages engaged in myelin breakdown. Ann Neurol 10:149–158. https://doi.org/10.1002/ana.410100205.

163. Razani B, Feng C, Coleman T, Emanuel R, Wen H, Hwang S, Ting JP, Virgin HW, Kastan MB, Semenkovich CF (2012) Autophagy links inflammasomes to atherosclerotic progression. Cell Metab 15:534–544. https://doi.org/10.1016/j.cmet.2012.02.011.

164. Reichert F, Rotshenker S (2003) Complement-receptor-3 and scavenger-receptor-AI/II mediated myelin phagocytosis in microglia and macrophages. Neurobiol Dis 12:65–72.

165. Reichert F, Slobodov U, Makranz C, Rotshenker S (2001) Modulation (inhibition and augmentation) of complement receptor-3-mediated myelin phagocytosis. Neurobiol Dis 8:504–512. https://doi.org/10.1006/nbdi.2001.0383.

166. Rosenson RS, Brewer HB Jr, Ansell BJ, Barter P, Chapman MJ, Heinecke JW, Kontush A, Tall AR, Webb NR (2016) Dysfunctional HDL and atherosclerotic cardiovascular disease. Nat Rev Cardiol 13:48–60. https://doi.org/10.1038/nrcardio.2015.124.

167. Rothhammer V, Borucki DM, Tjon EC, Takenaka MC, Chao CC, Ardura-Fabregat A, de Lima KA, Gutierrez-Vazquez C, Hewson P, Staszewski O, Blain M, Healy L, Neziraj T, Borio M, Wheeler M, Dragin LL, Laplaud DA, Antel J, Alvarez JI, Prinz M, Quintana FJ (2018) Microglial control of astrocytes in response to microbial metabolites. Nature 557:724–728. https://doi.org/10.1038/s41586-018-0119-x.

168. Ruckh JM, Zhao JW, Shadrach JL, van Wijngaarden P, Rao TN, Wagers AJ, Franklin RJ (2012) Rejuvenation of regeneration in the aging central nervous system. Cell Stem Cell 10:96–103. https://doi.org/10.1016/j.stem.2011.11.019.

169. Russell DG, Cardona PJ, Kim MJ, Allain S, Altare F (2009) Foamy macrophages and the progression of the human tuberculosis granuloma. Nat Immunol 10:943–948. https://doi.org/10.1038/ni.1781.

170. Sadler RH, Sommer MA, Forno LS, Smith ME (1991) Induction of anti-myelin antibodies in EAE and their possible role in demyelination. J Neurosci Res 30:616–624. https://doi.org/10.1002/jnr.490300404.

171. Salemi G, Gueli MC, Vitale F, Battaglieri F, Guglielmini E, Ragonese P, Trentacosti A, Massenti MF, Savettieri G, Bono A (2010) Blood lipids, homocysteine, stress factors, and vitamins in clinically stable multiple sclerosis patients. Lipids Health Dis 9:19. https://doi.org/10.1186/1476-511X-9-19.

172. Samson S, Mundkur L, Kakkar V (2012) Immune response to lipoproteins in atherosclerosis. Cholesterol 2012:571846. https://doi.org/10.1155/2012/571846.

173. Schulz C, Gomez Perdiguero E, Chorro L, Szabo-Rogers H, Cagnard N, Kierdorf K, Prinz M, Wu B, Jacobsen SE, Pollard JW, Frampton J, Liu KJ, Geissmann F (2012) A lineage of myeloid cells independent of Myb and hematopoietic stem cells. Science 336:86–90. https://doi.org/10.1126/science.1219179.

174. Shah AS, Tan L, Long JL, Davidson WS (2013) Proteomic diversity of high density lipoproteins: our emerging understanding of its importance in lipid transport and beyond. J Lipid Res 54:2575–2585. https://doi.org/10.1194/jlr.R035725.

175. Sheedy FJ, Grebe A, Rayner KJ, Kalantari P, Ramkhelawon B, Carpenter SB, Becker CE, Ediriweera HN, Mullick AE, Golenbock DT, Stuart LM, Latz E, Fitzgerald KA, Moore KJ (2013) CD36 coordinates NLRP3 inflammasome activation by facilitating intracellular nucleation of soluble ligands into particulate ligands in sterile inflammation. Nature Immun 14:812–820. https://doi.org/10.1038/ni.2639.

176. Shigeoka M, Urakawa N, Nishio M, Takase N, Utsunomiya S, Akiyama H, Kakeji Y, Komori T, Koma Y, Yokozaki H (2015) Cyr61 promotes CD204 expression and the migration of macrophages via MEK/ERK pathway in esophageal squamous cell carcinoma. Cancer Med 4:437–446. https://doi.org/10.1002/cam4.401.

177. Smith ME (1993) Phagocytosis of myelin by microglia in vitro. J Neurosci Res 35:480–487. https://doi.org/10.1002/jnr.490350504.

178. Smith ME (2001) Phagocytic properties of microglia in vitro: implications for a role in multiple sclerosis and EAE. Microsc Res Tech 54:81–94. https://doi.org/10.1002/jemt.1123.

179. Sommer MA, Forno LS, Smith ME (1992) EAE cerebrospinal fluid augments in vitro phagocytosis and metabolism of CNS myelin by macrophages. J Neurosci Res 32:384–394. https://doi.org/10.1002/jnr.490320310.

180. Spann NJ, Garmire LX, McDonald JG, Myers DS, Milne SB, Shibata N, Reichart D, Fox JN, Shaked I, Heudobler D, Raetz CR, Wang EW, Kelly SL, Sullards MC,

Murphy RC, Merrill AH Jr, Brown HA, Dennis EA, Li AC, Ley K, Tsimikas S, Fahy E, Subramaniam S, Quehenberger O, Russell DW, Glass CK (2012) Regulated accumulation of desmosterol integrates macrophage lipid metabolism and inflammatory responses. Cell 151:138–152. https://doi.org/10.1016/j.cell.2012.06.054.

181. Stys PK, Zamponi GW, van Minnen J, Geurts JJ (2012) Will the real multiple sclerosis please stand up? Nat Rev Neurosci 13:507–514. https://doi.org/10.1038/nrn3275.

182. Sun X, Wang X, Chen T, Li T, Cao K, Lu A, Chen Y, Sun D, Luo J, Fan J, Young W, Ren Y (2010) Myelin activates FAK/Akt/NF-kappaB pathways and provokes CR3-dependent inflammatory response in murine system. PLoS One 5:e9380. https://doi.org/10.1371/journal.pone.0009380.

183. Swift ME, Burns AL, Gray KL, DiPietro LA (2001) Age-related alterations in the inflammatory response to dermal injury. J Invest Dermatol 117:1027–1035. https://doi.org/10.1046/j.0022-202x.2001.01539.x.

184. Tabas I, Bornfeldt KE (2016) Macrophage Phenotype and Function in Different Stages of Atherosclerosis. Circ Res 118:653–667. https://doi.org/10.1161/CIRCRESAHA.115.306256.

185. Tacke F, Alvarez D, Kaplan TJ, Jakubzick C, Spanbroek R, Llodra J, Garin A, Liu J, Mack M, van Rooijen N, Lira SA, Habenicht AJ, Randolph GJ (2007) Monocyte subsets differentially employ CCR2, CCR5, and CX3CR1 to accumulate within atherosclerotic plaques. J Clin Invest 117:185–194. https://doi.org/10.1172/JCI28549.

186. Tettey P, Simpson S Jr, Taylor B, Blizzard L, Ponsonby AL, Dwyer T, Kostner K, van der Mei I (2014) An adverse lipid profile is associated with disability and progression in disability, in people with MS. Multiple Scler 20:1737–1744. https://doi.org/10.1177/1352458514533162.

187. Thamilarasan M, Koczan D, Hecker M, Paap B, Zettl UK (2012) MicroRNAs in multiple sclerosis and experimental autoimmune encephalomyelitis. Autoimmun Rev 11:174–179. https://doi.org/10.1016/j.autrev.2011.05.009.

188. Trapp BD, Peterson J, Ransohoff RM, Rudick R, Mork S, Bo L (1998) Axonal transection in the lesions of multiple sclerosis. N Eng J Med 338:278–285. https://doi.org/10.1056/NEJM199801293380502.

189. Tridandapani S, Siefker K, Teillaud JL, Carter JE, Wewers MD, Anderson CL (2002) Regulated expression and inhibitory function of Fcgamma RIIb in human monocytic cells. J Biol Chem 277:5082–5089. https://doi.org/10.1074/jbc.M110277200.

190. Trotter J, DeJong LJ, Smith ME (1986) Opsonization with antimyelin antibody increases the uptake and intracellular metabolism of myelin in inflammatory macrophages. J Neurochem 47:779–789.

191. Ullery-Ricewick JC, Cox BE, Griffin EE, Jerome WG (2009) Triglyceride alters lysosomal cholesterol ester metabolism in cholesteryl ester-laden macrophage foam cells. J Lipid Res 50:2014–2026. https://doi.org/10.1194/jlr.M800659-JLR200.

192. Ulvestad E, Williams K, Vedeler C, Antel J, Nyland H, Mork S, Matre R (1994) Reactive microglia in multiple sclerosis lesions have an increased expression of receptors for the Fc part of IgG. J Neurol Sci 121:125–131.

193. Vainchtein ID, Vinet J, Brouwer N, Brendecke S, Biagini G, Biber K, Boddeke HW, Eggen BJ (2014) In acute experimental autoimmune encephalomyelitis, infiltrating macrophages are immune activated, whereas microglia remain immune suppressed. Glia 62:1724–1735. https://doi.org/10.1002/glia.22711.

194. van der Laan LJ, Ruuls SR, Weber KS, Lodder IJ, Dopp EA, Dijkstra CD (1996) Macrophage phagocytosis of myelin in vitro determined by flow cytometry: phagocytosis is mediated by CR3 and induces production of tumor necrosis factor-alpha and nitric oxide. J Neuroimmunol 70:145–152.

195. van Rossum D, Hilbert S, Strassenburg S, Hanisch UK, Bruck W (2008) Myelin-phagocytosing macrophages in isolated sciatic and optic nerves reveal a unique reactive phenotype. Glia 56:271–283. https://doi.org/10.1002/glia.20611.

196. van Tits LJ, Stienstra R, van Lent PL, Netea MG, Joosten LA, Stalenhoef AF (2011) Oxidized LDL enhances pro-inflammatory responses of alternatively activated M2 macrophages: a crucial role for Kruppel-like factor 2. Atherosclerosis 214:345–349. https://doi.org/10.1016/j.atherosclerosis.2010.11.018.

197. van Zwam M, Huizinga R, Melief MJ, Wierenga-Wolf AF, van Meurs M, Voerman JS, Biber KP, Boddeke HW, Hopken UE, Meisel C, Meisel A, Bechmann I, Hintzen RQ, t Hart BA, Amor S, Laman JD, Boven LA (2009) Brain antigens in functionally distinct antigen-presenting cell populations in cervical lymph nodes in MS and EAE. J Mol Med 87:273–286. https://doi.org/10.1007/s00109-008-0421-4.

198. van Zwam M, Samsom JN, Nieuwenhuis EE, Melief MJ, Wierenga-Wolf AF, Dijke IE, Talens S, van Meurs M, Voerman JS, Boven LA, Laman JD (2011) Myelin ingestion alters macrophage antigen-presenting function in vitro and in vivo. J Leukoc Biol 90:123–132. https://doi.org/10.1189/jlb.1209813.

199. van Zwam M, Wierenga-Wolf AF, Melief MJ, Schrijver B, Laman JD, Boven LA (2010) Myelin ingestion by macrophages promotes their motility and capacity to recruit myeloid cells. J Neuroimmunol 225:112–117. https://doi.org/10.1016/j.jneuroim.2010.04.021.

200. Vogel DY, Vereyken EJ, Glim JE, Heijnen PD, Moeton M, van der Valk P, Amor S, Teunissen CE, van Horssen J, Dijkstra CD (2013) Macrophages in inflammatory multiple sclerosis lesions have an intermediate activation status. J Neuroinflammation 10:35. https://doi.org/10.1186/1742-2094-10-35.

201. Wang G (2002) How the lipid-free structure of the N-terminal truncated human apoA-I converts to the lipid-bound form: new insights from NMR and X-ray structural comparison. FEBS lett 529:157–161.

202. Wang M, Kaufman RJ (2016) Protein misfolding in the endoplasmic reticulum as a conduit to human disease. Nature 529:326–335. https://doi.org/10.1038/nature17041.

203. Wang X, Cao K, Sun X, Chen Y, Duan Z, Sun L, Guo L, Bai P, Sun D, Fan J, He X, Young W, Ren Y (2015) Macrophages in spinal cord injury: phenotypic and functional change from exposure to myelin debris. Glia 63:635–651. https://doi.org/10.1002/glia.22774.

204. Watkins LM, Neal JW, Loveless S, Michailidou I, Ramaglia V, Rees MI, Reynolds R, Robertson NP, Morgan BP, Howell OW (2016) Complement is activated in progressive multiple sclerosis cortical grey matter lesions. J Neuroinflammation 13:161. https://doi.org/10.1186/s12974-016-0611-x.

205. Weber MS, Hemmer B, Cepok S (2011) The role of antibodies in multiple sclerosis. Biochimica et biophysica acta 1812:239–245. https://doi.org/10.1016/j.bbadis.2010.06.009.

206. Weinger JG, Omari KM, Marsden K, Raine CS, Shafit-Zagardo B (2009) Up-regulation of soluble Axl and Mer receptor tyrosine kinases negatively correlates with Gas6 in established multiple sclerosis lesions. Am J Pathol 175:283–293. https://doi.org/10.2353/ajpath.2009.080807.

207. Weinstock-Guttman B, Zivadinov R, Mahfooz N, Carl E, Drake A, Schneider J, Teter B, Hussein S, Mehta B, Weiskopf M, Durfee J, Bergsland N, Ramanathan M (2011) Serum lipid profiles are associated with disability and MRI outcomes in multiple sclerosis. J Neuroinflammation 8:127. https://doi.org/10.1186/1742-2094-8-127.

208. Wermeling F, Karlsson MC, McGaha TL (2009) An anatomical view on macrophages in tolerance. Autoimmun Rev 9:49–52. https://doi.org/10.1016/j.autrev.2009.03.004.

209. Wickman G, Julian L, Olson MF (2012) How apoptotic cells aid in the removal of their own cold dead bodies. Cell Death Differ 19:735–742. https://doi.org/10.1038/cdd.2012.25.

210. Williams K, Ulvestad E, Waage A, Antel JP, McLaurin J (1994) Activation of adult human derived microglia by myelin phagocytosis in vitro. J Neurosci Res 38:433–443. https://doi.org/10.1002/jnr.490380409.

211. Wolvers DA, Coenen-de Roo CJ, Mebius RE, van der Cammen MJ, Tirion F, Miltenburg AM, Kraal G (1999) Intranasally induced immunological tolerance is determined by characteristics of the draining lymph nodes: studies with OVA and human cartilage gp-39. J Immunol 162:1994–1998.

212. Wong CK, Smith CA, Sakamoto K, Kaminski N, Koff JL, Goldstein DR (2017) Aging Impairs Alveolar Macrophage Phagocytosis and Increases Influenza-Induced Mortality in Mice. J Immunol 199:1060–1068. https://doi.org/10.4049/jimmunol.1700397.

213. Wouters K, van Gorp PJ, Bieghs V, Gijbels MJ, Duimel H, Lutjohann D, Kerksiek A, van Kruchten R, Maeda N, Staels B, van Bilsen M, Shiri-Sverdlov R, Hofker MH (2008) Dietary cholesterol, rather than liver steatosis, leads to hepatic inflammation in hyperlipidemic mouse models of nonalcoholic steatohepatitis. Hepatol 48:474–486. https://doi.org/10.1002/hep.22363.

214. Yamasaki R, Lu H, Butovsky O, Ohno N, Rietsch AM, Cialic R, Wu PM, Doykan CE, Lin J, Cotleur AC, Kidd G, Zorlu MM, Sun N, Hu W, Liu L, Lee JC, Taylor SE, Uehlein L, Dixon D, Gu J, Floruta CM, Zhu M, Charo IF, Weiner HL, Ransohoff RM (2014) Differential roles of microglia and monocytes in the inflamed central nervous system. J Exp Med 211:1533–1549. https://doi.org/10.1084/jem.20132477.

215. Yan Y, Jiang W, Liu L, Wang X, Ding C, Tian Z, Zhou R (2015) Dopamine controls systemic inflammation through inhibition of NLRP3 inflammasome. Cell 160:62–73. https://doi.org/10.1016/j.cell.2014.11.047.

216. Yang F, Wang Z, Wei X, Han H, Meng X, Zhang Y, Shi W, Li F, Xin T, Pang Q, Yi F (2014) NLRP3 deficiency ameliorates neurovascular damage in experimental ischemic stroke. J Cereb Blood Flow Metab 34:660–667. https://doi.org/10.1038/jcbfm.2013.242.

217. Yao S, Miao C, Tian H, Sang H, Yang N, Jiao P, Han J, Zong C, Qin S (2014) Endoplasmic reticulum stress promotes macrophage-derived foam cell formation by up-regulating cluster of differentiation 36 (CD36) expression. J Biol Chem 289:4032–4042. https://doi.org/10.1074/jbc.M113.524512.

218. Yuan XM, Li W, Brunk UT, Dalen H, Chang YH, Sevanian A (2000) Lysosomal destabilization during macrophage damage induced by cholesterol oxidation products. Free Radic Biol Med 28:208–218.

219. Zani IA, Stephen SL, Mughal NA, Russell D, Homer-Vanniasinkam S, Wheatcroft SB, Ponnambalam S (2015) Scavenger receptor structure and function in health and disease. Cells 4:178–201. https://doi.org/10.3390/cells4020178.

220. Zhang Z, Zhang ZY, Schittenhelm J, Wu Y, Meyermann R, Schluesener HJ (2011) Parenchymal accumulation of CD163+ macrophages/microglia in multiple sclerosis brains. J Neuroimmunol 237:73–79. https://doi.org/10.1016/j.jneuroim.2011.06.006.

221. Zhou J, Lhotak S, Hilditch BA, Austin RC (2005) Activation of the unfolded protein response occurs at all stages of atherosclerotic lesion development in apolipoprotein E-deficient mice. Circ 111:1814–1821. https://doi.org/10.1161/01.CIR.0000160864.31351.C1.

222. Zizzo G, Hilliard BA, Monestier M, Cohen PL (2012) Efficient clearance of early apoptotic cells by human macrophages requires M2c polarization and MerTK induction. J Immunol 189:3508–3520. https://doi.org/10.4049/jimmunol.1200662.

Permissions

All chapters in this book were first published in ANC, by BioMed Central; hereby published with permission under the Creative Commons Attribution License or equivalent. Every chapter published in this book has been scrutinized by our experts. Their significance has been extensively debated. The topics covered herein carry significant findings which will fuel the growth of the discipline. They may even be implemented as practical applications or may be referred to as a beginning point for another development.

The contributors of this book come from diverse backgrounds, making this book a truly international effort. This book will bring forth new frontiers with its revolutionizing research information and detailed analysis of the nascent developments around the world.

We would like to thank all the contributing authors for lending their expertise to make the book truly unique. They have played a crucial role in the development of this book. Without their invaluable contributions this book wouldn't have been possible. They have made vital efforts to compile up to date information on the varied aspects of this subject to make this book a valuable addition to the collection of many professionals and students.

This book was conceptualized with the vision of imparting up-to-date information and advanced data in this field. To ensure the same, a matchless editorial board was set up. Every individual on the board went through rigorous rounds of assessment to prove their worth. After which they invested a large part of their time researching and compiling the most relevant data for our readers.

The editorial board has been involved in producing this book since its inception. They have spent rigorous hours researching and exploring the diverse topics which have resulted in the successful publishing of this book. They have passed on their knowledge of decades through this book. To expedite this challenging task, the publisher supported the team at every step. A small team of assistant editors was also appointed to further simplify the editing procedure and attain best results for the readers.

Apart from the editorial board, the designing team has also invested a significant amount of their time in understanding the subject and creating the most relevant covers. They scrutinized every image to scout for the most suitable representation of the subject and create an appropriate cover for the book.

The publishing team has been an ardent support to the editorial, designing and production team. Their endless efforts to recruit the best for this project, has resulted in the accomplishment of this book. They are a veteran in the field of academics and their pool of knowledge is as vast as their experience in printing. Their expertise and guidance has proved useful at every step. Their uncompromising quality standards have made this book an exceptional effort. Their encouragement from time to time has been an inspiration for everyone.

The publisher and the editorial board hope that this book will prove to be a valuable piece of knowledge for researchers, students, practitioners and scholars across the globe.

Contributors

Michael W. Ronellenfitsch, Hans Urban and Joachim P. Steinbach
Dr. Senckenberg Institute of Neurooncology, University Hospital Frankfurt, Goethe University, Schleusenweg 2-16, 60528 Frankfurt am Main, Germany
German Cancer Consortium (DKTK), Partner Site Frankfurt/Mainz, Frankfurt am Main, Germany
German Cancer Research Center (DKFZ), Heidelberg, Germany

Pia S. Zeiner
Dr. Senckenberg Institute of Neurooncology, University Hospital Frankfurt, Goethe University, Schleusenweg 2-16, 60528 Frankfurt am Main, Germany
German Cancer Consortium (DKTK), Partner Site Frankfurt/Mainz, Frankfurt am Main, Germany
German Cancer Research Center (DKFZ), Heidelberg, Germany
Institute of Neurology (Edinger-Institute), University Hospital Frankfurt, Goethe University, Heinrich-Hoffmann-Str. 7, 60528 Frankfurt am Main, Germany

Patrick N. Harter
German Cancer Consortium (DKTK), Partner Site Frankfurt/Mainz, Frankfurt am Main, Germany
German Cancer Research Center (DKFZ), Heidelberg, Germany
Institute of Neurology (Edinger-Institute), University Hospital Frankfurt, Goethe University, Heinrich-Hoffmann-Str. 7, 60528 Frankfurt am Main, Germany

Michel Mittelbronn
Institute of Neurology (Edinger-Institute), University Hospital Frankfurt, Goethe University, Heinrich-Hoffmann-Str. 7, 60528 Frankfurt am Main, Germany
Luxembourg Centre for Systems Biomedicine (LCSB),University of Luxembourg, Dudelange, Luxembourg
Laboratoire national de santé (LNS), Dudelange, Luxembourg
Luxembourg Centre of Neuropathology (LCNP), Dudelange, Luxembourg

Torsten Pietsch
Department of Neuropathology, University of Bonn, Bonn, Germany

Dirk Reuter
Oncoscience GmbH, Schenefeld, Germany

Christian Senft
Department of Neurosurgery, University Hospital Frankfurt, Goethe University, Frankfurt am Main, Germany

Manfred Westphal
Department of Neurosurgery, University Hospital Hamburg Eppendorf, Martinistrasse 52, 20246 Hamburg, Germany

Melanie Hüttenrauch, Hans Klafki and Oliver Wirths
Department of Psychiatry and Psychotherapy, University Medical Center (UMG), Georg-August-University, Von-Siebold-Str. 5, 37075 Göttingen, Germany

Jens Wiltfang
Department of Psychiatry and Psychotherapy, University Medical Center (UMG), Georg-August-University, Von-Siebold-Str. 5, 37075 Göttingen, Germany
German Center for Neurodegenerative Diseases (DZNE), Göttingen, Germany

Isabella Ogorek and Sascha Weggen
Department of Neuropathology, Heinrich-Heine-University, Düsseldorf, Germany

Markus Otto
Department of Neurology, University of Ulm, Ulm, Germany

Christine Stadelmann
Department of Neuropathology, University Medical Center, Georg-August-University, Göttingen, Germany

Isabel Ortuño-Lizarán, Gema Esquiva, Pedro Lax and Nicolás Cuenca
Department of Physiology, Genetics and Microbiology, University of Alicante, 03690 San Vicente del Raspeig, Spain

Thomas G. Beach and Geidy E. Serrano
Banner Sun Health Research Institute, Sun City, AZ 85351, USA

Charles H. Adler
Mayo Clinic Arizona, Scottsdale, AZ 85259, USA

Rachel Jester, Iya Znoyko, Maria Garnovskaya, Joseph N Rozier, Ryan Kegl, Mary Richardson and Daynna J Wolff
Department of Pathology and Laboratory Medicine, Medical University of South Carolina, 171 Ashley Ave, Charleston 29425, SC, USA

Adriana Olar
Department of Pathology and Laboratory Medicine, Medical University of South Carolina, 171 Ashley Ave, Charleston 29425, SC, USA
Department of Neurosurgery, Medical University of South Carolina, 171 Ashley Ave, Charleston 29425, SC, USA
Hollings Cancer Center, 86 Jonathan Lucas Street, Charleston 29425, SC, USA

Sunil Patel
Department of Neurosurgery, Medical University of South Carolina, 171 Ashley Ave, Charleston 29425, SC, USA

Tuan Tran
Department of Pathology, Baylor University Medical Center, 3500 Gaston Ave, Dallas 75246, TX, USA

Malak Abedalthagafi
Genomics Research Department, Saudi Humane Genome Project, King Fahad Medical City and King Abdulaziz City for Science and Technology, Riyadh, Saudi Arabia

Craig M Horbinski
Department of Pathology and Neurosurgery, Feinberg School of Medicine, Northwestern University, 251 E. Huron St, Chicago 60611, IL, USA

Razvan Lapadat
Department of Pathology, Loyola University Medical Center, 2160 S 1st Ave, Maywood 60153, IL, USA

William Moore
Department of Radiology, UT Southwestern Medical Center, 5323 Harry Hines Blvd, Dallas 75390, TX, USA

Fausto J Rodriguez
Department of Pathology, Johns Hopkins Hospital, 1800 Orleans St, Baltimore 21287, MD, USA

Jason Mull
Department of Pathology, UT Southwestern Medical Center, 5323 Harry Hines Blvd, Dallas 75390, TX, USA

Myriam Vezain, Matthieu Lecuyer, Sophie Coutant, Isabelle Tournier and Bruno J Gonzalez
Normandie Univ, UNIROUEN, Inserm U1245, Normandy Centre for Genomic and Personalized Medicine, F 76000 Rouen, France

Thierry Frébourg and Pascale Saugier-Veber
Normandie Univ, UNIROUEN, Inserm U1245, Normandy Centre for Genomic and Personalized Medicine, F 76000 Rouen, France
Department of Genetics, Normandy Centre for Genomic and Personalized Medicine, Rouen University Hospital, F 76000 Rouen, France

Annie Laquerrière
Normandie Univ, UNIROUEN, Inserm U1245, Normandy Centre for Genomic and Personalized Medicine, F 76000 Rouen, France
Department of Pathology, Rouen University Hospital, F 76000 Rouen, France

Marina Rubio and Denis Vivien
Normandie Univ, UNICAEN, Inserm U1237, F 14000 Caen, France

Valérie Dupé, Leslie Ratié and Véronique David
Rennes1 University, Faculty of Medicine, UMR6290 CNRS IGDR, F 35000 Rennes, France

Sylvie Odent
Rennes1 University, Faculty of Medicine, UMR6290 CNRS IGDR, F 35000 Rennes, France
Department of Genetics, Rennes University Hospital, F 35000 Rennes, France

Laurent Pasquier
Department of Genetics, Rennes University Hospital, F 35000 Rennes, France

Laetitia Trestard
Belvedere Hospital, Department of Genetics, F 76130 Mont-Saint-Aignan, France

Homa Adle-Biassette
Lariboisière Hospital, APHP, Department of Pathology, F 75000 Paris, France
Paris Diderot University, Sorbonne Paris Cité, PROTECT INSERM, F 75019 Paris, France

Ayami Okuzumi, Taku Hatano, Takeshi Fukuhara and Nobutaka Hattori
Department of Neurology, Juntendo University Graduate School of Medicine, 2-1-1 Hongo, Bunkyo-ku, Tokyo 113-8421, Japan

Nobuyuki Nukina
Department of Neurology, Juntendo University Graduate School of Medicine, 2-1-1 Hongo, Bunkyo-ku, Tokyo 113-8421, Japan
Laboratory of Structural Neuropathology, Doshisha University Graduate School of Brain Science, 1-3 Tatara Miyakodani, Kyotanabe-shi, Kyoto 610-0394, Japan

Masaru Kurosawa
Institute for Environmental and Gender-specific Medicine, Juntendo University Graduate School of Medicine, 2-1-1 Tomioka, Urayasu-shi, Chiba 279-0021, Japan

Masashi Takanashi
Department of Neurology Juntendo University Koshigaya Hospital, 560 Fukuroyama, Koshigaya city, Saitama 343-0032, Japan

Shuuko Nojiri
Medical Technology Innovation Center, Clinical Research and Trial Center, Juntendo University Graduate School of Medicine, Tokyo, Japan

Tomoyuki Yamanaka, Haruko Miyazaki and Saki Yoshinaga
Laboratory of Structural Neuropathology, Doshisha University Graduate School of Brain Science, 1-3 Tatara Miyakodani, Kyotanabe-shi, Kyoto 610-0394, Japan

Yoshiaki Furukawa
Laboratory for Mechanistic Chemistry of Biomolecules, Department of Chemistry, Keio University, 3-14-1 Hiyoshi, Kohoku, Yokohama 223-8522, Japan

Tomomi Shimogori
Laboratory for Molecular Mechanisms of Brain Development, RIKEN Center for Brain Science, 2-1 Hirosawa, Wako, Saitama 351-0198, Japan

Jane Merlevede and Emilie Barret
UMR8203,Vectorologie et Nouvelles Thérapies Anticancéreuses, CNRS, Gustave Roussy, Univ. Paris-Sud, Université Paris-Saclay, 94805 Villejuif, France

David Castel, Thomas Kergrohen and Jacques Grill
UMR8203,Vectorologie et Nouvelles Thérapies Anticancéreuses, CNRS, Gustave Roussy, Univ. Paris-Sud, Université Paris-Saclay, 94805 Villejuif, France
Département de Cancérologie de l'Enfant et de l'Adolescent, Institut de Cancérologie Gustave Roussy, Université Paris-Sud, Université Paris-Saclay, 114 rue Édouard Vaillant, 94805 Villejuif Cedex, France

Cathy Philippe
UMR8203,Vectorologie et Nouvelles Thérapies Anticancéreuses, CNRS, Gustave Roussy, Univ. Paris-Sud, Université Paris-Saclay, 94805 Villejuif, France
NeuroSpin/UNATI, CEA, Université Paris-Saclay, Gif-sur-Yvette, France

Marie-Anne Debily
UMR8203,Vectorologie et Nouvelles Thérapies Anticancéreuses, CNRS, Gustave Roussy, Univ. Paris-Sud, Université Paris-Saclay, 94805 Villejuif, France
Université Evry, Université Paris-Saclay, 91057 Evry Cedex, France
Univ. Evry, Université Paris-Saclay, 91057 Evry Cedex, France

Martin Sill
Hopp Children's Cancer Center at the NCT Heidelberg (KiTZ), Heidelberg, Germany
Division of Pediatric Neurooncology (B062), German Cancer Research Center (DKFZ) and German Cancer Consortium (DKTK), Im Neuenheimer Feld 280, 69120 Heidelberg, Germany

Stefan M. Pfister
Hopp Children's Cancer Center at the NCT Heidelberg (KiTZ), Heidelberg, Germany
Division of Pediatric Neurooncology (B062), German Cancer Research Center (DKFZ) and German Cancer Consortium (DKTK), Im Neuenheimer Feld 280, 69120 Heidelberg, Germany
Department of Pediatric Hematology and Oncology, Heidelberg University Hospital, Heidelberg, Germany

David T. W. Jones
Hopp Children's Cancer Center at the NCT Heidelberg (KiTZ), Heidelberg, Germany
Pediatric Glioma Research Group, German Cancer Research Center (DKFZ) and German Cancer Consortium (DKTK), Im Neuenheimer Feld 280, 69120 Heidelberg, Germany

Stéphanie Puget and Christian Sainte-Rose
Department of Pediatric Neurosurgery, Hôpital Necker-Enfants Malades, Université Paris V Descartes, Sorbonne Paris Cité, Paris, France

Christof M. Kramm
Division of Pediatric Hematology and Oncology, University Medical Center Goettingen, Goettingen, Germany

Chris Jones
Divisions of Molecular Pathology and Cancer Therapeutics, The Institute of Cancer Research, Sutton, Surrey, UK

Pascale Varlet
Department of Neuropathology, Hôpital Sainte-Anne, Université Paris V Descartes, Sorbonne Paris Cité, Paris, France

Shannon L. Risacher and Eileen F. Tallman
Department of Radiology and Imaging Sciences, Indiana University School of Medicine, 355 West 16th Street, Suite 4100, Indianapolis, IN 46202, USA
Indiana Alzheimer Disease Center, Indiana University School of Medicine, Indianapolis, IN, USA

Andrew J. Saykin
Department of Radiology and Imaging Sciences, Indiana University School of Medicine, 355 West 16th Street, Suite 4100, Indianapolis, IN 46202, USA
Indiana Alzheimer Disease Center, Indiana University School of Medicine, Indianapolis, IN, USA
Department of Medical and Molecular Genetics, Indiana University School of Medicine, Indianapolis, IN, USA

Liana G. Apostolova
Department of Radiology and Imaging Sciences, Indiana University School of Medicine, 355 West 16th Street, Suite 4100, Indianapolis, IN 46202, USA
Indiana Alzheimer Disease Center, Indiana University School of Medicine, Indianapolis, IN, USA
Department of Neurology, Indiana University School of Medicine, Indianapolis, IN, USA
Department of Medical and Molecular Genetics, Indiana University School of Medicine, Indianapolis, IN, USA

Martin R. Farlow
Indiana Alzheimer Disease Center, Indiana University School of Medicine, Indianapolis, IN, USA
Department of Neurology, Indiana University School of Medicine, Indianapolis, IN, USA

Daniel R. Bateman and Frederick W. Unverzagt
Indiana Alzheimer Disease Center, Indiana University School of Medicine, Indianapolis, IN, USA
Department of Psychiatry, Indiana University School of Medicine, Indianapolis, IN, USA

Francine Epperson, Rose Richardson and Jill R. Murrell
Indiana Alzheimer Disease Center, Indiana University School of Medicine, Indianapolis, IN, USA
Department of Pathology and Laboratory Medicine, Indiana University School of Medicine, Indianapolis, IN, USA

Bernardino Ghetti
Indiana Alzheimer Disease Center, Indiana University School of Medicine, Indianapolis, IN, USA
Department of Neurology, Indiana University School of Medicine, Indianapolis, IN, USA
Department of Psychiatry, Indiana University School of Medicine, Indianapolis, IN, USA
Department of Pathology and Laboratory Medicine, Indiana University School of Medicine, Indianapolis, IN, USA
Department of Medical and Molecular Genetics, Indiana University School of Medicine, Indianapolis, IN, USA

Jose M. Bonnin
Department of Neurology, Indiana University School of Medicine, Indianapolis, IN, USA
Department of Pathology and Laboratory Medicine, Indiana University School of Medicine, Indianapolis, IN, USA

Angela N. Viaene, Mariarita Santi, Marilyn M. Li and Lea F. Surrey
Department of Pathology and Laboratory Medicine, Children's Hospital of Philadelphia, University of Pennsylvania Perelman School of Medicine, Philadelphia, PA, USA

Jason Rosenbaum
Department of Pathology and Laboratory Medicine, University of Pennsylvania Perelman School of Medicine, Philadelphia, PA, USA

MacLean P. Nasrallah
Department of Pathology and Laboratory Medicine, University of Pennsylvania Perelman School of Medicine, Philadelphia, PA, USA
Hospital of the University of Pennsylvania, FO6.089 3400 Spruce St, Philadelphia, PA 19104, USA

Maggie M. K. Wong, Stephanie D. Hoekstra, Lauren M. Watson and Esther B. E. Becker
Department of Physiology, Anatomy and Genetics, University of Oxford, Sherrington Road, Oxford OX1 3PT, UK

Jane Vowles and Sally A. Cowley
Sir William Dunn School of Pathology, University of Oxford, South Parks Road, Oxford OX1 3RE, UK

Geraint Fuller
Gloucestershire Hospitals, NHS Foundation Trust, Cheltenham General Hospital, Sandford Road, Cheltenham GL53 7AN, UK

Olaf Ansorge and Kevin Talbot
Nuffield Department of Clinical Neurosciences, University of Oxford, Level 6, West Wing, John Radcliffe Hospital, Oxford OX3 9DU, UK

Andrea H. Németh
Nuffield Department of Clinical Neurosciences, University of Oxford, Level 6, West Wing, John Radcliffe Hospital, Oxford OX3 9DU, UK
Oxford Centre for Genomic Medicine, ACE Building, Oxford University Hospitals NHS Trust, Nuffield Orthopaedic Centre, Windmill Road, Oxford OX3 7HE, UK

Jana Dautzenberg
Institute of Neuropathology, Faculty of Medicine, University of Freiburg, Freiburg, Germany

Marco Prinz
Institute of Neuropathology, Faculty of Medicine, University of Freiburg, Freiburg, Germany
BIOSS Centre for Biological Signaling Studies, University of Freiburg, Freiburg, Germany

Tuan Leng Tay
Institute of Neuropathology, Faculty of Medicine, University of Freiburg, Freiburg, Germany
Cluster of Excellence BrainLinks-BrainTools, University of Freiburg, Freiburg, Germany
Institute of Biology I, Faculty of Biology, University of Freiburg, Freiburg, Germany

Sagar and Dominic Grün
Max-Planck-Institute of Immunobiology and Epigenetics, Freiburg, Germany

Shaomin Li, Ming Jin, Lei Liu, Yifan Dang, Beth L. Ostaszewski and Dennis J. Selkoe
Ann Romney Center for Neurologic Diseases, Department of Neurology, Brigham and Women's Hospital and Harvard Medical School, 60 Fenwood Road, Boston, MA 02115, USA

Anthony P. Y. Liu, Yahya Ghazwani, Amar Gajjar and Ibrahim Qaddoumi
Department of Oncology, St. Jude Children's Research Hospital, 262 Danny Thomas Place, MS 260, Memphis 38105-3678, TN, USA

Julie H. Harreld
Department of Diagnostic Imaging, St. Jude Children's Research Hospital, Memphis, TN, USA

Lisa M. Jacola and Madelyn Gero
Department of Psychology, St. Jude Children's Research Hospital, Memphis, TN, USA

Sahaja Acharya
Department of Radiation Oncology, St. Jude Children's Research Hospital, Memphis, TN, USA

Shengjie Wu
Department of Biostatistics, St. Jude Children's Research Hospital, Memphis, TN, USA

Xiaoyu Li and Jason Chiang
Department of Pathology, St. Jude Children's Research Hospital, 262 Danny Thomas Place, MS 250, Memphis 38105-3678, TN, USA

Paul Klimo Jr
Department of Surgery, St. Jude Children's Research Hospital, Memphis, TN, USA
Department of Neurosurgery, University of Tennessee Health Science Center, Memphis, TN, USA
Le Bonheur Neuroscience Institute, Le Bonheur Children's Hospital, Memphis, TN, USA
Semmes Murphey Clinic, Memphis, TN, USA

Soheil Zorofchian
Department of Pathology and Laboratory Medicine, University of Texas Health Science Center at Houston, 6431 Fannin St., MSB 2.136, Houston, TX 77030, USA

Leomar Y. Ballester
Department of Pathology and Laboratory Medicine, University of Texas Health Science Center at Houston, 6431 Fannin St., MSB 2.136, Houston, TX 77030, USA
Department of Neurosurgery, University of Texas Health Science Center at Houston, 6431 Fannin St., MSB 2.136, Houston, TX 77030, USA
Memorial Hermann Hospital, Houston, TX 77030, USA

Guangrong Lu, Yuanqing Yan and Ping Zhu
Department of Neurosurgery, University of Texas Health Science Center at Houston, 6431 Fannin St., MSB 2.136, Houston, TX 77030, USA

Yoshua Esquenazi and Jay-Jiguang Zhu
Department of Neurosurgery, University of Texas Health Science Center at Houston, 6431 Fannin St., MSB 2.136, Houston, TX 77030, USA
Memorial Hermann Hospital, Houston, TX 77030, USA

Octavio Arevalo
Department of Radiology, University of Texas Health Science Center at Houston, Houston, TX 77030, USA

Roy F. Riascos
Department of Radiology, University of Texas Health Science Center at Houston, Houston, TX 77030, USA

Memorial Hermann Hospital, Houston, TX 77030, USA

Venkatrao Vantaku, Arun Sreekumar and Nagireddy Putluri
Department of Molecular and Cellular Biology, Baylor College of Medicine, 120D, Jewish Building, One Baylor Plaza, Houston, TX 77030, USA

Vasanta Putluri
Advanced Technology Core, Baylor College of Medicine, Houston, TX 77030, USA

Michaela Kerstin Müller and Eric Jacobi
Institute of Pathophysiology, University Medical Center of the Johannes Gutenberg University Mainz, 55128 Mainz, Germany

Jakob von Engelhardt
Institute of Pathophysiology, University Medical Center of the Johannes Gutenberg University Mainz, 55128 Mainz, Germany
Synaptic Signalling and Neurodegeneration, German Center for Neurodegenerative Diseases (DZNE), 53127 Bonn, Germany

Kenji Sakimura
Department of Cellular Neurobiology, Brain Research Institute, Niigata University, Niigata 951-8585, Japan

Roberto Malinow
Center for Neural Circuits and Behavior, Department of Neuroscience and Section for Neurobiology, Division of Biology, University of California at San Diego, San Diego, CA, USA

Sebok K. Halder, Ravi Kant and Richard Milner
Department of Molecular Medicine, MEM-151, The Scripps Research Institute, 10550 North Torrey Pines Road, La Jolla, CA 92037, USA

Tianhong Chen, Xinglong Shi and Cao Huang
Department of Pathology, Anatomy and Cell Biology, Thomas Jefferson University, 1020 Locust Street, Philadelphia, PA 19107, USA

Bo Huang
Laboratory Animal Center, Shanxi Provincial People's Hospital, Taiyuan, Shanxi 030012, People's Republic of China
Animal Laboratory of Nephrology, Shanxi Provincial People's Hospital, Taiyuan, Shanxi 030012, People's Republic of China

Limo Gao
Department of Ophthalmology, The Third Xiangya Hospital of Central South University, Changsha, Hunan 410013, People's Republic of China

Matthew P. Shaw, Adrian Higginbottom, Alexander McGown, Lydia M. Castelli, Evlyn James, Guillaume M. Hautbergue and Pamela J. Shaw
Sheffield Institute for Translational Neuroscience, University of Sheffield, 385a Glossop Road, Sheffield S10 2HQ, UK

Tennore M. Ramesh
Sheffield Institute for Translational Neuroscience, University of Sheffield, 385a Glossop Road, Sheffield S10 2HQ, UK
The Bateson Centre, Firth Court, The University of Sheffield, Western Bank, Sheffield S10 2TN, UK

Elien Grajchen, Jerome J. A. Hendriks and Jeroen F. J. Bogie
Biomedical Research Institute, Hasselt University, Diepenbeek, Belgium/School of Life Sciences, Transnationale Universiteit Limburg, Diepenbeek, Belgium

Index